PSYCHOLOGY: ⋄

A NATURAL SCIENCE

UNIVERSITY OF MISSOURI –
ST. LOUIS

MICHAEL GRIFFIN
GEORGE TAYLOR

PEARSON CUSTOM PUBLISHING

Copyright Acknowledgments

Copyright Acknowledgments

Contents

PART ONE:
INTRODUCTION TO THE FIELD

The word "psychology" conjures up many different visions in the minds of different laypeople, but none of the visions are likely to include the bulk of the topics in this book. A quick glance at the Table of Contents reveals chapters in each of the five Parts of this book that may leave the introductory student thinking he or she has picked up a biology text by mistake. Rest assured that this is a psychology textbook. More accurately it is a "behavior" textbook because behavior is the subject matter of psychology. Most people outside of academia have an idea of psychology that involves patients lying on a sofa and talking about very personal problems as a kindly looking therapist scribbles notes. Indeed, that has formed a segment of psychology for the past century, and it remains an important segment of the field today. Yet, there is another part of psychology, one that centers on the scientific study of normal, everyday behaviors. It is a study that has become more and more physiological as technology allows us to look deeper and deeper into the biological underpinnings of behavior, most important being the functioning of the brain. In Part One, we will see the history of why and how psychology has found itself near the end of the twentieth century as a branch of science that looks more like a natural science than a social science. At the end of Part One, there is the first "Classic Reading in Psychology" that will appear at the ends of each subsequent part, along with an article review form and a Practice Test. More in class about those items. In Chapters 2 and 3, the reader will find descriptions of the methods that allow us to call ourselves scientists. All this sets the stage for the underlying theme of the book, psychology as behavioral neuroscience. That is, our approach is one that acknowledges a biological basis of behavior and gives most attention to the great behavioral organ, the brain. We hope you will find this approach as exciting as we do.

∾ ∾ ∾ ∾ ∾ ∾

1
BEGINNINGS

M R. WILHELM VON OSTEN CUT QUITE A FIGURE IN THAT DUSTY BERLIN COURTYARD, STANDING DEFIANTLY IN HIS LONG WHITE SMOCK BESIDE the red brick buildings. Everyone called him *Mister* von Osten, partly in keeping with the formality of that day, partly out of respect for this elderly, rather eccentric, retired schoolteacher. He wore his long smock even on the warmest days, and a large black hat usually covered his head. His floppy white hair stuck out in all directions beneath its broad brim.

Privileged visitors and a few dignitaries waited expectantly in a small grandstand. For all other spectators, there was standing room only.

When all was quiet, Mr. von Osten moved to the center of the courtyard. Taking a position in front and just to the right of his pupil, he began the performance.

"How much is two and four?" he asked. Hans answered readily.

"How much is three *times* three?" Mr. von Osten spoke the *times* loudly, lest Hans fail to notice that the problem required multiplication. Again, Hans succeeded, and the audience murmured appreciatively.

"What is the square root of 16?" After the last of 4 steady taps, the spectators erupted into hearty applause. After all, Hans was a horse.

A large brown stallion with white socks, Hans could tell time, knew the value of German coins, and remembered the days of the week. He tapped out popular sayings and the answers to spectators' questions by using a special chart that Mr. von Osten had constructed, displaying the letters of the German alphabet in numbered rows and columns. By tapping a pair of numbers, Hans could indicate a specific letter; by tapping several pairs, he could spell a word. He also answered by shaking his head or pointing with his nose.

The horse had become known as Clever Hans, a celebrity throughout Europe and even in the United States, where the *New York Times* carried stories on the wonderful horse. In 1904, letters to the editor of the *Berliner Tageblatt*, the major newspaper in the city, arrived in overwhelming numbers. Readers of the newspaper demanded an explanation. *How* did Hans do it? What might he do next? Mr. von Osten explained that he had given Hans five years of intensive instruction, using the most modern methods available. The horse's ability lay in this careful training (Pfungst, 1911).

This challenge to explain Clever Hans offered early psychology a special opportunity. Psychology might demonstrate to an eager public the breadth and usefulness of its methods, focusing on an unusual problem, a horse in an open courtyard, rather than people in a private laboratory or clinic. In those early days, psychology was chiefly the study of human mental life, but partly through the case of Clever Hans, it began to expand considerably.

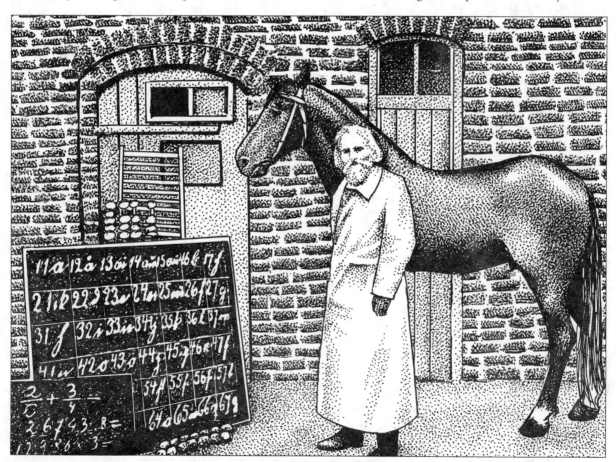

Today, the field of **psychology** is defined as the scientific study of human and animal behavior, experience, and mental processes. Its goals are to understand why organisms behave, feel, and think as they do and to apply this knowledge in diverse situations. Psychology is thus involved in all human concerns. It is devoted to creating peace and harmony in a troubled world, to helping the homeless and the underprivileged, to improving our schools, television, and legal systems.

This chapter begins with selected historical antecedents and afterward turns to the founding of psychology. Then, proceeding chronologically, it presents several views or systems of psychology and concludes with an emphasis on the diversity in psychology today.

• HISTORICAL ANTECEDENTS •

In introducing the story of Clever Hans, we are not horsing around. The animal had become a beastly problem in Berlin, disrupting people's thoughts about their universe, prompting nightmares about what might happen next. "Many a young lieutenant," wrote one reporter, "will be embarrassed to put his spurs to the nag which can add better than he" (Block, 1904). "We humans," he continued, "who put so much stock in our knowledge and progress, will do well to pack up our wisdom and with every passing coach horse doff our hats respectfully. Who can say whether or not some secret Socrates lies within that melancholy skull?"

Amid this turmoil, Count Otto zu Castell-Rüdenhausen entered the courtyard and asked Hans the date, thinking it was the seventh of September. Hans tapped eight times, and suddenly the embarrassed Count realized that Hans was right. It was indeed the eighth of the month. On another occasion, Hans was asked to spell a name, and his questioner interrupted, pointing out a mistake. Hans continued anyway, spelling the full name correctly. He was not wrong; the human being had erred. On these occasions, when Hans proved superior to his questioners, the celebrated horse greatly enhanced his reputation.

The exploits of Clever Hans, occurring early in the history of modern psychology, provoked a great deal of interest, but the subject matter of psychology has interested people throughout the ages. In fact, the word *psychology* is derived from two Greek words: *psyche*, meaning "soul," and *ology*, meaning "study." Prescientific psychology was the study of the soul. Scientific psychology has far broader concerns.

CONTRIBUTING FIELDS

Modern psychology emerged as a scientific enterprise just over a century ago, only a few years before Clever Hans. It appeared first in Germany, stimulated by developments in philosophy, biology, and other academic fields, as well as practical concerns.

PHILOSOPHICAL FOUNDATIONS. One prominent concept in nineteenth-century philosophy was empiricism, an idea many centuries old. According to **empiricism**, from the Greek word for "experience," all knowledge is gained through the senses, directly from experience. Empiricism stresses *observable* phenomena. It emphasizes that ideas are not innate or inborn but rather acquired during our lifetime. This viewpoint can be traced to Aristotle. In taking this position, Aristotle was speaking out against his teacher, Plato, who said that certain ideas are common to all people and thus must be innate.

For almost 2,000 years, the Aristotelian idea was virtually ignored. In the seventeenth century, an important British philosopher, John Locke, revived it. He described the human mind as a *tabula rasa*, a "blank sheet" at birth. The thoughts and ideas that arise during our lives are based on experience and written on this slate. Although this view does not seem new today, it was radical at that time.

An implication of this doctrine is that almost anyone can be made reasonably intelligent. Empiricism was therefore regarded with much favor by educators, including Mr. von Osten, who decided that with appropriate instructions even a horse could be made intelligent. He taught Hans with learning aids of all sorts, including a counting machine, colored cloths, cards with numbers, and cards with letters. He also used a very gradual method, beginning with a simple command, moving the horse's hoof himself, and then offering a carrot. After countless trials of this sort, he gave the command and just touched the hoof—which Hans promptly lifted, thereby receiving a carrot.

Eventually, Mr. von Osten simply spoke the command and pointed; Hans lifted his hoof and received his reward. Finally, much to the trainer's great joy, the command itself sufficed. Hans lifted the hoof and began to tap when the command alone was given (Figure I-I).

Empiricism also had enormous implications for science, including psychology. If the way to knowledge is through the senses, scientific knowledge must be pursued in this same manner. Observe the event and let the senses tell the story.

The importance of direct observation has been illustrated in a farcical story about another horse and a most controversial discussion in an ancient temple of learning. The quarrel arose over this question: How many teeth are there in a horse's

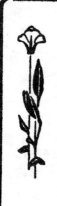
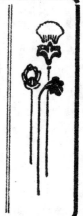

BERLIN'S WONDERFUL HORSE

He Can Do Almost Everything but Talk— How He Was Taught.

Special Correspondence THE NEW YORK TIMES. BERLIN, Aug. 23.—In an out-of-the-way part of the German capital a horse is now shown which has stirred up the scientific, military, and sporting world of the Fatherland. It should be said at the very outset that the facts in this article are not drawn from the imagination, but are based upon true observations and can be verified by Dr. Studt, Prussian Minister of Education; by the famous zoologist, Prof. Moebius, director of the Prussian

became signs for visible objects, and he used footsteps as signs for his perceptions, according to the same psychic laws as we use a language to make others understand.

After Herr von Osten had taught Hans this simple sign language, the foundation for further education was established. He put before him gold, silver, and copper coins, and taught him to indicate gold pieces by one movement of the foot, silver with two, and copper with three steps. When, for example, three coins were placed

FIGURE 1-1 BERLIN'S WONDERFUL HORSE. The *New York Times* special correspondent, Edward Heyn, visited Clever Hans in the courtyard and contributed this account, shown here only in part. The second column describes how Hans tapped with his foot.

mouth? The debate raged for 13 days with no resolution, although all important books and chronicles had been fetched and consulted. On the 14th day, a youthful newcomer called for his elders' attention and offered a preposterous way to answer the question: Go look in the mouth of a horse! Upon hearing this coarse suggestion, his learned superiors were deeply hurt, and they drove him from the temple for declaring such an unholy manner of finding the truth, one that might prove contradictory to the teachings of their forebears. Instead, after many days of strife, the assembly declared unanimously that the problem must remain an everlasting mystery due to the lack of historical, theological, and other evidence (Mees, 1934).

In this satire, the youth's empiricism offered a very different approach from common sense or the word of some authority. A cornerstone of modern science, empiricism is the first principle or theme in this book, appearing intermittently throughout the chapters. It emphasizes a basic aim in psychology: to obtain the answer "straight from the horse's mouth." This effort at direct observation is what separated the upstart friar from his unbending superiors.

EVOLUTIONARY BIOLOGY. One person who made careful observations a half century earlier was Charles Darwin. He completed a voyage around the world and wrote a book about what he had observed, *The Origin of Species* (1859). Specifically, Darwin noted the wide variations in structure and behavior among the species and observed the struggle for existence among them.

Darwin concluded that the organisms that survive are those with variations that enable them to adapt most adequately to their environment. The poorly adapted perish and produce no offspring. This process of natural selection, continued over millions of years, led to the appearance of distinctly different organisms. Darwin developed these ideas into his **theory of evolution,** which states that any given plant or animal species has developed through modifications of pre-existing species, all of which have undergone the process of natural selection.

The theory of evolution had an almost unprecedented influence on scientific and lay thought. It suggested that if human beings are descended from animals, there may be continuity from the animal to the human mind (Darwin, 1859, 1872). Furthermore, the idea of animal instincts led to the question of human instincts and the study of human motivation. If animals are our ancestors and they have instincts, perhaps we have instincts. By pointing out that our psychological as well as structural characteristics evolved from those prehuman organisms, Darwin stimulated enormous interest in the study of human and animal behavior (Innis, 1992).

Darwin's theory prompted Mr. von Osten to decide, quite erroneously, that many animals have a potentially high intelligence, as shown in his work with Clever Hans. This same intellectual capacity, Mr. von Osten added modestly, could be demonstrated in any horse of average ability (Pfungst, 1911).

PRACTICAL CONCERNS. In addition to philosophy and biology, other academic fields also influenced the founding of psychology, especially physics and physiology. Studies in vision and hearing, for example, emerged from investigations of light and sound in physics. Studies of the brain and other mechanisms of behavior evolved from physiology. However, amid these developments in the academic world, certain practical concerns cannot be overlooked.

Especially in the past two centuries, people who experience mental disorders have been regarded as ill or disturbed rather than possessed by the devil. The person first responsible for this change in attitude was a French physician,

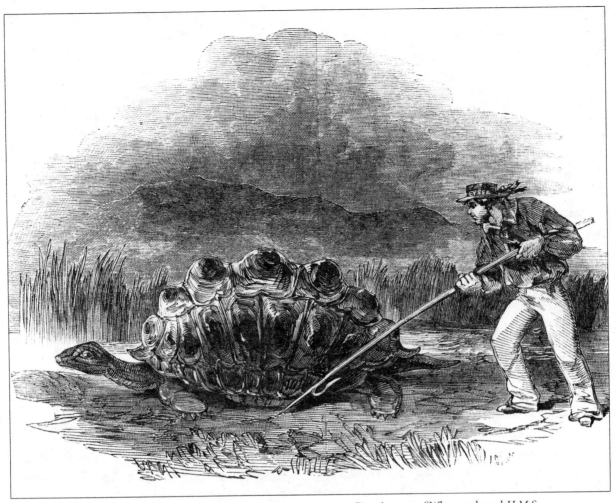

FIGURE 1–2 VOYAGE OF THE BEAGLE. Darwin wrote: "When on board *H.M.S. Beagle*, as naturalist, I was much struck with certain facts in the distribution of organic beings inhabiting South America…" Studying the giant tortoises in the Galapagos Islands, Darwin was assisted by sailors from his ship. For careful scrutiny, they used boathooks to turn over these creatures.

Philippe Pinel, who removed the chains from asylum inmates during the French Revolution. By this act, he stimulated a more humane treatment of these individuals and, at the same time, a more scientific approach to problems of personal adjustment.

A century later, another French physician advanced this perspective. Jean-Martin Charcot, a neurologist, reached the height of his practice in the years immediately following publication of the work by Darwin (Figure 1–2). Equally important, Charcot made a lasting impression on one of his students, a Viennese physician, Sigmund Freud (Figure 1–3).

Originally trained in a highly scientific orientation, Freud became a leader in the clinical study of psychological problems. As other physicians and practitioners became interested, they too contributed to the founding of scientific psychology.

But what is science? This term refers to more than the techniques and findings in biology, physics, and chemistry. In a general sense, **science** means "knowing" or "knowledge" but it implies that careful systematic procedures have been followed in obtaining that knowledge. Science is not a particular field of study; rather, it is a system for making discoveries.

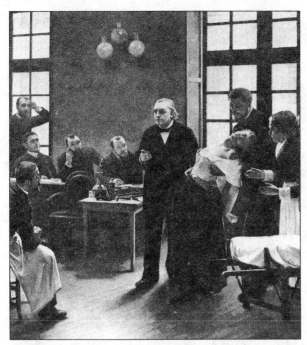

FIGURE 1–3 CHARCOT'S DEMONSTRATIONS. Using actual patients, Jean Martin Charcot showed physicians and medical students how to use hypnotic procedures. The bearded figure in the front row wearing an apron is presumed to be Sigmund Freud.

∾
SCIENTIFIC INQUIRY

This system of discovery is sometimes called the **scientific method,** an expression that can be misleading. There are many different scientific methods. One constant task of science is to develop improved methods of research. The fundamental characteristic of science is an attitude—one of demanding evidence. In idealized form, this evidence is obtained in three stages or steps.

STAGES OF THE SCIENTIFIC METHOD. In the conventional view, scientific research begins by **forming an hypothesis,** which involves making an educated guess or prediction. The investigator develops some tentative explanation about something. In Berlin, many observers hypothesized that Hans's performance was based on trickery by Mr. von Osten, his suspicious-looking owner.

The next stage, **testing the hypothesis,** involves collecting evidence in support or refutation of the prediction. The hypothesis is tested in a laboratory, clinic, or any other place where the behavior occurs. A zoologist named Carl Georg Schillings, widely respected for his adventures with animals and love of fair play, held the trickery hypothesis. He went into the courtyard and tested it by questioning Clever Hans alone, without Mr. von Osten. To his surprise, Hans performed all of the feats attributed to him. Trickery, Schillings concluded, was no longer a reasonable possibility.

In **replicating the result,** the investigation is repeated and the finding re–examined to confirm its accuracy. The essence of a scientific finding, according to many authorities, is that the same result is obtained over and over again in every repetition of the original research. Count zu Castell-Rüdenhausen, a prominent social figure, also tested Clever Hans alone. After a full session, he too declared that no tricks were involved (Pfungst, 1911).

Even these three broad steps are not always followed, however, as when a psychologist merely describes a crowd reaction or a zoologist examines an animal without any hypothesis in mind. Furthermore, some scientists contend that the first stage in research is observation, from which the hypothesis is developed. Others point to the difficulty in determining just when observation begins, for we are observing all our lives. Therefore, they restrict their definition of the scientific method to these three broad stages beyond observation: forming an hypothesis, testing the hypothesis, and replicating the result.

THE RESEARCH REPORT. Successful scientific inquiry also requires a *research report,* which presents in detail the method, results, and interpretations of the study. If the procedure has been carried out objectively and the report is explicit, other investigators can repeat the research and draw their own conclusions.

Without these reports, there would be no science of psychology, and without a standard format, their use would be greatly complicated. For this reason, guidelines have been prepared. For example, there is a convention for citing the sources used in any report or book in psychology. The author's name and the date of publication appear in parentheses following the material to which the citation refers. As the reader has perhaps noticed already, references to the story of Clever Hans have appeared in this way: (Pfungst, 1911).

Who was Pfungst? What did he do? He was a student in psychology with a special interest in Clever Hans. He appears later in this chapter.

• FOUNDING OF PSYCHOLOGY •

The event usually considered to mark the formal beginning of modern psychology occurred with little fanfare. In the late 1870s, Wilhelm Wundt, a German philosopher and physiologist, was gradually establishing a three-room research laboratory on the top floor of a building at the University of Leipzig. Looking back years later, he chose 1879 as the official date for the founding of his laboratory, not because it was constructed then but because a graduate student completed the first independent research in that year. Owing to his direction of that laboratory and his prodigious handbook on experimental psychology, historians credit Wundt with founding *scientific* psychology and regard his laboratory as its birthplace (Figure 1–4).

WUNDT AND STRUCTURALISM

A distinctive feature of Wundt's approach was its use of *introspection*, which involves contemplating and reporting on one's own experiences. Introspection itself was not new; anyone who examines or reflects on personal experiences is introspecting.

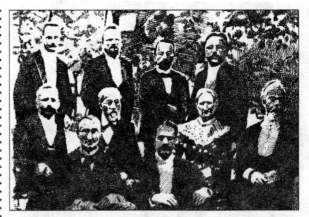

FIGURE 1–4 WILHELM WUNDT— (1832–1920). Seated with his wife in the middle of the second row, surrounded by psychologists from his laboratory, Wundt celebrated his 80th birthday.

But the people who made observations in Wundt's laboratory were specially trained in introspecting. First, they were instructed how to make their reports. Then they were exposed to some specific stimulation, such as a whirl of color, and afterward they were asked to describe the basic elements of their experience.

For Wundt and his followers, psychology was the study of immediate, conscious experience. Their aim was to analyze human experience much as the chemist analyzes matter into its elements. This psychology was referred to as **structuralism** or *structural psychology*, for its goal was to describe the basic units or structure of human consciousness. Through proper study, the fundamental elements of mental life would be disclosed.

Psychology at this time was defined as the science of conscious experience, and anything that did not lead in this direction was thought to be outside its sphere of interest. Most of the results were subjective, evident only to the experiencing individual, and there was great difficulty in establishing verifiable, repeatable observations. This approach excluded animals and young children, who could not give accurate reports of their experiences. In fact, structuralists would have no research interest in Clever Hans and little interest in the eccentric Mr. von Osten, who might give unreliable reports.

Strictly speaking, Wundt was not solely a structuralist, but his efforts spawned this laboratory work (Figure 1–5). There was a narrowness in this approach, but no comparable opportunity for research existed elsewhere. Thus it attracted students from all over Europe and the United States, making an indelible impact on early American psychology (Benjamin, Durkin, Link, Vestal, & Acord, 1992).

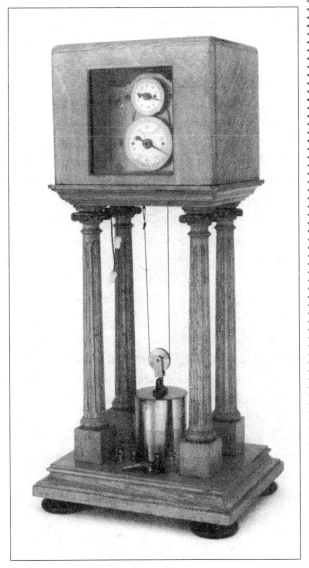

FIGURE 1–5 EARLY LABORATORY APPARATUS. This instrument, used to study reaction time, measured the speed with which a person could stop a falling weight. Prior to each trial, the weight in the center was pulled to its highest point. At a signal, it was released, moving the pointers as it fell, indicating the elapsed time before the person tugged on a wire to stop its fall.

JAMES AND FUNCTIONALISM

One early visitor to Wundt's lab was William James, a young American suffering from an identity crisis. Bright, personable, and witty, he had received an excellent education in the United States and Europe, but he could not decide what he wanted to do with his life. His efforts at finding a vocation ranged from art to zoology, and he wrote that he had four interests: "natural history, medicine, printing, and beggary" (Perry, 1935). College students today can perhaps appreciate his predicament.

After his short visit to Germany, while still preoccupied with the problem of "finding himself," James accepted a modest teaching position in physiology at Harvard University. He began as an unknown except for the growing fame of his brother, Henry, a novelist. Soon, however, William James shifted from physiology to psychology, and in 1875, four years before Wundt, he developed his own laboratory, used for demonstrations rather than research. Thus, the credit for founding scientific psychology is accorded to Wundt. Looking back on these early efforts, James wryly observed: "The first lecture I ever heard on psychology is the one I gave myself" (Perry, 1935).

With poor eyesight and a weak back, James was not inclined to laboratory work. He did studies on memory, thinking, and vision, usually with some practical goal in mind, and presented his views to diverse audiences. These lectures, within and outside the classroom, did a great deal to promote the new field.

Even more important to the future of psychology were James's accomplishments as a writer. When his two-volume textbook *The Principles of Psychology* appeared in 1890, it immediately earned him an international reputation, not only for its science but also for its literary style, and it did a great deal to stimulate interest in psychology. William James is rec-

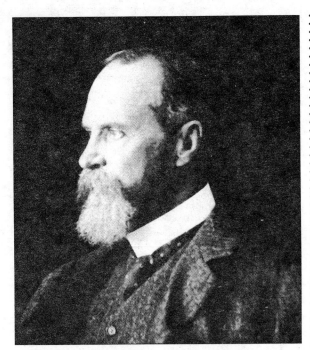

FIGURE 1–6 WILLIAM JAMES (1842–1910). Of the James brothers, it is said that William, the scientist, wrote like a novelist, and Henry, the novelist, wrote like a scientist.

ognized as the early leader of American psychology, largely because of his writings, which continue to influence the field (Estes, 1991b; Howard, 1993).

James could not find much value in Wundt's structural psychology. In America, he advocated a much broader approach, called **functionalism** or *functional psychology*, which emphasized the functions rather than the content of mental life (Figure 1–6). The concern was with the purposes of mental life, not its nature. The functionalists thought that consciousness should be studied from the standpoint of how its processes are related to the *adaptation* of *any* organism. Wundt asked, "What is mind?" James asked, "What is mind for?"

In short, functionalists were more interested in what mental life does than what it is, a natural view for practical-minded Americans. They used whatever method was helpful or necessary, rather than restricting themselves to a given procedure. Functionalism was a psychology of adjustment, clearly compatible with Darwin's theory of evolution.

Through James's functionalism, psychology gained much of its identity and gradually broadened in scope, for he wrote on such diverse topics as habit, reasoning, instinct, emotion, education, and hypnotism, in addition to mental disorders. His views on emotion still play a role in contemporary research (Mandler, 1990). Modern psychology is broadly functional, including all aspects of mental life and behavior, thanks in no small way to James's efforts. In turn, James found his own identity through his work in psychology.

CALKINS'S CONTRIBUTIONS

One of James's most celebrated students was a college professor, a young instructor at a nearby women's institution. Mary Whiton Calkins, while teaching Greek at Wellesley College, was offered an opportunity to teach psychology and to establish a psychology laboratory there, *if* she could obtain the proper training. Psychology in the 1890s was a new field, and opportunities for students and faculty were limited (Scarborough & Furumoto, 1987).

WOMEN'S ISSUES. Calkins found only two institutions open to graduate study for women, and neither gave access to a laboratory. At age 30, prohibited from entering a laboratory course with men, she obtained private lessons from an instructor at nearby Clark University. Later, as a woman at all-male Harvard University, she needed special permission to study psychology. Her request to work with William James was granted, and she faithfully attended his classes.

Calkins eventually completed all of the requirements for the doctoral degree at Harvard University, but in those days Harvard did not award degrees to women. Instead, it offered a degree from Radcliffe, an affiliated women's college. Calkins refused the award, pointing out that she had not earned the degree from Radcliffe. Even at the out-

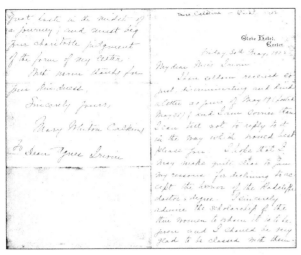

FIGURE 1-7 CALKINS AND WOMEN'S EDUCATION. In her letter of refusal to Dean Agnes Irwin of Radcliffe College, Calkins began: "I have seldom received so just discriminating and kind letter as yours of May 19 (posted May 21); and I am sorrier than I can tell not to reply to it in the way which would best please you...." After stating her view of "the best ideals of education," she added: "You will be quick to see that holding this conviction, I cannot rightly take the easier course of accepting the degree" (H.U. Archives, May 30, 1932).

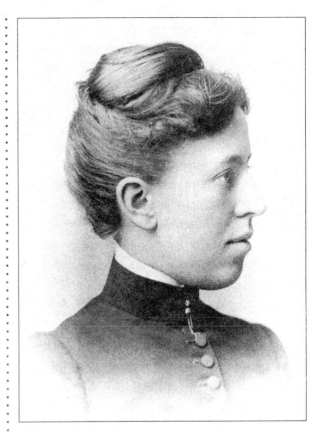

set of her career, she steadfastly resisted sexism (Figure 1–7).

ATTEMPT AT RECONCILIATION. Two years later, Calkins was elected to membership in the American Psychological Association (APA). This recognition was followed by considerable success in the field, including books and theoretical papers on the psychology of the self. In the process, she developed original experimental methods in the study of memory that are still employed today (Madigan & O'Hara, 1992).

A dozen years thereafter, she was awarded the highest honor in the American Psychological Association. She was elected to its presidency. In her inaugural address in 1905, she attempted to reconcile structural and functional psychology, using the concept of the self, or self-awareness, as the connecting link. The study of the self, she declared, is analyzable into basic elements, as the structuralists would have it, and it is also composed of complex relationships with the environ-

ment, social and physiological, which is the functionalists' perspective. In other words, the psychology of self-awareness requires both approaches, an understanding of the basic, structural elements and also a view of one's adjustment to the surroundings.

In Calkins's view, this focus on the self from two directions resolved the controversy: "It harmonizes the truth in the teachings of structural and of functional psychology" (Calkins, 1905).

CONTROVERSY AND SCIENCE. Controversy has played an important role throughout the history of psychology, and attempts to settle it are the basis of much research. Ideas are promoted; the debates begin; and investigations follow. Like the structural-functional dispute, many controversies are never clearly settled, but they serve to stimulate research activity.

While Mary Calkins sought to settle the structural-functional controversy in the United States, psychologists and newspapers in Berlin and America tried to resolve a smaller but more heated psychological question, the intelligence of Clever Hans. Finally, the newspapers invited Professor Carl Stumpf into the arena. As director of the Berlin Psychological Institute, he reluctantly agreed to study Clever Hans. For this purpose, he assembled 13 diverse but uniquely qualified citizens, ranging from schoolteachers to cavalry officers, promptly dubbed the Hans Commission. On September 12, 1904, after two days of questioning the horse in a very careful manner, with its owner sometimes present and sometimes absent, the commission announced its findings: It detected no tricks of any sort.

One disgruntled citizen insisted on another investigation. Someone should call the horse on the telephone (Block, 1904). Carl Stumpf also insisted on further study, this time without a committee of 13, which proved cumbersome. One or two well-trained investigators should be sufficient. Until that time, he was withholding judgment.

• SYSTEMS OF PSYCHOLOGY •

Particularly as seen in the efforts of Wundt and James, a new science often develops through competing theories and positions. Wundt's approach was extremely influential for a few decades, and then it disappeared rapidly as psychology developed different interests and methods.

When a certain broad perspective becomes prominent in psychology, it is often called a model or **system of psychology,** for it guides research and theory for many investigators. A system defines the field of inquiry for its advocates, identifying the problems to be studied and the methods to be used. A new system or model often develops in reaction to previous systems or is embedded in the

spirit of the times. It can attract a large group of adherents, especially if it is sufficiently open-ended to indicate all sorts of research questions for them to pursue (Kuhn, 1962).

Today there are distinctly different systems in psychology, just as there are different systems of religion, politics, economics, and other social institutions. No one perspective can embrace an entire field. Also, there are countless different theories. Somewhat smaller than a system, a **theory** is a set of principles with explanatory value. For example, psychoanalysis is a system of psychology; it offers a framework for approaching the whole field of psychology. Within psychoanalysis can be found a theory of dreams, a theory of neurosis, a theory of childhood sexuality, and so forth, all part of the larger system. Often the terms *systems* and *theories* are used interchangeably, for some theories are broad indeed. In the following discussion, the case of Clever Hans offers a basis for comparisons among five systems: the biological approach, psychoanalysis, behaviorism, humanistic psychology, and cognitive psychology.

BIOLOGICAL APPROACH

Wilhelm Wundt, the first person who, without reservation, could be called a psychologist, regarded the new field as physiological psychology. He considered psychology a descendant of physiology, although his interests and methods sometimes diverted him onto other paths. Even today, there is a tendency to emphasize the kinship of psychology with biology, occasionally to the detriment of psychology's independence and uniqueness (McPherson, 1992).

The basic premise in the **biological approach** is that behavior and experience are most usefully studied in terms of the underlying physical and biochemical structures. These are the mechanisms that

14

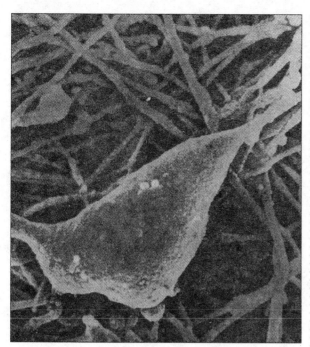

FIGURE 1–8 NEURAL STRUCTURES.
Enlarged many thousands of times, this photograph shows nerve cells in the human brain. Forming an exquisitely intricate network, they underlie the versatility of human behavior.

enable us to respond (Figure 1-8). All of our experiences and information from our own bodies, and all of our reactions to these experiences and sensations, can be studied in the context of brain structures, nerve impulses, genes, hormones, and so forth. Today there is considerable emphasis on neural mechanisms. Hence this approach is also known as *neurobehavioral psychology* or **neuropsychology,** recognizing the role of the nervous system, especially the central nervous system, in relation to behavior and experience.

In studying Clever Hans, the biological approach would focus on the physical structures of the animal and his master. Clever Hans read numbers and letters readily, even without moving his head. What characteristics of his eyes enabled the horse to do so? Hans tapped his answers in much the same way on each occasion, almost as a ritual. Which organs controlled this behavior? And most important, how was the horse able to think? Mr.

von Osten taught the horse. Which mechanisms played a role in this behavior? How did they function? These sorts of questions are prominent in the biological approach.

✍
ORIGINS OF PSYCHOANALYSIS

Some scholars say that Sigmund Freud's psychoanalysis arose as a grand intellectual protest against the rigid social code in his Vienna. A remark by his father illustrates the attitudes of the day and his son's capacities: "My Sigmund's little toe is cleverer than my head, but he would never dare to contradict me!" (Wittels, in Jones, 1957).

Psychoanalysis first appeared late in the 19th century. According to Freud, his most important book was *The Interpretation of Dreams*, published in 1900. Many people therefore regard this date as the beginning of psychoanalysis, although psychoanalytic theory gained a truly international reputation in 1909, when Freud gave five introductory lectures in America (Patterson, 1990).

Freud's basic premise was that behavior can be influenced by events of which we are no longer aware. Wundt claimed that psychology should study conscious experience, but Freud described an unconscious realm, one that could be understood only by careful examination of childhood experiences. For this purpose, he introduced a new method of therapy, the "talking cure," in which the person reclined on a couch and expressed whatever thoughts came to mind. The term **psychoanalysis,** originating with Freud, refers to a theory of personality that focuses on unconscious childhood conflict and also to a method of therapy that attempts to relieve these early conflicts, still influential in the individual's life.

A more recent term, *psychodynamic approach,* is used in both of these ways. It is particularly applicable to modifications of Freud's work, especially

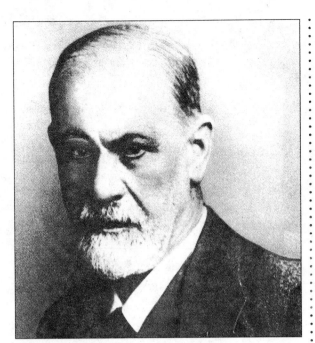

FIGURE 1–9 SIGMUND FREUD (1856–1939). He is shown here a few years after his trip to the United States in 1909, which gave international recognition to his work. It also enabled him to see a wild porcupine, which he claimed was the second purpose of his trip. Smoking as many as 20 cigars per day, he died from cancer of the jaw.

those approaches that, while recognizing the significance of past conflict, give increased emphasis to the person's *present* social environment.

Freud's revolutionary theory soon developed into a whole system of psychological thought, including many distinct concepts. The most fundamental principle, **unconscious motivation,** states that human behavior is significantly influenced by childhood events of which the individual is no longer aware. Hidden in the deep recesses of the mind, they motivate adult behavior in disguised ways, often sexual or aggressive (Figure 1–9).

Although hardly applicable to Clever Hans, psychoanalysis might have been of value in studying the eccentric Mr. von Osten. What was his motivation for these lonely hours in that dusty courtyard? Why was he so completely consumed with this tedious, forbidding task, shunning the neighbors and all other human contacts? Did the answers lie in long-forgotten childhood experiences, leaving him fearful,

unable to enjoy the company of human beings? Such questions illustrate the psychoanalytic perspective.

The theory of psychoanalysis has been enormously controversial and highly influential in psychology, as well as in medicine, the social sciences, art, literature, and other fields today. Also, it has been modified and adapted since Freud's time (Pedder, 1990). Anyone interested in the ideas that make our modern world distinct from earlier ages must give serious consideration to the psychoanalytic approach.

Psychoanalytic Theory

Contrary to popular thought, Sigmund Freud, founder of psychoanalysis, was not particularly interested in therapy. "I have never really been a doctor in the proper sense," he said. Then he added: "Nor did I ever play the doctor game." He practiced therapy for two reasons— to earn a living, which he could not do by research, and to gather the information necessary to build a theory. That information came from people who sought his therapeutic assistance. His basic goal in life was "to understand something of the riddles of the world in which we live . . . perhaps even to contribute something to their solution" (Freud, 1927).

As its founder, Freud spoke of psychoanalysis in two major ways. First, **psychoanalysis** is a theory of personality stating that unconscious conflict, usually from childhood, is a major force in the adult personality. This conflict arises largely through early sexual development and the individual's effort to deal with the resulting anxiety. In addition, psychoanalysis is a method of therapy based on Freud's theory and discussed in a later chapter (Figure).

Conflict was a central theme in Jenny's life, not only in day-to-day events but also in three dramatic instances. Jenny's father died when she was 18, leaving her as the chief source of support for six siblings. After they left home, Jenny left too, engaged to a man whom her father had disliked. Amid a quarrel with her mother and aunts and uncles, she married this man anyway, a divorced citizen from another country and a different religion. Following this upheaval, she broke connections with her family.

Two years later, when Jenny was pregnant with their first child, her young husband suddenly died. Once again, she became the head of a household, this time of her own family. After five years as a widow with a young son, Jenny returned to her sisters and brother. Once more a quarrel broke out, this one over her approach to childrearing. Jenny ended the conflict by severing relations again, this time for 25 years.

This pattern of conflict and rupture was repeated still again in her confrontation with Ross. Jenny disowned her only offspring. "The idea of my holding out the olive branch to Ross," she declared emphatically after that moment in her doorway, "is too disgusting for words" (Allport, 1965).

At that point in her life, Jenny had no close family relationships and no friends, for minor emotional breakups occurred regularly. As always, Jenny attributed them to the other person. She had no insight into her own behavior and how it might have contributed to the problem. According to psychoanalysis, Jenny lacked this insight because the earlier conflicts, responsible for precipitating this quarrelsome behavior, had been forgotten. They had been pushed into an unconscious realm, although they still influenced her behavior.

STRUCTURE OF PERSONALITY

In psychoanalytic theory, the building blocks of personality consist of three systems or psychic forces: the id, ego, and superego. They are called psychic forces because they are mental processes that influence the ways we think and behave. Sometimes they are said to represent, in a very loose way, the biological, psychological, and social elements of personality, respectively. Collectively, they constitute the basic structure of personality (Freud, 1923).

INBORN NATURE OF THE ID. The new baby is activated purely by innate impulses. It strives for physical satisfaction and nothing more. These inborn biological urges, present in all human beings, are collectively referred to as the id.

The id has complete disregard for anything except biological satisfaction, and it includes two fundamental impulses: sex and aggression. The sex impulse, called **eros** or the *life instinct,* concerns survival. It is love directed toward oneself and others. The needs for sustenance and sleep, as well as the desire for love and sexual experience, are all part of the life instinct. The other impulse, called **thanatos** or the *death instinct,* was a late addition to psychoanalytic theory and not as fully developed. Operating in a more subtle fashion, it involves aggression and destructive behavior toward the self and others. These two forces, eros and thanatos, are inseparable, one seeking creation, the other destruction. In referring to each of them as an instinct, however, Freud was not using the term in its conventional sense today. He was speaking instead of a broader, less well defined tendency, more like an inborn motivational or emotional disposition.

The newborn is "all id," wanting food right away when hungry, urinating without consideration of time or place, and so forth. The id follows the **pleasure principle,** which requires the immediate satisfaction of needs, regardless of the circumstances or consequences. The primary concern, in fact the only concern, is immediate gratification.

EMERGENCE OF THE EGO. As the growing infant learns to react to its environment, the expression of the id becomes modified. Partly out of the energy provided by the id, and partly from experiences in the environment, there emerges a new dimension called the **ego.** The ego, which in Latin means "I" or "self," becomes the executive or problem-solving dimension of the personality, operating in the service of the id. It assists the id in achieving its ends, taking into account the conditions of the external environment.

The ego follows the **reality principle,** which is the capacity to delay gratification in order to avoid an unpleasant outcome or to obtain a better outcome later. In the words of psychoanalysis, it requires a suspension of the pleasure principle according to the circumstances in the environment. Most infants soon discover that sucking on clothes does not satisfy hunger and that wet diapers are uncomfortable. As the baby calls for the mother and finds other ways to solve its problems, the ego emerges, especially through such psychological processes as perceiving, learning, remembering, and reasoning—all aspects of the ego. Under these influences, the child gradually refrains from acting solely according to biological impulses.

The relation between the ego and id has been compared with that between a rider and horse. All of the locomotive energy is provided by the id, or horse, while the rider, or ego, has the opportunity to determine the goal and guide his or her powerful mount toward it. But in these relations the picture all too often changes. The rider is obliged to direct the steed toward the goal that the animal itself wishes to pursue (Freud, 1933).

DEVELOPMENT OF THE SUPEREGO. Throughout life, the ego is confronted with another force in the personality, one that develops a bit later, through contact with various people. Especially through the influence of parents and teachers, the child acquires certain values and standards of behavior, known as the **superego.** These standards are learned. They represent the internalized values of the parents and, through them, of society.

One part of the superego, roughly comparable to a **conscience,** is critical and involves prohibitions; it discourages behavior deemed undesirable by parents and elders. It develops primarily under the influence of scorn and threats of punishment. The gradual development of the conscience is illustrated by the little girl who was dropping eggs from her high chair, one by one, observed surreptitiously by her mother. "Mustn't

dood it," said the child, shaking her head before each release. "Mustn't dood it." Splat! At that point in her life, the result was more intriguing than the strength of her conscience.

Another part of the superego, the **ego ideal,** has positive values, encouraging the goals of the parents and other elders. It too develops through experience, guilt, and the support of elders, as well as through imitation of them. Together, the conscience and ego ideal, formed early in life, make up the superego, the third basic dimension of personality.

THE EGO'S TASKS. As the self, or director of the personality, the ego is responsible for enabling the individual to take his or her place in society. In doing so, it operates in the service of the id, meeting the individual's biological requirements under the watchful eye of the superego. The id and superego, with their very different concerns, usually make separate demands on the ego, but they are not necessarily opposed to one another and the ego is not a referee. For example, a highly aggressive, despotic leader may decide that it is his duty to destroy a certain sect or group of people. Here the destructive impulses of the id and the conscience of the superego have the same goals, placing heavy pressure on the ego.

The ego must meet these demands in a particular context—that is, in a given reality, one that may not offer ready satisfactions for the id or superego. The ego is therefore beset with demands on all sides: biological urges, social prescriptions, and the limitations of the environment. A strong, effective ego is the essential ingredient in a mature personality.

Did Jenny possess a strong, well-formed ego? In some respects she did, for early in life she supported several sisters and a brother. Later, she alone supported her son, providing him with extensive care (Figure 2). In some respects she did not, for she was unable to manage her life to her own satisfaction. She was without friends, separated from all of her family, and without any meaningful activity.

PERSONALITY DEVELOPMENT
In the words of the poet John Milton: "The childhood shows the man, / As morning shows the day" *(Paradise Lost, IV).* After many years of studying adult men and women in his consulting room, Sigmund Freud agreed. A person's early experiences exert a profound influence on later behavior.

There are two reasons for the powerful influence of early experiences. First, the child is relatively helpless in the face of conflicts—too

18

weak to fight, too small to flee, too mute to explain, too ignorant to understand, too immature even to ask useful questions. At the mercy of his or her environment, the child must simply endure whatever happens. Second, the outcomes of these early conflicts set patterns that, once underway, are difficult to change. For better or worse, they become fixed or permanent.

What are these conflicts? They are the ego's struggles with the biological demands of the id, the social standards of the superego, and the constraints of the environment. When the ego cannot manage these pressures readily and directly, which is often the case for a child or even an adult, the conflict is resolved indirectly. Through the process of repression, the objectionable experience is excluded from awareness, banished from consciousness. It becomes unconscious, seemingly forgotten, as noted in further detail shortly. Certain cases of childhood sexual abuse seem to lend support to this view (Briere & Conte, 1993; Clark, 1993).

PSYCHOSEXUAL STAGES. In the childhood years, there is a steady physical unfolding in several areas. In locomotion, for example, the infant first raises its head, then sits with support, then without support, then stands with help, and so forth, until the child is able to run, skip, and move about in other complex ways. In grasping, the infant first waves the arms, then palms things using the whole hand, then opposes all of the fingers to the thumb, then just the index finger, and so forth. In sexual development, broadly defined to include sensual as well as explicitly sexual experiences, there is also a predictable sequence of unfolding. This growth of sensitivity occurs first in the mouth, then the anus, and finally the genitals.

These phases of sexual development are called psychosexual stages, meaning that psychological development is influenced by unfolding sexual interests. These sexual interests can become the source of exquisite pleasure and profound frustration. Thus, the child's early conflicts develop in the context of these stages (Freud, 1933).

ORAL STAGE. The infants first concern is to obtain food, and the body area of greatest sensitivity at this time is the mouth, especially the lips and tongue. Thus, this early task of ingesting food, together with the sensitivity of the mouth, prompted Freud to call this initial period the **oral stage.** If the caretaker regularly satisfies the infant's food requirements during this period, along with sucking and other oral needs, the experience is pleasurable and an

optimistic view of life begins to emerge. The child develops a trusting, confident outlook. Most important, this first relationship with a caretaker sets a pattern or model for all subsequent relationships. If the infant's needs are not met, feelings of uncertainty and dissatisfaction are likely outcomes and, if repressed, they may become manifest later, in the adult personality (Figure 3).

An adult with unresolved problems in this first stage may develop into an *oral character*, prone to excessive eating and drinking, sarcasm and arguing, or depression and pessimism. Dissatisfied with the love, food, and attention received in the first stage of life, the individual's psychological growth has been arrested at that point. The person unconsciously attempts to resolve the earlier problems by seeking extra love, attention, food, knowledge, and so forth, or perhaps through some less obvious fixation, such as gossip, argument, or biting remarks. This condition is known as a **fixation** because normal gratification has been blocked at an earlier stage and the individual remains preoccupied with achieving the pleasure denied earlier.

When we consider Jenny Masterson from the psychoanalytic perspective, we note immediately her adversarial, unfriendly relationships with essentially everyone she encountered. Even when she liked someone initially, she had a predictable tendency to turn against that person eventually her lawyer, physician, landlords, employers, postal clerks, sales clerks, a friend here, another there, and so forth, to say nothing of her parents, siblings and, alas, even her son. Looking backward in a psychoanalytic vein, we would speculate that Jenny's disrupted love relationships with Ross and virtually all other ' adults, including her family, reflected conflict and frustration in the very earliest stage of life, the oral stage, which set the pattern for later relationships.

ANAL STAGE. In the second and even the third year, the **anal stage,** a new sensitivity appears, in the anus, and the child is confronted with a very difficult task: toilet training. It can become a special problem because the child, perhaps for the first time, is expected to oppose or deny the demands of the id. Toilet training therefore plays a role in ego . development. If the training is smooth and successful, the child takes further pleasure in himself or herself and develops further confidence. But if the demands are too harsh, fixation may again occur.

In adulthood, the anal character may be incurably messy and disobedient, perhaps in continued defiance of an overly strict parental approach in earlier years. Or this person may be scrupulously neat, clean, prompt, and precise, attempting to make amends for childhood slips. Consider the once popular play and television show about a pair of mismatched bachelors who decide to live together, *The Odd Couple*. Dirty, rumpled Oscar uses his napkin to clean his shoes and his sleeve to wipe his mouth. Squeaky-clean Felix wears plastic Baggies on his hands when touching his own door knobs and incessantly sprays his home with disinfectant. These two men, so much at odds with one another, have the same underlying problem, according to psychoanalytic theory—an unresolved anal problem. As infants, they received toilet training that was too strict for their readiness at the time. As adults, they are fixated; their difficult earlier days are still with them.

These stereotyped descriptions of personality are regarded with skepticism by many modern psychologists, but many believe in the broader principle that adult life brings a symbolic re-enactment of childhood problems. In calling attention to the importance of childhood experiences in adult behavior, apart from these hypothesized outcomes, Freud made a most significant contribution to the study of personality.

PHALLIC STAGE. The period from three to six years is the phallic stage, a term that Freud used for both boys and girls, during which the child discovers pleasures associated with the genitalia, including various forms of masturbation. But more important for personality development is an increasing awareness of sex roles and an emerging interest in the parent of the opposite sex. Freud described this reaction with reference to King Oedipus, a figure in early Greek drama who unknowingly murdered his father and married his mother. In the **Oedipus complex,** a son regards his father as a rival and seeks intimate relations with his mother. Freud referred to the daughter's family position in the same way; she strives in particular for the love of her father and regards her mother as an obstacle to this goal. Other psychologists have labeled this condition of the daughter the **Electra complex** (Powell, 1993).

This rivalry with the same-sex parent causes anxiety, for that parent is big and powerful. The normal child therefore handles the Oedipus problem by a shift in outlook. In this process, called **identification,** the child adopts the manner, attitudes, and interests of the same-sex parent, attempting in this way to avoid the rivalry with that parent and, at the same time, to win the love and respect of the other parent. This process

is assumed to be particularly important for developing appropriate sex roles.

LATER STAGES. At the conclusion of the phallic stage, there is an apparent absence of sexual interests. They are present, Freud claimed, but he called this period of late childhood the **latency stage** because sexuality is not an overt concern. This stage, from age six to the onset of adolescence, may be a cultural artifact, however. In certain societies, including ours, there may be no decrease in sexual interests in late childhood.

With the beginning of adolescence and the **genital** stage, there is a reawakening of sexual interests and a search for people to provide sexual satisfaction. The individual becomes other-oriented as well as self-oriented, seeking to combine self-concerns with those of other people. Insofar as the earlier conflicts have been adequately resolved, the individual settles into the task of establishing mature relationships with other people, a stage that lasts throughout the adult years (Figure 4).

UNCONSCIOUS MOTIVATION

In psychoanalysis, the fundamental concept is the unconscious - or unconscious motivation - discussed in prior chapters on consciousness, memory, and motivation. In **unconscious motivation,** traumatic events earlier in life, seemingly forgotten, continue to influence behavior, but they do so without the individual's full awareness. Too difficult for the ego to manage, they never fully disappear.

To review earlier discussions succinctly, unconscious motivation can be viewed as developing in these stages: conflict, repression, and symbolic behavior. A *conflict* in the early years cannot be managed by the immature ego, thereby causing anxiety. To deal with this anxiety, the ego uses *repression,* by which memory of the conflict is pushed into the unconscious realm. Repression requires energy, however, and at various points in later life, especially when the individual is tired, annoyed, or ill, the repressed conflict reappears in *symbolic behavior,* as an expression but also a disguise of the underlying conflict. The disguise is part of the ego's work, keeping unwanted, repressed thoughts and feelings out of consciousness (Freud, 1900, 1938).

According to Freud, mental life actually occurs at several levels. The first, the *conscious,* consists only of an individual's current thoughts and feelings at any given moment. It is transitory. The next, the *preconscious,* can become conscious with some simple, direct effort at recall. For example, describe your first kiss. That should be possible, provided it was not too traumatic. If it were, then that experience should be buried in the third level, the unconscious. The contents of the *unconscious* have been repressed and cannot become conscious through ordinary efforts at recall. The special techniques of psychoanalytic therapy are necessary to retrieve these memories (Figure 5). Otherwise, the contents of the unconscious are revealed only occasionally and in disguise through symbolic behavior—in the form of dreams, errors in everyday life, defense mechanisms, maladjustment, and even lifestyle.

ERRORS IN EVERYDAY LIFE. The symbolism in dreams has been considered already, in the chapter on consciousness, and it is still debated today. However, Freud's view of errors in everyday life has become so popular that a minor error in speech, writing, memory, or the performance of some task is often called a *Freudian slip*, meaning that it is a symbolic expression of some unconscious motive. The slip partially reveals some repressed impulse or conflict. A man contemplating a diet asked a woman for a good seducing plan. A woman, not wanting her daughter to leave home, injured herself in a highly unusual manner, requiring her daughter to stay home and assume the burden of care. Freud noticed such mistakes in his own and others' lives, speculated on their origins, and wrote at length about their significance in *The Psychopathology of Everyday Life* (1914), a book that played an enormous role in the acceptance of Freud's initially shocking theories (Gay, 1990).

At a party, Freud once surprised himself in offering his hand to his hostess, as a polite greeting. Aware of no dishonorable intent, he suddenly found that he had untied the bow at the front of her gown "with the dexterity of a conjurer" (Freud, 1914).

Carl Gustav Jung on several occasions had forgotten to mail a particular letter lying on his desk. Then he tried to mail it, and he discovered that it had no address. One day, he finally did mail it, and the post office sent it back—for it had no stamp (Freud, 1914). It seemed to Jung that he had a strong unconscious resistance to sending that letter.

The evidence for Freudian slips is largely anecdotal because it is difficult to study small mistakes in everyday life, but experimental studies have provided some support. In a typical investigation, two groups of men performed the same simple task, reciting pairs of words. This task was explained to one group by a male experimenter who attached electrodes to their bodies in preparation for unpredictable electric

shocks— which were never administered. The task was explained to the other group by a seductive female experimenter dressed in a distinctly provocative manner. Word pairs were then flashed on a screen for one second each, such as *shamdock* and *brood-nests*. At the sound of a buzzer, the men spoke aloud whatever pair had just appeared on the screen. The men in the fear-arousal condition showed a tendency to pronounce the first pair as *damn shock;* those in the sexual-arousal condition, if they made a mistake on the second example, were most likely to say *nude breasts*. Similarly, *worst-cottage* became *cursed wattage* for the first group; *past-fashion* became *fast passion* in the second group. Still further, the men most anxious about sexual issues in general made a distinctly higher number of sex-related slips than others in the second group (Motley, 1987).

Of course, not all slips and bungled actions seem to involve unconscious urges. Many of them can be more reasonably explained on the basis of habit or faulty thinking. In January, for example, we often write the date incorrectly, referring to the old year. In these instances, habit seems to be the primary factor, not unconscious motivation.

DEFENSE MECHANISMS. Another manifestation of symbolic behavior, popular in the public domain, is the *defense mechanism*, a method used by the ego in dealing with anxiety aroused by the id or the superego. The primary defense mechanism is *repression*, for that is the ego's basic defense against overwhelming anxiety. Then, to aid the repression and often to disguise further the real problem, the ego may use additional mechanisms. In the defense mechanism of *rationalization*, for example, the individual is not only unaware of repressed thoughts but also substitutes false reasons for real ones. A man applies unsuccessfully for a job and responds with a sour-grapes attitude: "Who'd want to work for that so-and-so anyway?" He offers an alibi for a situation that he finds threatening to his self-esteem—being rejected for the position.

Throughout adulthood, Jenny engaged in confrontations with almost everyone she met. She failed to understand her constant fighting stance and its detrimental effects, apparently because its origins in childhood conflict had been pushed into the unconscious. The ego, through repression, had rejected awareness of this conflict and, through rationalization, had cast the resulting hostile impulses into a favorable light instead, claiming that they produced a useful outcome: "They clear the air." This rationalization served a dual purpose. It allowed Jenny to go on picking fights and also enabled her to avoid rejection, for she spurned others before they might reject her.

In another defense mechanism, called *reaction formation*, the individual adopts attitudes and behaviors that are the opposite of those judged to be unacceptable. These opposed reactions, it is hypothesized, also aid repression. After a narrow escape on one of his missions, a wartime flyer declared that he never feared anything. He fainted, however, after each of his next two flights. Later, following administration of sodium Pentothal, the so-called truth drug, he revealed more basic feelings. He said, "I was scared. Me scared! I didn't think I'd ever be scared" (White, 1964).

Rather than adopting false reasons or reasons that are the opposite of our repressed feelings, we sometimes attribute the unwanted feelings, behavior, or problem to someone else, in which case we may be engaging in *projection*. Again, there are two phases: repressing unacceptable thoughts and, in this case, ascribing them to others, which promotes the repressive process.

In a classic study of projection as a defense mechanism, college men rated themselves and others on four socially undesirable traits: stinginess, obstinacy, disorderliness, and bashfulness. Some students gave themselves high ratings on traits for which they received high ratings from their friends. Other students gave themselves low ratings on traits for which they received high ratings from friends; furthermore, they rated other people higher on these undesirable traits than did the rest of the group (Sears, 1936). These students lacked insight into their own undesirable qualities and falsely saw them in others instead. They engaged in projection, one of the predominant defense mechanisms in late adolescence (Cramer, 1991).

Other behaviors often considered symbolic, and therefore evidence of unconscious motivation, include adjustment disorders, many of which Freud called neuroses, and various lifestyles. A Lifestyle is a way of living which reflects certain attitudes, motives, values, or other personal concerns. According to psychoanalysis, repressed childhood conflict may become manifest not only in the lifestyles of oral and anal characters but also, for example, in the behavior of a *Don Juan,* a man obsessed with the seduction of women, presumably owing to a fixation at the phallic stage. Extreme fears, addictions, hostilities, and other preoccupations, including excessive hobbies and pleasures, also may be regarded in this way (Figure 6).

This assumption, that long-forgotten childhood trauma may be responsible for unusual adult behavior, has become increasingly accepted in modern research, especially in investigations of amnesia, phobias, psychophysiological disorders, and aggressive behaviors. It shows Freud's unquestionable influence not only on our ideas about adjustment and psychological disorders, the topics of the next chapter, but also on the formulations of other leading theorists.

Summary
PSYCHOANALYTIC THEORY
1. Personality is generally defined as the unique and characteristic ways in which an individual reacts to his or her surroundings. The fundamental elements in the structure of personality in psychoanalytic theory are the id, ego, and superego.
2. Early experiences are emphasized in psychoanalytic theory, particularly the psychosexual stages: oral, anal, and phallic. The oral stage involves the first love relationship. The anal stage concerns the formation of habits. The phallic stage emphasizes interpersonal relations and the Oedipus-Electra complex.
3. According to psychoanalytic theory, early conflicts and frustrations may be repressed and later reappear in symbolic form, often sexual or aggressive in nature. This sequence of conflict, repression. and symbolic behavior is known as unconscious motivation.

∾

RISE OF BEHAVIORISM

Somewhat later, another system of psychology arose as a protest against the study of consciousness as developed by Wundt. In simplest terms, the basic premise of early, radical **behaviorism** was that overt behavior is the only suitable topic for study in psychology. Psychologists must concern themselves exclusively with observable phenomena. The study of consciousness is wrong because it is subjective— known only by the experiencing individual. It exists only in someone's mind and cannot be verified by others.

As the leader of this protest movement in 1913, John B. Watson was a colorful, active personality, able to promote the new outlook in diverse ways—through research, a textbook, and the lecture platform. He argued that physicists study phenomena that any trained physicist can observe, not just privately but in common with others of this training. Likewise, biologists study what other biologists can observe. Watson urged psychologists to look outward, like natural scientists, rather than inside their skulls, and to study human beings as objects in nature.

Later, behaviorism acquired another controversial spokesperson, B. F. Skinner, known for his research with rats and pigeons and often misunderstood for his ideas on human learning

(Figure 1–10). He studied animals not to learn about them but to learn about the learning process. Animals are suitable, convenient subjects, especially when their background and environment can be controlled. Skinner continued the behavioristic emphasis on objectivity and stressed the ways in which behavior is developed and sustained by external events (Skinner, 1990). The appearance of food, a smile, or some other favorable event following a certain behavior increases the likelihood that the behavior will be repeated. Such events are called **reinforcement** because they strengthen the behavior that precedes them, increasing the likelihood that the behavior will reappear.

A traditional behaviorist studying Clever Hans or his trainer would focus on observable events, avoiding speculation on what might be happening

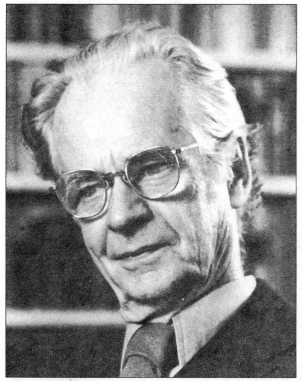

FIGURE 1–10 B. F. SKINNER
(1904–1990). Even in the later years of his career, Skinner arose at 4:30 a.m., fresh and rested, and immediately resumed research and writing. Accomplishing most of his day's work by midmorning, he enjoyed classical music in the afternoons and evenings.

inside their skulls. In particular, the behaviorist would look for the reinforcements that kept both of these creatures at their seemingly impossible tasks. Mr. von Osten continued his instruction, the behaviorist would argue, because his efforts were reinforced. Step by step, Hans mastered one task, then another, and then another. Hans, in turn, kept on tapping because he received carrots or bread after each correct answer. In short, the behaviorist would emphasize that a system of reinforcement supported the persistent efforts of Wilhelm von Osten, his horse, and anyone else who happened to be involved in this enterprise.

The details of the behavioristic outlook are considered throughout this book, especially in connection with an approach to learning called *conditioning*. For now, it is sufficient to note that there are many behavioristic psychologists today and many opponents of this view, both inside and outside the field. Many modern behaviorists, furthermore, are more willing than Watson and Skinner to consider unobservables, including the workings of the mind (Rachlin, 1991).

HUMANISTIC PSYCHOLOGY

Behaviorism was not the only protest movement. Humanistic psychology arose in the 1960s as a protest against both behaviorism and psychoanalysis. The emphasis in **humanistic psychology** is on the complexity, subjectivity, and capacity for growth of human beings, features often ignored in other systems. In this view, human beings are not ruled by the reinforcement principle in their daily behavior, as behaviorism would have it, and they are not exclusively controlled by deep inner forces dating to bygone years, as suggested in psychoanalysis. Instead, they have free will. They are an extraordinary species with capacities and awareness not found in other animals. Especially significant is the capacity for personal growth.

According to humanistic psychology, human beings must be studied as a unique development on the evolutionary scene, emphasizing the actualizing tendency. The **actualizing tendency** is a fundamental, inborn motivation for growth and fulfillment, arising because human beings, among all species, have a special capacity for controlling their own actions, making choices, and growing from their experiences. Choice is at the very center of human existence, responsible for humanity's greatest achievements—and its most penetrating moments of anxiety. This emphasis on choice and free will stands in marked contrast to the uncontrollable influences postulated in behaviorism and psychoanalysis. Led in this country by Carl Rogers and Abraham Maslow, the roots of this system are deep and diverse (Figure 1–11).

The concern in humanistic psychology is with conscious experience, meaning one's feelings at the present moment, not the unconscious and the past, as in psychoanalysis. And the most important viewpoint is that of the individual, not some particular system of psychology (De Carvalho, 1991). Many contemporary humanistic psychologists regard subjective reality as the only certain reality and therefore the proper topic of study in psychology. To understand a person's response, one must understand how that individual perceives the reality of that particular situation.

The humanistic psychologist would have had no research interest in the wonderful Berlin horse. Concerned with the special capacities and predicaments of human beings, it would not even focus on Mr. von Osten's rewards from training the horse, as in behaviorism, or on his childhood experiences, as in psychoanalysis. Both of these concerns lead in the wrong direction. Humanism instead would attempt to understand Mr. von Osten's thoughts and feelings at the moment, his capacity for making choices, and the ways in which the actualizing tendency was thwarted or enhanced. The human capacity to choose and make plans is a unique endowment, allowing us to select our own way of life. It is also a singular burden, causing anxiety about these choices.

The humanistic trend at times has been called *third-force psychology*, meaning that it represents the most significant system of psychology after behaviorism and psychoanalysis (Smith, 1990). But only history can confirm such a description.

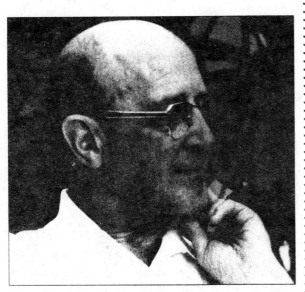

FIGURE 1–11 CARL ROGERS (1902–1987). Raised in rural Minnesota without close friends, Rogers regarded himself as peculiar and a loner. In pursuing these personal issues and his career, he increasingly emphasized the forces of growth within human beings.

COGNITIVE PSYCHOLOGY

Still another approach, the cognitive model, has been highly influential in American psychology in recent decades, despite its lack of a unifying theory. The basic concern in **cognitive psychology** is with mental processes; the focus is on perceiving, remembering, and thinking. Cognition is concerned with knowledge or understanding; cognitive psychology studies the mental processes by which we understand our world. It therefore stands in opposition to traditional behaviorism, which concentrates on overt acts rather than mental processes.

Modern cognitive psychology does not have a single, obvious leader in the sense that Freud promoted psychoanalysis and Skinner guided behaviorism. Nevertheless, a Swiss psychologist, Jean Piaget, became an early, inspirational figure in the study of human cognitive development. He began his academic career as a biologist with a special interest in birds and concluded it as a psychologist-philosopher, interested in the origins of knowledge (Figure 1–12). His pioneering studies of cognition in children have been regarded as lasting contributions to psychological theory (Hilgard, 1993).

Cognitive psychology has been stimulated by advances in computer technology and simulations of human thought, but it is broadly based. Today a guiding principle in cognitive psychology is the concept of **information processing,** which refers to the ways in which human beings and other species obtain, retain, and use information about their world. In the past quarter century, this approach has evolved into a sophisticated experimental science (Leahey, 1992).

Cognitive psychologists would approach Clever Hans as a set of problems in information processing. To what extent could Hans perceive the questions posed by his master? How successful was his memory? Could he actually manipulate symbols? And what about his master, who read the works of Charles Darwin and Annie Sullivan, teacher of Helen Keller? He had a great storehouse of information on horses, mathematics, evolution, and education, all intermixed. How did he retain it? Why did he sometimes become confused? Cognitive psychologists would study Hans and Mr. von Osten in

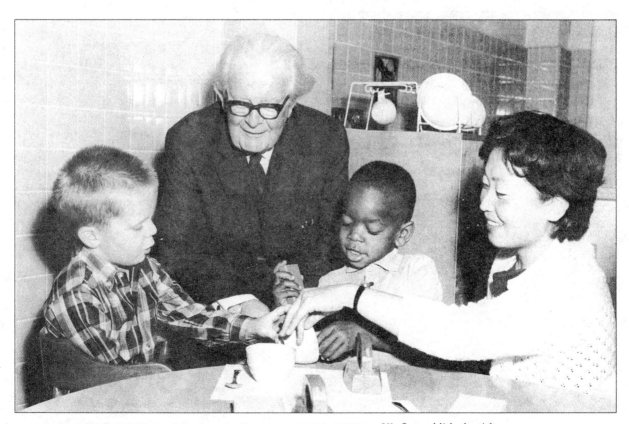

FIGURE 1–12 JEAN PIAGET (1896–1980). His first published article, on a rare albino sparrow, was well received. Piaget was pleased; he was only eleven years old at the time.

25

terms of the mental schemes or systems they employed in acquiring, storing, and using information.

Compared to the humanistic approach, cognitive psychology is more scientific and less philosophical. It differs from psychoanalysis in its greater concern with conscious mental life. And cognitive psychology, emphasizing mental processes, differs sharply from traditional behaviorism, which is concerned only with directly observable phenomena.

And here we arrive at the second principle in this book. Psychology is guided not only by empiricism but also by *various theories.* Psychology recognizes and encourages diverse interpretations of its observations. The human condition is far too complex to be encompassed by any single system or theory. Instead, each perspective makes its own special contribution (Table 1-1).

• DIVERSITY IN PSYCHOLOGY •

To satisfy the public and perhaps his own curiosity as well, Carl Stumpf selected two graduate students, Oskar Pfungst and Erich von Hornbostel, to make a more thorough investigation of Clever Hans. Still in his 20s, just beginning a career, Pfungst did not use any particular system of psychology. The different systems were just emerging at that time, and many psychologists today do not limit themselves to one or another.

After assuring themselves that Hans could indeed perform the tasks attributed to him, Pfungst and von Hornbostel turned to their first question. Did Clever Hans produce these answers *by himself?* In other words, they prepared to test the hypothesis that Clever Hans possessed a special intelligence.

This investigation illustrates a fundamental aim in contemporary psychology. Called **basic research,** it seeks to increase our understanding of the world in which we live. The goal is to find out about things. Did Clever Hans have a special mental ability? Can horses really see color? How do human beings think? Why do we forget? In basic research, the focus is on knowledge. Let there be light!

A second aim, called **applied psychology** or *applied research,* attempts to solve practical problems and improve conditions of life. The aim is to make things better for all. How can an understanding of Clever Hans improve the conditions of human life? Of animal life? What are the best ways to teach animals— and children? Applied psychology is concerned with the fruits of science. What is its practical value?

Thus science has a dual aim. Through it, we seek both light and fruit. "Most of us," observed Lord Adrian, "would like both if we can get them."

Today there are approximately 90,000 psychologists in the United States, seeking light or fruit or both. Their work is diverse, but most are employed in one of four settings: academic, medical, private practice, or business and government. The range of interests, abilities, and responsibilities among psy-

SYSTEM	EARLY LEADER	FOCUS
Biological	Wilhelm Wundt	All bodily mechanisms, especially the nervous system
Psychoanalysis	Sigmund Freud	Unconscious conflicts, dating from childhood, influencing adult life
Behaviorism	B. F. Skinner	Development of habits in all species, based on reinforcement
Humanistic	Carl Rogers	The actualizing tendency and capacity to choose a way of life
Cognitive	Several	Perceiving, remembering, thinking; information processing

TABLE 1-1 SYSTEMS OF PSYCHOLOGY

chologists is as broad as society itself. In fact, maintaining the unity of the field stands as a challenge for the whole discipline of psychology (Wand, 1993).

≈

BASIC RESEARCH

Psychologists in basic research obtain and disseminate psychological information. In this country, many of them are members of the American Psychological Association or a newer organization, the American Psychological Society (APS), devoted specifically to the advancement of psychology as a science (Bower, 1992). Psychologists from both organizations have conducted most of the investigations in the body of knowledge now called psychology.

FIELD EXPERIMENTS. When Pfungst and his assistant began work, their aim was pure research—to discover whether the horse truly had the abilities attributed to him. Thus they established two conditions and compared them. In one, called "with knowledge," the questioner always knew the answer to the problem presented to the horse, such as the number printed on a placard. And Hans answered with 98% success. In the other, called "without knowledge," the cards were scrambled face down. The questioner selected a card and, without looking at its other side, held up the card for the horse to tap the number. In these instances, Clever Hans began tapping, then faltered and stopped, tossed his head, and sometimes reared into the air. His overall success on these trials fell to 8%.

Next Pfungst tested Clever Hans in daylight and in darkness. Later he tested him in the open and behind a screen. By these comparisons, Pfungst determined that the correct answer did not come from the horse. Clever Hans knew nothing whatsoever of numbers, letters, coins, or musical tones. When denied a view of his questioner, Hans did not even know his own name.

In fact, Hans was responding to totally unintentional, very tiny visual cues. Exceedingly slight, these subtle signals had completely escaped even the careful scrutiny of the Hans Commission (Pfungst, 1911).

Each questioner, Pfungst discovered, bent forward ever so slightly after presenting the horse with a question and bent backward and upward ever so slightly when the correct tap was reached. Hans was simply responding to these minute visual cues, the start and stop signals. The chief explanation for the horse thus lay with the basic principles of behaviorism. A forward tilt of Mr. von Osten's head was the signal for Hans to start tapping, a backward tilt was the signal to stop, and a carrot or crust of bread was Hans's reward, or reinforcement, for doing so correctly.

In more general terms, Mr. von Osten's head movement was a **stimulus,** the Latin word for "spur," meaning that it initiates some activity. The resulting activity, or consequent event, is called a **response,** which was Clever Hans's tapping or the cessation of tapping. In much of psychology, including behaviorism, the aim is to understand stimulus–response relationships. The research problem is to discover which stimulating conditions lead to which responses.

So perceptive was Hans in noticing these signals, including head movements from side to side and slight turns in one direction or another, that he gave his name to this phenomenon. Communication through slight, unintentional, nonverbal cues is now called the **Clever Hans effect.** Prior to Pfungst's work, these cues had not been reported in scientific research. Yet they are recognized today as unconscious signals in posture, gesture, and vocal tone emitted by all of us in speaking our language (Ambady & Rosenthal, 1992; Scheflen, 1964).

The answer that was sought in the horse was found in his questioner—and in the careful training by Mr. von Osten. In this story of unconscious signaling, we must pin the tale on the horse's past.

If the horse's answer lay with his questioner, then how do we explain those celebrated moments when he proved superior to his human examiner? Further research showed that in these instances, two human errors occurred at the same time, one precisely compensating for the other. A flustered questioner had the wrong answer in mind and gave the signal for it at the wrong time, which was the right moment for the correct answer. These few coincidences greatly enhanced the horse's reputation, and eventually all of this research was reported in a book under the title *Clever Hans: The Horse of Mr. von Osten* (Pfungst, 1911).

LABORATORY INVESTIGATIONS. In one modern study of these unconscious cues, several people were asked to act out six different moods—anger, fear, indifference, seductivity, sadness, and happiness—each of which was videotaped. The tapes were shown to large audiences, who tried to identify the emotion being portrayed. Sometimes the actors were successful, but sometimes their emotional intentions were not at all in harmony with their behavior. One woman tried to display all six moods, but the judges in every instance decided she was angry. Another invariably impressed the judges as seductive, even when

she tried to be indifferent. Imagine how difficult life must have been for both of these women if their behavior outside that contrived situation always suggested to others a mood they did not feel (Beier, 1974).

When verbal and nonverbal messages are inconsistent, the nonverbal communication may be closer to the true message. This outcome apparently arises because we can listen to our own words more readily than we can monitor our movements and vocal tones. Thus underlying thoughts and feelings are more likely to emerge in nonverbal ways (Ambady & Rosenthal, 1993).

A detailed analysis of 44 separate research studies showed that successful judgments of the honesty, competency, biases, and effectiveness of others can sometimes be made through very brief nonverbal cues, lasting no more than 30 seconds (Ambady & Rosenthal, 1993). To paraphrase Ralph Waldo Emerson: "What you are speaks so loudly I cannot hear what you say." Or, rather, I know all too well what you are *really* saying.

These laboratory and field studies give only the barest hint of their diversity. Psychologists in basic and applied areas possess markedly varied interests (Figure 1–13). The growth of all specialties during this century has been remarkable (Figure 1–14).

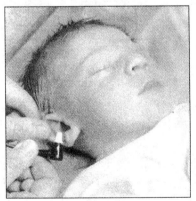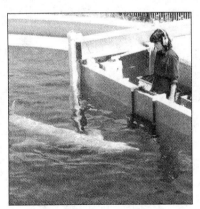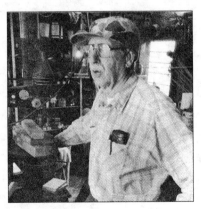

FIGURE 1–13 BASIC RESEARCH. People and animals are studied across the lifespan, as in this example of hearing. The infant's hearing is tested by inserting a probe into the ear. Dolphins are studied for their ability to maintain contact with one another by high-pitched cries, inaudible to the human ear. Among elderly people, hearing loss is studied to understand the effect of aging on the auditory mechanisms.

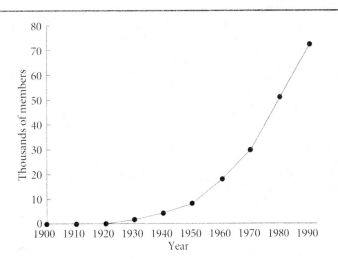

General Psychology	1	Community Psychology	27
Teaching of Psychology	2	Psychopharmacology & Substance Abuse	28
Experimental Psychology	3	Psychotherapy	29
Evaluation, Measurement, & Statistics	5	Psychological Hypnosis	30
Physiological & Comparative Psychology	6	State Association Affairs	31
Developmental Psychology	7	Humanistic Psychology	32
Personality & Social Psychology	8	Mental Retardation & Disabilities	33
Study of Social Issues	9	Population & Environmental Psychology	34
Psychology & The Arts	10	Psychology of Women	35
Clinical Psychology	12	Psychology of Religion	36
Consulting Psychology	13	Child, Youth & Family Services	37
Industrial & Organizational Psychology	14	Health Psychology	38
Educational Psychology	15	Psychoanalysis	39
School Psychology	16	Clinical Neuropsychology	40
Counseling Psychology	17	Psychology-Law Society	41
Public Service	18	Independent Practice	42
Military Psychology	19	Family Psychology	43
Adult Development & Aging	20	Lesbian & Gay Issues	44
Engineering Psychology	21	Ethnic Minority Issues	45
Rehabilitation Psychology	22	Media Psychology	46
Consumer Psychology	23	Exercise & Sport Psychology	47
Theoretical & Philosophical Psychology	24	Peace Psychology	48
Experimental Analysis of Behavior	25	Group Psychology & Psychotherapy	49
History of Psychology	26	Addiction	50

FIGURE 1–14 GROWTH OF PSYCHOLOGY. Since mid-century, membership in the American Psychological Association has increased sevenfold. Divisions of special interest have grown accordingly; there are no divisions numbered 4 or 11 (American Psychological Association, 1994).

~
APPLIED PSYCHOLOGY

The aim in applied psychology is to use psychological principles for the improvement of the human condition. For instance, our understanding of the Clever Hans effect has been usefully applied in a wide variety of situations: improving family relations, analyzing business negotiations, teaching human language to animals, and studying the cuing of subjects in a research setting (Sebeok, 1985). Most recently, it has proved useful in understanding the seemingly incredible performance of autistic children receiving instruction by means of electronic devices for word processing (Silliman, 1992).

A fuller understanding of applied psychology can be gained from specific examples. These range from peace psychology to sports psychology, from social issues to cultural differences. In recent years, *cultural psychology* has experienced a reemergence in national and international spheres as the need for greater cultural understanding has become increasingly obvious (Shweder & Sullivan, 1993). Among dozens of applied specialties currently recognized by the American Psychological Association, the following concern our environment, health, education, media, and law.

ENVIRONMENTAL PSYCHOLOGY. Among the many people today who pursue careers in environmental protection and maintenance, some have a background in psychology. This specialty, called **environmental psychology,** aims to design physical settings appropriate to successful human living, making them functional and comfortable in a mental, physical, and ecological sense (Stokols, 1992; Sundstrom, Bell, Busby, & Asmus, 1996).

The focus of environmental psychologists can be as specific as a bathroom appliance or as broad as a national forest. In the human-made environment, they work with architects and city planners; in the natural environment, they are involved with biologists and conservationists (Figure 1-15). This diverse employment shows that the traditional boundaries between various fields are becoming less and less distinct (Strathman, Baker, & Kost, 1991).

HEALTH PSYCHOLOGY. Some years ago, psychologists decided that heart disease is related to twentieth-century work habits, and they proposed to test this idea. Specifically, they hypothesized that heart attack was related to the *type A personality,* in which the individual's behavior is generally characterized by ambition, a sense of urgency, and rapid performance of tasks. People lacking in these behaviors were considered the *type B personality,* showing less ambition and only a minor concern with competition or deadlines. More than 250 employed men between the ages of 40 and 60 were identified in one early study, and after 8½ years, follow-up investigations showed that cardiovascular disease was significantly associated with type A

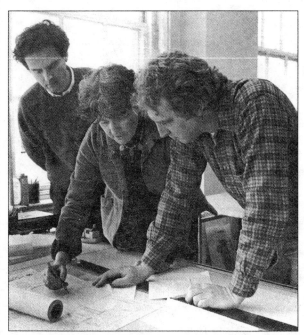

FIGURE 1-15 ENVIRONMENTAL PSYCHOLOGY. Psychologists in city planning distinguish between density, which is the number of people per unit of space, and crowding, which is a feeling of stress in the presence of others. The aim is to make life in high-density areas as comfortable as possible, partly by designing these areas to avoid the sense of crowding.

individuals. They had twice as many fatal heart attacks and five times as many heart problems as type B people (Rosenman et al., 1975). Some later studies confirmed this finding; others did not, pointing instead to the influence of smoking, eating habits, family history of heart disease, and underlying anger, more than ambition. Collectively, these studies show that the social and emotional components of heart disease are highly complex and interrelated. As they become more fully identified, the fundamental goal of prevention becomes more attainable (Strube, 1991b).

The specialty of **health psychology** concerns not only diagnosis, treatment, and prevention of illness but also the critical issue of health education. Heart disease and cancer, the two leading causes of death in the United States, are influenced by smoking, alcohol consumption, and obesity. These risks have been markedly reduced through the contributions of health psychology in changing the norms and attitudes toward risk-related behaviors (Levine, Toro, & Perkins, 1993). Known earlier as *medical psychology* and *behavioral medicine*, health psychology is rapidly becoming a worldwide enterprise (Kinoshita, 1990).

In the future, even humor may find its way into the domain of health psychology, both for prevention and treatment. Laughter decreases stress and also seems to play a role in recovery from disease, relieving symptoms and even diminishing pain. "There isn't much fun in medicine," Josh Billings joshed, "but there is a heck of a lot of medicine in fun."

Like physical exercise, laughter stimulates various internal organs through its vibrations and other movements. The huffing and puffing in a half minute of hearty laughter may even be the equivalent of that in three minutes of rowing (Fry, 1986). Especially among older people, unable to exercise and sometimes beset with unpleasantness, humor may be a matter of laugh or death (Goodman, 1994).

EDUCATIONAL PSYCHOLOGY. "Children are tyrants," one prominent educator has declared, thinking of the crisis in the schools. "They contradict their parents, gobble their food, and tyrannize their teachers." These words were spoken more than two thousand years ago by Socrates.

Subsequent centuries have not changed the view of many educators, who have made numerous suggestions for improvement: deregulate teaching, let students tutor one another, use experts as teachers, diversify the schools, and recognize individual learning styles (Satin, 1990). Among them, the approach that perhaps offers the best chance of encompassing the others is simple and demanding: Make classes smaller. Students in large classes do not receive the attention they need.

The specialty of **educational psychology** seeks to expand knowledge and concern about the teaching–learning process and to apply this knowledge in school and work settings. The focus is on improving instruction and curriculum at all levels, kindergarten through college, as well as in the workplace. Allied professionals in *school psychology* work directly with individual students, particularly those with special needs, usually at the primary and secondary levels.

MEDIA PSYCHOLOGY. Children begin to watch television before they are one year old. By age three they spend an average of four hours per day in this activity. Television is the child's early window to the world outside the home.

What do children learn from looking out this window? The average unrestricted viewer eventually receives more detailed information in how to commit assassination, burglary, and rape than in any other class of activities. By the teenage years, the typical American adolescent has observed several thousand violent assassinations on television. Meanwhile, the research linking television violence and aggressive behavior in viewers has become convincing. Media portrayals of violence influence *both* the attitudes and behavior of youth (Comstock & Strasburger, 1990; Dorr, 1986; Hoberman, 1990).

For children, *all* television is educational. The question is: What are we going to teach? Our great need is for a less violent, more cooperative world, and one way to achieve that society will be through appropriate media for children, especially children's television programs (Comstock & Paik, 1991). The aim of **media psychology** is to understand how electronic and printed information can be used for the public good.

LEGAL PSYCHOLOGY. Psychologists are also employed in diverse ways in the field of law. This work, called **legal psychology,** uses the science of human behavior to improve our system of laws, making them more humane and just. The idea is that a background in psychology can offer an empirical perspective that cannot be obtained through the study of law alone (Small, 1993).

The jury, for example, is often the core of the legal process, and yet it is composed of ordinary citizens unfamiliar with the law. Before each case, they receive standard instructions from the judge's handbook, phrased in legal jargon. How useful are these instructions?

In one instance, college undergraduates simulated jury members exposed to trial proceedings. One group received the standard legal instructions; another received instructions rewritten for greater juror comprehension; and still another group received no instructions. After the trial, all jury members completed a questionnaire based on the facts of the trial and on legal negligence, the issue on which the verdict was to be based. It was found that the decisions of the jurors receiving the rewritten instructions were most in agreement with the intent of the law. Regrettably, the jurors exposed to the standard instructions performed no better than those with no instructions at all (Elwork, Sales, & Alfini, 1977).

Given the existence of so many homeless people today, for example, there is a clear need to improve social institutions. Like all other fields, the law has numerous defects, depicted for centuries by poets and social philosophers. As Anatole France pointed out: "The law, in its majestic equality, forbids the rich as well as the poor to sleep under the bridges" (1894, *The Red Lily*).

These applications of psychology, ranging from law to the media, education, health, and so forth, together with the many areas of basic research, are just a few of the diverse interests in the field today. The numbers and endeavors of psychologists have increased precipitously since the beginning of this century.

～

ETHICS AND PRINCIPLES

Attempts to understand human behavior have existed since earliest recorded history. Some of them are essentially naïve, as when people explain behavior by reliance on gossip, a fable, or some striking personal characteristic, such as the distance between a person's eyes, the size of the head, or the shape of the body. Mr. von Osten claimed that Hans was particularly intelligent because he had an unusually large forehead, even for a horse. He believed in *phrenology*, which states that a person's character and intelligence can be understood by examining the bumps and contours of the skull. This approach came to a bumpy end; it claimed too much, demonstrated too little, and was abandoned as a useful theory long before Mr. von Osten's day. "Bumpology" had no scientific validity.

How was it determined to be invalid? It was simply a matter of employing the scientific method. Phrenologists hypothesized that agreeableness lay in a bump high on the forehead, memory at the intermediate level, and language close to the eyes. Skeptical investigators tested these hypotheses with various people and found them to be false. Further tests replicated these results. Phrenology's downfall lay not just in the fact that its hypotheses were wrong—but also in the fact that they were testable. They could be *proved* wrong; they were falsifiable.

A theory or explanation that is **falsifiable** at least has the potential to be proved incorrect. It is not so broad and all-encompassing that it covers all possibilities or so vague that it cannot be tested. Some theories of astrology, using the stars, and numerology, using numbers, are not falsifiable. As scientific explanations, they have little value.

FRAUDULENT PRACTICES. It is one matter to adopt an incorrect theory or have an honest misunderstanding of established facts. It is quite another to misrepresent oneself intentionally as a psychologist or other expert, claiming a certain title or background. Unethical practices of this sort are considerably more common than one might expect.

In most states, clinical and counseling psychologists must be certified or licensed by law. The work of **clinical psychology** deals with maladjustment of all sorts, including the diagnosis and treatment of mental disorders. As a specialty within the field of psychology, it shares certain characteristics with *psychiatry*, a specialty within the field of medicine (Table 1–2). In contrast, **counseling psychology** deals with problems in the more normal range, such as vocational problems, adjustment to retirement, and school progress. People misrepresenting themselves as psychologists run the risk of legal penalties, but often they circumvent this legality by adopting some other professional-sounding title. At present, extensive public education seems to be the most promising approach to such problems.

FALSE CLAIMS. Fraud also occurs in manufacturers' claims for products and services, such as tapes for sleep learning, seminars for firewalking,

> *Psychology:* the study of all forms of behavior, experience, and mental life.
>
> *Clinical psychology:* the diagnosis, treatment, and prevention of mental disorders, often emphasizing insight therapy, behavior therapy, and research.
>
> *Medicine:* the study and treatment of all forms of illness and disease.
>
> *Psychiatry:* the diagnosis, treatment, and prevention of mental disorders, often emphasizing insight therapy and the prescription of drugs.
>
> **TABLE 1–2 CLINICAL PSYCHOLOGY AND PSYCHIATRY.** A clinical psychologist earns a Ph.D. in psychology. A psychiatrist, trained in medicine, earns an M.D. Both are concerned with diverse problems of adjustment, offering similar services with somewhat different emphases.

and self-help subliminal messages. All of us would like to improve ourselves with little or no effort. Why not, for example, turn on a tape recorder and learn while asleep?

Several early studies of sleep learning produced promising results, and the mass media quickly publicized these claims. Later investigations showed an important shortcoming: The sleepers, who were supposed to be dozing on the job, were not fully asleep. Instead, they had been partially awakened by the recordings. In studies designed to correct this defect, the tape recordings remained on only when patterns of brain waves showed that the subjects were truly asleep. Under these conditions, the sleepers showed no evidence of learning (Emmons & Simon, 1956).

A recent confirmation of these findings showed no memory for lists of words presented during sleep. Partial recall sometimes occurred, but only when the presentation of words was followed immediately by arousal (Wood, Bootzin, Kihlstrom, & Schacter, 1992). One general conclusion remains from most research on topics of this sort: Self-improvement is typically proportional to the effort. Claims to the contrary, whether they concern subliminal messages or psychic secrets, are typically made by unethical people who profit from the false impressions of a gullible public (Moore, 1992).

FALLACY OF THE SINGLE CAUSE. A warning about simple solutions to complex problems is in order here. The **fallacy of the single cause** states that one condition or factor leads to one or more specific outcomes—for example: "Early to bed, early to rise makes a person healthy, wealthy, and wise." In fact, several factors besides one's habitual bedtime inevitably are involved in health, wealth, wisdom, and other conditions of life.

We can express this caution differently. Behind every complex problem there is one answer that is simple, efficient, attractive—and probably wrong. In the study of human behavior and experience, we need great respect for the complexity of the issues.

MULTIPLE BASES OF BEHAVIOR. This concept of multiple causation can be expressed in more positive terms. Known as the **multiple bases of behavior,** it states that behavior is typically influenced by many factors, both within and outside the individual, often in interaction with one another. It is assumed that there is an orderliness among these factors and that their number in any one instance is not infinite. Hence, they are potentially discoverable.

This emphasis on the multiple bases of behavior is the third and final principle in this book. Indeed, it is the *central* principle. Psychology as a field of study is guided by these three principles: empiricism, various theories, and a conviction in the multiple bases of behavior. This textbook describes the factors that seem most important in any given instance and, as far as possible, indicates how they have been identified. In fact, Clever Hans's ability to answer questions of all sorts, even

from spectators, demonstrates the multiple bases of behavior in three realms—physical, personal, and social.

The physical factor lay in the nature of his eyes. How did the *horse* notice the signals when all around him were human beings, their eyes darting hither and yon, unsuccessful in their efforts to find out what was happening? The answer is that Hans's eyes, much larger than ours, contained a larger retina, which was very well suited to the detection task that Mr. von Osten unintentionally had set for him. Like those of any horse, Hans's large eyes also were especially adapted to noticing sudden, slight movements, a vital capacity for wild horses escaping predators. Further, the location of Hans's eyes, one on each side of the head, allowed him to scrutinize the entire scene around him, almost 360 degrees, without moving his eyes or his head and thereby disclosing the direction of his gaze (Figure 1-16).

The personal factor lay in Mr. von Osten's preference for clothes, specifically his broad-brimmed hat. This headgear apparently brought to Hans's attention the slightest change in Mr. von Osten's posture. Any movement of the trainer's head was greatly magnified in the arc transcribed by the edge of his hat. This movement was obvious in the first stages of training, when Mr.

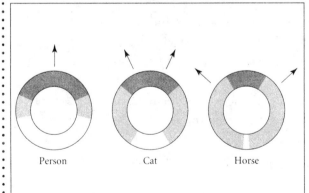

FIGURE 1–16 VISUAL FIELD. The light gray areas show monocular vision; the dark areas show binocular vision; and the arrows show the direction of normal gaze (Walls, 1942).

von Osten bent over to lift or touch Hans's hoof. It was still obvious when he bent forward and pointed. But it went unnoticed by all except the horse when Mr. von Osten, or anyone else, merely asked the question and thought of the correct answer. In certain respects, that hat was the thin thread by which hung this unusual tale (Fernald, 1984).

The social factor lay in the convention that most of us follow whenever we have finished asking a question: tipping the head forward unconsciously, ever so slightly. It is a signal learned from our elders, indicating that we expect a reply, after which we tip it backward again.

And at this point we follow another social convention, giving a tip of the hat to Mr. von Osten for his prodigious effort. He could lead his horse to water but he could not make him think, at least not in the human sense.

• SUMMARY •

HISTORICAL ANTECEDENTS

1. Psychology is defined as the scientific study of human and animal behavior, experience, and mental processes. It emerged as a clearly formulated science just a century ago, stimulated by: empiricism in philosophy, evolutionary biology, and experimental methods in physics and physiology. In addition, there were factors of practical significance, especially attempts to deal with behavior disorders.
2. There is no one scientific method, but the various stages in the scientific process are sometimes identified as forming hypotheses, testing hypotheses, and replicating the results.

FOUNDING OF PSYCHOLOGY

3. The founding of modern psychology is credited to Wilhelm Wundt, who established the first laboratory. He was interested in the study of feelings and sensations, and his students, intending to discover the structure of the mind, developed an early approach to psychology called structuralism.
4. William James, the early leader of American psychology, stimulated the new field by his creative writing and teaching. He inspired the broad development of psychology, emphasizing the functions rather than the structure of mental life, and therefore his approach was called functionalism.

5. Mary Calkins, a student of William James, founded an early laboratory and, through the concept of the self, attempted to resolve the differences between structuralism and functionalism. Amid these activities, she remained a significant advocate for improved educational opportunities for women.

SYSTEMS OF PSYCHOLOGY

6. There are different systems or models of psychology, one of which is the biological approach, based on the view that behavior can be most readily understood by examining neurons, hormones, genes, and other structures of the body. Underlying all behavior are the mechanisms that enable us to respond.
7. Another system, psychoanalysis, states that human behavior is influenced by past events in a person's life of which that individual is no longer aware. The basic concept is unconscious motivation; the basic concern is with childhood conflict.
8. In behaviorism, the emphasis is on an objective approach, stressing the study of overt behavior and its consequences in the environment. This system states that certain events in the environment, called reinforcement, strengthen or support the behavior that precedes them.
9. Another model, humanistic psychology, arose more recently in resistance to both behaviorism and psychoanalysis. Emphasizing humanity's unique capacity for growth and choice, as reflected in the

actualizing tendency, it states that the study of subjective reality in the present moment is the proper topic for psychology.

10. Still another system, cognitive psychology, focuses on the role of mental processes in human behavior, especially perceiving, remembering, and thinking. The chief aim is to understand information processing—the ways in which people obtain, retain, and utilize information about their world.

∾

DIVERSITY IN PSYCHOLOGY

11. There are two different aims in much of modern psychology. In basic research the aim is to increase our understanding of ourselves and the world in which we live. Research psychologists want to find out about human and animal behavior, experience, and mental processes.

12. Another aim in modern psychology is the betterment of humankind, to be achieved through practical applications of psychological knowledge. This approach, called applied psychology, includes many diverse specialties: environmental, health, educational, media, and legal psychology.

13. The central theme of this book, the multiple bases of behavior, states that a given response typically is influenced by a variety of factors. Psychology, as a field of study, is guided by three fundamental principles: empiricism, various theories, and a conviction in the multiple bases of behavior.

• WORKING WITH PSYCHOLOGY •

∾ REVIEW OF KEY CONCEPTS ∾

psychology

Historical Antecedents
empiricism
theory of evolution
science
scientific method
forming an hypothesis
testing the hypothesis
replicating the result

Founding of Psychology
structuralism
functionalism

Systems of Psychology
system of psychology

theory
biological approach
neuropsychology
psychoanalysis
unconscious motivation
behaviorism
reinforcement
humanistic psychology
actualizing tendency
cognitive psychology
information processing

Diversity in Psychology
basic research
applied psychology
stimulus
response

Clever Hans effect
environmental psychology
health psychology
educational psychology
media psychology
legal psychology
falsifiable
clinical psychology
counseling psychology
fallacy of the single cause
multiple bases of behavior

∾ CLASS DISCUSSION/CRITICAL THINKING ∾

A NARRATIVE TWIST
Mr. von Osten's broad-brimmed hat signaled to the horse the slightest movements of the man's head. Suppose the retired schoolmaster had never worn such a hat. Would we know today about the effect named for Clever Hans? If so, how might we have learned about it and what might the effect be called? If not, why not? Defend your answer by citing your own ideas and, if possible, relevant information from the text. ∾

• *Historical Antecedents.* Should the real beginnings of psychology be attributed to the musings of Aristotle on the nature of the soul or to developments in evolutionary biology in the nineteenth century? Explain the reasons for your answer.

• *Founding of Psychology.* What might be some differences between a structuralist's and functionalist's commentary on a baseball game?

• *Systems of Psychology.* Would a person charged with assaulting an abusive spouse want a jury of behaviorists, psychoanalysts, or humanists? Why?

• *Diversity in Psychology.* Describe some specific problem on which psychologists might well work with physicians, lawyers, or educators to improve the public welfare. Focus on joint problem solving rather than on solutions.

❧ TOPICS OF RELATED INTEREST ❧

The major systems of psychology are discussed in several chapters of this book. The biological approach is considered under the biological foundations of behavior (3); psychoanalysis appears in the discussions of memory (8), personality (14), and therapy (16); behaviorism is discussed in the context of conditioning (7), as well as in personality (14) and therapy (16); humanistic psychology appears in personality (14) and therapy (16); and cognitive psychology is the basic perspective in perception (5), memory (8), and thought and language (9).

2

RESEARCH METHODS

IN HIGH SCHOOL, THEY CALLED HIM SMART STANLEY. HE
READ THE *NEW YORK TIMES,* EDITED THE SCIENCE MAGA-
ZINE, AND KNEW THE ANSWERS TO QUESTIONS THAT PUZ-
zled his classmates.

A lean teenager full of ambition, he was intellectual more than social.
Early in life, he began to study questions for which there were no answers
(Zimbardo, 1992).

Growing up in New York City, Stanley Milgram was a city person.
He loved cities. He observed the movement of crowds, behavior of
bystanders, and reactions of strangers. He marveled at the coordination
among millions of city dwellers as they read the morning newspapers
simultaneously, walked the streets together, and arrived at places on time,
all in a relatively confined area. He watched people compete for seats on
the subway, positions in waiting lines, machines at the laundromat and, of
course, parking spaces.

Growing up during World War II, Milgram was deeply concerned about human aggression, grieving over the destruction of millions of people in Nazi concentration camps. At age 16, just three years after the war, he demonstrated his concern, as well as his capacity for finding out about things. He published his first research article, describing the effects of radiation from the atomic bomb. "It was as easy as breathing," he said of his research. "I tried to understand how everything worked" (Milgram, 1992).

Afterward, Milgram became a part-time photographer, amateur songwriter, inventor of gadgets, and finally a social psychologist. Observing people became his life's work. No matter where he traveled, he used his inquiring mind and roving eye, the tools of his trade. He studied people on the sidewalks, in the streets, and at cafes, as well as in the laboratory. People in any context could serve as his subjects.

In planning an investigation, Milgram sought direct, simple procedures, approaching research as an excursion into the unknown. "It is tentative, indeterminate, something that may fail," he said. It might yield only a confirmation of the obvious, reflecting what we think we already know through common sense. Or it might yield highly significant, unexpected insights (Milgram, 1992).

For two reasons, important research findings in psychology are often considered common sense. First, we are all amateur psychologists more than

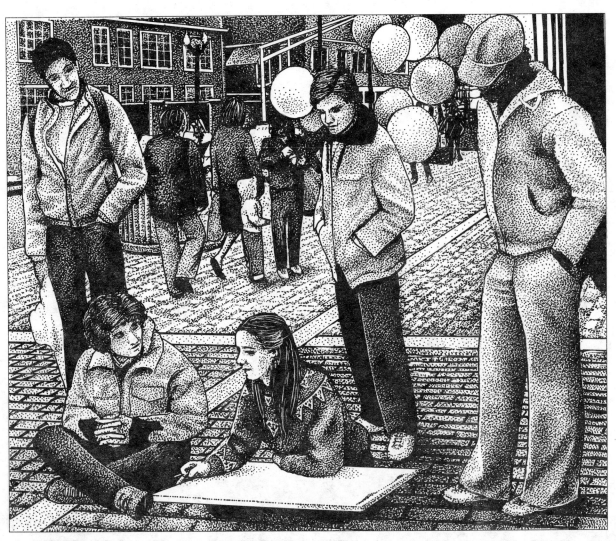

we are amateur physicists, chemists, or biologists because psychological issues—our personal relations, individual achievements, emotional experiences, and so forth—are generally more important to us than are the impersonal elements of our environment. Second, common sense supplies several answers for most psychological questions. In most situations, almost any human reaction is conceivable. Thus, the task for scientific psychology is to determine which common sense beliefs are relevant, which are not, and to reconcile contradictions among them. Common sense is *sometimes* supported by research (Kelley, 1992).

This chapter concerns the ways in which psychologists conduct research, showing how they collect or gather information. Specifically, it describes four basic methods: naturalistic observation, the survey method, case study, and the experimental method. As noted in the closing discussion on research in perspective, each of them makes its own special contribution. This chapter does not include the so-called correlational approach, which is *not* a method for collecting information. It is a later phase of the research process, a statistical procedure for analyzing and interpreting information after it has been gathered. Correlation is therefore considered briefly at the end of this chapter and extensively in a later chapter on statistics.

• NATURALISTIC OBSERVATION •

In **naturalistic observation,** the most basic of the four methods, the aim is to study behavior in its usual setting, without asking the subjects any questions or administering any tests. The investigator simply observes and records what happens in the natural environment. For this reason, naturalistic observation is often the first step in a research program.

Each morning for several years, Milgram awaited the commuter train to New York City, and there he observed the same people at the same time, standing in the same places every day. Yet they almost *never* spoke to each other. Fellow commuters, he decided, are like trees, posts, and billboards—regarded as scenery, not as people with whom to talk and exchange greetings. Milgram called these people *familiar strangers,* for they encountered each other daily but never introduced themselves. Instead, they stood in clusters, back to back, staring straight ahead. "I found a particular tension in this situation," he confessed (Milgram, 1992).

TYPES OF OBSERVATION

The basic technique in naturalistic observation is to be a very careful observer. As an eager tourist noted: "You can observe an awful lot just by watching." Yet there are important decisions to be made and subtle procedures to be followed. Among these, the most basic is whether to acknowledge or disguise the research purpose.

OVERT OBSERVATION. In overt observation, the subjects are aware that they are being studied; the research purpose is acknowledged. Milgram sometimes studied familiar strangers by taking photographs of people at train stations, later showing them to commuters, and then asking them whom they recognized. From their responses, he determined that the typical commuter encountered four or five familiar strangers at the station compared with only one or two speaking acquaintances.

Milgram's finding gave a specific, quantified answer. The average New York City commuter had 4.5 familiar strangers in his or her life. As Milgram explained, city people must discourage many potential relationships. "If you live on a country road, you can say hello to each of the occasional persons who passes by; you can't do this on Fifth Avenue" (Milgram, 1992).

But the focal point here is that these commuters knew they were being observed and photographed. Milgram and the other researchers even stated their purpose. Hence, this investigation was an instance of overt observation.

Overt observation may not influence subjects at some distance or subjects who are sleeping, for example, but in other instances this research procedure could be disruptive. Commuters might alter their behavior to impress the observer, or they might avoid the observer, taking a different train. To deal with this problem, the investigator might spend time helping them become accustomed to his or her presence and the research procedure. After the subjects seem to be behaving naturally once again, the actual research begins.

From these observations, Milgram drew a conclusion about familiar strangers. When making a small request, such as asking the time of day, a person is more likely to ask a complete stranger than a familiar stranger—someone never spoken to but seen regularly for years. "Each of you is aware that a history of noncommunication exists between you," he said, "and both of you have accepted this as the normal state." Requesting even a small favor would disrupt this well-established, tacit agreement (Milgram, 1992).

COVERT OBSERVATION. To ensure that the subjects behave in a natural manner, the investigator sometimes uses **covert observation,** in which the individuals being studied do not know they are part of a research project. The investigator can mingle openly with the subjects and then make notes secretly or remain hidden in some way. Of course, this effort to hide one's work may restrict the range of observation.

A question of research ethics emerges immediately. To what extent is a researcher justified in secretly studying commuters, coworkers, or even neighbors? The answer is complex, but it depends on the way in which the unsuspecting individuals are involved, the extent to which they may be affected, whether recordings are made, and so forth. We shall return later to this issue, noting in passing

that even overt observation raises questions about subjects' rights (Pope & Vetter, 1992).

Both methods, overt and covert, are used with animals. Field studies have stimulated much interest in chimpanzees, owing partly to certain similarities to human beings (Figure 2–1). Of course, the most celebrated naturalistic studies are those of Charles Darwin, whose trip aboard the *Beagle* enabled him to make observations of plants and animals around the globe.

USES AND CAUTIONS

Naturalistic observation serves two purposes. It provides an excellent description of certain phenomena, and it can be a rich source of hypotheses. As one investigator commented: "I find that during

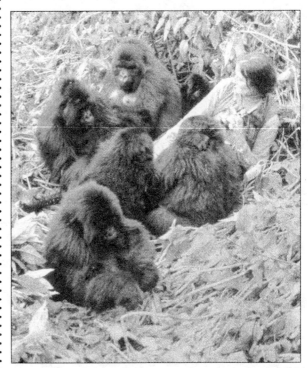

FIGURE 2–1 OBSERVATION OF ANIMALS. Dian Fossey conducted extensive studies of wild gorillas in the mountains of Rwanda, Africa. Spending months at the edge of their territory, until they were comfortable in her presence, she gained their confidence by imitating their vocalizations and adopting a submissive posture. Ultimately, she assembled a large mass of information on gorilla habits and characteristics. She found, in fact, that individual adult gorillas possessed quite distinctive personalities (Fossey, 1983).

the long hours of observation in the field, I not only learn about behavior patterns, but I get ideas, 'hunches,' for theories, which I later test by experiments whenever possible" (Tinbergen, 1965).

There is a drawback, however. Naturalistic observation is not notably useful as a source of explanation. It does not identify cause-and-effect relations with any certainty. These must be examined in a more controlled setting, typically with the experimental method. In the study of memory, for example, there has been recent debate over the most fruitful approach, some urging naturalistic observations, others advocating controlled laboratory conditions. This difference of opinion is partly resolved when naturalistic observation is regarded as a good starting point for research but not as a substitute for controlled experiments to reveal the underlying causal factors (Roediger, 1991).

Even as a starting point, the process of naturalistic observation is not as simple and straightforward as it may seem. It presents the investigator with some difficult questions and the constant problem of bias.

QUESTION OF PARTICIPATION. Some years ago, a small religious group in Chicago believed that the world would be destroyed by a series of floods and earthquakes on December 21. They would be saved by flying saucers, they decided, if they followed appropriate rituals, such as removing all metal from their clothing, remaining indoors, and reading the sacred writings. A team of psychologists and sociologists wanted to study them, but the cult did not permit outsiders to observe its activities. Thus, the investigators used their only recourse: They became cult members. Their research method was **participant observation,** in which an investigator joins the people being studied and takes part in their activities, living with them for an extended period, if necessary.

These investigators used *covert* participant observation out of necessity. If they had used *overt*

participant observation, they would have been banished from the premises as disbelievers. If they had not participated, they would not have gained access to the group's activities. They knew their mere presence in the group would tacitly support the members' convictions about world destruction, but there was no alternative.

Our interest here lies in research methods, not the findings, but in passing the reader will be relieved to learn that the world was not destroyed on that December day. And the faith of the cult members was not destroyed either. On December 22 and 23, after some doubt, delay, and debate, the members decided that their Creator had not destroyed the world precisely *because* they had maintained their faith in the face of skepticism from others. Their unwavering loyalty had saved the whole world from destruction (Festinger, Reicken, & Schachter, 1956).

As a rule, researchers do not engage in the daily activities of their subjects. They generally remain apart from the people they are observing, a research procedure called **nonparticipant observation.** Stanley Milgram once observed crowds of pedestrians from a sixth-floor window. These people did not know they were being studied, and Milgram did not participate in their activities. His method was *covert* nonparticipant observation. Later, he stood in the street and openly made notes about the pedestrians: *overt* nonparticipant observation.

PROBLEM OF BIAS. Recognizing several difficulties in naturalistic observation, William James stated that exact procedures for observation could not be established in advance. Rather, he advised the observer: "Use as much sagacity as you possess." He also warned of the great sources of error in this method, especially the intrusions of personal bias (James, 1890).

A **bias** is a preference or inclination that

		ACTIVITY	
		PARTICIPANT	**NONPARTICIPANT**
	OVERT	Waiting with other commuters, taking notes obviously	Standing aside from commuters, taking notes obviously
DISCLOSURE			
	COVERT	Waiting with other commuters, taking notes secretly	Hiding from commuters, taking notes secretly

TABLE 2–1 TYPES OF OBSERVATION. Two decisions, overt or covert, and participant or nonparticipant, yield four research strategies. The chief issues are ease of observation and disruption of the subjects' behavior.

inhibits objective observation. It results in an inaccurate judgment. A man who is suspicious of people may make biased judgments about strangers. One method for dealing with this problem is to use several observers, assuming their biases are randomly distributed. Another is to train observers carefully. Still another involves the use of remote recording equipment (Pepler & Craig, 1995).

Concerned about this problem, Stanley Milgram had his city observers work in pairs. Sometimes a newcomer and a long-term resident toured the area together, walking side by side down the street, but they made their recordings separately. This way, Milgram had a check or verification on what had taken place, for he believed that the long-term resident, while sensitive to nuances, might have the habit of tuning out many events noticed by the newcomer. City life perhaps required that sort of adaptation (Milgram, 1992).

Using naturalistic observation, Milgram identified the phenomenon of familiar strangers and other habits of city dwellers. But he could not, through observation alone, determine the underlying causal factors. And he typically could not study significant moral issues in detail (Table 2–1).

• SURVEY METHOD •

A research psychologist collecting information may intrude beyond naturalistic observation. Usually the next step is to ask questions. What do you think about this? Why do you do that? When many people are questioned, often by mail, telephone, or in a large group, the procedure is called the **survey method,** which has the advantage of including a large number of subjects.

The origins of this method are usually credited to two illustrious English cousins, Charles Darwin and Sir Francis Galton, the latter well known for his practical discoveries in testing the sensory abilities of human beings and animals. Here, too, William James had a warning: "Messrs. Darwin and Galton have set the example of circulars of questions sent out by the hundreds to those supposed able to reply. The custom has spread, and it will be well for us in the next generation if such circulars be not ranked among the common pests of life" (James, 1890).

USE OF QUESTIONNAIRES

In addition to his studies of conformity among commuters, Milgram's curiosity turned to questions of obedience, and he began giving lectures on this topic. In some lectures, he described a hypothetical situation that involved taking orders for administering electrical shocks to another person. Following the lecture, he employed the survey method with the audience. He wanted to find out what the members thought they would do in that situation. Under orders, how much punishment would they administer to a person who constantly made mistakes in learning a certain task? Here Milgram was asking: What does common sense tell you?

This method of collecting information of course depends heavily on the questions that are asked. A **questionnaire** is a printed form with questions of all sorts, often administered by mail or telephone, sometimes in a direct interview. It is intended to be answered by many people. Some questionnaires are simply a list of reminders to be checked as applicable or not.

TYPES OF ITEMS. These questions or reminders can vary from highly specific to broad and vague. Milgram's questions were specific, for people were asked to indicate how long they would follow orders—that is, how much shock they would administer to someone, under the condition that the strength of the shock would be increased by 15 volts each time the learner performed incorrectly. An exact answer was requested, using a numerical scale on the questionnaire.

In a survey on dental care, specific questions might include: "How many times per day do you clean your teeth?" and "Do you brush with a vertical, horizontal, or circular motion—or with more than one motion?" Each of these is a *structured item*, for there is little leeway in answering. Or the question might be an *open-ended item*, which can be answered in a wide variety of ways, such as: "What is your approach to dental care?" On an open-ended item, people are more likely to reveal what is important to them, but they may include endless details of no significant value. In either case, variations in the wording of the item may substantially influence the response (Table 2–2).

DEVELOPING NORMS. When Milgram administered his questionnaire to college students in New Haven, Connecticut, most of them stated that they would refuse to give any punishment stronger than 150 volts. Middle-class adults and psychiatrists responded the same way. All people in all groups indicated that they would disobey the orders eventually. None would administer the full shock of 450 volts; in fact, no one would proceed beyond 300 volts.

These results can serve as norms, for they are the responses from a large number of subjects. In short, **norms** show how people perform, indicating what is common and rare in a given population. Norms provide a means for interpreting a person's results. We can compare the response of that subject with those of the group to find out whether that subject's response is highly typical, somewhat typical, or rather deviant. Usually, a person's response is most

YEAR	DESCRIPTIVE PHRASE	LABEL
	"HALT RISING CRIME RATE"	"LAW ENFORCEMENT"
1984	69.3%	56.5%
1985	67.3%	57.8%
1986	66.8%	52.9%
	"ASSISTANCE TO THE POOR"	"WELFARE"
1984	64.1%	25.2%
1985	65.2%	19.8%
1986	62.8%	23.1%

TABLE 2–2 WORDING OF QUESTIONNAIRES. During a three-year period, a descriptive phrase *or* a label was used to ask opinions about government spending on law enforcement and welfare. For both topics in all three years, the descriptive phrase generated more public support than the label (Rasinski, 1989).

appropriately evaluated with the norms for his or her age, sex, economic status, and so forth.

SAMPLING PROCEDURES

A critical issue in the survey method is the people asked to respond. These people are typically called a **sample,** which is a number of subjects drawn from some larger group. This larger group, known as the **population,** includes all the people, objects, or events in a particular class. It might be all students in a certain college, as defined by the registrar's office; the general population of the United States, as defined by the census; or all red marbles in a certain toy store, as defined by a count of all the marbles in stock. When any sample accurately reflects the characteristics of a certain population, it is called a **representative sample.** It includes appropriate proportions of tall students, sophomores, men, and so forth, in comparison with the college population.

RANDOM SAMPLING. The most common means of obtaining a representative sample is to develop a **random sample,** in which each subject in the population has the same chance of being included. To obtain a random sample of 20 students, for example, each student in the college is designated by a different number. Then 20 numbers are selected by random drawings or random-digit dialing on the telephone.

While there are other methods, random sampling is the basic procedure for obtaining a representative sample. In fact, randomization is a fundamental principle in any research, from naturalistic observation to the experimental method. As any sample is increased in size, the influence of chance factors generally becomes less. In other words, a large random sample is more likely to be representative of the population than is a small one.

INCIDENTAL SAMPLE. In predicting the outcome of an election or testing a new drug, a representative sample is indispensable. The investigator must know the extent to which the sample reflects the population. In the early phases of some research, however, or if individual differences are not important, the investigator may use an **incidental sample,** which includes anyone who happens to be available and willing to respond. It is for this reason that so much psychological research is based on college sophomores and white rats. An incidental sample is relatively easy to obtain; the danger lies in the conclusions drawn from such a sample.

In administering his questionnaire at his lectures, Milgram obtained incidental samples. Anyone who came to a lecture could complete the questionnaire. To ensure representative samples in other instances, he used a telephone book and city records for the general population of New Haven, culling thousands of names and addresses by random methods.

Even when the sample is representative, some people do not return the questionnaire or refuse to give an interview. Unless adequate substitutes are found, these situations may produce a *nonresponse bias,* in which the findings are invalid or biased due to the lack of returns from the full sample. The people who fail to respond may be against the whole issue, or they may simply have different reactions than those who do reply. These difficulties have prompted considerable research aimed at improving the survey method (Dillman, 1991).

UNOBTRUSIVE MEASURES

Besides the sampling question, there is also the problem of reliability. The investigator cannot be certain that all subjects have responded honestly and carefully to all of the questions. The results merely show what people *say* about their dreams, cereals, sex life, or electric shocks, not what they actually *do*.

In thinking about his questionnaire results, Milgram was impressed by the extent to which college students, psychiatrists, and middle-class adults all said they would disobey orders. They would not administer the highest shock available or even a dangerous shock. "But," Milgram noted, "they show little insight into the web of forces that operate in a real social situation" (Milgram, 1992).

TYPES OF UNOBTRUSIVE MEASURES.

Subjects in survey research may try to please the investigator, present themselves in a favorable manner, or complete the task as soon as possible. This problem is called the *guinea pig effect*, meaning that the subjects know they are "guinea pigs"—participants in a research situation. To deal with this problem, survey researchers sometimes employ unobtrusive measures, rather than questionnaires. In **unobtrusive measures,** the investigator collects information from people without disturbing them in any significant way—and without even observing them directly. The subjects do not know they have been included in a research project. The investigator simply examines the traces of their behavior.

For example, some unobtrusive procedures are called *erosion measures*, for they indicate the ways in which people use and wear out the environment. In a library, the dirty, wrinkled, and torn pages tell a story. Those magazines are used. Clean pages and stiff bindings give a very different impression. Investigators also use *accretion measures*, examining the materials people leave behind in corridors and restrooms, such as wrappers, graffiti, and empty bottles and cans. In short, our refuse can be revealing (Figure 2–2).

The use of *archival data* offers still another unobtrusive measure, for an investigator can consult institutional files for all sorts of information, ranging from births and marriages to thefts and accidents. Retrieving this information is unobtrusive, although

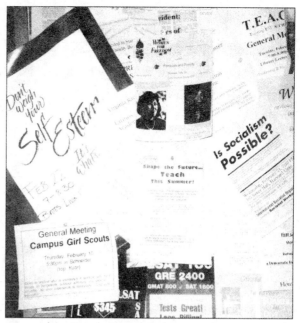

FIGURE 2–2 ACCRETION MEASURES.
An observer might make hypotheses about the background and interests of people who read and post notices on this bulletin board.

the process of obtaining it originally perhaps was quite intrusive for the subjects, as when the census taker appeared at the front door. Institutional files have been used, for example, to study the outcome of legal proceedings and techniques of control with disruptive children (Himelein, Nietzel, & Dillehay, 1991; Skiba & Raison, 1990).

The use of unobtrusive measures stands somewhere between naturalistic observation and the survey. It is not traditional naturalistic observation, for the behavior is never observed. It is not a traditional survey either, for the subjects do not know that they have participated in research. Except for the archival method, it offers little information on the people who serve as subjects.

USING UNOBTRUSIVE MEASURES.

Bothered by the guinea pig effect with questionnaires, Milgram employed an unobtrusive measure known as the *lost-letter technique*, in which many letters are distributed throughout a city, stamped and addressed but unposted. Anyone who finds one must decide what to do. Mail it? Destroy it? Ignore it? By varying the addresses on the envelopes and calculating the proportion mailed, this survey technique can be used to measure attitudes toward the addressees (Milgram, 1992).

In one instance, Milgram distributed 400 letters in parking lots, streets, shops, and phone booths throughout the city of New Haven. Each letter was addressed to a medical research group, a private individual, or the Communist or Nazi party. Each envelope was coded and sealed in a manner to indicate later where it had been dropped and whether it had been opened. For most Americans, common sense would have predicted that the letters addressed to the Nazi and Communist parties would be least often mailed and most often opened. Milgram's returns showed these results (Milgram, 1992; Table 2–3).

The use of this unobtrusive measure is not as simple as it may seem. First, all letters must be "lost" separately, requiring hundreds of different locations. Milgram once tried dropping them from an airplane, and many never reached a proper destination, landing instead on roofs and in trees. He tried throwing them from cars, only to have many fall in the gutters or be blown away. Moreover, the letters were sometimes found by people who did not read the address—children, illiterates, street cleaners, and some college sophomores.

Second, the method is not useful for asking subtle questions. The finder simply shows an overall attitude, favorable or unfavorable, by mailing or not mailing the letter. This technique is appropriate for measuring positions on either-or questions, such as the abortion issue and sexual orientation (Kunz & Fernquist, 1989; Levinson, Pesina, & Rienzi, 1993). It is not suitable for determining *why* people take one stand or the other.

Milgram was much impressed by the extent to which people mailed the letters, even though no letter contained any such request. These results showed a widespread compliance with an unstated invitation—far greater than he might have anticipated. But again, he could not, through the survey method alone, determine the underlying causal factors. Then he thought again about his questionnaire on electric shocks. When confronted with the actual situation, would these people disobey the order?

• CASE STUDY •

Those answering Milgram's questionnaire said they would refuse to punish the learner. They also believed that other people would disobey. Most people reject unnecessary pain and therefore would not follow brutal orders. The responses of college students, psychiatrists, and middle-class adults all predicted that only 1% or 2% of the general population would obey such orders fully, administering the highest shock available.

In pursuing this question further, we turn to a line of inquiry quite different from naturalistic observation and the survey. It takes place not only in clinics and hospitals but also in businesses, schools, and a wide range of other institutions. Called the **case study,** or the *clinical approach* due to its origin in hospitals and clinics, it refers to diverse psychological techniques carried out with the aim of examining a specific person, group of people, or event in considerable detail.

ADDRESSEE	TOTAL
Medical Research Associates	72
Mr. Walter Carnap	71
Communist Party	25
Friends of the Nazi Party	25

TABLE 2–3 RETURN OF "LOST" LETTERS   Letters to the Communist and Nazi parties were least mailed and most often opened: 40% and 32%, respectively (Milgram, 1992).

The case study may concern almost anyone or anything—a religious group, dangerous expedition, or the mayor's office. While it commonly focuses on a problem of personal adjustment, it provides an opportunity to examine relevant factors in the widest possible context (Bromley, 1990).

These procedures for collecting psychological information show two distinct differences from the other research methods. First, the study of the individual plays a more central role. In fact, the case study is sometimes erroneously thought to be concerned exclusively with the individual. Second, this approach usually involves more direct contact with the subjects, as readily reflected in the chief procedures: interviews, psychological tests, and case histories.

INTERVIEWS AND TESTS

In Milgram's research, a woman given the pseudonym Gretchen Brandt was particularly memorable during two long interviews, partly because she spoke with a thick German accent. She had immigrated to the United States several years earlier, but even at age 26 her pronunciation of English often made her words unintelligible.

INTERVIEW PROCESS. Perhaps the most fundamental technique in the case study, the *interview* is a conversation between two people, variously called the *counselor* and *client, interviewer* and *interviewee,* or *therapist* and *patient.* In various ways, the counselor aims to assist the client with some personal problem. In thinking of the interview, we should never overlook the power of words—not only to express our own thoughts and feelings but also to learn about other people and even to influence them. Words, observed Rudyard Kipling, are the most powerful drug used by humanity.

When Milgram interviewed Gretchen Brandt, she showed no signs of tension either by what she said or what she did, such as fidgeting, shifting her position, averting her gaze, or attempting to withdraw from the interview. She spoke of herself only when asked directly and did so in a firm, simple manner, without stammering or making unwarranted claims or irrelevant comments. She said she was not tense or nervous in any way, and her appearance corresponded well to this claim.

Another interviewee, Morris Braverman, proved to be quite different. Under the same circumstances, his brow furrowed constantly, suggesting that he carried with him many burdens. Throughout most of the interview, he behaved in a carefully controlled, serious fashion. In moments of tension, however, he began to snicker, then laugh, and then wheeze with uncontrollable laughter. At one point, he became visibly agitated trying to stifle his nervous laughter. Almost the same age as Gretchen Brandt, he seemed a great deal older because of his lined face and typically serious manner (Milgram, 1974).

As these descriptions indicate, people in interviews communicate not only with words but also by their actions. The skillful, experienced interviewer uses all available evidence in reaching conclusions based on this method.

PSYCHOLOGICAL TESTS. Perhaps the best-known devices in psychology are psychological tests. For many, they should be classified with taxes, traffic lights, and television, unwanted by-products of an advanced society. For others, they are simply an additional means of gathering information about someone, helping that individual to find his or her most appropriate place in our highly complex society. We shall return to this controversy in later discussions of intelligence.

The reader is undoubtedly familiar with **group tests,** also called *pencil-and-paper tests,* which are administered to many people simultaneously and scored by machine. Each answer is indicated by selecting one of three or four choices and marking it on the printed form.

Most group tests have two significant limitations. The first concerns the test questions, which examinees must read and answer without individual attention from the test administrator. These questions are largely *verbal items*, placing heavy emphasis on the ability to use words, which does not always reflect an individual's personal characteristics or mental ability. In fact, it may simply indicate the person's subculture (Table 2–4). Second, the test administrator cannot be sure that each subject understands the instructions, has suitable motivation, and is in a proper condition to take the test. Such problems can lead to spuriously low test scores.

There is a simple rule for interpreting the results of group tests. High scores probably represent a high level of the trait in question. Low scores do not necessarily indicate a low level. For various reasons, a person may perform far below his or her true capacity.

Less familiar are the **individual tests,** administered to one person at a time. These include inkblots and ambiguous pictures, as well as the more traditional questions. A highly trained examiner observes as the subject responds by speaking or by some other overt actions, rather than by writing. On *nonverbal items*, which do not require the use of words, the subject manipulates puzzles, blocks, and pictures, an approach that can be used to test people with language deficits (Figure 2–3).

Which person has not become an eponym?
    Achilles
    Charles Darwin
    Earl of Sandwich
    Puskas

TABLE 2–4 VERBAL TEST ITEM. To answer this test item, a person must know the meaning of the word *eponym* and possess a background in Western history and culture.

Answer: An eponym is someone whose name is given to something. The tendon connecting the heel bone to the calf muscle is named for Achilles, a hero in Greek mythology; Darwin's name has been given to the evolutionary approach in biology; and the Earl's name is attached to what we now call the sandwich. Puskas, a former Spanish soccer player, is not an eponym.

The advantages of individual tests reflect the drawbacks of group tests. A wide variety of items can be employed, and the examiner can note the subject's efficiency, conviction, and mode of answering. The examiner observes behavior, not pencil marks on an answer sheet, perhaps discovering that the subject is correct but without confidence, brashly incorrect, or has obtained the correct answers for the wrong reasons. To the extent that the test is used in these additional ways, test administration is a time-consuming, expensive, and exacting task.

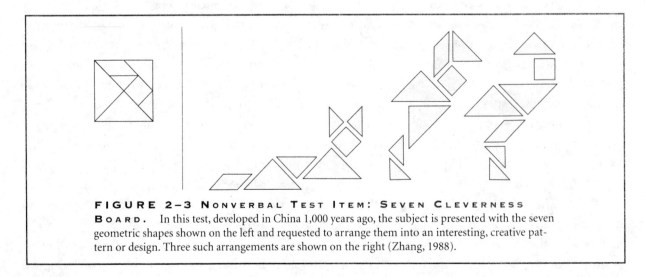

FIGURE 2–3 NONVERBAL TEST ITEM: SEVEN CLEVERNESS BOARD. In this test, developed in China 1,000 years ago, the subject is presented with the seven geometric shapes shown on the left and requested to arrange them into an interesting, creative pattern or design. Three such arrangements are shown on the right (Zhang, 1988).

CASE HISTORY

Sometimes the investigator collects information from several outside sources, such as family, friends, schools, business accounts, and medical records. Whenever detailed social and medical information is combined with an extensive psychological background and assembled in some chronological order, it is known as a **case history**. This history is almost a biography of an individual or, in the case of an event, an account of all relevant incidents.

STUDYING AN INDIVIDUAL. From a research perspective, the intensive study of one individual or event is sometimes known as **idiographic research,** for it attempts to describe the special "lawfulness" of just one person or case. It focuses on the predictable behaviors of *that* individual. Even when several people are studied in this way, individual differences are emphasized; uniformities among people are of less concern (Pelham, 1993).

With Gretchen Brandt, the aim was to understand the ways in which her behavior marked her as different from all other people. Working as a technician in a local medical school, she showed poise and satisfaction with her life. She grew to adolescence in Nazi Germany and World War II, and yet she lived easily within her new culture. This reaction was especially interesting in view of her exposure to Nazi propaganda during her youth. She seemed quite capable of resisting authority that she regarded as evil or wrong.

STUDYING SEVERAL CASES. Sometimes a psychologist conducts a series of studies for some practical purpose and later examines them again, searching for basic principles among them. The aim here is to discern common or universal themes. These studies are called **nomothetic research** because their purpose is to discover general laws of behavior applicable to all human beings in varying degrees. Several case histories, or complete case studies, considered collectively, may reveal unexpected findings about people in general. Most of this book, and indeed most of psychology, is devoted to discovering and understanding these general principles.

Earlier in the history of psychology, controversy arose over the respective merits of the idiographic and nomothetic approaches. Today they are recognized as complementary rather than antagonistic. The idiographic approach develops clinical insights; the nomothetic approach serves in the broader domains of personality, adjustment, and therapy (Lamiell, 1991; Fraenkel, 1995). Both contribute to our knowledge of human behavior.

• EXPERIMENTAL METHOD •

In his naturalistic observations, Milgram noted a high degree of conformity among commuters. In the survey method, he found that almost all subjects claimed they would disobey malevolent authority. Through case studies, he discovered that people differed sharply in response to questions of compliance and obedience, as illustrated by Gretchen Brandt and the others. However, none of this research allowed him to draw conclusions about the *causes* of conformity, compliance, and obedience. For this purpose, he needed still another method—one that would enable him to collect information about cause-and-effect.

The most promising answers to cause-and-effect questions are found in the **experimental method,** in which the chief factors in a research problem are manipulated or controlled in precise ways. For this reason, the experimental method is often considered to stand foremost among the various research techniques in psychology.

CLASSICAL EXPERIMENT

In his effort to accomplish morally significant research in social psychology, Milgram placed an announcement in a New Haven newspaper. It offered a reasonable sum of money for participation in a laboratory study of memory. People with all sorts of occupations returned the newspaper coupon and participated in this research. Among them was a 35-year-old drill-press operator named Jack Washington, a pseudonym.

Unknown to Jack and the others, the true purpose of this research was not to study memory but to identify factors that influence obedience and disobedience. To investigate them, Milgram designed a classical laboratory experiment.

In the **classical experiment,** all potentially influential factors are controlled or held constant except one, which is manipulated. What happens when it is manipulated? One by one, each presumably important factor is tested in this way. In modern multifactor studies, to be considered later, several factors can be examined simultaneously.

MANAGEMENT OF VARIABLES. Any changeable factor or element in research is called a **variable.** It is some condition that the investigator wishes to study. In the classical experiment, the investigator selects for study only one variable at a time. This method follows the **rule of one variable,** in which just one factor is manipulated, or examined, at any given moment. If an effect is observed—that is, if some specific event takes place—it is regarded as a result of the manipulated factor, assuming that other potentially influential factors are held constant.

Milgram studied obedience this way, using three people and an important deception. The real subject, such as Jack Washington, arrived at the laboratory prepared to engage in a study of memory, unaware of any deceit. In a rigged drawing, Jack drew the role of "teacher" and was given the task of administering punishment to a person trying to memorize a list of words. This second person, the "learner," was an accomplice of the experimenter, and he made many mistakes, for which he had agreed to receive electric shocks as punishment. In fact, he never received any shocks—none were administered. But by complaining and pounding the wall he acted as if he were in pain. The third person, the investigator, served as the authority figure, requesting Jack, as the teacher, to administer stronger and stronger shocks for successive mistakes by the learner. These shocks began at 15 volts and ranged up to 450 volts, each labeled with a verbal description on the shock generator (Figure 2–4).

To what extent would Jack Washington and other subjects obey the orders? We have already noted what common sense suggested to most people. On the basis of the questionnaire responses, it seemed that essentially all subjects would disobey the authority.

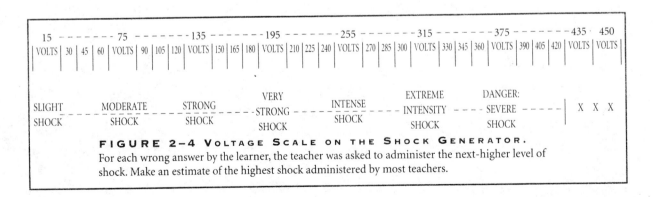

FIGURE 2–4 VOLTAGE SCALE ON THE SHOCK GENERATOR.
For each wrong answer by the learner, the teacher was asked to administer the next-higher level of shock. Make an estimate of the highest shock administered by most teachers.

With the learner strapped to a chair in the next room, Jack began the procedure, shocking the learner for his occasional errors. At the beginning, these errors were infrequent and the shocks mild. At 75 volts, the learner grunted, and at 150 volts his first protests were heard. Jack looked sadly at the authority figure but continued to obey. At 300 volts, the learner hollered: "I absolutely refuse to answer any more. Get me out of here." Yet Jack, following orders, continued to administer stronger and stronger punishment, even when the learner no longer answered.

Finally, when he reached the 450-volt level, the maximum shock available, Jack once again turned to the investigator across the room and asked what to do. He was told: "Continue using the 450-volt switch for each wrong answer. Continue, please." With a dejected expression on his face, Jack resumed his difficult task (Milgram, 1974).

Jack had been completely obedient. He followed all orders—but he was not alone. In several repetitions of this procedure with various subjects, 60% of *all* subjects eventually shocked the learner with the maximum voltage available. They obeyed all orders, showing a wide range of emotions, attitudes, and styles. Some were humble, some were self-assured, and most were deeply concerned about the learner. A minority of subjects resisted the orders before reaching the maximum voltage available. One of them was Gretchen Brandt, who disobeyed at 210 volts. At that point, in a calm but resolute manner, she refused to proceed further, thereby placing herself among the first quarter of all subjects in resisting malevolent authority.

Using this situation and many subjects, Milgram then designed a series of experiments to examine the causal factors in this astonishing obedience. One by one, he manipulated these variables: proximity of the learner, closeness of authority, prestige of the setting, and presence of rebellious peers.

INDEPENDENT AND DEPENDENT VARIABLES. The variable to be manipulated is called an **independent variable** because changes in it are independent of any other aspect of the experiment. It is varied in accordance with the investigator's purpose. If the aim is to discover the influence of the proximity of the learner on the obedience of the teacher, the investigator places the learner at various distances from the teacher. This factor, the distance between learner and teacher, is the independent variable (Table 2–5).

In addition to introducing an independent variable, the experimenter observes and measures the subject's response. This response is referred to as the **dependent variable** because it is the result of the manipulation; its presence or intensity depends

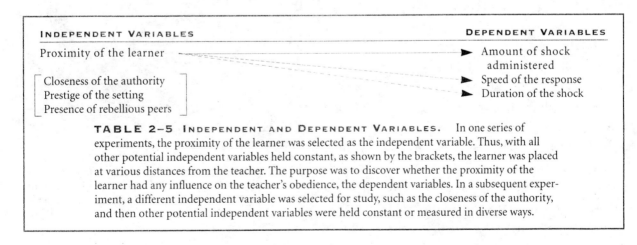

INDEPENDENT VARIABLES	DEPENDENT VARIABLES
Proximity of the learner	Amount of shock administered
Closeness of the authority Prestige of the setting Presence of rebellious peers	Speed of the response Duration of the shock

TABLE 2–5 INDEPENDENT AND DEPENDENT VARIABLES. In one series of experiments, the proximity of the learner was selected as the independent variable. Thus, with all other potential independent variables held constant, as shown by the brackets, the learner was placed at various distances from the teacher. The purpose was to discover whether the proximity of the learner had any influence on the teacher's obedience, the dependent variables. In a subsequent experiment, a different independent variable was selected for study, such as the closeness of the authority, and then other potential independent variables were held constant or measured in diverse ways.

on the independent variable. In most of Milgram's experiments, the dependent variable was the amount of shock the teacher administered. Instead, it might have been the teacher's speed in administering the shock or the duration of the shock.

As a rule, the independent variable is some stimulus; the dependent variable is some response. A word of caution is in order, however. In many experiments, the independent and dependent variables are more complex and cannot be so readily identified in terms of stimuli and responses.

OPERATIONAL DEFINITIONS. In any research, the variables must be clearly defined. As a rule, scientists use operational definitions for this purpose. An **operational definition** indicates the specific procedures by which something is measured; it depicts the meaning of something in highly explicit, usually *quantifiable* terms.

To study obedience, for example, Stanley Milgram did not use a dictionary definition: "following orders" or "carrying out commands." He devised an experiment with a fake shock generator, explicitly defining obedience as the highest amount of electric shock administered by the subject. Someone who administered 450 volts was more obedient then someone who administered only 300 volts, and so forth. The merit in this definition lies in its clarity and quantification.

Milgram might have studied obedience in other ways. Using the method of naturalistic observation, he might have observed people on city streets, defining obedience as discarding waste in refuse receptables, following pedestrian signals, or obeying laws about public transportation. He might even have used all of these measures together, employing a composite definition. Using the survey method, he could have consulted public records, defining obedience as timely payment of city and state taxes. In another experiment, he could have requested each subject to engage in an extremely boring task, defining obedience as the length of time the subject persisted in that task (Figure 2–5).

Operational definitions do not necessarily require quantification. For example, how might cohabitation be defined? You may say: "Oh, that's easy—unmarried people living together." But how long must they live together? How regularly?

Instead of setting a time limit, some surveys of cohabitation have used marriage applications to create an operational definition. If the partners for a license gave the same address, their living condition was considered cohabitation. If they gave different addresses, they were not considered cohabitants (Reimann-Marcus, 1992). With this definition there may be some false positives, partners considered cohabitants who were not together

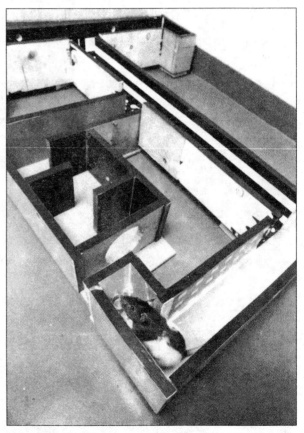

FIGURE 2–5 OPERATIONAL DEFINITION OF INTELLIGENCE. The animal learning this maze begins in the start box, at the upper right end of the maze, and finishes in the goal box, as shown, where it obtains food. Its speed in completing the maze and number of wrong turns are measures of its performance—that is, they m†ay constitute an operational definition of intelligence.

very much, very long, or in a very loving way. And there may be false negatives, partners who lived together romantically but gave different addresses. However, the definition is precise, which is a requirement of scientific research, and no definition can readily satisfy all potential criteria for a complex concept.

This use of operational definitions restricts the scope of any research and the conclusions that can be drawn from the findings. For example, Milgram's research has been questioned on this basis, though studies using a different operational definition have confirmed the overall outcome (Meeus & Raaijmakers, 1986).

DESIGN OF EXPERIMENTS

Following the rule of one variable, subjects in experiments are often studied under two contrasting conditions. There is the **experimental condition,** in which the independent variable is present or manipulated in some degree. There is also the **control condition,** equivalent to the experimental condition except for the independent variable, which is absent or held constant under its normal, nonexperimental circumstances. It is not manipulated. Thus, the control condition provides a basis for comparison. The investigator assesses the influence of the independent variable by comparing the outcomes under the experimental and control conditions. Unwanted influences should have occurred equally in both conditions, and therefore any difference in the subjects' response must have been due to the independent variable (Table 2–6).

In Milgram's early studies, the learner was placed in another room, where he could not be seen or heard by the teacher. He simply flashed his answers on a screen. This condition can be regarded as the control condition. Then, in successive experimental conditions, the learner was located closer and closer to the teacher. For example, when Jack Washington participated as a subject, the learner sat in an adjacent room, but his cries of pain and resistance were distinctly audible through the wall. For other subjects, the learner sat in the same room, readily visible to the teacher. And in still another condition, the learner sat next to the teacher and received a shock only if the teacher pressed the learner's hand against the shock plate. This tactile condition required the obedient teacher to have physical contact with the learner. These different experimental conditions, in which the proximity of the learner was varied, were compared with the remote or control condition, in which there was no

1. Establish the research question: Does proximity of the learner influence obedience?
2. Assign subjects randomly to an experimental or a control condition:

VARIABLES

	Independent Variable	Dependent Variable
Experimental	Learner's cries can be heard	Amount of shock administered
SUBJECTS		
Control	No cries can be heard	Amount of shock administered

3. Collect the results from the experimental group, which heard the learner's cries, the independent variable, and from the control group, which heard no cries.
4. Determine the difference in obedience between the two groups; obedience is the dependent variable.

TABLE 2–6 DESIGN OF AN EXPERIMENT These steps are followed in a traditional experiment. In Milgram's studies, the proximity of the learner made a marked difference. The closer the learner, the less was the obedience.

contact of any sort with the learner. In this way, Milgram investigated the influence of the proximity of the learner on the obedience of the teacher (Figure 2–6).

This overall plan for different conditions is called the *design* of the experiment. It includes the choice of subjects and apparatus, as well as the manipulation of the independent variable, but no issue is more important than the control condition. The chief concern here is control of confounding variables. An *extraneous* or **confounding variable** is any factor that may exert an unwanted influence on the dependent variable, giving the experiment an uninterpretable result.

In Milgram's studies on proximity, suppose the learner in some instances was a child and in others an adult. Then both variables, the learner's age and the learner's proximity, might influence obedience. In this poorly designed experiment, the learner's age would be a confounding variable, producing results which might be confused with those produced by the learner's proximity, the independent variable.

TYPES OF DESIGN. In addition to identifying and manipulating variables, experimenters need to decide how to use their subjects. In one common experimental design, all subjects serve in

both conditions, experimental and control. Each subject in the experimental condition is compared with himself or herself in the control condition. In this way, the two conditions should be equal, except for the key factor, the independent variable. This procedure is called the *within-subject design* or *own-control design* because comparisons are made within each subject, who serves under different conditions, providing his or her own control condition.

Sometimes the same subjects cannot serve in both conditions. This restriction often occurs when the independent variable extends over a long period of time, as in a program of therapy. If the therapy lasts for two years, the experimental subjects will be two years older and wiser, and they will have completed a program of therapy before beginning the control condition. Hence, the subjects in the two conditions will not be equal. The major method for dealing with this problem involves multiple sets of subjects matched for important characteristics, such as age and sex, each group serving in one condition or the other, experimental or control. This procedure is called the *between-groups design* because the subjects are *randomly* assigned to the experimental *or* control group; then their results are compared.

Milgram debriefed all subjects immediately after the experimental hour, for he did not want them to leave the research thinking that they had really administered pain to someone. Thus, his subjects could not serve as their own control; his method here involved the between-groups design.

Using such procedures, he found that the closeness of the authority also made a great deal of difference. When the experimenter sat just a short distance away, 65% of the subjects obeyed all commands. When the experimenter left the laboratory and gave instructions by telephone or a tape recording, obedience diminished sharply. Only 23% of subjects delivered the highest level of shock, and many subjects surreptitiously administered lower shocks than required, assuring the experimenter by telephone that they were proceeding according to

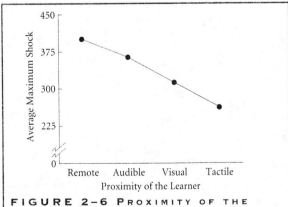

FIGURE 2–6 PROXIMITY OF THE LEARNER. As proximity to the learner increased, obedience to the malevolent authority decreased (Milgram, 1974).

the original plan (Milgram, 1974).

In the same way, Milgram found that the presence of rebellious peers greatly influenced the subject's obedience. These peers, pretending to be assistant teachers, in fact were accomplices of the experimenter. When they refused to follow orders, the subject refused too. "The effects of peer rebellion are very impressive in undercutting . . . authority," Milgram concluded.

CONTROL OF EXPECTATIONS. In many experiments, the subjects have an expectation about what should happen. Controlling expectations is especially important, for example, in testing the physiological effect of drugs, for the investigator wants to know what benefits are available *apart from* the knowledge that treatment has been received. The experimental group therefore receives the actual drug, and the control group receives a sugar pill, identical in appearance, with no medical properties. This pill, with no active ingredients, is called a **placebo,** which, freely translated, means "I shall please." The aim is to give the control subjects the same set or expectation as that in the experimental group (Figure 2–7).

The placebo effect also occurs in daily life, as well as in research. One former student had been asked to make a mixed drink each evening for his grandfather, who enjoyed the warm, relaxed feeling it provided. One day he confided that, per the doctor's orders, he never spiked the drink, but the thought of vodka certainly satisfied his grandfather.

There is evidence, nevertheless, that a placebo may not be purely psychological. The thought of receiving a certain medication may prompt activity within the nervous system, releasing neurotransmitters that can influence the subject's reactions in significant ways, especially regarding the perception of pain. Further research on the placebo effect is underway in diverse areas of psychology, ranging from education to health (Adair, Sharpe, & Huynh, 1990; Jensen & Karoly, 1991).

Similarly, the experimenter's expectations can be a concern. The experimenter's hopes, habits, and personal characteristics can influence the results of the investigation without his or her knowledge, a condition referred to as **experimenter effects.** The experimenter unconsciously signals to the subjects the response he or she hopes to obtain from them. This unintentional cuing is also known as the *Clever Hans effect,* named for the presumably intelligent Berlin horse that tapped out answers by observing subtle cues from people around him (Pfungst, 1911).

When the subjects' expectations are controlled by preventing them from knowing which treatment they have received, the procedure is called a **single-**

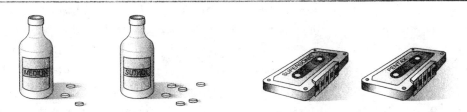

Which pills have medicinal properties?   Which tape allegedly contains a subliminal message?

FIGURE 2–7 USE OF PLACEBOS.   One pill has medicinal properties; the other is merely a salt pill. One tape allegedly contains a subliminal message; the other makes no such claim. The concept of placebo, derived from drug studies, now applies to any object, event, or other treatment used to control expectations in research.

blind design. It is illustrated in the use of the placebo. Instead, the experimenter may not know which subjects have received which treatments, again a single-blind design. Sometimes both the experimenter and subjects do not know their treatments, a procedure called a double-blind design. In the latter design, neither the investigator nor the subject knows to which group the subject belongs. A third party decides which subjects receive what treatment and codes them so that the experimenter can evaluate each subject's responses without knowing the treatment received. Under these conditions, expectancy cannot create a bias in the research outcomes.

The study of animals offers special possibilities for research design, which is one reason for psychologists' interest in animals. Genetic factors can be manipulated through selective breeding. Environmental conditions can be managed in ways not possible at the human level. Comparisons across species and among different research designs offer a powerful technique for disentangling the diverse determinants of behavior (Timberlake, 1993). Still another advantage is the animals' faster maturation rates. Studies of growth and development often can be completed in a year or two, as opposed to several decades with human beings.

❧

MULTIFACTOR STUDIES

The research procedures just described illustrate the classical experimental design, so called because the earliest experiments were conducted in this fashion, following the rule of one variable. But modern science also recognizes that behavior typically is influenced by more than one factor. For this reason, psychologists often study two or more independent variables together, a procedure made possible with the use of refined statistical methods. Many contemporary investigators prefer these investigations, known as multifactor studies, because of their capacity to identify relationships among several different factors or variables. However, the basic procedure is similar to that of the single-factor model.

The interest in multifactor studies lies in their greater efficiency and in the capacity to discover what happens when two or more factors are combined. Sometimes the result is an additive effect, meaning that the total influence of all the factors is the sum of their separate influences. No independent variable influences the effect of any other independent variable; the final result is simply their cumulative sum. In Milgram's experiments, the subjects were moderately obedient when the authority figure was nearby and moderately obedient when the learner was in another room. If these effects were additive, both factors together would produce even greater obedience.

In other instances, the result is an interactive effect, meaning that the influence of one variable depends on other variables or that the influence of one variable changes with alterations in other variables. Milgram did not examine interaction effects in these experiments, but a dramatic example can be observed in everyday life with the consumption of alcoholic beverages. Mild consumption of alcohol before going to sleep may have no significant effect on a person's health. Similarly, ingestion of phenobarbital, taken to induce sleep, may have no significant effect. But when taken together, even in moderate amounts, they can be fatal (Figure 2–8).

Outside an experimental situation, these mutual influences among variables are known as the *interaction principle*, and their subtleties sometimes escape notice in daily life. In supermarkets, for example, baggers and produce clerks sometimes experience an itch or a rash, especially on the hands and forearms. People working with dairy products or stocking shelves are not afflicted. The reason? Chemicals from certain vegetable products, such as celery and parsnips, are deposited on the skin in minute amounts. But that is not all. The problem appears largely in the summer, occurring through a

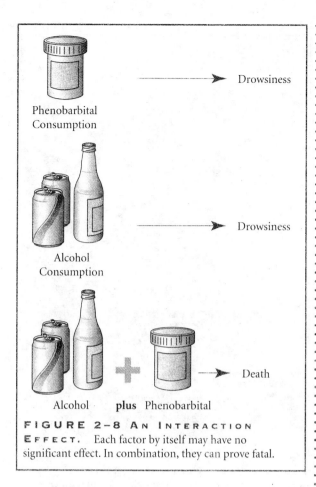

FIGURE 2-8 AN INTERACTION EFFECT. Each factor by itself may have no significant effect. In combination, they can prove fatal.

combination of the chemical deposits *and* exposure to sunlight. The name of this disorder might cause anyone to itch or scratch: phytophotodermatitis. *Phyto* indicates the plant, *photo* the light, and *dermatitis* the resulting rash. To avoid it, one should work with canned goods, wear long gloves, or stay out of the hot sun.

• RESEARCH IN PERSPECTIVE •

Psychiatrists had predicted that only 1/10 of 1% of Milgram's subjects would give the maximum shock. Instead, approximately 60% did so, obeying fully. Is there any doubt that common sense gave an incorrect answer here? One, of course, might doubt the common sense of psychiatrists. However, graduate students and faculty, college sophomores, and middle-class adults had predicted that only 1% or 2% of subjects would obey completely. The common sense of all these groups was very wrong.

The research subjects, Milgram emphasized, were ordinary people—typical citizens from the professional and working classes. And they obeyed even when no further reason was given except these statements: "The experiment requires that you go on. . . . It is absolutely essential that we continue."

On publication, Milgram's findings generated a wide range of commentary. Many readers thought about the astonishing obedience of the Nazis in carrying out brutal, inhumane orders. More than one critic decided that Milgram had accomplished some of the most morally significant investigations in modern psychology (Elms, 1972). Another described Milgram's work as "a momentous and meaningful contribution to our knowledge of human behavior" (Erikson, 1968). In sharp contrast, another decided that Milgram himself had behaved immorally, duping his subjects and persuading them to perform this distasteful task. No matter what they revealed, his findings were not worth the tension and self-doubt they created in his subjects (Baumrind, 1964). Many others have voiced opinions between these extremes or contributed different interpretations of his findings (Nissani, 1990).

These diverse views offer an opportunity to examine research methods from a broader perspective, focusing on ethical issues and comparisons among the different methods. Depending on the situation, each method has special assets and limitations.

RESEARCH ETHICS

Earlier we asked: To what extent is a researcher justified in secretly studying commuters awaiting their train? Is it acceptable to induce people to mail "lost" letters? Here we ask: Was Milgram's experimental study of obedience justifiable and ethical?

This question of research ethics concerns the

experience of subjects participating in a scientific investigation. It requires the humane and just treatment of all subjects. This issue is regularly raised in animal research by psychologists and the lay public (Timberlake, 1993; Ulrich, 1991). It is also confronted in the clinic, usually by the investigators themselves (Hall, 1991a).

People commuting to work may become subjects in naturalistic observation, but they do not alter their behavior in any way. Ethics should not become an issue, *provided* that the results are managed with discretion and confidentiality. People mailing lost letters go out of their way, but they do so voluntarily, just as they do to assist an elderly person, use a trash can, or help someone with parking. The general rule is that the subject's explicit consent to participate is not required if the behavior in question occurs as part of a normal routine, if there is no coercion, and if the findings are handled in a manner that fully respects the right to privacy.

BASIC ETHICAL QUESTIONS. When Jack Washington participated in Milgram's experiment, he went out of his way, was duped by a rigged drawing for the teacher and learner roles, and received false information about the electrical shocks. These are more fundamental ethical issues.

Such issues are not unique to psychology; they occur in all disciplines. For some people, the entire field of nuclear physics is an ethical issue. In biology, animals are confined to cages and subjected to surgery solely for research purposes. In legal and psychiatric research, ethical issues arise over the question of clients' rights. Even educational research involves ethical considerations, for the procedures sometimes impose researchers' values on the students in the study (Figure 2–9).

The issues in animal rights, for example, are more complex than might be readily apparent, as demonstrated when a cat lover complained that her neighbor's pet boa constrictor devoured kittens. The neighbor replied that the snake merely ate

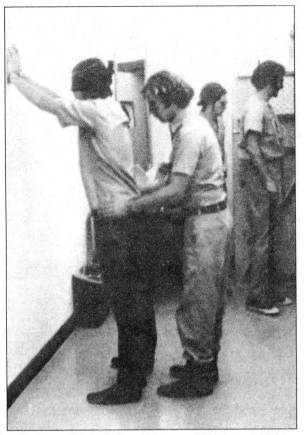

FIGURE 2–9 RESEARCH ETHICS. Issues of moral values and moral behavior underlie all research. When research subjects are exposed to a prison environment, for example, questions immediately arise concerning their physical and mental welfare.

mice and pointed out an advantage of snakes as pets. Having extraordinarily low metabolism, they consume far fewer fellow creatures than the approximately 54 million pet cats in this country. One reason for the cat lover's complaint, of course, is that cats rank higher than snakes on the human list of pet preferences. In killing and preparing cats' food, human beings make attractive packages out of the dead fish, horses, rats, and other animals fed to felines. In short, the animal world pays a high price for our pets, which we keep chiefly for one purpose—affection (Herzog, 1991). And the proper relation of human beings to lower animals, whether in research or relaxation, remains a perplexing ethical issue (Locke, 1992).

One **basic ethical question** in research seems to be this: Does any possible discomfort incurred by all subjects collectively outweigh the gain in alleviation of human and nonhuman problems? Many of Milgram's subjects experienced tension, doubt, and self-recrimination, clearly signs of discomfort. On the other side of the ledger, the obedience of the Nazis played an important role in the pain experienced by millions of people in World War II, and after their capture they did not appear to be cruel and sadistic. Instead, they seemed like ordinary citizens who did what they thought was their duty, which is the way many of Milgram's subjects characterized themselves. After the experiment, they decided that they had to resist authority more effectively in the future. Thus, the question still stands: On balance, was this research justifiable? Was the suffering of Milgram's subjects offset by the gain in understanding obedience to malevolent authority?

This ethical question involves value judgments about the feelings of research subjects. It also involves value judgments about the role of research in society. It extends beyond obedience and disobedience to include legitimate versus illegitimate authority and even benevolent versus malevolent orders (Saks, 1992). Taking a thoughtful ethical stand is a challenging task.

INFORMED CONSENT. Throughout his research, Milgram employed certain procedures to protect the subjects and to provide them with maximum benefit from their participation. These precautions, implemented in all proper investigations today, include informed consent before participation, privacy during participation, and confidentiality on completion of the research (Korn, 1988).

Among these, the most important is **informed consent,** which means that the general nature, risks, and benefits of research participation are explained to each subject before the procedures begin. The subjects are told about the tasks they will be expected to perform, and if they agree to participate, they do so giving informed consent. In Milgram's work, all subjects were informed of the basic experimental procedures at the outset. Each of them signed a consent form, indicating voluntary participation in this research.

An obvious question in informed consent concerns the complexity of the explanation and, in some cases, the need for deception about underlying purposes. Sometimes a less-than-full explanation may be acceptable, providing the subject incurs no other risk by participation. Still another issue is the subject's ability to give informed consent, especially in three populations: elderly people, the mentally disabled, and children. Investigators studying young children typically rely on a proxy from their parents, but each research project, with its unique characteristics, requires special steps to ensure that children's rights are respected (Hughes & Helling, 1991; Krener & Mancina, 1994).

For these reasons, an interdisciplinary ethics committee now must evaluate all federally funded psychological research. The goal is to permit the most useful, productive research without endangering the subjects in any way. The ideal solution to this problem, and one toward which many psychologists are working, is the development of research techniques that rely on the subjects' usual behavior and naturally occurring events rather than on contrived situations and misleading information (Huntingford, 1984; Kelman, 1967).

DEBRIEFING INTERVIEW. At the close of each research session, Milgram interviewed the subject. This procedure is called a **debriefing interview,** and it has a dual purpose: to ensure the maximum benefit for the subject and to obtain any further information that might be useful. Concern for the subjects is paramount, directed not only to ensuring that they are as fit and healthy as they were before the research but also to enable them to profit as much as possible from the experience.

Milgram's debriefing instructions included a meeting between the teacher and the un-harmed learner, as well as extended discussion with the authority figure. During his debriefing interview, Jack Washington explained that he would have discontinued the shocks if he had received a signal from the experimenter. "I did not get a cue to stop," he emphasized. Then he added that he knew the shocks were painful but not dangerous. Earlier in life he had received a very strong, accidental shock to his hand, causing him pain but no permanent damage, and thus he believed the investigator's contention that the shocks were not harmful.

Some weeks later, all subjects received a five-page report, including a questionnaire asking them to express once again their thoughts and feelings about the experience. Altogether, 80% of the subjects recommended more experiments of this nature, and 74% replied that they had learned something important to them personally. For Milgram, this finding constituted the central justification of this research: The participants judged it as acceptable and worthwhile (Milgram, 1974).

∾

COMPARISON OF METHODS

The system that we call science is unfinished—always aimed at evaluating and extending the ideas it has generated. Conducting research is like fighting the many-headed hydra of Greek mythology. For every head that is cut off, two more grow in its place. In science, the price of getting a head is more work to be done.

This work is accomplished by all four methods, combined and modified in various ways to fit the requirements of a particular research question. We know about Milgram's use of these methods through his collected reports, *The Individual in a Social World* (1992), and his book with a single focus,

Obedience to Authority (1974). In response to continued interest 15 years after publication of the former volume, two of Stanley Milgram's followers, John Sabini and Maury Silver, edited and republished that book as a second edition under his name (Milgram, 1992). These works show how Milgram found ways to collect research information by using an original mix of methods: observation, the survey, the case study, and, of course, laboratory experiments (Zimbardo, 1992).

STATISTICAL ANALYSES. After collecting the information, the investigator's next task is to analyze and interpret it. Sometimes qualitative analysis is involved, requiring considerable wisdom on the part of the investigator. Especially in naturalistic observation and case studies, subjective judgments and verbal descriptions may be the only recourse for depicting the findings. More often, quantitative analysis is included, meaning that the information is expressed in numerical units and statistical techniques are employed to assess them. These techniques, discussed in detail in the final chapter, can be categorized as descriptive, correlational, and inferential statistics.

Utilized in all research methods, *descriptive statistics* characterize or summarize a group of scores, often by presenting just a few numerical values. Usually they include some typical score, such as an average, and some measure of variability, indicating the extent to which other scores differ from the typical score. For example, Milgram found that commuters in New York City had an average of 4.5 familiar strangers in their lives. In one instance, the range was from zero, for a commuter new at the depot, to more than 12 for long-time commuters who recognized almost every "regular" at the station. These numerical values are descriptive statistics.

Instead, an investigator may want to know about the relationship between two sets of scores.

In his studies of pedestrians, Milgram noted that the size of crowds varied considerably according to several factors. We might wonder about the relationship between pedestrians and sidewalk performers. When pedestrians increase or decrease in number, do sidewalk performers also increase or decrease? Answers to such questions involve *correlational statistics*, which indicate the association between two sets of scores. They show whether there is a relationship between the number of pedestrians and the number of sidewalk performers.

Numerically, these relationships can vary from 0.00, meaning no correlation, to +1.00, a perfect positive correlation, or to -1.00, a perfect negative correlation. A correlation of +.60, for example, indicates a direct, rather strong association. As pedestrians increase in number, so do sidewalk performers. A correlation of -.10 indicates a weak, indirect association. As the number of pedestrians increases, the number of sidewalk performers tends to decrease mildly. However, correlational statistics do *not* indicate causality. Both factors *may* be influenced by a third variable, such as the weather or a holiday season.

Finally, *inferential statistics* are used to make a guess, an inference, or a statement of probability about one or several groups of scores. In Milgram's studies of obedience to authority, the subjects were asked to use a 14-point scale to estimate the amount of pain experienced by the learner. For a sample of obedient subjects, the mean was 11.36; for defiant subjects, it was 11.80. Is there a statistically significant difference between these two means? Expressed differently, what might be found with other samples of obedient and defiant subjects? Clearly, Milgram could not test all possible subjects. Inferential statistics allow the investigator to estimate the probability that the same findings would occur if the same experiment were repeated over and over again. Inferential statistics are common in the experimental and other research

methods as the investigator tries to determine the reliability of the findings.

To emphasize the basic point once again: Research methods are used to collect information. Diverse statistical methods are used afterward to analyze and interpret this information.

CONTINUUM OF METHODS. When these research methods are compared, they fall to some degree on a continuum of intervention or control. That is, they differ in the extent to which the investigator intervenes in the subjects' lives.

In naturalistic observation, at one end of this continuum, the subjects are studied in their own environment, unaffected by the investigator insofar as possible. In the survey, further along the continuum, the subjects' privacy is invaded to some degree by mail or telephone. Toward the opposite end of the continuum, case studies often take place in a clinic or comparable institution. At the far end of this continuum, opposite from naturalistic observation, the experimental method involves the fullest control and the most intervention. The subject usually enters a laboratory setting, and the investigator manipulates this environment in varying degrees, permitting the most definitive study of cause-and-effect relations.

There are innumerable variations in these methods. A study of animal migration might involve a combination of naturalistic observation and the survey method. Experiments can be conducted in school, at work, and elsewhere in the natural environment. Called *field experiments*, they reflect modifications in the basic experimental design. The overall aim is to find the most useful integration of methods for any topic of inquiry (Banaji & Crowder, 1989; Conway, 1991).

Collectively, these different methods provide a variety of useful approaches to the study of psychological problems. Each has advantages and disadvantages, and each makes a special contribution

METHOD	DESCRIPTION	MILGRAM EXAMPLE	CHIEF ADVANTAGE	CHIEF DISADVANTAGE
Naturalistic Observation	Studying behavior in its usual setting	Observing conformity among commuters at a railway station	Deals with everyday situations and events	May have high potential for investigator bias
Survey	Obtaining information from many subjects by mail, phone, or letters	Administering an obedience questionnaire; distributing "lost" letters	Allows access to a large number of subjects	May yield unreliable or unrepresentative data
Case Study	Conducting an interview, administering tests, preparing a case history	Interviewing Gretchen Brandt, testing her, and developing a case history	Offers opportunity to deal with practical problems and individual cases	May be expensive and not generalizable
Experimental Method	Manipulating and controlling relevant factors for study	Varying the proximity of the learner, closeness of authority, and so forth	Provides for the study of cause-and-effect relations	May involve artificial environments and manipulations

TABLE 2–7 METHODS OF RESEARCH

(Table 2–7). As these diverse methods become more fully developed and integrated, through psychologists' continual search for improved research techniques, we should become more and more skillful in understanding all sorts of behavior, including conformity, compliance, and obedience.

IN CONCLUSION. Milgram's studies prompted him to develop two hypotheses about the performance of women. Traditionally more compliant than men, they might show more obedience. Traditionally more empathic too, they might display more resistance to shocking someone. What do you think? Choose one of these hypotheses before reading further.

When Milgram performed these experiments with women, he found that the level of obedience was virtually identical to that of men. When these experiments were repeated by other investigators in Italy, Australia, Germany, and South Africa, each time with a somewhat different sample of subjects, the level of obedience was as high as that found by Milgram. In one instance, the subjects were required to administer psychological punishment, rather than physical punishment, harassing and berating an interviewee. Once again, the level of obedience was comparable to that in Milgram's work (Meeus & Raaijmakers, 1986).

These replications have essentially verified Milgram's findings on obedience to authority. Scientists within and outside of psychology therefore regard this work as a rare integration of the humanistic and empirical perspectives and as an extraordinary contribution to the study of moral issues. Panels of experts have selected this research as one of the most important investigations in modern psychology. With the exception of Darwin's book, it was the only single piece of research included in a comprehensive list of terms and concepts depicting basic psychological information (Boneau, 1990).

Milgram showed that what subjects say on a questionnaire may be very different from what they actually do. Further, he showed that social situations can powerfully override personal dispositions in influencing behavior. This conclusion is widely accepted, although personal factors cannot be entirely discounted (Blass, 1991). Finally, he showed that what people do is not necessarily predictable through common sense (Milgram, 1974).

Sometimes common sense is supported by psychological research. These occasions are gratifying, indicating that we learn something about human behavior and experience through daily life. Sometimes common sense is contradicted by psychological research. These occasions are important because scientific research is generally considered the most rigorous and reliable pathway to knowledge. A psychology that consistently opposed common sense would be disturbing, apparently concerned with a different reality than the one we think we know. A psychology that merely supported common sense would be a waste of time. The value of employing diverse research methods in modern psychology is that they increase our chances of distinguishing one from the other.

For his simple, elegant research methods, Stanley Milgram became internationally famous. For his studies of obedience, he was awarded numerous honors, including the prize in socio-psychology offered by the American Association for the Advancement of Science. This series of experiments has been described as one of the few classic studies in social psychology, containing all the elements of a parable: a story line, conceptual simplicity, vivid imagery, and an unexpected outcome (Kotre, 1992).

Stanley Milgram completed these obedience studies while he was still in his twenties. Sadly, this early success was followed by an untimely death many years before it might have been expected. His genius is now to be found frozen in his published works (Sabin & Silver, 1992). He has left us an inspirational legacy in research methods, morally significant findings, and a reminder about our own lives: "We are all fragile creatures, entwined in a cobweb of social constraints."

EXTRASENSORY PERCEPTION

For many years in the United States, fire walking has been considered a psychic activity, along with postmortem survival, water dowsing, and other allegedly occult phenomena. One reason is that fire walking was practiced only in distant lands. Not much was known about it in this country. Another reason is that the mind can influence experience. There is no doubt about that. It can make us more tolerant of pain through spiritual, mystic, and other beliefs — although it cannot make the feet invulnerable to intense heat.

Among all claims of psychic phenomena, the most popular and widely debated is extrasensory perception, or ESP, which is awareness without any sensory basis. Information is obtained without the use of our normally recognized senses. Fire walking is not an instance of ESP, for no special awareness is claimed. In fact, almost the opposite is true: There is lack of awareness of the heat of the coals. Nevertheless, the concept of ESP is widely used for almost any inexplicable event or special awareness. It therefore merits attention in the context of sensation.

ANECDOTES, FRAUD, AND PROBABILITIES.

In one of their first meetings, Sigmund Freud and Carl Gustav Jung were discussing psychic phenomena when suddenly the bookcase made a noise. Then, for some reason that he was never able to explain, Jung predicted another loud noise. Bang! It occurred just as he spoke, and this event made a profound impression on both of them (Jung, 1963).

Such reports are impressive, especially when given by respected individuals, but the problem with anecdotes is that we do not know the full details. Was the original perception accurate? Has the anecdote been distorted in retelling? Noting the unreliability of anecdotal evidence, William James, a very strong believer in psychic experience, lamented his inability to discover an absolutely irrefutable case of ESP. To demonstrate the existence of the supernatural, he pointed out, just one good instance is needed. In more colorful language, he emphasized: To upset the law that all crows are black, we need just one white crow.

Another difficulty in claims of ESP is the widespread incidence of obvious fraud. For this reason, Randi, a nationally recognized magician, has written books, given lectures, and received large grants to expose fraudulent psychics. He has offered $10,000 to any psychic performing a feat that he, Randi, cannot duplicate. To this date, no psychic has even accepted the challenge, much less proved him wrong (Rand, 1982).

More serious cases of fraud have occurred in ESP laboratories. Two decades ago, J. B. Rhine, the foremost American investigator of ESP, declared that dishonesty was no longer an issue in this research (Rhine, 1974b). Three months later, Rhine's successor in the ESP movement, the director of one of the world's leading ESP laboratories, was discovered to be falsifying research results (Rhine, 1974a).

Also, probabilities are used skillfully. One self-proclaimed psychic takes a "psych-up walk" before each ESP performance, and he uses probabilities very cleverly later. In the parking lot before the show, he notes all sorts of telltale signs: a license plate here, a baseball sticker there, twin infant seats in another car. Afterward, in front of the audience, he makes his psychic claims: "I have the feeling there is someone in the audience from Maryland." "Who roots for the Tigers?" "One of you has a special interest in twins." When probabilities are used in this way, augmented by assistance from accomplices and trick equipment, faking ESP is not a difficult task.

Did you know, for example, that with just 30 people in a room, the chances are better than two to one that at least two of them will have birthdays on the same day of the year? And the odds rise above 90% in a group of 50 people (Bergamini, 1971).

AN UNSETTLED ISSUE.

A major obstacle in the scientific study of ESP is the lack of a conceptual framework. Despite a century of scientific investigation, there is no useful theory, not even according to the leading figures in this field. The field, in fact, is defined by what it is not; it is anything not otherwise explainable by science. If ESP does exist, we have no adequate approach to interpreting such phenomena, despite continuing efforts to test ESP hypotheses (Gissurarson, 1990; Walther, 1986).

This lack of a theoretical basis has implications for the research methods, which must be aimed at excluding any known sensory channel. As the controls against normal sensory awareness increase, the evidence for ESP usually becomes weaker, a circumstance that is contrary to what one finds elsewhere in science. Usually the expected effect grows stronger as extraneous variables are eliminated.

A notable exception involved a study in mental telepathy with "senders" and "receivers" isolated from one another. In contrast to earlier investigations, the sender viewed highly dramatic images, such as a crashing tidal wave or wildly animated cartoon, while the receiver sat quietly in another room, trying to apprehend this visual image. Later, when shown four different images and asked to select the one that was transmitted, the receiver chose it with a success rate of approximately 32%, well above the expected level of 25%. The probability of a difference this large occurring by chance is extremely low (Bem & Honorton, 1994). This finding, defying statistical odds and using stimulating visual images rather than the geometric patterns of earlier years, will make ESP research more intriguing and perhaps more creative in the future.

A survey of college psychologists showed that they were equally divided on the ESP issue. Approximately one-third viewed ESP as essentially impossible; one-third were uncertain; and one-third regarded ESP as a likely or established fact. But compared with professors in other fields, including other scientists, psychologists were much more doubtful. Only 3% of the natural scientists decided that ESP is impossible (Wagner & Monnet, 1979). Clearly, people from different backgrounds, including different research experience, have very different views of ESP.

As these investigations continue, we need to remind ourselves of the implications of the ESP perspective. Accepting its underlying assumptions and applying them broadly to the human condition would radically alter the content of modern thought. It would generate a fundamentally different set of explanations about human behavior, profoundly changing our thinking about religion, education, law, medicine, and virtually all other areas of human existence (Adams, 1991).

IN CONCLUSION. With Bernie and Bill safely back at the university, beyond the glowing coals, we should acknowledge another principle of physics and one from physiological psychology as well. In the *Leidenfrost Effect*, protection from heat is provided by a thin, watery layer, basically a form of thermal insulation produced naturally through perspiration or artificially by wetting the skin. For this reason, people spit on their fingers before touching a hot iron. For human feet, perspiration is often sufficient to produce this minimal insulation, but for insurance the workers at the fire walking seminar kept the sod around the pits rather damp (Leikind & McCarthy, 1985).

The principle of physiological psychology concerns the timing of the whole event, which began late in the evening and included 2 hours of instruction, used for raising motivation, enlisting cooperation, and, of course, justifying the expense of the seminar. The actual fire walking took place at 1:00 A.M., long past our usual bedtime, and therefore when we are probably less aware of pain. The responsiveness of our bodies is significantly governed by the circadian rhythm, meaning that our bodies exhibit a cycle of approximately 24 hours, completing a full wake-sleep span within that period. When it is well past our usual bedtime, bodily functions become depressed, as though the body is trying to sleep. People walking on hot coals in the wee hours of the morning are less likely to feel pain than those hearty souls doing so at high noon.

In addition, responsiveness to pain is governed by endorphins, the body's own pain killers, released at abnormally high levels during times of stress. The presence of all of these factors shows once again the multiple bases of behavior.

However, people who stand or walk barefoot on hot coals for more than a few seconds will get burned regardless of what they are thinking, how deeply they breathe, how much they are sweating, where they walk, when they walk, or what they believe. So, please be careful. And be courteous! Let someone else go first.

Finally, we must add a warning about quick fix seminars. These brief encounters may temporarily enhance self-esteem or prepare people to ignore pain, and there may be other gains too, but without more extensive practical counseling a long-term benefit is unlikely. Worse yet, participants may experience adverse reactions later. Those who attend the seminar but forego the fire walking may develop increased self-doubts. Those who trust their soles to the coals may develop false notions about themselves. Whatever happens, do not go home, call everyone into the kitchen, and take hot pans out of the oven bare-handed. Instead, take a reputable course in physics, psychology, or the sociology of crowds.

Summary

1. Awareness usually involves internal or multisensory perception. Our information about the world at any given moment is based on several sense organs typically seeking information and also on data previously stored in the brain. The various sensory systems operate in an interrelated and active manner.
2. Extrasensory perception (ESP) implies perception without the use of any currently known sense organs. This phenomenon has been questioned on the basis of anecdotal reports, the problem of fraud, use of probabilities, and difficulty in establishing useful theory and research procedures.

NATURALISTIC OBSERVATION

I. Naturalistic observation involves the study of behavior in its usual setting. In overt observation the researcher's presence is known to the subjects; in covert observation it is concealed.

2. Naturalistic observation may not appear complex, but it requires considerable training. The investigator must decide whether to participate in the subjects' activities and how to minimize personal bias. This approach is useful for generating hypotheses.

SURVEY METHOD

3. The purpose of the survey is to obtain information from a large number of subjects in an efficient manner. A questionnaire, containing structured or open-ended items, is used and the results may provide norms indicating what is normal or expected for a certain group.

4. The people to whom the questionnaire is administered constitute a sample, which is a group of subjects drawn from a larger group called the population. When a sample accurately reflects the characteristics of a certain population, it is called a representative sample. As a rule, a large random sample is more likely to be representative than a small one.

5. Some surveys are based on unobtrusive measures, in which the subjects never know that they have been included in a research project. The lost-letter technique is a modified unobtrusive measure because the investigator presents potential subjects with a specific stimulus. Most unobtrusive measures provide little knowledge of the sample of subjects.

CASE STUDY

6. The case study describes one person, a group of people, or an event in detail. Extensive information is gained through a series of interviews. Psychological tests also are useful for gathering information.

7. The case history includes social, educational, and medical information, as well as the psychological background, obtained from all available sources. Case histories, interviews, and psychological tests may involve idiographic analysis, concerned with discovering the underlying principles in a given case. They also may involve nomothetic research, which has the purpose of discovering general laws of behavior.

EXPERIMENTAL METHOD

8. The experimental method, involving control or manipulation of variables, is concerned with cause-and-effect relationships. In the classical experiment the investigator manipulates an independent variable, usually a stimulus, and notes its influence on the dependent variable, usually a response.

9. To control disruptive influences, subjects are studied under two conditions, experimental and control, which are equal except for the presence of the independent variable. This variable is manipulated, and then the two conditions are compared. Sometimes the same subjects are used for the experimental and control conditions. In another design, two sets of subjects are used, and they are placed in comparable groups by matching or procedures for randomization.

10. The multiple bases of behavior prompt some psychologists to study the influence of several independent variables simultaneously. These multifactor studies can reveal additive effects, in which the influences are simply cumulative, and interactive effects, in which the influences are interdependent.

RESEARCH IN PERSPECTIVE

11. Research ethics with human beings require informed consent prior to participation, privacy during participation, and complete confidentiality of records at all times. At the end of the research, debriefing is required, in which the aim and research procedures are explained to the subject as fully as possible, and a written report is prepared, designed to enhance the value of the experience for all participants.

12. Each research method has advantages and disadvantages and makes its own contribution to our understanding of human and animal behavior, experience, and mental processes. These methods are used in complementary ways as investigators examine complex psychological questions.

• WORKING WITH PSYCHOLOGY •

✦ REVIEW OF KEY CONCEPTS ✦

Naturalistic Observation
naturalistic observation
overt observation
covert observation
participant observation
nonparticipant observation
bias

Survey Method
survey method

questionnaire
norms
sample
population
representative sample
random sample
incidental sample
unobtrusive measures

Case Study
case study

group tests
individual tests
case history
idiographic research
nomothetic research

Experimental Method
experimental method
classical experiment
variable

rule of one variable
independent variable
dependent variable 0
operational definition
experimental condition
control condition
confounding variable

placebo
experimenter effects
single-blind design
double-blind design
multifactor studies
additive effect
interactive effect

Research in Perspective
basic ethical question
informed consent
debriefing interview

∾ CLASS DISCUSSION/CRITICAL THINKING ∾

A NARRATIVE TWIST

The subjects in Stanley Milgram's obedience studies reacted in a surprising manner—not at all as psychiatrists had predicted. Suppose instead that they had behaved according to expectations. Would Milgram's research then have been largely meaningless? Explain the reasons for your view, including a discussion of psychology and common sense. Would this research have raised ethical issues? Again, explain the reasons for your view.

TOPICAL QUESTIONS

• *Naturalistic Observation.* Suppose that you want to study jaywalking in a moderately large city. Decisions about revealing your purpose offer two approaches to observation, overt and covert. Which approach would you use? Explain your reasons. ∾

• *Survey Method.* Sometimes surveys are administered to college students, and the results are reported as representative of the general population. Are students sufficiently different from one another and sufficiently similar to the general population that they adequately reflect our society? Explain your answer.

• *Case Study.* It has been said that a test merely provides a sample of the subject's behavior. If, instead, the examiner had the opportunity to accompany the subject for 24 hours in daily life, that opportunity would yield more useful information than the test. Do you agree or disagree? Why?

• *Experimental Method.* To what extent are confounding variables part of every type of investigation? Explain the reasons for your view.

• *Research in Perspective.* Describe how each of the four basic research methods might be used in studying the effectiveness of a new pill for the common cold.

∾ TOPICS OF RELATED INTEREST ∾

The design of research includes correlational studies, described in detail in the chapter on statistics (18). Research methods and instruments are also described in the context of biological foundations (3), intelligence and testing (13), and therapy (16).

3
STATISTICAL METHODS

EXAMINE THE KEYS ON YOUR COMPUTER OR TYPE-
WRITER KEYBOARD. NOTICE THAT *E*, THE MOST COM-
MON LETTER IN ENGLISH, HAS AN INCONVENIENT
location. It requires a s–t–r–e–t–c–h.

The letter *A*, also frequently used, is a bit hard to reach. With small hands or short fingers, that must be exasperating.

The consonants, alphabetized in the home row, are not alphabetical elsewhere. And the vowels are scattered unpredictably throughout the keyboard. Why?

This keyboard is one of the most important tools in modern society. Could it be improved? Should it be redesigned for today's high-tech workplace?

Back in the 1930s, a pair of brothers-in-law, August Dvorak and William Dealey, decided to study typing behavior. Both psychologists, they began by observing people using the early typewriting machines. Then they filmed typists in action and viewed these films in slow motion. Convinced

71

by these films that further studies would be worthwhile, they planned hundreds of statistical tests of various letter and finger combinations. To accomplish this goal, they added other psychologists to their team (Dvorak, Merrick, Dealey, & Ford, 1936).

Without knowing it, this group at the University of Washington, working partly under the auspices of the U.S. Navy, had entered a race against time, for the winds of World War II had already swept across parts of Western Europe. And without knowing it, they were in competition with corporate America, which had its own interests to protect.

We shall follow their surprising, bittersweet story throughout this chapter, for it shows how statistics can be used to answer research questions. It also illustrates the human-factors approach in psychological investigations.

These psychologists, men and women, worked in **human-factors psychology,** a specialty devoted to the design of tools and procedures well suited to human use, especially in the work environment. Employing diverse research techniques, including statistical methods, human-factors psychologists have studied jobs of all sorts, from bricklaying to using the computer keyboard. This interdisciplinary field today is composed largely of psychologists and engineers (Howell, 1994). As our society continues to evolve, human-factors psychologists will face many challenges,

including those posed by the new technologies, our longer life span, and their interactions (Nickerson, 1992).

In Europe, where this specialty has an industrial background, it is known as *ergonomics,* meaning the study of work or energy expenditure. In both instances, the concern is not only with physical equipment, such as tools and machines, but also with the psychological environment, including personnel and management policies (Page, 1995).

Especially in the design of computer equipment, there is a growing awareness of human-factors issues, most evident in the popular label *user friendly.* Manufacturers' failure to attend to this issue today usually results in the loss of sales. Sometimes it becomes the basis of litigation in liability for health and safety. As a lure for buying countless products, advertisers now proclaim that their products have an *ergonomic design* (Howell, 1994).

This chapter begins by illustrating quantification in psychology, using examples from human-factors research. Then it turns to three major topics: descriptive statistics, which characterize a group of scores; correlational statistics, which indicate relationships among scores; and inferential statistics, used to make guesses about scores that are not available. The chapter closes with a statement about statistics as a tool in science.

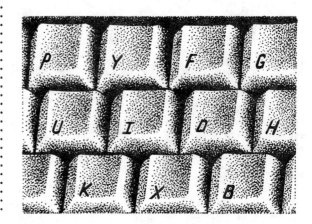

For hundreds of years, progress in science has been closely linked to developments in mathematics and statistics. Tremendous advances in astronomy occurred in the eighteenth century after the mathematical laws of celestial motion were established. Developments in probability theory played an indispensable role in the growth of physics. The potential uses of statistical procedures in sociology and anthropology were first realized in the nineteenth century. And Sir Francis Galton, late in that century, brought statistical methods into psychology through his studies of physical and psychological differences among people. These successive developments reflect Galton's view, shared by many scholars: Until the observations in any field of study have been quantified, that branch of knowledge cannot be considered science.

STATISTICS IN RESEARCH

The term **statistics** refers to the collection and evaluation of numerical information, including methods for demonstrating facts and the relations among them. This meaning, emphasizing methods, is intended throughout this chapter. The term also has a second meaning; it refers to the results of using these methods—the numerical values themselves. This second meaning is implied whenever someone says: "Statistics show that . . ."

PRODUCTIVITY AT WORK. Early in this century, a young college dropout found work in the coal mines and a place for himself in the history of psychology—by using simple statistical methods. Shortly after his arrival at the Bethlehem Steel Company, Frederick Taylor noticed that most of the workers shoveled heavy iron ore, up to 38

pounds per shovelful, and they tired quickly. Or they shoveled rice coal, with less than 4 pounds in each shovelful, and they exerted themselves relatively little, even after several hours. Intrigued with this information, Taylor decided to find out the most appropriate load for a worker shoveling all day—that is, the poundage per shovelful that would permit him to do the most work.

Assigning shovelers to different parts of the yard, Taylor appointed observers to study them with watches and weighing scales. At the outset, all of these workers used shovels with large blades, and the weight of the material they shoveled each day was carefully noted. Then part of the blade was cut off, making a smaller load and, after another period of shoveling, the total weight of the shoveled material was noted once more. By this process, cutting the blade again and again, making the loads lighter and lighter, Taylor discovered the optimal shovelful: 22.5 pounds. That amount enabled the average man to do the most work per day.

That finding prompted Bethlehem Steel Company to change its procedures. Thereafter, the company distributed each day to each worker a shovel of a certain size, depending on the material that worker would be lifting. Respect for that new policy enabled Taylor to receive a promotion, and respect for that investigation, demonstrating the value of statistics in research, helped inaugurate the field of human-factors psychology (Taylor, 1911).

The workplace has changed considerably since Frederick Taylor's day, but human factors psychologists still study lifting of all sorts. They measure strain, fatigue, and energy expenditure, all to make the work easier and more productive (Gallagher, 1991; Mital, 1992).

COMFORT IN THE HOME. Human-factors psychology is not limited to the work environment. On awakening in the morning, you look at the clock, fill the bathtub, check the thermometer, and seat yourself in a chair for breakfast. The shape, size, and design of each of these devices have been influenced by human-factors psychologists.

In the bathroom, if the tub is too small, you are uncomfortable. If it is too big, it requires unnecessary space and hot water. What is the preferred shape and size for most people? Here human-factors psychologists have been interested in comfort rather than work, and they answer such questions by modifying bathtubs in various ways, asking subjects to bathe, and then assessing their comfort. But despite their findings, bathtubs today often use conventional designs (Figure 18–1).

HEALTH AND THE KEYBOARD. In most settings, productivity and comfort are dual considerations, accompanied by another factor, health. These three issues, readily evident in the use of the computer keyboard, account in a general way for most of the specific goals in human-factors psychology.

When the typewriter was invented almost 125 years ago, little thought was given to productivity. Rather, it was believed that the machine would give a neater, cleaner result than the usual handwriting, which certainly has been the case. Workers might use the machine with one finger, two fingers, or whatever way they wished. Hand movements were not an issue.

By the time the human-factors team from the University of Washington entered the scene, touch typing had become the predominant mode of operation and hand movements had become a concern. The University of Washington, incidentally, is known around Seattle as UW or, more colloquially, U Dub. When the UW team examined its films of typists at work, these pictures showed the hands

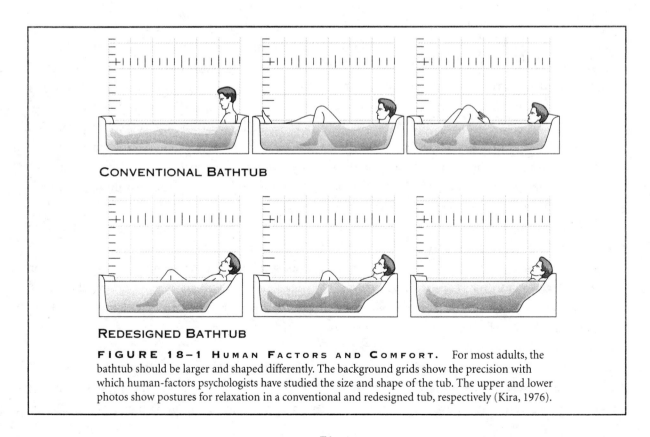

CONVENTIONAL BATHTUB

REDESIGNED BATHTUB

FIGURE 18–1 HUMAN FACTORS AND COMFORT. For most adults, the bathtub should be larger and shaped differently. The background grids show the precision with which human-factors psychologists have studied the size and shape of the tub. The upper and lower photos show postures for relaxation in a conventional and redesigned tub, respectively (Kira, 1976).

moving far more than appeared necessary. The rhythm essential for fast typing often seemed disrupted by awkward movements.

Today, with still greater speed and massive use of the keyboard throughout the workplace, operators using the standard electronic keyboard are producing many hand movements and finger movements per hour. In short, they are overtaxing themselves, resulting in a dramatic rise in injuries (Figure 18–2). Caused by constant, similar movements, *repetitive strain injuries* from the keyboard include pain in the wrist, fingers, and elbows, accompanied sometimes by swelling or numbness in the hands. The data entry operator, who may stroke the keys up to 200,000 times per day, is especially prone to this disorder. In terms of movement, this work is perhaps the equivalent of walking with the fingers across the keyboard for about 10 miles (Jones, Burnsed, & Marquardt, 1991).

What can be done about this problem? The answer to that question appears later in this chapter, derived largely through statistical methods. The UW team of course never anticipated this problem, although its members did their unknowing best to offer a solution based on statistical analyses.

∾
MISUSE OF STATISTICS

Responsibility for the successful use of statistical information lies largely with the producer, but it also falls to the consumer, who must develop statistical literacy. A major approach to knowledge, **statistical literacy** is the ability to make sound judgments about the quality and usefulness of numerical information. It is acquired slowly, but the appropriate attitude—a cautious interpretation of the evidence—is readily illustrated.

In 1936, at just the time the UW team was conducting investigations of typing behavior, the *Literary Digest*, a national magazine, was conducting the first major poll in a national presidential election. Over two million voters were sampled from lists in telephone directories and automobile registrations, and the results predicted an overwhelming victory for the Republican candidate, Alfred Landon. However, Franklin Delano Roosevelt, the Democratic candidate, won easily in almost every state. Then it was discovered that in those years of the Great Depression the lists did not represent Republicans and Democrats equally. Far more

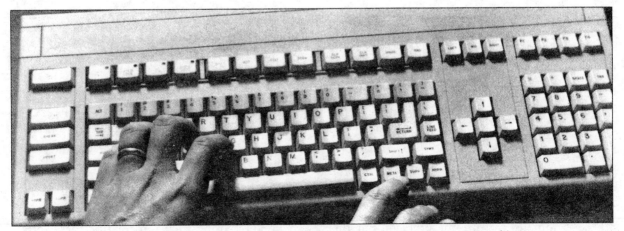

FIGURE 18–2 HAND MOVEMENTS ON THE KEYBOARD. As this photo indicates, the hands must move rapidly into many different positions while typing on the standard keyboard. If continued for extended periods, these movements can result in tendinitis and other repetitive strain injuries.

Republicans owned cars and telephones, and shortly after this massive, embarassing error, the *Literary Digest* became defunct.

Although telephones may be more equally distributed among members of the political parties today, this problem has not disappeared. Many households now have unlisted telephones; others have no telephones. Telephone directories still do not include the entire population. Mail surveys have a low response rate because people do not want to take the time or trouble to answer. Even in-person surveys have limitations, due chiefly to the potential for interviewer bias.

In viewing the results of any poll or survey, a statistically literate person will be cautious. He or she will ask how the subjects were chosen, how the data were collected, by whom, with what instrument, and so forth. If these procedural details are not available, then the results themselves must be regarded with considerable skepticism.

Even when the information is correct, the presentation may give a wrong impression. Consider further examples, again from very different settings.

During World War II, the Office of Strategic Services carried out an elaborate series of tests for selecting men and women to serve as spies, counterspies, and undercover agents. In one of many tests, groups of four to seven candidates were assembled separately beside a secluded brook that was to be regarded as a raging torrent so fast and deep that nothing could rest on the bottom. The task was to transport equipment and personnel to the other side as quickly as possible within one hour. In this situation, the examiners looked for signs of cooperation, resistance, leadership, impulsive behavior, and so forth (OSS Assessment Staff, 1948).

The candidates required, on the average, about 30 to 45 minutes to solve the problem. But this statement gives an incomplete, distorted picture of what really happened. Many groups failed to solve the problem at all. A few did so very rapidly, one in just four minutes (OSS Assessment Staff, 1948).

Thus, the average time required for the solution does not provide a satisfactory understanding of the overall performances.

Statistical findings are also presented visually. Misleading graphs are sometimes created by using pictures to distort the real differences between quantities (Figure 18–3).

One broad aim of this chapter is to encourage a critical attitude toward statistics. Even without impressive statistical literacy, we can still be cautious about the interpretation of numerical information.

• DESCRIPTIVE STATISTICS •

After reviewing their films of the typing process, the UW team decided that the standard keyboard was the typist's "first difficult problem . . . a crazy patchwork put together long ago" (Dvorak, Merrick, Dealey, & Ford, 1936). Hence, this human-factors team abandoned their investigation of the learning process to confront more directly the problem of fitting the machine to the worker. Here the first step was simply to measure the efficiency of the standard keyboard. If this efficiency was found to be low, as expected, then the team would pursue a second goal, the development of an improved design.

To assess the standard keyboard, the UW team needed information on two sets of variables—the work to be performed and the workers' capabilities. The work to be performed is a transcription skill; visual or auditory signals must be accurately and rapidly transformed into letters on a screen or page. The capabilities of the worker are chiefly finger and hand dexterity, as well as knowledge of the language.

For presenting such information, descriptive statistics are extremely useful. In **descriptive statistics,** the aim is to describe or characterize a set of scores, usually by indicating the typical score and differences among the scores. Descriptive statistics

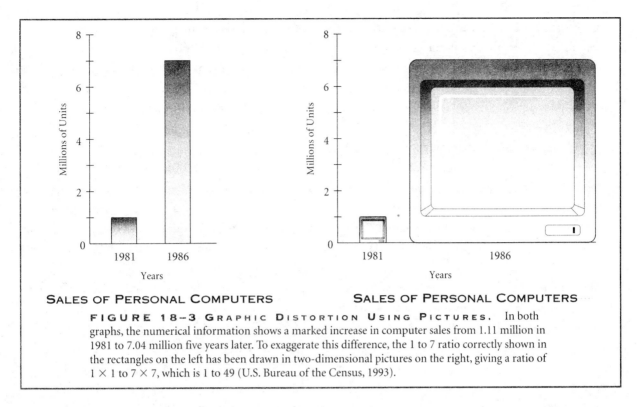

FIGURE 18-3 GRAPHIC DISTORTION USING PICTURES. In both graphs, the numerical information shows a marked increase in computer sales from 1.11 million in 1981 to 7.04 million five years later. To exaggerate this difference, the 1 to 7 ratio correctly shown in the rectangles on the left has been drawn in two-dimensional pictures on the right, giving a ratio of 1 × 1 to 7 × 7, which is 1 to 49 (U.S. Bureau of the Census, 1993).

show in a relatively simple manner the overall trends in a group of scores.

GRAPHS AND NUMBERS

The UW team commenced with the question of letter frequencies. Which letter of the alphabet is most commonly used in English? Which is next, and so forth? Which letter is least used? Samples of written English from diverse sources revealed the frequencies for the 26 letters and four punctuation marks: the period, comma, colon, and semicolon.

A	*B*	*C*	*D*	*E*	*F*	*G*	*H*
684	160	231	261	1,000	102	99	402
I	*J*	*K*	*L*	*M*	*N*	*O*	*P*
484	23	41	349	198	469	561	158
Q	*R*	*S*	*T*	*U*	*V*	*W*	*X*
10	423	486	685	223	66	132	20
	Y	*Z*	.	,	:	;	
	175	9	86	115	11	16	

The following scores were obtained:

These scores are called **raw scores** because they are original scores, just as they were obtained from the original measurement. In other words, raw scores are untreated; they have not been submitted to any statistical analysis. But with a large number of raw scores, as in this case, the major characteristics cannot be readily perceived. The scores are too numerous. Some *general* description is needed, and here we turn to two ways of summarizing results: graphs and numerical values.

USE OF GRAPHIC DISPLAYS. One method for presenting any group of scores is to construct a **graph**, which is a visual display of numerical values made by connecting lines or geometric figures. Graphs are pictures of a sort.

They show the frequency with which scores or other items occurred, or they display the relationship between sets of scores. Generally, the scores or items appear on the horizontal axis, and the frequencies or performances are indicated on the vertical axis. The vertical axis should begin at zero and accomodate all possible scores.

One graph constructed with bars, the **bar graph**, shows the frequency of the different scores or items by using rectangles of appropriate heights. The width of the rectangle is arbitrary, but the height is proportional to the frequency of the scores it represents.

When the scores for all 26 letters are displayed in a bar graph, the differences become readily apparent. The letter *E* is by far the most frequently used letter, outscoring not only its nearest rivals but almost half of the alphabet. It occurs more often than the 12 least-used letters combined (Figure 18–4).

Which finger of a trained keyboard operator types the letter *E?* The left middle finger, which is not as agile as the left index finger. And for most people, the left is not as agile as the right. So *E* does not appear to be well assigned. And where is it placed? It is not even in the home row—but we are getting ahead of ourselves.

Using this graph, an observer can tell at a glance the most common scores, least common scores, and those of intermediate frequency. Graphs truly provide a quick picture. Here it can be readily observed that the letters *J, X, Q,* and *Z* are rarely used. In all such cases, an old saying must be modified: A well-constructed graph is worth a thousand numbers.

USE OF NUMERICAL VALUES. The second major method for describing a group of raw scores is the use of numerical values. A few such values can summarize the performance of the whole group, commonly by providing two types of information: the typical scores and the extent to which all scores differ from the typical scores.

For example, the frequency counts for the 26 letters show that scores of 198 and 223 are in the middle of the distribution. In this respect, they are typical scores. The letters *E* and *Z* include the highest and lowest scores, 1,000 and 9, respectively. They are extreme scores. Collectively, these numerical values give some idea of the full distribution,

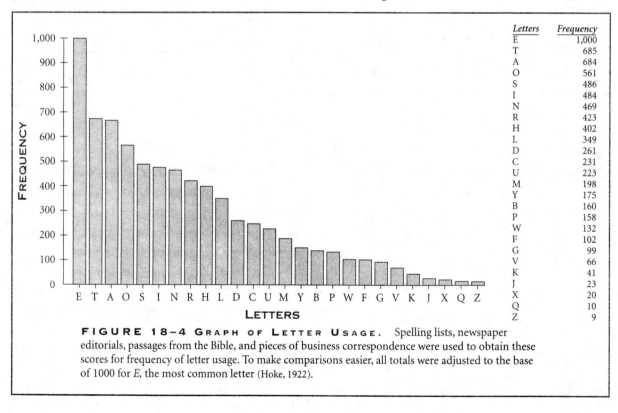

Letters	Frequency
E	1,000
T	685
A	684
O	561
S	486
I	484
N	469
R	423
H	402
L	349
D	261
C	231
U	223
M	198
Y	175
B	160
P	158
W	132
F	102
G	99
V	66
K	41
J	23
X	20
Q	10
Z	9

FIGURE 18–4 GRAPH OF LETTER USAGE. Spelling lists, newspaper editorials, passages from the Bible, and pieces of business correspondence were used to obtain these scores for frequency of letter usage. To make comparisons easier, all totals were adjusted to the base of 1000 for *E,* the most common letter (Hoke, 1922).

but they can be supplemented by other values, to which we now turn.

MEASURES OF CENTRAL TENDENCY

The most obvious values for describing a group of scores indicate the central tendency. They are called **measures of central tendency** because they indicate the performance of typical subjects or items, near the *center* of the group. For the letters of the alphabet, inspection suggests that the central or typical score is around 200 or so, but this answer is just a guess. To be more precise, three different measures are available.

MODE, MEDIAN, AND MEAN. One measure of central tendency is called the **mode** because it is the score that occurs most frequently. It can be remembered by thinking of pie à la mode, which literally means "pie in the current fashion." The score most in fashion, or most frequent, is the mode. Among the 26 raw scores tabulated for the letters, no score occurred more than once. Thus, there is no mode, or modal score.

Another measure of central tendency, the **median,** is the middle point in a distribution when all scores have been ranked according to size. It has half of the scores above it and half below it. The meaning of this term can be remembered by thinking of a highway where the sign says: "Keep Off the Median Strip." This strip divides the highway in half, just as the median divides the ranked scores in half.

When there is an odd number of cases, the median is the middle of the ranked scores; with even-numbered groups, it is that point equidistant between the two middle scores. In the group of 26 raw scores, the median is halfway between the scores for *M* and *U,* as evident when all 26 scores are ranked in order of magnitude. These middle scores are 198 and 223, giving a median of 210.5.

The most useful measure of central tendency is generally the **mean,** which is remembered simply as the arithmetic average. It is obtained by adding all of the scores and dividing by the number of scores. For the 26 raw scores, the sum is 7,451 and the mean is 286.6.

INTERPRETATION OF MODE, MEDIAN, AND MEAN. For practice, consider the following scores made by ten male keyboard operators in a typing pool. They show typing speed expressed as words per minute:

58 42 52 40 59 46 54 50 41 58

What is the mode? It is the most frequent score, which is 58. Two operators made this score.

What is the median? It is the middle point when all ten scores are ranked by size. In this case, it is 51.

What is the mean? It is the average for all scores. The sum of the scores is 500. When divided by 10, it gives a mean of 50.

When comparisons are made among these measures of central tendency, certain conclusions can be drawn. The mode is the least reliable measure, particularly when the number of scores is small. It may change markedly when just one score is added, subtracted, or altered in any way because it represents only the most frequent score. If one of the keyboard operators who achieved 58 words per minute had been ill on the day of the test and scored 41, the mode for the whole group would have become 41, decreasing by 17 points.

The median is more reliable, or stable, because it represents the ranks of all scores. Changing one score from 58 to 41 would lower the median by only 3 points because only the position of that one score in the ranked group would be changed. It would move from the high end of the distribution to the low end, making the median 48 instead of 51. The median is a better measure of central tendency because the *ranks* of all scores are considered.

The mean, based on the *values* of all scores, not just the ranks, is generally the most reliable measure of central tendency. It is the only measure that takes into account all of the information about each score. If any score is changed at all, the mean is always changed somewhat. For this reason, the mean is a basic point of departure for further statistical analysis. In the change just mentioned, the mean would have been altered by less than two points, from 50 to 48.3.

One caution is in order. When some scores are quite deviant, the mean is more affected than either the median or mode. In these instances, the median may be the most useful measure of central tendency.

Suppose an eleventh keyboard operator, for some reason, typed only six words per minute. Including this score lowers the mean by 4 points, making it 46. The mode remains unchanged at 58, and the median is changed by only one point, decreasing from 51 to 50. Thus, the three measures vary in stability depending on the distribution of scores in the group. *Usually* the mean is most descriptive, or most stable, but its use in unusual distributions may be debatable.

THE NORMAL DISTRIBUTION. When the distribution is completely symmetrical, these three measures of central tendency all have the same value. For example, when the scores for 100 typists in a pool are presented in graphic form, they accumulate in the center and decline on both sides at a decreasing rate. Whenever many factors act in a complex, often unknown, way to determine a single event, the symmetrical, bell-shaped distribution, with moderate variation among the scores, is called a *normal curve* or **normal distribution**. With large samples, many human characteristics, such as height, weight, intelligence, and typing speed, appear as approximately normal distributions (Figure 18–5).

All normal distributions are symmetrical and bell-shaped, but all symmetrical distributions are not necessarily normal. Sometimes the symmetrical distribution does not look much like a bell. The scores are too tightly clustered, making the distribution too tall, or they are too spread out, making it too flat to constitute a normal, bell-shaped distribution.

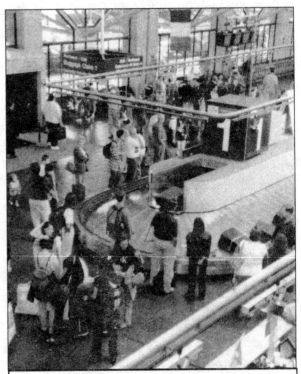

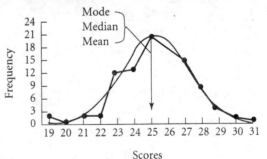

FIGURE 18–5 NORMAL DISTRIBUTION. The black figure presents 100 typing scores according to the number of typists who made each score. If more scores were obtained, this figure would approach even more closely the symmetrical, bell-shaped pattern of the normal curve, shown in color.

SKEWED DISTRIBUTIONS. At other times, the scores pile up at one end or the other, and the distribution is clearly not normal. In a **skewed distribution,** which has a spread of exceptionally high scores, or low scores, the three measures of central tendency provide different indications of the typical score. With a skewed distribution, care must be taken in selecting any measure of central tendency as representative of the entire group.

A number of unusually low scores produces a **negatively skewed distribution,** observed in arrival times at concerts, ball games, and similar events. A few people may arrive an hour or more before the performance, enjoying the players' warm-up and one another's company. Others arrive well ahead; most appear just before the show begins; and there are always a few latecomers, usually by only a few minutes. The latecomers are rarely as tardy as the early arrivals are ahead of the starting time.

In a **positively skewed distribution,** a spread of scores extends in the direction of high scores. For example, the distribution of departure times after a theatre performance or athletic contest produces a positive skew. Most people leave promptly, but a number linger for varying lengths—chatting, resting, reminiscing, or simply waiting for the crowd to disappear (Figure 18–6).

In both skewed distributions, the spread of extreme scores always pulls the mean in its own direction. Thus, in comparison to the other measures of central tendency, a negative skew lowers the mean; a positive skew raises the mean.

MEASURES OF VARIABILITY

In addition to the average or typical score for the letters of the alphabet, the UW team was interested in differences among them. Were the scores for the various letters much alike, or did they vary markedly? The mean score for all letters and punctuation marks was 286.6. Were the scores for the individual letters clustered nearby, or did they range widely?

Similarly, were the typing scores much like one another? The mean typing score for ten men was 50 words per minute. Were most scores close to 50 or did they differ markedly?

To understand any group of scores, we need not only some measure of central tendency but also some measure of difference or dispersion. These latter measures, called **measures of variability,** indicate the degree to which the scores in a group *differ* from some typical score. The usual measures of variability are the range and standard deviation.

RANGE AND STANDARD DEVIATION. The simplest indicator of variability is the **range,** which is the difference between the lowest and

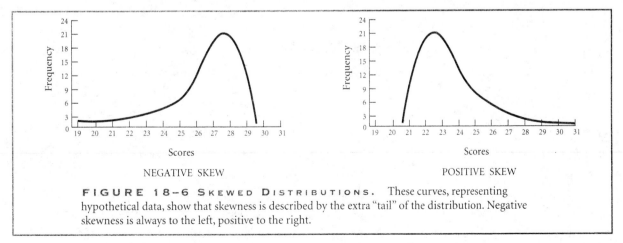

NEGATIVE SKEW   POSITIVE SKEW

FIGURE 18–6 SKEWED DISTRIBUTIONS. These curves, representing hypothetical data, show that skewness is described by the extra "tail" of the distribution. Negative skewness is always to the left, positive to the right.

highest scores. The range for letter frequencies was calculated in this way, as noted already. The score of 1,000, for *E*, minus 9, for *Z*, gave a range of 991. Like the mode, the range is unstable, for it takes into account only two scores in the group. Without the *E*, the highest score would have been for *T*, at 685, and the range would have been reduced to 676, a difference of over 300 points.

Another measure of variability, less well known and more complex, is preferred in science because, like the mean, it is based on *every* value in the group. It is therefore more reliable than the range. Called the **standard deviation** (SD), it indicates the degree of deviation of all the scores from the mean. In a sense, it is a sort of average deviation except that squaring and a square root are involved. Addressing the question of dispersion or variability, it shows whether the scores are close to the mean or widely dispersed.

For ease of understanding, consider two sets of hypothetical scores. For the Reds, they are: 2, 14, 25, 39, and 45. The mean of these scores is 25. For the Blues, they are: 109, 109, 110, 111, and 111. The Blues' mean is 110. Obviously, the scores for the Reds are more widely dispersed than those for the Blues. Thus, the standard deviation for the Reds will be larger than that for the Blues. This fact can be confirmed by noting the deviation of each score from its mean:

	Reds				
Raw Scores	2	14	25	39	45
Deviations	−23	−11	0	+14	+20

	Blues				
Raw Scores	109	109	110	111	111
Deviations	−1	−1	0	+1	+1

One might hastily conclude that the standard deviation is simply the mean of these deviations, but that is not the case. The rules of mathematics and the intricacies of the standard deviation require one further step, partly because the sum of the positive deviations is always equal to the sum of the negative deviations, giving an overall sum of zero. For this reason, among others, we square the deviations. Then we sum them and divide by their number, obtaining the average of these squared deviations. Finally, we take the square root of that number because earlier, we squared the deviations. As the last step, they must be unsquared. This procedure returns the standard deviation to the same units as the original scores.

In summary, the standard deviation is calculated in the following manner. Find the deviation of each score from the mean. Square each deviation. Find the average of these squared deviations by adding them and dividing by their number. Then obtain the square root.

As a further illustration of the range and standard deviation, consider once again the scores from the typing pool, this time involving ten women as well as the ten men. The lowest score for the women is 45 and the highest is 56, giving a range of 11 words per minute. For the men, the range is from 40 to 59, or 19 words per minute. On this basis, the men differed from one another more than did the women, although both groups achieved a mean score of 50 words per minute:

Women 51 48 45 49 53 52 50 47 49 56
Men 58 42 52 40 59 46 54 50 41 58

The standard deviation provides a similar conclusion but on a much firmer and more precise basis. For the ten women's scores, the sum of the squared deviations from the mean is 90. Hence, the standard deviation is the square root of 90/10, which is the square root of 9, or 3. For the ten men's scores, the sum of the squared deviations is 490. Thus, the standard deviation is the square root of 490/10, which is the square root of 49, or 7 (Figure 18–7).

| | | WOMEN | | | | MEN | |
SUBJECT	SCORE	DEVIATION (D)	DEVIATION SQUARED (D^2)	SUBJECT	SCORE	DEVIATION (D)	DEVIATION SQUARED (D^2)
1	51	+1	1	1	58	+8	64
2	48	−2	4	2	42	−8	64
3	45	−5	25	3	52	+2	4
4	49	−1	1	4	40	−10	100
5	53	+3	9	5	59	+9	81
6	52	+2	4	6	46	−4	16
7	50	0	0	7	54	+4	16
8	47	−3	9	8	50	0	0
9	49	−1	1	9	41	−9	81
10	56	+6	36	10	58	+8	64
Sums	500	0	90	Sums	500	0	490

Mean = 50
Computation:

$$SD = \sqrt{\frac{sum\ D^2}{N}} = \sqrt{\frac{90}{10}} = \sqrt{9} = 3$$

Mean = 50
Computation:

$$SD = \sqrt{\frac{sum\ D^2}{N}} = \sqrt{\frac{490}{10}} = \sqrt{49} = 7$$

FIGURE 18–7 COMPUTATION OF STANDARD DEVIATION.
Calculation of the standard deviation (SD) involves the number of scores (N) and the deviation of each score from the mean (D). It is simply the average deviation of the scores from the mean—except that squaring and a square root are involved. These examples illustrate use of the formula.

INTERPRETATION OF STANDARD DEVIATION. The standard deviation of 7, compared with 3, indicates more variability among the men than among the women. In this instance, as in all others, the larger the standard deviation, the greater is the variability.

Boxes of cereal seem to be highly variable in the amounts they contain. When newly opened, some are almost half empty. Others are moderately full. A few are filled to the top. In contrast, dollar bills are minted with extremely little variation in size, color, and so forth, partly to prevent counterfeiting. People on the street show more variability in dress than people in church. There is more variability in sexual behavior among human beings than among animals. All of these differences are most accurately and usefully reflected in the standard deviation.

In personality, one individual may be steady and impassive, showing little emotion of any sort. Another person may be sometimes calm, sometimes highly emotional, openly displaying markedly positive and negative feelings. If we were to quantify the degree of expressed emotion in these two people, they would produce very different standard deviations. The first individual would show a distinctly lower mean and a smaller standard deviation than the second person.

The standard deviation is useful in several ways, especially in a *normal* distribution. With large samples of subjects, the scores for most human characteristics are distributed approximately according to the normal distribution. In these distributions, the standard deviation identifies a certain proportion of the scores and even the positions of individual scores within the group.

The scores between one standard deviation below the mean and one standard deviation above the mean always comprise 68% of all scores in the group. Similarly, 95% of the scores are included between two standard deviations below the mean and two standard deviations above the mean. Finally, the distance between three standard deviations below and three standard deviations above the mean includes approximately 99% of all the scores. This relationship between standard deviation units and percentage of cases under the normal distribu-

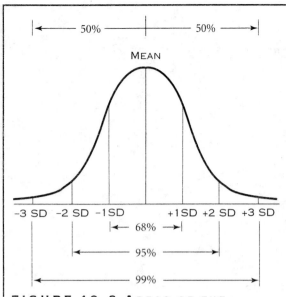

50% ← MEAN → 50%

-3 SD -2 SD -1 SD   +1 SD +2 SD +3 SD

← 68% →

95%

99%

FIGURE 18-8 AREAS OF THE NORMAL DISTRIBUTION. As indicated above the figure, a normal distribution has half of the scores on each side of the mean. The percentages below the figure show the proportion of scores between the mean and various standard deviations. These properties of the normal distribution play a central role in estimating probabilities.

tion is basic to inferential statistics, which we shall consider later (Figure 18–8).

DESCRIBING SETS OF SCORES

With the information about letter usage in English, the UW human-factors team turned to the next question, the capability of the worker. Their aim was to discover the dexterity of the different fingers. For this purpose, they studied several groups of subjects, male and female, all potential typists. In one instance, investigators measured finger dexterity by requesting 54 subjects to tap with each finger separately as rapidly as possible on a table. The wrist and nontapping fingers were held stationary, using a 30-second interval for each finger (Hoke, 1922).

To describe these scores, measures of central tendency and variability are needed. Together they indicate the typical performance and deviations from the typical performance.

For central tendency, the mean was employed, calculated separately for each finger, excluding the thumb, and separately for each hand. In this way, it was found that the right index finger was most capable, followed by the left index finger. Next were the middle fingers, then the little fingers, and finally the ring fingers, again right and left, respectively (Hoke, 1922). It appears no accident that the two index fingers are used in the hunt-and-peck method of typing.

Then came the question of variability. How consistent were the different fingers? Did the index finger vary more in its performance than the middle finger or ring finger? These data could be influential in designing a new keyboard.

As it turned out, consistency was not an issue. The standard deviations among the fingers were similar. No one finger was markedly less predictable than the others. They all displayed about the same amount of variability in performance (Table 18–1).

Examples of the value of taking into account both measures, means and standard deviations, are evident throughout human behavior. One golfer,

FINGER	MEAN	STANDARD DEVIATION
Right index	161.2	25.0
Left index	149.9	24.6
Right middle	134.3	25.9
Left middle	120.8	26.0
Right little	114.8	27.5
Left little	105.9	29.7
Right ring	101.4	29.9
Left ring	98.6	25.5

TABLE 18-1 FINGER ABILITIES. When ranked from fastest to slowest according to mean rate of tapping, there were marked differences among the fingers. However, the fingers did not differ significantly in variability, as shown by the standard deviations (Hoke, 1922).

with an average score of 82, is *always* in the low eighties. The other, a far better player, often comes close to par, but on bad days he becomes upset and scores in the nineties. He too has an average score of 82, but these two golfers are very different types of players.

With this information on finger ability, the human-factors team then turned to finger workload. What was the workload for each finger? These workloads were determined by noting the keys assigned to each finger and the frequencies with which they were typed. When these frequencies were summed for all keys for each finger, the left index finger scored highest, the left middle next, then the right index, and so forth (Table 18–2).

The total workload for each finger was the only concern. Hence, there was no calculation of central tendency or variability.

• CORRELATIONAL STATISTICS •

The first recorded typewriter patent was registered in London in 1714, and for the next century and a half inventors attempted to build a machine that would work. All sorts of contraptions were tried, including typewriters for use on horseback. All sorts of keyboards were designed, intended for use by the hunt-and-peck method. But all of these early machines failed. One major difficulty was the constant jamming of the keys. These failures were widely ridiculed, and attempts to modify the keyboard to present jamming were regularly ineffective.

Finally, in 1873, Christopher Sholes and his coworkers in Milwaukee solved the problem. They developed a successful machine, chiefly by constructing a keyboard on which the keys did not interfere with one another. This keyboard became widely popular. Universally accepted as the *QWERTY* or *standard keyboard*, it was the design investigated by the UW human-factors team 60 years later. *QWERTY* refers to the first letters in the upper row.

The UW team knew about the work to be performed on this keyboard. It had been determined by the frequencies of letter usage in English. This team also knew about the abilities of the fingers, discovered by the tapping test. The next step was to discover whether the most work was assigned to the most capable fingers, a critical issue in typing efficiency.

To achieve this goal, they turned to a second major method, **correlational statistics,** describing the *relationship between two sets* of scores. The concern was no longer with describing one or several sets of scores. The team was interested instead in determining the *association between pairs* of scores, each pair generated by the same subject or source. This association is referred to as *correlation.*

The term **correlation,** coming from *co-relation,* indicates the extent to which two variables are related.

FINGER	KEYS TYPED: LETTERS AND PUNCTUATION						WORKLOAD
Left index	*r* 423	*f* 102	*v* 66	*t* 685	*g* 99	*b* 160	1,535
Left middle	*e* 1000	*d* 261	*c* 231				1,492
Right index	*y* 175	*h* 402	*n* 469	*u* 223	*j* 23	*m* 198	1,490
Right ring	*o* 561	*l* 349	. 86				996
Left little	*q* 10	*a* 684	*z* 9	*shift* 100			803
Left ring	*w* 152	*s* 486	*x* 20				658
Right middle	*i* 484	*k* 41	, 115				640
Right little	*p* 158	; 16	: 11	? 11	*shift* 100		296

TABLE 18–2 FINGER WORKLOADS. The workload for each finger was determined by adding the frequencies of the letters and punctuation marks it typed. Responsibilities for the shift key were divided equally between the left and right little fingers (Hoke, 1922).

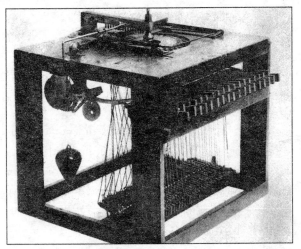 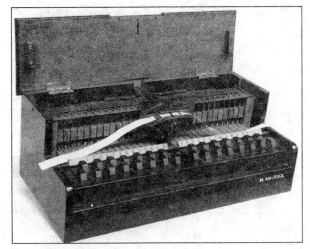

FIGURE 18-9 EARLY TYPEWRITERS. These early machines developed mechanical failures of all sorts, including the persistent problem of a workable keyboard.

Among adults, age and illness are related. Older adults are more likely than younger adults to have physical disorders. Typing speed and hat size are not correlated. Fast typists do not wear larger or smaller hats than slow typists. Temperature and aggression are mildly related. The higher the temperature, the greater are the chances of a riot or mob reaction.

❧ TYPES OF CORRELATION

Specifically, the UW team was confronted with this question: What was the correlation between finger ability and workload? Were the strongest, most capable fingers doing the most work? Were the weakest, least capable fingers doing the least work? If the most capable fingers were carrying the heaviest loads, the correlation would be high, and the keyboard was reasonably well designed. If not, if some of the less capable fingers were carrying heavy loads and vice versa, then the correlation would be low. The keyboard would be laid out poorly (Figure 18–9).

Correlations have two characteristics, size and direction. In size, they can range from high to low; in direction, they can be positive or negative. If the standard keyboard is efficient, the correlation between finger ability and finger workload should be high *and* positive.

SIZE OF CORRELATION. In numerical value, or size, the correlation can range from 0 to +1.00 or from 0 to -1.00. No correlation can exceed a value of 1.00, which indicates a perfect relationship, something rarely found in psychological studies. A statistical computation that yields a larger result must be in error.

Correlations close to 1.00, positive *or* negative, are regarded as high; those near 0 are described as low; and those in between are considered mild or moderate. Among adult human beings, the relationship between weight and height is moderate to high, perhaps in the vicinity of .60 to .80, depending on the composition of the group. The relationship between weight and intelligence is low, essentially 0. And the relationship between weight and strength is intermediate, the exact value varying with the individuals in the sample.

DIRECTION OF CORRELATION. The direction of correlation can be positive or negative. When it is positive, both scores in each pair tend to go in the same direction, increasing together or

86

decreasing together. Among older adults, age and illness are said to be positively correlated. When age is high, the probability of illness is high. When age is low, the probability of illness is low. The pairs of scores increase or decrease together in a **positive correlation.** For a given individual, *both* scores tend to be low or moderate or high. Expressed differently, we can say that there is a direct relationship between the two variables.

In negative correlation, a high score on one variable is associated with a low score on the other. The two members of each pair of scores go in opposite directions in a **negative correlation;** if one score is high, the other tends to be low, and vice versa. Among adults, age and health are negatively correlated. As they grow older, adults tend to be less healthy. Among children, interest in reading and the tendency to drop out of school are also negatively correlated. The higher the interest in reading, the lower is the dropout problem. There is an inverse, or negative, relationship between these variables (Figure 18–10).

Provided that the variables are understood, no particular merit is attached to a positive or negative correlation. Both indicate a relationship. Among adults, the correlation between exercise and health is positive; the correlation between exercise and disease is negative. This issue is the way the second variable is expressed, as health or illness.

DETERMINING RELATIONSHIPS

Earlier, we saw that raw scores can be presented visually, as a graph, or numerically, by indicating an overall score or value. These same two approaches can be used for correlation, but two sets of scores are involved. For the keyboard, these scores describe finger ability and finger workload.

Finger ability was determined by tapping tests, as indicated earlier. The right index finger scored highest, the left index finger next, and so forth through the left ring finger, which ranked lowest in ability.

The scores for finger workload were developed by noting the letters for which each finger was responsible and the frequency with which these letters were typed. Thus, the next task was to depict the relationship between these two sets of scores, using a graphic display or numerical calculation.

USE OF SCATTERGRAMS. In a graphic display, each entry is shown according to both scores. One score is plotted on the horizontal axis, the other on the vertical axis. The result, when all pairs of scores have been plotted, is called a **scattergram,** which shows the distribution, or scatter, among the plotted points. It gives some idea of the relationship between the two sets of scores.

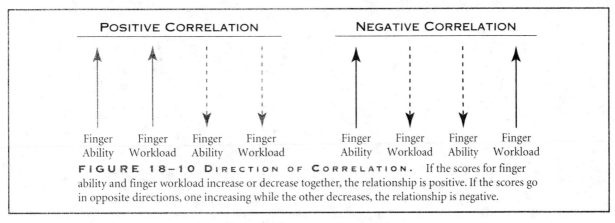

FIGURE 18–10 DIRECTION OF CORRELATION. If the scores for finger ability and finger workload increase or decrease together, the relationship is positive. If the scores go in opposite directions, one increasing while the other decreases, the relationship is negative.

The less the scatter, the stronger the relationship. In fact, if the correlation is perfect, the points fall in a straight diagonal line, and this condition is called a straight-line or **linear relationship.** If the points are widely scattered, the relationship is close to zero. Furthermore, if the slope of the scatter is upward, left to right, the relationship is positive. If it is downward, left to right, the relationship is negative (Figure 18–11).

In constructing the scattergram for finger ability and finger workload, the ability score for each finger was plotted on the horizontal axis and the workload score on the vertical axis. Inspection of the resulting scatter showed that the plotted points did not form a straight line. They fell in a mildly diffuse pattern, indicating only a moderate positive relationship (Figure 18–12).

OBTAINING A COEFFICIENT. The scattergram gives a visual representation, not a numerical value. For greater precision, and for use with further statistical methods, a coefficient is calculated.

This **coefficient of correlation** is a numerical value between 0.00 and ±1.00 showing the degree of relationship between two sets of scores. The closer the coefficient is to 1.00, the higher is the relationship between the sets of scores.

There are several methods for finding the coefficient of correlation. One frequently used procedure, the *product-moment method,* takes into account the deviations of scores from the mean of each variable. Developed by an Englishman, Karl Pearson, and therefore called the Pearson product-moment, the resulting numerical value, or coefficient, is symbolized as *r.* In another method, called the *rank-difference method,* the basic procedure is to find the difference in ranks for each pair of scores. Also called the Spearman rank-difference, after another Englishman, Charles Spearman, the resulting numerical value is *rho.*

Using the scores indicated earlier, the ranks for finger ability and finger workload were entered into the rank-order formula. The result was a coefficient of correlation of +.43.

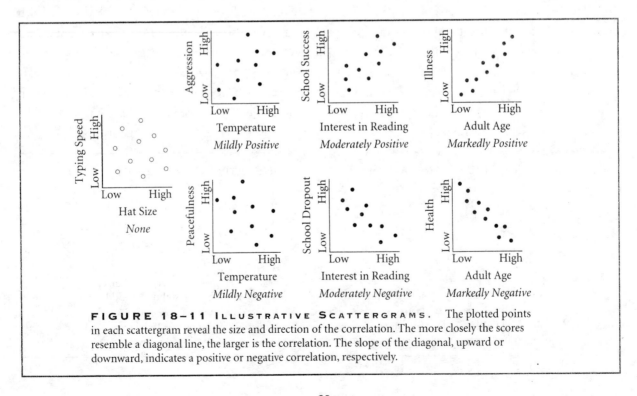

FIGURE 18–11 ILLUSTRATIVE SCATTERGRAMS. The plotted points in each scattergram reveal the size and direction of the correlation. The more closely the scores resemble a diagonal line, the larger is the correlation. The slope of the diagonal, upward or downward, indicates a positive or negative correlation, respectively.

FINGER	ABILITY	WORKLOAD
Right index (RI)	161.2	1,490
Left index (LI)	149.9	1,535
Right middle (RM)	134.3	640
Left middle (LM)	120.8	1,492
Right little (RL)	114.8	296
Left little (LL)	105.9	803
Right ring (RR)	101.4	996
Left ring (LR)	98.6	658

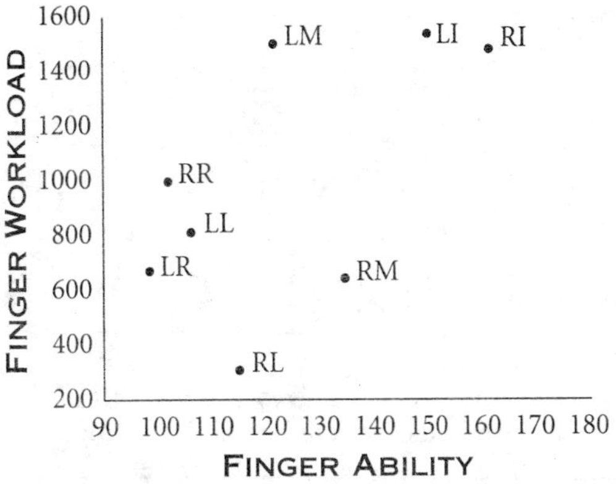

FIGURE 18–12 SCATTERGRAM OF FINGER ABILITY AND WORKLOAD. The scores for finger ability and finger workload are scattered, indicating a moderate correlation. The slope is slightly upward, left to right, indicating a positive relationship.

INTERPRETATION OF THE COEFFICIENT. In evaluating this finding, note first that the correlation is positive, meaning that high scores on one variable are associated with high scores on the other; low scores on one variable are associated with low scores on the other. But note also the size of the coefficient. It shows only a moderate relationship between finger ability and workload. Considering the extremely wide usage of this standard keyboard, this relationship of +.43 is not impressive. In several instances, less capable fingers do more work than more capable ones. The middle finger of the right hand is third in ability, yet it has the next to lowest workload of all eight fingers.

This correlation, or any other, does not indicate that one variable causes the other. It does not mean that finger ability causes workload or vice versa. Among children, weight and memory are positively correlated, but one would not reasonably conclude that gaining weight improves a child's memory or that improvement in memory causes weight gain. Both conditions increase with a third variable, age. The influence of age becomes evident when we correlate weight and memory in children of the same age, for then the relationship is negligible. In short, a correlation merely shows a relationship; it does *not* demonstrate a causal relationship.

Although one may exist, cause and effect cannot be assumed.

Furthermore, a correlation does not indicate a percentage. A coefficient of +.43 does *not* mean that one variable accounts for 43% of the other variable. And it does not mean that these two variables have 43% in common. Rather, the mutual dependence between them is considerably less than might be expected from a casual glance. If the correlation coefficient is .40, for example, then squaring it gives: $.40 \times .40 = .16$. Only 16% of the variability on one measure can be explained by variations in the other (Evans & Waites, 1981). Similarly, a correlation of +.50 indicates only 25% interdependence. In other words, correlation shows the degree of agreement between two variables, not their common properties.

This relationship between finger workload and finger ability suggests that the standard keyboard is not well designed. It could be more efficient. Ask any of today's million keyboard operators to type the word *million*. Imagine typing it yourself, if you know this keyboard.

As the UW team pointed out, this word is typed entirely with the right hand. Such a discovery was disappointing. Imagine typing: *Afterwards we were sadder.* Like that italicized phrase, thousands of

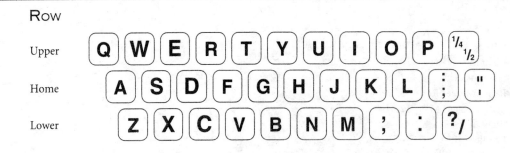

FIGURE 18–13 STANDARD KEYBOARD. The hands are positioned on the home row with the index fingers on *F* and *J*. Most typing occurs in the upper row.

words are typed entirely with the left hand, which does the most work. The standard keyboard is not the *greatest*, overtaxing the left hand (Figure 18–13). There are many one-handed sequences, in which one hand types several consecutive letters while the other remains idle, thereby limiting typing speed to one-half its maximum pace. Without alternation of the hands, efficiency is at a *minimum*.

• INFERENTIAL STATISTICS •

One early supporter of the new "type-machine," as he called it, was Mark Twain. In fact, he claimed to be the first person ever to write a book with it, using it for the last half of the manuscript for *The Adventures of Tom Sawyer*. Nevertheless, he found it full of devilish defects (Figure 18–14).

These defects included the keyboard design, which later offered a subtle benefit for crafty salespersons. Using just the index fingers, as was the habit in those earlier days, they could readily demonstrate to prospective customers the promise of their product. Perhaps the keyboard was planned this way—so that they could type the name of the machine in the upper row: T Y P E W R I T E R (Gould, 1987).

With clear evidence of the inappropriate workload for the different fingers and the numerous one-handed sequences in English, August Dvorak

took a strong stand against the standard keyboard: "This 'universal keyboard' tosses the typing into an upper row of keys. . . . overburdens the lesser fingers and . . . forces frequent idling of one hand while the other types entire words" (Dvorak, Merrick, Dealey, & Ford, 1936). Faced with this discouraging design after two years of evaluation, the UW team took a new direction. They began to prepare an improved keyboard.

To achieve this purpose, they gathered more statistical information on letter usage; they experimented with many different locations for the keys; and they studied the relationships among finger movements. They assessed error rates, speed of typing, and even the rhythms reported by experienced typists. Gradually, they developed a completely new keyboard, known as the *Dvorak* or *simplified keyboard*.

To assess the effectiveness of this simplified keyboard, they used typing speed as the chief criterion of success, measuring words per minute. There were thousands of keyboard operators in the United States, however, and all of these people could not be included in their various tests. Here they were faced with the third and final major problem in statistics, the problem of statistical inference.

In *descriptive statistics*, a group of scores is described, and all of them are available. Certain values, such as the mean and standard deviation, indicate the performance of the whole group. In

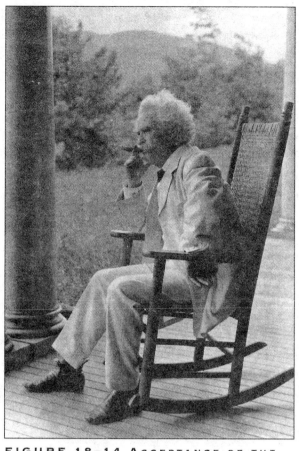

FIGURE 18–14 ACCEPTANCE OF THE TYPEWRITER. Mark Twain used the typewriter in 1874 and then ignored it for 30 years, until he wrote his autobiography in 1904. At the beginning of this interval, he noted, the machine was a curiosity, and people who used it were a curiosity, too. But by the turn of the century, he decided, the situation had been reversed. People who did *not* own it were a curiosity (Twain, 1906).

correlational statistics, the purpose is to discover the relationship between two sets of scores. The aim is to show the degree of association, if any, between one variable and another. In **inferential statistics,** an inference, or educated guess, is made about the probability of obtaining the observed scores and scores *not* observed. Inferential statistics concern *probability,* meaning the chances that a certain event will occur. In the case of the keyboard, the scores of a sample of typists using the simplified keyboard can be used to make an inference or statement of probability about the scores that might be obtained from all typists using this simplified keyboard.

In studying their keyboard, the human-factors psychologists selected a **sample** of subjects, which is only a portion of all possible subjects. A sample is a subgroup; it is part of a larger group. The sample of typists might have included 10, 100, or 1,000 subjects, depending on the ease of obtaining them and the sampling method employed. All possible subjects in the larger group comprise the **population,** a term that does not refer exclusively to animals or human beings. A population includes *all* possible cases in any particular class or category: aggressive behaviors, athletic shoes, abdominal pains, or albino rats, as well as typists using the simplified keyboard. All typists using the simplified design could not be tested; therefore, estimates about the whole population were made by testing just some of them—a sample.

It should be emphasized that the larger the sample—that is, the more subjects from the population included in the sample—the greater is the probability that the sample will reflect the characteristics of the population. In other words, increasing the size of the sample increases the chances for reaching correct conclusions about the population.

When a sample reflects the characteristics of the population from which it has been selected, it is called a **representative sample.** It accurately depicts the population; it shows what is fundamentally true about that larger group. When it does not, it is a *biased sample,* meaning that it is prejudiced or inclined in one way or another. The usual way of obtaining a representative sample is through random sampling. In a **random sample,** every person or item in the population has an equal chance of being included. This condition is often achieved by using random numbers, assigning one number to each subject, and then drawing the numbers in such a way that no number is more likely to be chosen than any other number.

In studies of the simplified keyboard, samples of various sizes were obtained. One sample included 44 college students and adults. Another included 83 college students. After testing these beginning typists on the simplified keyboard, the investigators inferred how the *whole population of beginning typists* might perform while typing the same material on this same keyboard. The mean score for one sample was approximately 41.5 words per minute after 45 hours of instruction. Thus, it might be inferred that the whole population would perform at this speed after the same instruction.

POINT ESTIMATION

One form of inferential statistics is called **point estimation** because a score obtained with a few subjects is used to estimate a score that might be obtained with many subjects. Forty people might be tested on the simplified keyboard, for example, and their mean score might be used to estimate the mean for all simplified keyboard users. This procedure involves point estimation because the purpose is to estimate one point or value in a population—such as the mean—by using information from a sample.

Point estimation is widely used in political polls. A few voters are questioned, and these results are used to predict the winner. In all such cases, the accuracy of the estimate depends significantly on which subjects are included in the sample. Sampling techniques are now so sophisticated that predictions can be highly accurate, even with relatively small samples.

THE STANDARD ERROR. But with the beginning typists, no one could be certain that the sample mean, 41.5 words per minute, truly represented the mean of the whole population of people beginning to use the simplified keyboard. The only way to know for certain would have been to test all beginning operators, but that was impossible. Thus, steps were taken to deal with the uncertainty, using a procedure for estimating the probable error. This procedure is possible because *chance errors* in sampling, in the long run, tend to be distributed according to the normal distribution. As noted earlier, many factors acting in a complex, unknown way on a single event often produce a normal distribution.

The sample mean for the typing test was 41.5 words per minute. For other samples, the means might have been higher, lower, or the same. We simply do not know. But if the investigators continued taking samples from the entire population of beginning simplified keyboard users and continued finding their means, eventually they would have discovered that this distribution of sample means was nearly a normal distribution. Furthermore, the *mean of these sample means* would have been close to the population mean. It would have reflected the true mean of the population of all beginning simplified keyboard operators.

The problem was that these investigators, like others, could not take endless samples. In fact, they had only a few samples. But fortunately, statisticians have developed a method for determining how much any one sample mean may be in error. This measure, called a **standard error,** is used in determining the amount of error likely in a sample statistic. An extension of the concept of standard deviation, the standard error provides an estimate of the amount that a sample mean varies by chance from the true mean of the population.

FACTORS INFLUENCING THE STANDARD ERROR. By now, you may be approaching the standard error with some shortness of breath and moist palms. Relax. It is not necessary to calculate the standard error here, and this statistic does not involve any new concepts. The aim in this context is simply to understand how it operates, and you can be assured that it is essentially a function of just two factors, both encountered already. The standard error depends on the size of the sample and the standard deviation of that sample.

The larger the sample, the smaller is the standard error. A moment's reflection shows why this is true. Suppose an entire population consisted of 1,500 people using the simplified keyboard. A sample of 1,499 subjects would contain very little error, for only one keyboard operator would be missing. That person's typing score, even if by chance it were extremely high or low, would have little influence on the mean score made by 1,499 other people. But if the sample were 150 typists, constituting just 10% of the whole population, chance factors in that sample might give a false impression of the population. And if the sample included only three or four subjects, chance factors probably would give a wrong impression (Figure 18–15).

The other factor influencing the standard error, besides the size of the sample, is its standard deviation. For samples of at least moderate size, such as 30 or more entries, the smaller the standard deviation, the smaller is the standard error. In other words, the more closely the scores cluster around the sample mean, the more likely it is that the sample mean adequately represents the population mean.

In summary, when there are many scores, and when the deviation among them is small, the standard error is small. Under these conditions, the sample mean is likely to reflect the population mean.

When the standard error was obtained for one sample of simplified keyboard operators, it was found to be 1.5 words per minute. When this value was applied to the sample mean of 41.5 words per minute, probability statements

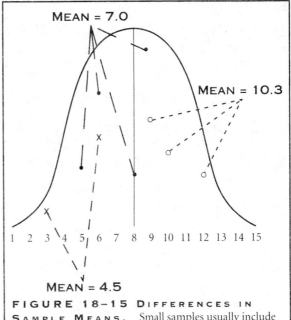

MEAN = 7.0

MEAN = 10.3

MEAN = 4.5

FIGURE 18–15 DIFFERENCES IN SAMPLE MEANS. Small samples usually include different subjects from the population, producing different sample means. These samples of two, four, and three subjects resulted in very different sample means. If, instead, they had comprised one sample of nine subjects, that sample mean would have been a more accurate representation of the population mean, which is eight.

could be made about the population mean. One standard error subtracted from the mean was equal to 41.5 minus 1.5, or 40. One standard error added to the mean was equal to 41.5 plus 1.5, or 43. Hence, the true mean score for the population of beginning Dvorak typists probably lay somewhere in the interval from 40 to 43 words per minute. The chances of the true mean falling within this interval, as evident in our earlier discussion of the standard deviation and the normal distribution, were approximately 68 out of 100. This statement of probability was the best estimate of the performance of the whole population of simplified keyboard users. For a higher degree of confidence, a still wider interval would have been necessary. For example, the chances were 95 out of 100 that it fell approximately between 38.5 and 44.5 and 99 out of 100 that it falls between 37.0 and 46.0. Stated in more general terms, it appeared likely that the population mean was a value close to 41.5 words per minute.

STUDY OF DIFFERENCES

All normal keyboards have three rows of letters, and obviously it is easier to use the home row, where the fingers are stationed initially, than to use either of the other rows. With the QWERTY or standard keyboard, more than half of the work is done on the row *above* the home row, which includes the letters *E* and *T*, two of the most frequently used letters. Slightly less than one-third of the work occurs in the home row.

For the Dvorak simplified keyboard, the human-factors psychologists placed the most common letters in the home row. They assigned the moderately used letters to the top row and the least-used letters to the bottom row, for it is easier to reach above than below the home row. This design distinctly favored the home row, where almost three-quarters of all typing is accomplished (Table 18–3).

To compare this model with the standard keyboard, we must go beyond point estimation. Instead, we want to know about the *difference* between two sample means, comparing the simplified keyboard with the standard keyboard. Thus, we want to estimate two points, one in each popula-

ROW	KEYBOARD	
	STANDARD	SIMPLIFIED
Upper	52	22
Home	32	70
Lower	16	8

TABLE 18–3 ROW WORKLOADS. The table shows the percent of typing in each row. With the typist's fingers so often in the home row of the simplifed keyboard, it almost seems that the hands are not moving at all.

tion. This question, determining whether a difference between two or more sample means represents a difference between the population means, is called the **study of differences** or *testing an hypothesis*.

The essential feature of much psychological research, evident in the study of differences, is a comparison between experimental and control groups. The question here is: Which subjects type faster, those with the simplified keyboard or those with the standard keyboard? At this point, in this last portion of the last chapter in this book, we encounter once again a recurrent theme: the effort to answer psychological questions through empiricism rather than by speculation, common sense, or even pure reasoning.

TESTING AN HYPOTHESIS. Answering this question empirically requires an appropriate experimental design. In the traditional approach, the experimental and control groups are as equal as possible in all relevant respects—age, experience, intelligence, motivation, and so forth—except one. This factor, the independent variable, is present or manipulated for the experimental group but not for the control group. In the case at hand, the independent variable is the keyboard design. If a difference in performance is found between the two groups, it is attributed to this variable.

On these bases, the UW group formed and tested their hypothesis: Operators using the experimental or simplified keyboard would learn faster than those using the standard design.

STATISTICAL SIGNIFICANCE. In early studies of the standard keyboard using hundreds of beginning operators, the mean score was 25.0 words per minute after one course of instruction. For two dozen beginning operators learning the simplified keyboard during less than half that period, the mean score was approximately 41.5

words per minute. The length of instruction was markedly shorter with the simplified design, and yet there was a difference of 16.5 words per minute in favor of that keyboard (Dvorak, Merrick, Dealey, & Ford, 1936).

This difference between samples of typists using the standard or simplified keyboard seems large, but would it have appeared if both populations had been tested instead? In other words, does this difference between the sample means reflect a true difference between the population means? Would another test, with different samples of subjects drawn from the same populations, have produced a similar difference?

The statistic of interest here is partly familiar, for it is again a standard error—this time the standard error of the *difference* between the means, rather than the standard error of just one mean. As we approach this new concept, there is again no need for heart palpitations and knocking knees. Calculations are not important. It is sufficient merely to appreciate that the procedure goes one step beyond the calculation of the standard error for a single mean. It is the difference between two sample means divided by the probable error in determining that difference. Once more, the normal distribution is relevant, and the probability again is expressed in terms of chances out of 100.

When the probability is low that a finding is due to chance, it is considered to have statistical significance. It might have occurred through chance factors, but the investigator is confident at a high level that it was due instead to the influence of the specific factor under investigation, in this case the keyboard design. As a rule, **statistical significance** is considered to be present when the probability of obtaining a certain result by chance is very small, typically less than 5 chances out of 100.

With statistical significance, if the experiment were repeated 100 times, for example, in only 5 instances would a difference of this magnitude be due to chance. This result is described as $p < .05$, which means that the probability of finding a difference this large or larger on the next trial, if there is really no difference between the populations, is less than 5 in 100.

To be even more stringent, the standard could be raised to $p < .01$, meaning that the probability of finding a difference this large on a chance basis, when there really was no difference, is 1 in 100, or less. In studies of difference, just as in point estimation, the true difference cannot be known for certain because all members of both populations cannot be tested. The conclusion remains a statement of probability.

In the case of the two keyboards, it was very unlikely that the difference of 16.5 words per minute between the sample means occurred on a chance basis ($p < .01$). In short, we are quite confident that it was due instead to the simplified design.

• STATISTICS AS A TOOL •

This difference of 16.5 words per minute, when calculated for a workday of seven or eight hours, represented a difference of several thousand words each day. It demonstrated rather clearly the advantage of the simplified keyboard. More important in the present context, it showed the value of statistical methods. They served as tools for the evaluation of the old keyboard and later for developing a new, simplified design.

Statistical methods are no different from other human tools. They can be used improperly; just like a hammer, violin, or ice skates, they are no better than their users. Whether statistics are beneficial or harmful, or whether a particular potential is achieved, depends in a large measure on who compiles and interprets them.

In constructing this simplified keyboard, the UW psychologists first placed the most frequently used letters in the home row. Then they assigned the most work to the most capable fingers. Finally, and most important, they assigned the letters for alternate use by the two hands, thereby diminishing one-handed sequences. To achieve this alternation, the UW team assigned the five vowels to the left hand and the five most common consonants to the right hand. Since consonants typically follow vowels and vice versa in English, alternation is maximized, and the amount of typing is approximately balanced between the two hands. On the simplified keyboard, one hand moves down to strike a letter while the other moves up into position to strike the next letter (Figure 18–16).

With this new keyboard, typists won seven first places in an international typing contest; the UW team achieved their research goal; and the members published their findings in a book entitled *Typewriting Behavior* (Dvorak, Merrick, Dealey, & Ford, 1936). Shortly thereafter, their keyboard was banned as unfair competition in typing contests, much like a curved stick in ice hockey or a deep pocket in lacrosse, making high scoring too easy. This decision did not deter Barbara Blackburn, who could barely type 50 words per minute on the standard keyboard. At the suggestion of her typing instructor, she turned to the Dvorak simplified model and has been listed in the *Guinness Book of World Records* as typing 150 words per minute for 50 consecutive minutes (Larsen, 1985). Unofficially, she has exceeded 200 words per minute (Cassingham, 1986).

If the simplified keyboard becomes widely accepted, the diminished effort of the operators may become a decisive factor, not only for increasing speed and comfort but also for decreasing the risk of repetitive strain injuries. The distance traveled by the fingers on the standard keyboard is 10 to 16 times greater than on the simplified design (Katzeff, 1983; Lamb, 1983). Many people who are not data entry personnel spend three or four hours per day at the keyboard, becoming susceptible to these injuries, including carpal tunnel syndrome, a painful disorder that can lead to permanent damage of the hand. It is caused by pressure on the nerve extending through the passage formed among the carpal bones of the wrist; more than 700,000 cases were diagnosed in 1988 (Oransky, 1994).

The increase in these injuries presents a challenging problem for human-factors psychologists (Howell, 1993). Even with the standard keyboard, this problem can be diminished by very different keyboard designs, including chorded keyboards, on which combinations of keys are pressed simultane-

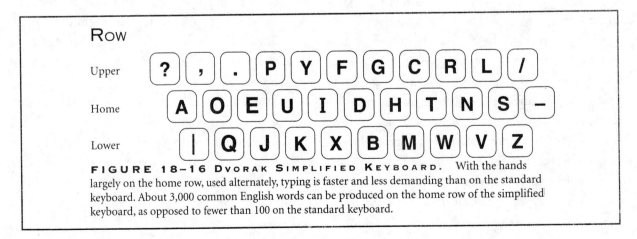

FIGURE 18–16 DVORAK SIMPLIFIED KEYBOARD. With the hands largely on the home row, used alternately, typing is faster and less demanding than on the standard keyboard. About 3,000 common English words can be produced on the home row of the simplified keyboard, as opposed to fewer than 100 on the standard keyboard.

ously, or by a split keyboard, with the two halves comfortably apart, providing each hand with its own, spatially separate set of keys (Gopher & Raij, 1988; Kroemer, 1992).

Statistics will be used in this research, just as they were employed in the design of the simplified keyboard. There they served to describe data, such as letter frequencies and typing speeds; to determine the association between sets of data, such as the correlation between finger ability and finger workload; and to test hypotheses about the success of the new keyboard. In the latter case, typists using the simplified design were much faster than those using the standard model.

This quantification of data does not provide incontestable evidence of any general phenomenon. It merely indicates in objective fashion what was found in a particular set of circumstances and the probability of obtaining the same findings in the future. The concept of **probability** concerns the likelihood that a particular event will appear or reappear, as opposed to a different event. It is a comparison of alternatives. All scientific statements are, in the last analysis, probability statements.

And at this point, with a head full of statistics, you may wonder why the standard keyboard was so poorly designed in the first place. There are two competing explanations. According to one, the so-called *random explanation,* the standard keyboard arose haphazardly, with no thought of touch typing until almost a quarter of a century later. Placement of the keys was determined by a random selection of the letters as they were taken from the printer's font, partly alphabetized. While the hunt-and-peck method prevailed, placement of the keys was relatively unimportant. The standard keyboard was satisfactory.

According to the other view, sometimes known as the *intentional explanation,* the standard keyboard was purposely scrambled in the early machines. The aim was to prevent collisions among the long levers on which the letters were mounted. If the typist worked rapidly, the keys jammed. An awkward keyboard design impeded typing speed, thereby offering a machine that worked. Intentionally scrambling the letters solved a nasty problem, one that baffled typewriter manufacturers at the time.

We do not know which explanation is correct, but we do know that the simplified keyboard was developed at the wrong time for its acceptance. The Great Depression, followed by World War II, and then the quickly formed habits in the rising economies of the 1950s and 1960s all became obstacles to change. There may have been another reason too—a commercial concern, less widely recognized. The potential manufacturers of the new keyboard were diverted from their usual commercial goals during World War II and became munitions manufacturers instead. After the war, one of them purchased the rights to this design and yet did nothing with them, perhaps because by that time the standard model was selling so well (Dvorak, 1985). Manufacturers generally do not make significant changes in products with brisk sales.

The simplified keyboard has been approved by the American National Standards Institute, an endorsement that provides official recognition (Lamb, 1983). It is faithfully employed by a number of private citizens and institutions but rarely found in the broader commercial world.

Statistical methods showed its success. Statistics also show that most keyboard operators today continue to use the old model. That model is something like an irregular verb. People may dislike it, but no one can seem to change it. Observing this neglect of his work, August Dvorak recalled the words of Ralph Waldo Emerson: "If a man builds a better mousetrap, the world will beat a path to his door." Then he added with a wry smile, "Emerson never said how long it would take."

QUANTIFICATION IN PSYCHOLOGY

1. Throughout its history, scientific progress has been closely linked with advances in statistical methods. The field of psychology is no exception. Use of statistical methods in psychological research is readily evident in human-factors psychology, a specialty devoted to the design of tools and procedures well suited to human use.

2. When properly employed, statistics can demonstrate certain facts more accurately than words. When misused in the collection and presentation of data, statistics can create a distorted impression.

DESCRIPTIVE STATISTICS

3. The aim of descriptive statistics is to present a group of scores clearly and simply. One approach involves pictorial methods, especially the use of graphs. They illustrate the results but do not permit further statistical analyses.

4. A more common approach is based on two numerical values, measures of central tendency and measures of variability. The three widely used measures of central tendency are: the mode, median, and mean. These measures are identical in a normal distribution.

5. Measures of variability indicate the extent to which scores in a group differ from one another. The simplest measure is the range, which includes only the lowest and highest scores and therefore is unreliable. The standard deviation, based on the values of all the scores, is used in most statistical analyses.

6. A group of scores can be analyzed and summarized by descriptive statistics, usually by presenting the mean and standard deviation.

CORRELATIONAL STATISTICS

7. Statistics also can be used to study the relationship between two sets of scores. In this case, a coeffi-cient of correlation is computed; it can be positive, meaning that high scores on one trait are associated with high scores on the other, or negative, meaning that high scores on one trait are associated with low scores on the other.

8. The magnitude of this relationship can be indicated by plotting all the entries on a scattergram. When this relationship is indicated by computing a coefficient of correlation, which gives a numerical result, it does not indicate a percentage, and it does not imply causality.

INFERENTIAL STATISTICS

9. For practical purposes, an investigator generally cannot study all potential subjects. Instead, a sample is selected and studied and, by use of this information, estimates are made about characteristics of the larger population. This process is called inferential statistics.

10. One form of inferential statistics is known as point estimation because a score obtained with a sample of subjects is used to estimate a score that might be obtained from the larger population.

11. In the study of differences, an inference is made about the difference between two or more population values, judging from the difference between sample values. These samples might represent experimental and control groups in research.

STATISTICS AS A TOOL

12. Statistical methods are important research tools, but like any other human tool they can be misused. The quantification of data can be used to describe findings in an objective fashion and to determine the probability of obtaining the same findings in the future.

❧ REVIEW OF KEY CONCEPTS ❧

human-factors psychology

Quantification in Psychology
statistics
statistical literacy

Descriptive Statistics
descriptive statistics
raw scores
graph
bar graph
measures of central tendency
mode
median
mean

normal distribution
skewed distribution
positively skewed distribution
negatively skewed distribution
measures of variability
range
standard deviation (SD)

Correlational Statistics
correlational statistics
correlation
positive correlation
negative correlation
scattergram
linear relationship

coefficient of correlation

Inferential Statistics
inferential statistics
sample
population
representative sample
random sample
point estimation
standard error
study of differences
statistical significance

Statistics as a Tool
probability

❧ CLASS DISCUSSION/CRITICAL THINKING ❧

A NARRATIVE TWIST

Rather than investigating the keyboard and developing a new design, the UW team might have studied the bathroom shower or bathroom sink instead, making one or the other more useful and pleasant for most people. Indicate the people they might have studied, variables they might have examined, statistical data they might have obtained, and some of the changes in the shower or sink they might have suggested as a result of their investigations. ❧

TOPICAL QUESTIONS

• *Quantification in Psychology.* Suggest a topic for a one-hour lesson to promote statistical literacy in elementary school. Describe how this lesson will develop an interest in

statistics, rather than competence in statistical calculations.

• *Descriptive Statistics.* To obtain an approximate measure of children's height in a remote school district without measuring every child, a researcher lined them up in order, from tallest to shortest, and then noted the height of each child at the end of the line and the one in the middle. Discuss the descriptive statistics obtained in this instance. Describe the reliability of these measures.

• *Correlational Statistics.* In discussing diet and health, Mr. Black says there is a high positive correlation; Mr. White says the correlation is high but negative; and Mr. Brown says the correlation is not just high but also causal. Who is right? Must

someone be wrong? Explain your reasons in each case.

• *Inferential Statistics.* Imagine that you are investigating racial attitudes among students at a city high school. You conduct the study with a sample of subjects and conclude that there is no racial tension. A week later, several interracial disruptions occur. Explain this apparent contradiction, using the concept of inferential statistics.

• *Statistics as a Tool.* Investigators point out that their results *show* or *demonstrate* such-and-such. Rarely do they claim that their results *prove* such-and-such. Why do they take this position? Explain your answer in the context of probability.

Sampling techniques are discussed in the context of research methods (2). Statistical methods are essential in the construction and use of psychological tests, especially the concept of correlation (13). The topic of experimental design is closely tied to testing hypotheses and using inferential statistics (2).

CLASSIC PSYCHOLOGY READING

∾

BEHAVIORAL STUDY OF OBEDIENCE

Stanley Milgram

Obedience is as basic an element in the structure of social life as one can point to. Some system of authority is a requirement of all communal living, and it is only the man dwelling in isolation who is not forced to respond, through defiance or submission, to the commands of others. Obedience, as a determinant of behavior, is of particular relevance to our time. It has been reliably established that from 1933–1945 millions of innocent persons were systematically slaughtered on command. Gas chambers were built, death camps were guarded, daily quotas of corpses were produced with the same efficiency as the manufacture of appliances. These inhumane policies may have originated in the mind of a single person, but they could only be carried out on a massive scale if a very large number of persons obeyed orders.

Obedience is the psychological mechanism that links individual action to political purpose. It is the dispositional cement that binds men to systems of authority. Facts of recent history and observation in daily life suggest that for many persons obedience may be a deeply ingrained behavior tendency, indeed, a prepotent impulse overriding training in ethics, sympathy, and moral conduct. C. P. Snow points to its importance when he writes:

> "When you think of the long and gloomy history of man, you will find more hideous crimes have been committed in the name of obedience than have ever been committed in the name of rebellion. If you doubt that, read William Shirer's Rise and Fall of the Third Reich. The German Officer Corps were brought up in the most rigorous code of obedience . . . in the name of obedience they were party to, and assisted in, the most wicked large scale actions in the history of the world."[1]

While the particular form of obedience dealt with in the present study has its antecedents in these episodes, it must not be thought all obedience entails acts of aggression against others. Obedience serves numerous productive functions. Indeed, the very life of society is predicated on its existence. Obedience may be ennobling and educative and refer to acts of charity and kindness, as well as to destruction.

∾

GENERAL PROCEDURE

A procedure was devised which seems useful as a tool for studying obedience.[2] It consists of ordering a naive subject to administer electric shock to a victim. A simulated shock generator is used, with 30 clearly marked voltage levels that range from 15 to 450 volts. The instrument bears verbal designations that range from Slight Shock to Danger: Severe Shock. The responses of the victim, who is a trained confederate of the experimenter, are standardized. The orders to administer shocks are given to the naive subject in the context of a "learning experiment" ostensibly set up to study the effects of punishment on memory. As the experiment proceeds the naive subject is commanded to administer increasingly more intense shocks to the victim, even to the point of reaching the level marked Danger: Severe Shock. Internal resistances become stronger, and at a certain point the subject refuses to go on with the experiment. Behavior prior to this rupture is considered "obedience," in that the subject complies with the commands of the experimenter. The point of rupture is the act of disobedience. A quantitative value is assigned to the subject's performance based on the maximum intensity shock he is willing to administer before he refuses to participate further. Thus for any particular subject and for any particular experimental condition the degree of obedience may be specified with a numerical value. The crux of the study is to systematically vary the factors believed to alter the degree of obedience to the experimental commands.

The technique allows important variables to be manipulated at several points in the experiment. One may vary aspects of the source of command, content and form of command, instrumentalities for its execution, target object, general social setting, etc. The problem, therefore, is not one of designing increasingly more numerous experimental conditions, but of selecting those that best illuminate the *process* of obedience from the sociopsychological standpoint.

RELATED STUDIES

The inquiry bears an important relation to philosophic analyses of obedience and authority (Arendt,[3] Friedrich,[4] Weber[5]), an early experimental study of obedience by Frank,[6] studies in "authoritarianism" (Adorno, Frenkel-Brunswik, Levinson, and Sanford,[7] Rokeach[8]), and a recent series of analytic and empirical studies in social power (Cartwright[9]). It owes much to the long concern with *suggestion* in social psychology, both in its normal forms (e.g., Binet[10]) and in its clinical manifestations (Charcot[11]). But it derives, in the first instance, from direct observation of a social fact; the individual who is commanded by a legitimate authority ordinarily obeys. Obedience comes easily and often. It is a ubiquitous and indispensable feature of social life.

METHOD

SUBJECTS: The subjects were 40 males between the ages of 20 and 50, drawn from New Haven and the surrounding communities. Subjects were obtained by a newspaper advertisement and direct mail solicitation. Those who responded to the appeal believed they were to participate in a study of memory and learning at Yale University. A wide range of occupations is represented in the sample. Typical subjects were postal clerks, high school teachers, salesmen, engineers, and laborers. Subjects ranged in educational level from one who had not finished elementary school, to those who had doctorate and other professional degrees. They were paid $4.50 for their participation in the experiment. However, subjects were told that payment was simply for coming to the laboratory, and that the money was theirs no matter what happened after they arrived. Table 1 shows the proportion of age and occupational types assigned to the experimental condition.

PERSONNEL AND LOCALE: The experiment was conducted on the grounds of Yale University in the elegant interaction laboratory. (This detail is relevant to the perceived legitimacy of the experiment. In further variations, the experiment was dissociated from the university, with consequences for performance.) The role of experimenter was played by a 31-year-old high school teacher of biology. His manner was impassive, and his appearance somewhat stern throughout the experiment. He was dressed in a gray technician's coat, the victim was played by a 47-year-old accountant, trained for the role; he was of Irish-American stock, whom most observers found mild-mannered and likable.

PROCEDURE: One naive subject and one victim (an accomplice) performed in each experiment. A pretext had to be devised that would justify the administration of electric shock by the naive subject. This was effectively

OCCUPATIONS	20–29 YEARS N	30–39 YEARS N	40–50 YEARS N	PERCENTAGE OF TOTAL (OCCUPATIONS)
Workers, skilled and unskilled	4	5	6	37.5
Sales, business, and white-collar	3	6	7	40.0
Professional	1	5	3	22.5
Percentage of total (age)	20	40	40	

Note: Total *n* = 40.

TABLE 1 DISTRIBUTION OF AGE AND OCCUPATIONAL TYPES IN THE EXPERIMENT

accomplished by the cover story. After a general introduction on the presumed relation between punishment and learning, subjects were told:

> But actually, we know *very little* about the effect of punishment on learning, because almost no truly scientific studies have been made of it in human beings.
>
> For instance, we don't know how *much* punishment is best for learning—and we don't know how much difference it makes as to who is giving the punishment, whether an adult learns best from a younger or an older person than himself—or many things of that sort.
>
> So in this study we are bringing together a number of adults of different occupations and ages. And we're asking some of them to be teachers and some of them to be learners.
>
> We want to find out just what effect different people have on each other as teachers and learners, and also what effect *punishment* will have on learning in this situation.
>
> Therefore, I'm going to ask one of you to be the teacher here tonight and the other one to be the learner.
>
> Does either of you have a preference?

Subjects then drew slips of paper from a hat to determine who would be the teacher and who would be the learner in the experiment. The drawing was rigged so that the naive subject was always the teacher and the accomplice always the learner. (Both slips contained the word "Teacher.") Immediately after the drawing, the teacher and learner were taken to an adjacent room and the learner was strapped into an "electric chair" apparatus.

The experimenter explained that the straps were to prevent excessive movement while the learner was being shocked. The effect was to make it impossible for him to escape from the situation. An electrode was attached to the learner's wrist, and electrode paste was applied "to avoid blisters and burns." Subjects were told that the electrode was attached to the shock generator in the adjoining room.

In order to improve credibility the experimenter declared, in response to a question by the learner: "Although the shocks can be extremely painful, they cause no permanent tissue damage."

LEARNING TASK. The lesson administered by the subject was a paired-associate learning task. The subject read a series of word pairs to the learner, and then read the first word of the pair along with four terms. The learner was to indicate which of the four terms had originally been paired with the first word. He communicated his answer by pressing one of four switches in front of him, which in turn lit up one of four numbered quadrants in an answer-box located atop the shock generator.

SHOCK GENERATOR. The instrument panel consists of 30 lever switches set in a horizontal line. Each switch is clearly labeled with a voltage designation that ranges from 15 to 450 volts. There is a 15-volt increment from one switch to the next going from left to right. In addition, the following verbal designations are clearly indicated for groups of four switches going from left to right: Slight Shock, Moderate Shock, Strong Shock, Very Strong Shock, Intense Shock, Extreme Intensity Shock, Danger: Severe Shock. (Two switches after this last designation are simply marked XXX.)

Upon depressing a switch, a pilot light corresponding to each switch is illuminated in bright red; an electric buzzing is heard; an electric blue light, labeled "voltage energizer," flashes; the dial on the voltage meter swings to the right; various relay clicks are sounded.

The upper left-hand corner of the generator is labeled Shock Generator, Type ZLB, Dyson Instrument Company, Waltham, Mass. Output 15 Volts–50 Volts.

Details of the instrument were carefully handled to insure an appearance of authenticity. The panel was engraved by precision industrial engravers, and all components were of high quality. No subject in the experiment suspected that the instrument was merely a simulated shock generator.

SAMPLE SHOCK. Each naive subject is given a sample shock on the shock generator, prior to beginning his run as teacher. This shock is always 45 volts, and is applied by pressing the third switch of the generator. The shock is applied to the wrist of the naive subject, and has its source in a 45-volt battery wired into the generator. This further convinces the subject of the authenticity of the generator.

SHOCK INSTRUCTIONS. The subject is told to administer a shock to the learner each time he gives a wrong response. Moreover—and this is the key command—the subject is instructed to "move one level higher on the shock generator each time the learner flashes a wrong answer." He is also instructed to announce the voltage level before administering a shock. This serves to continually remind subjects of the increasing intensity of shocks administered to the learner.

PRELIMINARY AND REGULAR RUN. Pretests revealed that the procedure of reading words and administering shocks requires some practice before it can be handled smoothly. Therefore, immediately preceding the regular run, the teacher is given a preliminary series of 10 words to read to the learner. There are 3 neutral words in the practice series (i.e., words that the learner answers correctly), so that shocks are administered for 7 of the words, with the maximum shock at 105 volts (moderate shock). Almost all subjects master the procedure by the time the preliminary run is over.

Subjects are then presented with a second list, and are told that the procedure is the same as for the first list; the experimenter adds, however: "When you get to the bottom of the list, repeat it over again, and continue giving shocks, until the learner has learned all the pairs correctly." The experimenter instructs the subject to "start from 15 volts and increase the shock level one step each time the learner gives a wrong answer."

FEEDBACK FROM THE VICTIM. In all conditions the learner gives a predetermined set of responses to the word pair test, based on a schedule of approximately three wrong answers to one correct answer. In the present experimental condition no vocal response or other sign of protest is heard from the learner until Shock Level 300 is reached. When the 300-volt shock is administered, the learner pounds on the wall of the room in which he is bound to the electric chair. The pounding can be heard by the subject. From this point on, the learner's answers no longer appear on the four-way panel.

At this juncture, subjects ordinarily turn to the experimenter for guidance. The experimenter instructs the subject to treat the absence of a response as a wrong answer, and to shock the subject according to the usual schedule. He advises the subjects to allow 5–10 seconds before considering no response as a wrong answer, and to increase the shock level one step each time the learner fails to respond correctly. The learner's pounding is repeated after the 315-volt shock is administered; afterwards he is not heard from, nor do his answers reappear on the four-way signal box.

EXPERIMENTER FEEDBACK. At various points in the experiment the subject may turn to the experimenter for advice on whether he should continue to administer shocks. Or he may indicate that he does not wish to go on. It was important to standardize the experimenter's responses to these inquiries and reactions.

If the subject indicated his unwillingness to go on, the experimenter responded with a sequence of "prods," using as many as necessary to bring the subject into line.

Prod 1: Please continue, *or* Please go on.
Prod 2: The experiment requires that you continue.
Prod 3: It is absolutely essential that you continue.
Prod 4: You have no other choice, you *must* go on.

The prods were always made in sequence: Only if Prod 1 had been unsuccessful could Prod 2 be used. If the subject refused to obey the experimenter after Prod 4, the experiment was terminated. The experimenter's tone of voice was at all times firm, but not impolite. The sequence was begun anew on each occasion that the subject balked or showed reluctance to follow orders.

SPECIAL PRODS. If the subject asked if the learner was liable to suffer permanent physical injury, the experimenter said: "Although the shocks may be painful, there is no permanent tissue damage, so please go on." [Followed by Prods 2, 3, and 4 if necessary.]

If the subject said that the learner did not want to go on, the experimenter replied: "Whether the learner likes it or not, you must go on until he has learned all the word pairs correctly. So please go on." [Followed by Prods 2, 3, and 4 if necessary.]

DEPENDENT MEASURES: The primary dependent measure for any subject is the maximum shock he administers before he refuses to go any further. In principle this may vary from

0 (for a subject who refuses to administer even the first shock) to 30 (for a subject who administers the highest shock on the generator). A subject who breaks off the experiment at any point prior to administering the thirtieth shock level is termed a *defiant* subject. One who complies with experimental commands fully, and proceeds to administer all shock levels commanded, is termed an *obedient* subject.

FURTHER RECORDS. With few exceptions, experimental sessions were recorded on magnetic tape. Occasional photographs were taken through one-way mirrors. Notes were kept on any unusual behavior occurring during the course of the experiments. On occasion, additional observers were directed to write objective descriptions of the subjects' behavior. The latency and duration of shocks were measured by accurate timing devices.

INTERVIEW AND DEHOAX. Following the experiment, subjects were interviewed; open-ended questions, projective measures, and attitude scales were employed. After the interview, procedures were undertaken to assure that the subject would leave the laboratory in a state of well being. A friendly reconciliation was arranged between the subject and the victim, and an effort was made to reduce any tensions that arose as a result of the experiment.

RESULTS

PRELIMINARY NOTIONS: Before giving an account of the experimental results, it is instructive to consider how persons predict others will perform when commanded to administer powerful shocks to another person. Fourteen Yale seniors, all psychology majors, were provided with a detailed description of the experimental situation. They were asked to reflect carefully on it, and to predict the behavior of 100 hypothetical subjects. More specifically, they were instructed to plot the distribution of obedience of "100 Americans of diverse occupations, and ranging in age from 20 to 50 years," who were placed in the experimental situation.

There was considerable agreement among the respondents on the expected behavior of hypothetical subjects. All respondents predicted that only an insignificant minority would go through to the end of the shock series. (The estimates ranged from 0 to 3 percent; i.e., the most "pessimistic" member of the class predicted that of 100 persons, 3 would continue through to the most potent shock available on the shock generator—450 volts.) The class mean was 1.2 percent. The question was also posed informally to colleagues of the author, and the most general feeling was that few if any subjects would go beyond the designation Very Strong Shock.

RESULT OF EXPERIMENT 1: *SUBJECTS ACCEPT SITUATION.* With few exceptions subjects were convinced of the reality of the experimental situation, that they were administering shocks to another person, and the most potent shocks were extremely painful. In the post experimental interview subjects were asked: "How painful to the learner were the last few shocks that you administered to him? Subjects were instructed to indicate their answers on a printed 14-point scale ranging from "Not at all painful" to "Extremely painful." The modal response was 14 (Extremely painful) with the mean at 13.42.

SIGNS OF EXTREME TENSION. Many subjects showed signs of nervousness in the experimental situation, and especially upon administering the more powerful shocks. In a large number of cases the degree of tension reached extremes that are rarely seen in sociopsychological laboratory studies. Subjects were observed to sweat, tremble, stutter, bite their lips, groan, and dig their fingernails into their flesh. These were characteristic rather than exceptional responses to the experiment.

One sign of tension was the regular occurrence of nervous laughing fits. Fourteen of the 40 subjects showed definite signs of nervous laughter and smiling. The laughter seemed entirely out of place, even bizarre. Full-blown, uncontrollable seizures were observed for 3 subjects. On one occasion we observed a seizure so violently convulsive that it was necessary to call a halt to the experiment. The subject, a 46-year-old encyclopedia salesman, was seriously embarrassed by his untoward and uncontrollable behavior. In the postexperimental interviews subjects took pains to point out that they were not sadistic types, and that the laughter did not mean they enjoyed shocking the victim.

DISTRIBUTION OF SCORES. It had been conjectured that persons would not, in general, agree to administer shocks beyond the level designated as Very Strong Shock. The distribution of maximum shocks for this experiment is shown in Table 2. The obtained distribution of scores deviates radically from the prediction.

Upon command of the experimenter, each of the 40 subjects went beyond the expected breakoff point. No subject stopped prior to administering Shock Level 20. (At this level—300 volts—the victim kicks on the wall and no longer provides answers to the teacher's multiple-choice questions.)

Of the 40 subjects, 5 refused to obey the experimental commands beyond the 300-volt level. Four more subjects administered one further shock, and then refused to go on. Two broke off at the 330-volt-level, and 1 each at 345, 360, and 375 volts. Thus a total of 14 subjects defied the experimenter. It is instructive to reprint their remarks at the point of defiance, as transcribed from the tape recordings:

"[0124] I think he's trying to communicate, he's knocking. . . . Well it's not fair to shock the guy . . . these are terrific volts. I don't think this is very humane. . . . Oh, I can't go on with this; no, this isn't right. It's a hell of an experiment. The guy is suffering in there. No, I don't want to go on. This is crazy. [Subject refused to administer more shocks.]"

"[0123] He's banging in there. I'm gonna chicken out. I'd like to continue, but I can't do that to a man. . . . I'm sorry I can't do that to a man. I'll hurt his heart. You take your check. . . . No really I couldn't do it."

These subjects were frequently in a highly agitated and even angered state. Sometimes, verbal protest was at a minimum, and the subject simply got up from his chair in front of the shock generator, and indicated that he wished to leave the laboratory.

Of the 40 subjects, 26 obeyed the orders of the experimenter to the end, proceeding to punish the victim until they reached the most potent shock available on the shock generator. At that point, the experimenter called a halt to the session. (The maximum shock is labeled

VERBAL DESIGNATION AND VOLTAGE INDICATION	NUMBER OF SUBJECTS FOR WHOM THIS WAS MAXIMUM SHOCK	VERBAL DESIGNATION AND VOLTAGE INDICATION	NUMBER OF SUBJECTS FOR WHOM THIS WAS MAXIMUM SHOCK
Slight Shock:		Intense Shock:	
15	0	255	0
30	0	270	0
45	0	285	0
60	0	300	5
Modern Shock:		Extreme Intensity Shock:	
75	0	315	4
90	0	330	2
105	0	345	1
120	0	360	1
Strong Shock:		Danger: Severe Shock:	
135	0	375	1
150	0	390	0
165	0	405	0
180	0	420	0
Very Strong Shock:		XXX	
195	0	435	0
210	0	450	26
225	0		
240	0		

TABLE 2 DISTRIBUTION OF BREAKOFF POINTS

450 volts, and is two steps beyond the designation: Danger: Severe Shock.) Although obedient subjects continued to administer shocks, they often did so under extreme stress. Some expressed reluctance to administer shocks beyond the 300-volt level and displayed fears similar to those who defied the experimenter; yet they obeyed.

After the maximum shocks had been delivered, and the experimenter called a halt to the proceedings, many obedient subjects heaved sighs of relief, mopped their brows, rubbed their fingers over their eyes, or nervously fumbled cigarettes. Some shook their heads, apparently in regret. Some subjects had remained calm throughout the experiment, and displayed only minimal signs of tension from beginning to end.

DISCUSSION

The experiment yielded two findings that were surprising. The first finding concerns the sheer strength of obedient tendencies manifested in this situation. Subjects have learned from childhood that it is a fundamental breach of moral conduct to hurt another person against his will. Yet, 26 subjects abandon this tenet in following the instructions of an authority who has no special powers to enforce his commands. To disobey would bring no material loss to the subject; no punishment would ensue. It is clear from the remarks and outward behavior of many participants that in punishing the victim they are often acting against their own values. Subjects often expressed deep disapproval of shocking a man in the face of his objections, and others denounced it as stupid and senseless. Yet the majority complied with the experimental commands. This outcome was surprising from two perspectives: first, from the standpoint of predictions made in the questionnaire described earlier. (Here, however, it is possible that the remoteness of the respondents from the actual situation, and the difficulty of conveying to them the concrete details of the experiment, could account for the serious underestimation of obedience.)

But the results were also unexpected to persons who observed the experiment in progress, through one-way mirrors. Observers often uttered expressions of disbelief upon seeing a subject administer more powerful shocks to the victim. These persons had a full acquaintance with the details of the situation, and yet systematically underestimated the amount of obedience that subjects would display.

The second unanticipated effect was the extraordinary tension generated by the procedures. One might suppose that a subject would simply break off or continue as his conscience dictated. Yet, this is very far from what happened. There were striking reactions of tension and emotional strain. One observer related:

"I observed a mature and initially poised businessman enter the laboratory smiling and confident. Within 20 minutes he was reduced to a twitching, stuttering wreck, who was rapidly approaching a point of nervous collapse. He constantly pulled on his earlobe, and twisted his hands. At one point he pushed his fist into his forehead and muttered: 'Oh God, let's stop it.' And yet he continued to respond to every word of the experimenter, and obeyed to the end."

Any understanding of the phenomenon of obedience must rest on an analysis of the particular conditions in which it occurs. The following features of the experiment go some distance in explaining the high amount of obedience observed in the situation.

1. The experiment is sponsored by and takes place on the grounds of an institution of unimpeachable reputation, Yale University. It may be reasonably presumed that the personnel are competent and reputable. The importance of this background authority is now being studied by conducting a series of experiments outside of New Haven, and without any visible ties to the university.

2. The experiment is, on the face of it, designed to attain a worthy purpose—advancement of knowledge about learning and memory. Obedience occurs not as an end in itself, but as an instrumental element in a situation that the subject construes as significant and meaningful. He may not be able to see its full significance, but he

may properly assume that the experimenter does.

3. The subject perceives that the victim has voluntarily submitted to the authority system of the experimenter. He is not (at first) an unwilling captive impressed for involuntary service. He has taken the trouble to come to the laboratory presumably to aid the experimental research. That he later becomes an involuntary subject does not alter the fact that, initially, he consented to participate without qualification. Thus he has in some degree incurred an obligation toward the experimenter.

4. The subject, too, has entered the experiment voluntarily, and perceives himself under obligation to aid the experimenter. He has made a commitment, and to disrupt the experiment is a repudiation of this initial promise of aid.

5. Certain features of the procedure strengthen the subject's sense of obligation to the experimenter. For one, he has been paid for coming to the laboratory. In part this is canceled out by the experimenter's statement that: "Of course, as in all experiments, the money is yours simply for coming to the laboratory. From this point on, no matter what happens, the money is yours."[12]

6. From the subject's standpoint, the fact that he is the teacher and the other man the learner is purely a chance consequence (it is determined by drawing lots) and he, the subject, ran the same risk as the other man in being assigned the role of learner. Since the assignment of positions in the experiment was achieved by fair means, the learner is deprived of any basis of complaint on this count. (A similar situation obtains in Army units, in which—in the absence of volunteers—a particularly dangerous mission may be assigned by drawing lots, and the unlucky soldier is expected to bear his misfortune with sportsmanship.)

7. There is, at best, ambiguity with regard to the prerogatives of a psychologist and the corresponding rights of his subject. There is a vagueness of expectation concerning what a psychologist may require of his subject and when he is overstepping acceptable limits. Moreover, the experiment occurs in a closed setting, and thus provides no opportunity for the subject to remove these ambiguities by discussion with others. There are few standards that seem directly applicable to the situation, which is a novel one for most subjects.

8. The subjects are assured that the shocks administered to the subject are "painful but not dangerous." Thus they assume that the discomfort caused the victim is momentary, while the scientific gains resulting from the experiment are enduring.

9. Through Shock Level 20 the victim continues to provide answers on the signal box. The subject may construe this as a sign that the victim is still willing to "play the game." It is only after Shock Level 20 that the victim repudiates the rules completely, refusing to answer further.

These features help to explain the high amount of obedience obtained in this experiment. Many of the arguments raised need not remain matters of speculation, but can be reduced to testable propositions to be confirmed or disproved by further experiments.[13]

The following features of the experiment concern the nature of the conflict which the subject faces.[13]

10. The subject is placed in a position in which he must respond to the competing demands of two persons: the experimenter and the victim. The conflict must be resolved by meeting the demands of one or the other; satisfaction of the victim and the experimenter are mutually exclusive. Moreover, the resolution must take the form of a highly visible action, that of continuing to shock the victim or

breaking off the experiment. Thus the subject is forced into a public conflict that does not permit any completely satisfactory solution.

11. While the demands of the experimenter carry the weight of scientific authority, the demands of the victim spring from his personal experience of pain and suffering. The two claims need not be regarded as equally pressing and legitimate. The experimenter seeks an abstract scientific datum; the victim cries out for relief from physical suffering caused by the subject's actions.

12. The experiment gives the subject little time for reflection. The conflict comes on rapidly. It is only minutes after the subject has been seated before the shock generator that the victim begins his protests.

   Moreover, the subject perceives that he has gone through but two-thirds of the shock levels at the time the subject's first protests are heard. Thus he understands that the conflict will have a persistent aspect to it, and may well become more intense as increasingly more powerful shocks are required. The rapidity with which the conflict descends on the subject and his realization that it is predictably recurrent may well be sources of tension to him.

13. At a more general level, the conflict stems from the opposition of two deeply ingrained behavior dispositions: first, the disposition not to harm other people, and second, the tendency to obey those whom we perceive to be legitimate authorities.

∾
NOTES

1. C. P. Snow, "Either/Or," *Progressive*, Feb., 1961, p. 24.

2. S. Milgram, "Dynamics of Obedience" (Washington, D.C.: National Science Foundation, January 25,1961), mimeo.

3. H. Arendt, "What Was Authority?" in *Authority*, C. J.. Friedrich (ed.) (Cambridge, Mass.: Harvard University Press, 1958), pp. 81–112.

4. C. J. Friedrich (ed.), *Authority* (Cambridge, Mass.: Harvard University Press, 1958).

5. M. Weber, *The Theory of Social and Economic Organization* (Oxford: Oxford University Press, 1947.

6. J. D. Frank, "Experimental Studies of Personal Pressure and Resistance," *J. Gen. Psychol.*, Vol. 30 (1944), pp. 23-64.

7. T. Adorno, Else Frenkel-Brunswik, D. J. Levinson, and R. N. Sanford, *The Authoritarian Personality* (New York: Harper, 1950).

8. M. Rokeach, "Authority, Authoritarianism, and Conformity," in *Conformity and Deviation*, I. A. Berg, and B. M. Bass (eds.) (New York: Harper, 1961), pp. 230-257.

9. D. Cartwright (ed.), *Studies in Social Power* (Ann Arbor: Univ. of Michigan Institute for Social Research, 1959).

10. A. Binet, *La Suggestibilité* (Paris: Schleicher, 1900).

11. J M. Charcot, *Oeuvres Complètes* (Paris: Bureaux du Progres Medical, 1881).

12. Forty-three subjects, undergraduates at Yale University, were run in the experiment without payment. The results are very similar to those obtained with paid subjects.

13. A series of recently completed experiments employing the obedience paradigm is reported in S. Milgram, "Some Conditions of Obedience and Disobedience to Authority," *Human Relations*, 1964.

❧ Journal Article Review Form ❧

Name _____ Date _____

Article Name: _____

Article Authors: _____

1. Why did the authors perform this study? (What question(s) did the authors want to answer?)

2. Identify the IV(s) and the DV(s) used in this study (Note: there may be more than one of each).

3. How was the welfare of human subjects or animal subjects safeguarded?

4. What were the major findings of this study?

5. Why were these results significant?

6. What would be a good follow-up to this study? (What study should be done next?)

1. Psychology as a separate field of study began with:
   a. Descartes
   b. Wundt
   c. Freud
   d. Watson
2. The field of Psychology is approximately _____ years old:
   a. 100
   b. 200
   c. 300
   d. 400
3. Descartes:
   a. suggested only humans have a mind.
   b. speculated that humans were simply a more intelligent animal.
   c. tried to undermine credibility of the bible and religion.
   d. suggested that a person's mind could not be perceived by his/her senses.
4. Who suggested that observable behavior is the only appropriate subject matter for psychological study?
   a. Freud
   b. Wundt
   c. Watson
   d. James
   e. All of the above
5. In which of the Freudian Stages of Development is the Oedipus complex expressed:
   a. oral
   b. anal
   c. phallic
   d. genital
6. What form of psychological practice stemmed from Freud's theory of the unconscious mind?
   a. psychoanalysis
   b. clinical psychology
   c. counseling psychology
   d. experimental psychology
7. In the Freudian system, the id and the superego:
   a. often make opposite demands on the ego
   b. are responsible for anxiety arising from conflict
   c. are unconscious
   d. All of the above
   e. None of the above
8. Which of the Freudian Personality Systems is (are) conscious?
   a. id
   b. ego
   c. superego
   d. both id and superego
   e. both ego and superego
9. Consider a study of the effects of outside-class reading on IQ in middle-school students. In this study, outside-class reading is the _____ and IQ is the _____.
   a. control variable; effect variable
   b. effect variable; cause variable
   c. independent variable; dependent variable
   d. dependent variable; independent variable
10. The crucial difference between the experiment and other methods of gathering data is:
    a. there are more variables in other methods than in the experimental method.
    b. the experiment only has two variables and so is easier to do.
    c. the experimental method controls potentially confounding variables.
    d. the experiment establishes a cause-effect relationship between the variables.

The World Wide Web (WWW) has become a major souce for information on virtually any topic. The Web has an enormous amount of information available related to the field of psychology. To view these sites you will need an Internet connection (you can get one for free through the University) and a web browser such as Netscape Navigator or Microsoft Internet Explorer. There is also a web site for this course that contains information about the course and an introduction to the World Wide Web. The Web address for the course is:

http://www.umsl.edu/~mgriffin/genpsych/

GENERAL PSYCHOLOGY STUDENT WEBSITE POINTERS

- Psychology Web Pointer
  http://www.coil.com/~grohol/web.htm
  compilation of psychology websites pertaining to various psychological disorders, support services, professional affiliations, etc.

- MegaPsych Home Page
  http://members.gnn.com/user/megapsych.htm
  compilation of Internet resources for psychology students

PSYCHOLOGY GRADUATE SCHOOL INFO

- Listing of U.S. Psychology Ph.D. Programs
  http://www.wesleyan.edu/psyc/psyc260/ranking.htm

- U.S. News & World Report: America's Best Graduate Schools
  http://www.usnews.com/usnews/fair/gpsych.htm

- Psychology Department Gopher
  gopher://unix1.utm.edu:70/11/departments/psych/depts
  listing of links to various psychology departments

BASIC PSYCHOLOGY INFO

- Psych Web by Russ Dewey
  http://www.gasou.edu/psychweb/psychweb.htm
  good info for psychology undergraduate students including class info, an APA format "crib sheet," tips for getting into graduate school, self-help, etc.

- American Psychological Association's (APA) PsychNET
  http://www.apa.org/

- American Psychology Society (APS)
  http://psych.hanover.edu/APS/

- Einet Search for Psychology Resources
  http://www.einet.net/galaxy/Social-Sciences/Psychology.html
  a search vehicle for finding specific psychology related websites

- Recommended Popular Books on Psychology
  http://www.personal.umich.edu/~tmorris/goodbook.html
  annotated compilation of psychology-related books

PSYCHOLOGY RESEARCH SITES

- APA Guide to Library Research in Psychology
  http://www.apa.org/science/lib.html

- Psychiatry On-Line
  http://www.priory.com/journals/psych.htm
  electronic psychiatry journal on web (graduate level)

- New England Journal of Medicine On-Line
  http://www.nejm.org/

- The Census Bureau
  http://www.census.gov/

- Inter-University Consortium for Political & Social Research (ICPSR)
  http://www.icpsr.umich.edu/archive1.html
  database of archival social science research; includes reference, abstract and data for each study searched

FUN PSYCHOLOGY SITES

- Personality Modeling
  http://sunsite.unc.edu/personality/faq-mbti.html
  test yourself to determine your Myers-Briggs personality type

- Emotional Intelligence
  http://www.utne.com/cgi-bin/eq
  contains a 10-item test to determine your emotional IQ

- Today in the History of Psychology
  http://www.cwu.edu/~warren/today.html
  find out what historical event happened in the world of psychology on any particular day

- Journal of Irreproducible Results
  http://www.reutershealth.dom/jir/
  online journal of research studies that will make you smile

PSYCHOLOGY DISCUSSION GROUPS

- Psych LISTSERVS
  gopher://unix1.utm.edu:70/11/departments/psych/list
  Listing & descriptions of various psychology related LISTSERV discussion groups.

- Research Methods Discussion
  send e-mail to LISTSERV@UNMVMA.UNM.EDU including the following:
  in body, type SUBSCRIBE METHODS Yourname (e.g., SUBSCRIBE METHODS Sigmund Freud) under subject (in the e-mail heading), leave blank mailing list that discusses social science research methods, statistics, etc.

- PSYCHTALK
  send e-mail to LISTSERV@FRE.FSU.UMD.EDU including the following:
  in body, type SUBSCRIBE PSYCHTALK Yourname (e.g., SUBSCRIBE PSYCHTALKTukey) under subject (in the e-mail heading), leave blank.
  World-wide discussion group especially for undergrads; covers topics such as stress, grades, graduate schools, ideas for term papers, etc.

- APSSCNET
  send e-mail to LISTSERV@CMUVM.CSV.CMICH.EDU including the following: in body, type SUBSCRIBE APSSCNET Yourname (e.g., SUBSCRIBE APSSCNET Abraham Maslow) under subject (in the e-mail heading), leave blank
  Forum for discussions re: scholarships, educational opportunities, and research issues for psychology students.

The following are a list of Web sites related to various chapters in the book:

CHAPTER 1: BEGINNINGS

- American Psychological Association
  (http://www.apa.org/)

- American Psychological Society
  (http://ww.hanover.edu/psch/APS/aps.html)

- PsyScope
  (http://poppy.psy.cmu.edu/psyscope/)

- Compsych
  (gopher://baryon.hawk.platts.burgh.edu::70/11/.ftp/pub/compsych)

- MacPsych Archive
  (gopher://gopher.stolaf.edu/11/Internet%20ResourcesS\ st.%olaf%20Sponsored%20Mailing%20Lists/MacPsych)

- Psych Web
  (http://www.gasou.edu/psychweb/psychweb.htm)

CHAPTER 2: RESEARCH METHODS

- Treatment of Human Subjects
  http://www.psych.bangor.ac.uk/deptpsych/Ethics/HumanResearch.html

- Research Ethics
  http://xerxes.nas.edu/nap/online/obas

CHAPTER 4: CONDITIONING AND LEARNING

- Psycholoquy—Pavlov-Bell
  http://cogsci.ecs.soton.ac.uk/~lac/topics.html#Pavlov-bell

- Journal of the Experimental Analysis of Behavior (JEAB)
  http://www.envmed.rochester.edu/wwwrap/behavior/jabahome.htm

- Journal of Applied Behavior Analysis (JABA)
  http://www.envmed.rochester.edu/wwwrap/behavior/jeab/jeabhome.htm

- Behavior analysis—Technical Terms
  gopher://alpha1.csd.uwm.edu/Oftp%3aalpha1.csd.uwm.edu%40/pub/ Psychology/Behavior Analysis/educational/course/eab-tech-terms-dermer

- The Behavior Analysis Home Page at the University of South Florida
  http://www.coedu.usf.edu/behavior/behavior.html

- Experimental Analysis of Behavior at Auburn
  http://www.duc.auburn.edu/~newlamc/

CHAPTER 5: MEMORY

- Mind Tools
  http://www.demon.co.uk/mindtool/memory.html

- Memory Reading Lists
  http://www.york.ac.uk/depts/psych/web/ug/course/core/rlcogch.html

- Journal of Experimental Psychology: Learning, Memory, Cognition
  (http://www.apa.org/journals/jeplmc.html)

- Amnesia Research Lab
  (http://hermes.cns.uiuc.edu/ARLHomePage.html)

- False Memory Syndrome Foundation
  (http://iquest.com/~fitz/fmsf)

CHAPTER 8: HUMAN DEVELOPMENT

- PEDINFO
  (http://www.1h1.uab.edu:80/pedinfo/Diseases.html)

- The Jean Piaget Society
  (http://www.wimsey.com/~chris1/JPS/JPS.html)

- The In Home Speech and Language Checklist
  (http://www.xmission.com/~kjay/)

- Adolescence Directory On-Line
  (http://education.Indiana.edu/cas/adol/adol.html)

- Facts for Families
  (http://www.psych.med.umich.edu/web/aacap/factsFam/)

- Institute for Brain Aging and Dementia
  (http://teri.bio.uci.edu/)

CHAPTER 11: I.Q. AND TESTING

- Introduction to 21st Century Problem Solving
  (http://www2.hawaii.edu/suremath/home.html)

- Conflict, Cooperation, & Rationality: An Introduction to Game Theory
  (http://william-king.www.drexel.edu/top/class/game.html)

- The Emergence of Intelligence
  (http://weber.u.washington.edu/~wcalvin/sciamer.html)

- Frequently Asked Questions (FAQ) on Psychological Tests
  (http://www.apa.org/science/test.html)

- School Psychology Resources On-Line
  (http://mail.bcpl.lib.md.us/~sandyste/school_psych.html)

- Skeptic Magazine Interview with Robert J. Sternberg Regarding The Bell Curve
  (http://www.skeptic.com/03.3fm-sternberg-interview.html)

- Two Views of The Bell Curve
  (http://www.apa.org/journals/bell.html)

- ERIC Clearinghouse on Assessment and Evaluation
  (http://www.cua.edu/www/eric_ae/)

- The Arc, a National Organization on Mental Retardation
  (http://www.metronet.com/~thearc/welcome.html)

CHAPTER 12: ADJUSTMENT AND DISORDER

- Internet Mental Health
  (http://www.mentalhealth.com/p.html)

- Cyber-Psych
  (http:://www.charm.net/~pandora/psych/index/html)

- Teaching Clinical Psychology
  (http://www1.rider.edu/~suler/tcp.html)

- Psychiatry On-Line
  (http://www.cityscape.co.uk/users/ad88/psych.htm)

- Electro-Convulsive Therapy
  (htttp://text.nlm.nih.gov/nih/cdc/www/51txt.html)

- The Efficacy of Psychotherapy
  (http:www.apa.org/practice/peff.html)

CHAPTER 15: SOCIAL BEHAVIOR

- Social Cognition-Social Osychology Paper Archive
  (http://www.psych.purdue.edu/~esmith/scarch.html)

- Social Psychology at the Australian National University
  (http://online.anu.edu.au/psychology/socpsych/socpsych.html)

CHAPTER 16: EMOTIONS AND STRESS

- Stress Pamphlet
  (http://ccserver.uoregon.edu/~dvb/pamstr.htm)

- Stress Busters
  (http://www.cts.com/~health/strssbus.html)

- Stress Management
  (http://www.ivf.com/stress.html)

- The Science of Obesity and Weight Control
  (http://www.loop.com/~bkrentzman/)

CHAPTER 17: BIOLOGICAL BASES OF BEHAVIOR

- Neurosciences Internet Resource Guide
  (http://http2.sils.umich.edu:80/Public/nirg/nirg1.html#alpha)

- Psych Web's list of Psychology Resources
  (http://www.gasou.edu/psychweb/resource/bytopic.html)

- Basic Neural Processes Tutorial
  (http://psych.hanover.edu/Krantz/neurotut.html)

- Neurosciences on the Internet
  (http:www.lm.com:80/~nab/

- Psycholoquy—Split-Brain Patients
  (http://cogsci.ecs.soton.ac.uk/~lac/topics.html#split-brain)

CHAPTER 18 SENSATION AND PERCEPTION

- Sensation and Perception Tutorial
  (http://psych.hanover.edu/Krantz/sen_tut.html)

- Audition Tutorial
  (http://lecaine.music.mcgill.ca/~welch/auditory/Auditory.html)

- Vision and Color Vision Phenomena
  (http://www.exploratorium.edu/imagery/exhibits.html)

- Sound Perception
  (http://sln.fi.edu/~helfrich/music/psychaco.html)

- Berkeley Psychophysiology Laboratory
  (http://violet.berkeley..edu/~lorenmc/bpl.html)

Please Note: These Web addresses were all viable sites when this book was organized. However, due to the dynamic nature of Web-based content some sites may no longer contain the information as it is specified here. If you get an error message when you try to link to a site it may mean that the site has moved or the information has been removed from that site. If this happens please let your instructor know, as we will continue to update the material in this book.

PART TWO: THE NATURE-NURTURE CONTROVERSY

Are our personalities a result of characteristics inherited directly from our parents or do they come exclusively from the environments in which we are raised? In the words of a scientist, is our behavior a product of nature (genes, inheritance, evolutionary history of a species) or nurture (environments, learning, conditioning)? No more fundamental question exists in psychology, nor is there a question that is more influential in shaping the way a scientist studies behavior or the way a non-scientist views fellow human beings. In fact, no one seriously doubts that the environments of our youth play a significant role in determining our adult behaviors. Evidence for the ubiquitous influence of learning is in everything we do each day, from the foods we choose to the music, readings and friends we prefer. That explains the chapters on learning and memory appearing in every Introductory Psychology textbook, including this text. The controversial proposition of the nature-nurture controversy is more about inheritance of behavior. Do genes contribute to any of our adult behaviors and, if yes, how much of a role does inheritance play? The chapter included in this section on Darwinian evolution suggests the answer to the first part of the question is almost surely yes. The chapter on the social behavior of animals, especially the last section on Human Ethology, gives reasons to suspect the hereditary influence may be substantial. Still, there are many scientific, as well as socio-political, reasons to "go slowly" on the temptations to generalize to human behavior. All this will become even clearer to the student near the end of the course after new ways of looking at the controversy are presented in Parts Three and Four. For now, let us take a look in Part Two at the nature-nature controversy as it has been debated over the past 150 years.

ॐ ॐ ॐ ॐ ॐ ॐ

4

CONDITIONING AND LEARNING

THE BELLS HAD STOPPED RINGING. THE MEN HAD MOVED SILENTLY INTO THE GREAT HALL, AND THEY WERE STANDING AT THEIR PLACES IN FRONT OF oaken tables, burnished and smooth from scrubbing and use. Suddenly they filled the hall with a song of grace, in perfect unison, giving thanks and proclaiming their faith. A moment later, the scraping of benches, again in unison and without a word, signaled the start of the evening meal.

This scraping of benches evoked the attention of a very different element of monastic life, a society of scavenger cats. Sleeping and resting on the warm hearths, they were quick to raise their heads and twitch their tails at this familiar sound, which meant that a tender morsel might fall from the tables. Always hungry, they licked their chops in anticipation of raw fish or some other delicacy.

As the brothers consumed bean soup, fish cakes, and ale, Saint Ildefonso rose to make the evening announcements. Among them was a statement about Brother Mendo. A Latin phrase had burst from his lips during the silence of predawn prayers. For this transgression, Brother Mendo would receive the usual punishment in the kitchen, but no mention was made of its length. That would be announced later, leaving Brother Mendo and the reader to contemplate for a while his misdeed and its possible consequences.

During the silent meal, almost imperceptible movements occurred among the brethren in that dining hall: a slow nod here, a half-wink there, a seemingly inward smile. These acts almost seemed like the exchange of friendly greetings. In any case, along with their vows of poverty, chastity, and obedience, the brethren were bound together by thoughts and feelings about communal living.

Monastery life in the Renaissance has been depicted by many writers, but none with more flair for the serious and humorous than Lope de Vega, a seventeenth-century Spanish author recognized as one of the world's most eminent and productive dramatists. He wrote 1,500 plays, often completing one in merely a day. He also fell in love with many women, was imprisoned, then banished from Madrid, and on 29 May 1588 sailed with the Spanish Armada, composing poetry while heading into battle. Later, he briefly pursued the priesthood and, perhaps on this basis, described the forthcoming punishment for Brother Mendo in *El Capellán de la Virgen* (1615). The instructional value of this drama was first brought to attention by a pair of professors at the University of Connecticut, one in Spanish literature, the other in psychology (Bousefield, 1955).

They showed that Lope de Vega's work antedated by more than 300 years psychological concepts reported in this chapter.

With its focus upon life in a Spanish kitchen centuries ago, this narrative serves as a reminder of cultural differences, and it offers a comparison with a kitchen in twentieth-century America and the events that took place there, reported in a term paper by a young woman called Dolores (Pinto, 1992). The occupants of these kitchens lived on different continents, in different eras, with different goals and interests in life, and yet one can propose that their different behaviors, reported in the following pages, arose *in the same ways,* similarly shaped by their very different environments. These environmental influences are prominent in animal behavior as well, as illustrated by the cats in both settings.

In short, this narrative emphasizes that forces in the environment are fundamental factors in human behavior. Specifically, the process of **conditioning,** which is a relatively simple form of learning, arises through associations among stimuli and responses, either accidental or intentional. Conditioning stresses events in the environment, not thought processes inside the head. The term **learning,** much broader in scope, includes conditioning and cognitive processes; it refers to any enduring change in behavior that is the result of experience, rather than illness, maturation, or various physiological adjustments. We shall return to this broader concept of learning at the end of this chapter.

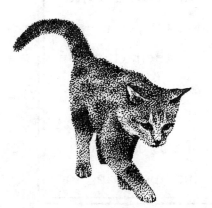
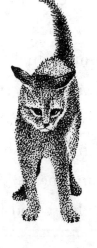
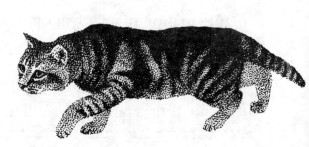

Conditioning processes, because they describe behavior as the function of stimulus–response associations, have been known as *S–R psychology.* Today they are more commonly regarded as part of **behaviorism,** noted for its concern with overt responses and external stimuli rather than internal processes. From this perspective, conditioning is the foundation of human learning, ranging across all cultures.

We begin this chapter with the study of classical conditioning, a relatively simple form of learning. Then, after defining two important concepts, respondent and operant behavior, we examine operant conditioning, which underlies the learning of basic habits and skills. At the close of the chapter, we focus on the learning of complex responses. Thus, the full discussion progresses from relatively simple to higher-level learning.

• CLASSICAL CONDITIONING •

Our modern understanding of classical conditioning began with a Russian physiologist interested in the study of gastric secretions. In fact, he received a Nobel Prize for his work on digestion. Does the name Ivan Pavlov ring a bell?

To study salivation in a live dog, Pavlov and his assistants made an incision in the dog's cheek and inserted rubber tubing, through which the saliva passed into a glass container. In this way, the amount of salivation could be measured in a precise, objective manner. When food was presented, the dog naturally salivated, and studies were made of these physiological processes.

Eventually something happened that caused Pavlov to redirect his interests. As these experiments progressed, the sight of the bowl, the sight of the experimenter, and eventually even the sound of the experimenter's footsteps produced salivation. Pavlov called these learned reactions in the dog *psychic*

secretions to distinguish them from the inborn physiological ones elicited by the food itself, and because they were interfering with his purpose, he felt they should be eliminated or studied directly. Deciding to study them, he changed the focus of his research from physiology to psychology. Today he and his numerous coworkers are generally regarded as psychologists in the Western world, although their work is considered part of physiology in the former Soviet Union (Windholz, 1990).

It had long been known that one's mouth waters at the sound of a dinner bell or some other stimulus related to food, but Pavlov saw in this circumstance a controlled method for investigating mental phenomena in live animals and perhaps human beings. The term *classical* means "in the established manner," which in this case refers to Pavlov's approach to these psychological processes. In **classical conditioning,** a previously neutral stimulus becomes capable of eliciting a certain involuntary response. This common definition serves adequately at this point, although closer inspection shows greater complexity (Rescorla, 1988, 1992). The function of classical conditioning, as will become evident later in the chapter, is primarily to assist the organism in preparing for some forthcoming important event (Kohn & Kalat, 1992).

PROCESS OF CLASSICAL CONDITIONING

Classical conditioning involves a relatively simple modification of involuntary behavior. This behavior is known as *respondent* behavior because the individual responds in an automatic, involuntary manner. Pavlov once referred to this conditioning process as "stimulus substitution": A previously neutral stimulus is substituted for a stimulus that originally elicited the response. The sound of the experimenter's footsteps became a substitute for the food; it too evoked the salivary response. This idea of stimulus substitution is helpful but not entirely accurate because the response to the new stimulus is not necessarily identical to the original response. It may be delayed, more abbreviated, less intense, or slightly different in other ways (Figure 7–1).

CONDITIONING PROCEDURES. In the laboratory, before the conditioning process begins, the new stimulus is tested to ensure that it is neutral. If, by itself, it elicits the response in question, then it is not a neutral stimulus for that response. Pavlov used the sound of a bell as a neutral stimulus for salivation. It did not elicit salivation but perhaps, through conditioning, it could develop the capacity to do so.

The conditioning process began when the bell was sounded on a number of occasions, each time followed by the appearance of food, which evoked the inborn, automatic salivary response. As this pairing was repeated, the sound of the bell developed the capacity to evoke salivation. Conditioning had occurred when this sound alone, a previously neutral stimulus, elicited the salivary response.

How might this process have influenced the monks at the monastery? At the sound of the bell for dinner, they experienced a mildly pleasant reaction, including salivation and other anticipatory responses. Over the years, the ringing of the bell had become a signal or temporary substitute for the food itself, evoking these reactions. For the scavenger cats, the scraping of the benches as the brethren sat down to dinner had become an even more powerful signal, for it immediately preceded a possible meal, intentionally or accidentally dropped from the table. On hearing this sound, they salivated, licked their lips, and twitched their tails in reflexlike fashion (Table 7–1).

A modern factory worker experienced this

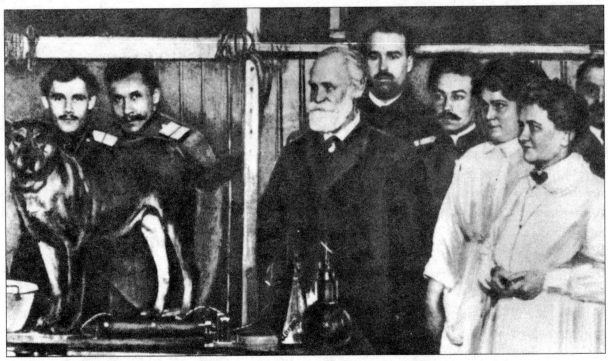

FIGURE 7–1 IVAN PAVLOV AND ASSOCIATES. Third from the left, not counting the dog, Pavlov was a professor of physiology in a military school before his appointment to the Russian Academy of Sciences where he studied the principles of classical conditioning.

SUBJECTS	SIGNALS
Pavlov's dogs	Experimenter's footsteps
Monks in the monastery	Dinner bell
Scavenger cats	Scraping of benches

TABLE 7-1 LEARNING SIGNALS. The dogs, monks, and cats all learned different signals, but the process was the same. A previously neutral stimulus, immediately preceding the appearance of food, became a signal for that event.

outcome—with an unusual twist. A freight train went by his workplace each morning at 11:30, just before his lunch break, and eventually he felt the desire for lunch whenever he heard the train. Then he was transferred to a factory 80 miles north, alongside the same railroad track. The same train passed each day two hours earlier. Whenever he heard it, he felt hungry, although he had never considered eating lunch at 9:30 in the morning.

BASIC TERMS. Food automatically elicits salivation, and therefore Pavlov called this stimulus the *unconditional stimulus,* meaning that no learning, or conditioning, was required. It led naturally to the salivary response, which he called the *unconditional reflex.* But when the sound of the bell prompted the dog to salivate, he designated salivation as a *conditional reflex,* which emphasized that it depended on a certain process—the pairing of the neutral stimulus with an automatic or natural one (Pavlov, 1927).

In translation, the Russian word *ouslovny* became "conditioned" rather than "conditional," leading to widespread use of the adjective *conditioned.* In later research it became apparent that many conditioned reactions, strictly speaking, are not reflexes. For these reasons, the following terms have come into general usage today: There is the natural or **unconditioned stimulus** (US), which automatically evokes a certain response, without prior learn-

ing, and there is the **unconditioned response** (UR), elicited by the unconditioned stimulus. The unconditioned stimulus automatically evokes that response. No learning is required.

In addition, there is a neutral stimulus; it has no original capacity to elicit the response in question. Through pairing with the unconditioned stimulus, eventually it becomes a **conditioned stimulus** (CS), capable itself of eliciting the response. That response is then called the **conditioned response** (CR) because it is elicited by the newly developed conditioned stimulus.

One statement depicts this process: In classical conditioning, a previously neutral stimulus acquires the capacity to evoke a certain response.

An example should provide further clarification. Walking in the woods in a foreign country, you encounter this sign: SREGNITS. It means nothing to you. It is a neutral stimulus for anxiety or fear. Almost immediately, you are stung by a swarm of bees. The next day you pass this sign elsewhere, and again you are stung by bees. On the third day, you become anxious as soon as you see the sign, and yet you are stung again. Do you need more trials? No! That sign has changed from a neutral stimulus to a conditioned stimulus, and your anxiety on viewing it is a conditioned response.

The unconditioned stimulus in this instance is the bee sting. It automatically causes anxiety and discomfort, without learning of any sort.

Notice the timing. The neutral stimulus, the meaningless sign, appears first, *before* the sting of the bees. Thus, it becomes a signal for what will happen next, an attack by the insects. This process is normal or forward conditioning, and learning is often rapid. If the sign appeared instead at the moment when the bees began to sting, eventually you might become afraid of it, but learning would be slower. And if you encountered the sign only *after* being ravaged by the bees, it would hardly function as a signal!

CLASSICAL CONDITIONING PRINCIPLES

The early findings from Pavlov's laboratory have been amplified by modern research that focuses on how this form of learning originates, how it is modified, and how it disappears. The primary concern is with the principles in the learning process, not with salivation or any other response used for studying it. Pavlov's expectation, borne out in much subsequent research, was that many physiological and emotional reactions are acquired in this way (Pavlov, 1927; Figure 7–2).

Pavlov's dog learned to salivate to the sight of the bowl and to the experimenter's footsteps, but no conditioning was intended. These responses arose by chance, through accidental conditioning. Many such responses are acquired by human beings and animals in this way. It was partly through classical conditioning that the monks in the monastery, including Brother Mendo, experienced a pleasant reaction when they viewed the oaken tables. This furniture had been paired with many a happy feast. The garden gate, too, evoked a pleasant feeling. After passing through it, the monks each day enjoyed a half hour of warm sunlight and the chirping of birds in the beautiful flower garden. The table, gate, and other objects, presumably neutral stimuli before these pairings, thus became conditioned stimuli.

TIME SEQUENCES. Any one of three sequences can result in classical conditioning. In one, called **simultaneous conditioning**, the neutral and unconditioned stimuli are present only at the same time. For example, the bell is rung only when food is present. The stimuli commence and cease simultaneously.

In another sequence, **delayed conditioning**, the neutral stimulus appears first and continues to be present during the appearance of the unconditioned stimulus. The bell is rung, and while it is ringing the food is presented. This sequence is the most common form of classical conditioning.

In **trace conditioning**, the neutral stimulus does not appear with the unconditioned stimulus. It appears first, then disappears, and then the unconditioned stimulus appears. In Pavlov's laboratory and at the monastery, the bell was rung and then, some moments after it had stopped ringing, the meal was served. A memory or *memory trace* of the sound remained in the listener's mind when the meal became available, and the conditioning process depended on this trace.

Considerable research has shown that the delayed and trace procedures result in faster and stronger learning than does simultaneous conditioning. The most effective CS–US interval, measured from the onset of each stimulus, has been said to be approximately one-half second, though it varies considerably with different responses and different species (Hill, 1981; Tarpy, 1975). Among

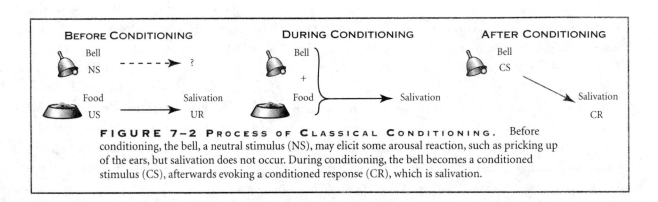

FIGURE 7–2 PROCESS OF CLASSICAL CONDITIONING. Before conditioning, the bell, a neutral stimulus (NS), may elicit some arousal reaction, such as pricking up of the ears, but salivation does not occur. During conditioning, the bell becomes a conditioned stimulus (CS), afterwards evoking a conditioned response (CR), which is salivation.

human beings the timing is not as important as among animals, for human beings have greater ability to make mental connections between temporally distant stimuli (Figure 7–3).

In this context, we should mention **backward conditioning,** in which the unconditioned stimulus precedes the neutral stimulus. The dog is fed and *then* the bell is rung. The bees sting you, and then the sign appears. This procedure does not produce significant conditioning, showing that the sequence of presentation is important. The primary factor in all conditioning is that the conditioned stimulus becomes a *signal* that the unconditioned stimulus is about to occur. In backward conditioning there is no signal.

STIMULUS GENERALIZATION.

Suppose the monastery bell developed a crack. Would its slightly different sound evoke a salivary reaction among the brethren? Suppose Pavlov used a different bell? Would it still evoke this reaction? If so, stimulus generalization would have occurred. In **stimulus generalization,** a conditioned response is evoked by a stimulus that is not identical but merely similar to the conditioned stimulus.

In this case, the magnitude of the response depends on the characteristics of the new stimulus. The greater the similarity between the new and conditioned stimuli, the larger will be the response.

Pavlov found that a certain buzzer produced much the same reaction as the bell, and he attributed this reaction to a spread of effects from one region of the brain to other parts not previously excited.

A baby with a bladder ailment was taken regularly for painful medical treatments. She became quite fearful of doctors, especially those in long white coats, which she associated with the examinations and treatments. One day her sister took her to a restaurant where the busboys wore short white coats. As soon as she saw them, she began screaming and crying. She was too young to know about stimulus generalization and other psychological terms. She simply knew that she did not like white coats of any sort. That was the long and short of it.

DISCRIMINATION.

In the process of **discrimination,** an individual learns the difference between two or more stimuli, responding only to the correct stimulus, not to others that may be similar. Pavlov taught his laboratory animals to make a discrimination between a large black *T,* the conditioned stimulus, and similar but not identical geometric patterns. When one of the similar patterns was presented, the dog at first salivated, but when this figure appeared several times without being followed by food, salivation gradually disappeared (Pavlov, 1927).

Discrimination eventually takes place whenever

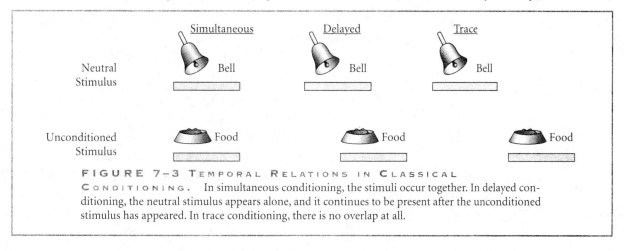

FIGURE 7–3 TEMPORAL RELATIONS IN CLASSICAL CONDITIONING. In simultaneous conditioning, the stimuli occur together. In delayed conditioning, the neutral stimulus appears alone, and it continues to be present after the unconditioned stimulus has appeared. In trace conditioning, there is no overlap at all.

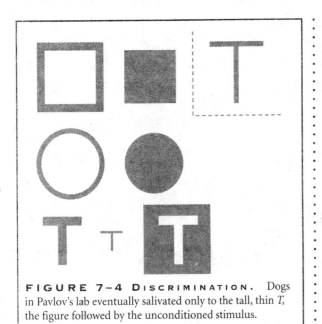

FIGURE 7–4 DISCRIMINATION. Dogs in Pavlov's lab eventually salivated only to the tall, thin *T*, the figure followed by the unconditioned stimulus.

the unconditioned stimulus always follows the conditioned stimulus but never follows other stimuli. After a while, the other stimuli cease to elicit a response (Figure 7–4). At the monastery, the brethren salivated to the dinner bell but not to the prayer bell, which was never followed by food. In other words, discrimination is essentially the opposite of stimulus generalization (Figure 7–5).

EXTINCTION AND SPONTANEOUS RECOVERY.

Once a conditioned response has been formed, how can it be eliminated? The most widely used method is to present the conditioned stimulus repeatedly without the unconditioned stimulus, a process called **extinction.** Gradually, the conditioned stimulus loses its acquired capacity. Pavlov's dog, after continued exposure to the bell without food, ceased to salivate to the bell. The conditioned response disappeared.

If the monks at the monastery became scrupulously careful about not dropping food, and yet the cats were exposed daily to their scraping benches, eventually this sound would lose its significance. The cats' reflexlike reactions of licking their chops and twitching their tails would not be elicited.

After a response has undergone extinction, it has not necessarily disappeared. Following an interval when the conditioned stimulus is not presented, the previously extinguished response may reappear, an outcome called **spontaneous recovery.** It is an inhibition, or forgetting, of extinction, showing that extinction is not necessarily permanent. For example, a child's fear of barking dogs may reappear after it has been extinguished if the child has not been in contact with dogs for an extended period. As Pavlov noted, however, spontaneous recovery grows weaker after each extinction. Continued extinction of a conditioned response produces less and less spontaneous recovery, until eventually the conditioned response fails to appear at all.

HIGHER-ORDER CONDITIONING. In his laboratory, Pavlov found that a conditioned stimulus could serve as an "unconditioned stimulus." In this process, called **higher-order conditioning,** a neutral stimulus becomes a conditioned stimulus *without* ever being paired with an unconditioned stimulus; instead, it is paired with a conditioned stimulus.

In Pavlov's laboratory, the sound of a bell was paired with food, and it became a conditioned stimulus, leading to salivation in the dog. This procedure was *normal, first-order conditioning* because an *un*conditioned stimulus, the food, was used. In the next phase, called *second-order conditioning,* a light was employed as the neutral stimulus, and it was paired with the bell, which was not an unconditioned stimulus. Rather, it had just become a conditioned stimulus through pairing with the food. After being paired with the bell on several occasions, the light also became a conditioned stimulus sufficient to elicit the salivary response. Second-order conditioning had occurred, for a second conditioned stimulus had been developed, this one *without* the use of an unconditioned stimulus.

Suppose that a tap on the nose is then paired with the light. It too is *never* paired with food. If

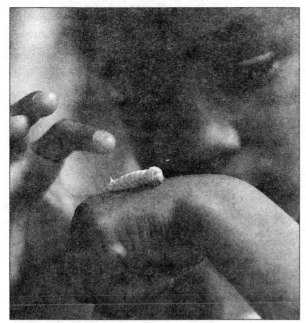

FIGURE 7–5 GENERALIZATION AND DISCRIMINATION. A child stung by a bee often fears other flying, buzzing insects. This outcome is efficient; through generalization, the child need not learn that the horsefly, for example may be dangerous. If the child fears all other insects, that response is inefficient. The child needs to develop a discrimination, learning that caterpillars and related creatures are not dangerous.

the tap eventually becomes effective in eliciting salivation, that process would be known as *third-order conditioning*, for it results in a third conditioned stimulus, again without using the unconditioned stimulus (Figure 7–6).

The key point in higher-order conditioning is that a neutral stimulus becomes a conditioned stimulus through pairing with a *previously conditioned stimulus* rather than with an unconditioned stimulus. Otherwise, the process is no different from first-order conditioning.

Pavlov experienced difficulty in obtaining more than second-order conditioning in dogs because the conditioned stimulus became extinguished after being used many times without the unconditioned stimulus. Pavlov believed that third-order, fourth-order, and higher levels of conditioning are possible with human beings. There is still debate on this issue, but most contemporary experts accept the concept of at least second-order conditioning in human beings and various animals (Barnet, Grahame, & Miller, 1991; Rescorla, 1988).

Higher-order conditioning also illustrates that a given stimulus cannot be identified as an unconditioned stimulus or a conditioned stimulus without reference to the way in which it is used. A bell can serve as a neutral stimulus in salivary conditioning; it can become a conditioned stimulus for salivation; and it can serve as an unconditioned stimulus for awakening someone.

ONE-TRIAL CONDITIONING. The conditioned response is usually built up gradually, but it also can develop through a single pairing of two stimuli, called **one-trial conditioning**. In these cases, the unconditioned stimulus may be of high intensity or prolonged, which is what happened in the case of Brother Mendo.

Saint Ildefonso finally announced his sentence: a week on the cold, hard kitchen floor. Apart from

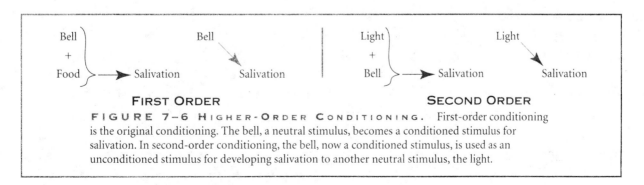

FIRST ORDER

SECOND ORDER

FIGURE 7–6 HIGHER-ORDER CONDITIONING. First-order conditioning is the original conditioning. The bell, a neutral stimulus, becomes a conditioned stimulus for salivation. In second-order conditioning, the bell, now a conditioned stimulus, is used as an unconditioned stimulus for developing salivation to another neutral stimulus, the light.

131

the humiliation of sitting at everyone's feet, the damp chill would make Brother Mendo shiver and shake constantly, and those unrelenting stones would make him ache and feel stiff. After his release from this one-trial conditioning, admittedly a long trial, just the sight of the floor would make him shiver and shudder a bit. All of the brothers punished in this manner detested that spot in the center of the floor.

Accidents commonly result in one-trial conditioning. In 20th-century America, a college student went for a drive in the country to celebrate the beginning of summer. While she was enjoying the fresh air and heavy fragrance of yellow jasmine, an oncoming car careened directly into her lane. There was a collision. The driver of the other car had fallen asleep, and the impact sent both cars into a field of yellow jasmine. Dazed and injured in the crash, for a long time afterward the young woman experienced a conditioned response. Her stomach tightened and she felt a bit queasy whenever she smelled yellow jasmine.

MULTIPLE CONDITIONED STIMULI. In his laboratory, Pavlov rang the bell to provide a specific stimulus, but he recognized that all sorts of stimuli can become conditioned, including the experimenter's footsteps and the dish containing the food. When we speak of *a* conditioned stimulus or *the* conditioned stimulus, we are simply citing a prominent stimulus that became conditioned. Modern research indicates that numerous associations can be formed in the conditioning process (Rescorla, 1988).

The ease with which certain stimuli become conditioned has interested experimental psychologists. Some become strongly conditioned on a single trial; others become conditioned weakly or not at all. According to this view, human beings and certain animals have a *biological preparedness* for certain instances and forms of conditioning (Seligman, 1970). For example, stimuli associated with

snakes are more fear-arousing and more resistant to extinction than stimuli associated with flowers (McNally, 1987). This difference in the acquisition and extinction of conditioned stimuli suggests that there is an evolutionary basis in the human predisposition to shun snakes and smell flowers.

To explore this hypothesis, several groups of water-deprived rats were treated in various ways, two of which deserve special attention. Both groups drank sweetened water from a spout that gave off a bright light and a clicking sound whenever it was licked. Thus, all rats drank "sweet, bright, noisy" water. Afterwards, the members of one group received an electric shock to the feet whenever they were drinking. The others received radiation poisoning that induced nausea an hour later.

The rats in each group were then tested with two different kinds of water. Some of those that received the shock were offered sweetened water, which they drank. Others were offered bright-noisy water, which they refused. Those that received the poison were tested in the same way, and they responded in the opposite manner, refusing the sweetened water and drinking the bright-noisy water (Figure 7–7). In other words, light and sound became conditioned when the stimulus was electric shock; the flavor became conditioned when the stimulus was nausea from the poison (Garcia & Koelling, 1966).

These outcomes confirmed the view that the associations in classical conditioning are not arbitrary. Some connections are more readily formed than others, perhaps because natural selection favors certain outcomes, as when wild rats become bait shy. They learn to avoid the poisoned food, but they do not avoid the place where they became poisoned. In other words, numerous stimuli may become conditioned stimuli, but we must also recognize a biological preparedness. When the unconditioned stimulus produces illness, flavors

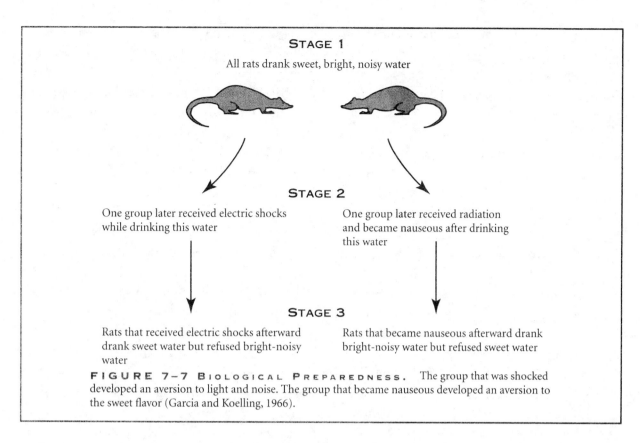

STAGE 1

All rats drank sweet, bright, noisy water

STAGE 2

One group later received electric shocks while drinking this water

One group later received radiation and became nauseous after drinking this water

STAGE 3

Rats that received electric shocks afterward drank sweet water but refused bright-noisy water

Rats that became nauseous afterward drank bright-noisy water but refused sweet water

FIGURE 7-7 BIOLOGICAL PREPAREDNESS. The group that was shocked developed an aversion to light and noise. The group that became nauseous developed an aversion to the sweet flavor (Garcia and Koelling, 1966).

and odors apparently become the conditioned cues. When the unconditioned stimulus produces pain, sights and sounds may become the important cues.

INFLUENCE OF CLASSICAL CONDITIONING

Ivan Pavlov's confidence in his studies led him to declare that "different kinds of habits based on training, education and discipline . . . are nothing but a long chain of conditioned reflexes" (1927). Most psychologists consider this statement oversimplified, although the influence of classical conditioning is widely recognized in a broad array of human activities. Practical applications have been found in such diverse problems as gambling, disease, and drug tolerance (Ban & Guy, 1985; Brown, 1986; Siegel, 1983). Probably the most common use occurs in advertising.

In the modern view, classical conditioning serves a broad signaling function. By this process, an organism learns about its environment; it prepares itself for some impending event (Kohn & Kalat, 1992).

In the monastery, the cats twitched their tails at the sound of the scraping benches. Formerly punished brethren, whenever they passed the kitchen floor, shuddered a bit, reliving their confinement. In our era, as just indicated, the sound of a train, the sight of busboys' coats, and the odor of yellow jasmine all have served in this same way, eliciting responses associated with an earlier event.

TESTING SENSORY ABILITIES. With this potential, classical conditioning procedures have been used to assess the sensory ability of infants, some handicapped people, and animals. In a clinic for hearing and speech disorders, suppose that an infant does not respond to certain sounds. How can we decide whether the child, too young to talk, has normal hearing?

While more modern methods are available, the use of classical conditioning is readily illustrated. We can gently prick the infant's foot and find that it is withdrawn. If so, the pinprick is an unconditioned stimulus for foot withdrawal. If we ring a bell in advance of the pinprick on each of several occasions, eventually the child with normal hearing withdraws the foot at the sound of the bell alone. We thus know that the infant's auditory mechanisms are functioning satisfactorily for this sound; some other factor must be causing its lack of reaction to certain sounds. There are, of course, certain constraints in using this procedure, but the conditioning process is successful even with very young infants.

TRAINING ANIMALS. To test for drugs after a horse race, for example, the animal must urinate, and yet no inspector wants to stand around, bottle in hand, waiting for that moment. Instead, at the horse trainer's whistle, the beast responds—usually. How does that happen? The answer lies in early conditioning. Soon after the animal's birth, the trainer whistles every time the newborn urinates naturally, and this practice of simultaneous conditioning is continued for months. As an adult, the horse cannot be made to urinate if it has no need to do so, but it can be helped to relax, and thereby to behave reflexively, by whistling the appropriate tune.

Classical conditioning is widely used for teaching animals the meaning of a verbal signal, such as "Bad Charlie." The words are spoken and then the dog perhaps is struck with a newspaper, causing it to cower and tremble. In the same manner, the animal learns "Good Charlie." The words are uttered and then the dog is fed and hugged. After several pairings, the dog wriggles or cowers at these previously neutral words. The dog does not understand language in any significant way; the hugging and swatting simply serve as unconditioned stimuli following the vocal tone, which becomes a conditioned stimulus.

Many household animals also become trained unintentionally in this way, responding to the can opener, the sound of keys, or even the mail carrier's footsteps. Signal learning of this sort goes on throughout the lives of many domesticated animals.

DEVELOPMENT OF EMOTIONAL REACTIONS. The most widespread influence of classical conditioning lies in the development of attitudes and feelings among human beings. Conditioned responses of this sort pervade everyday life, as readily evident in the foregoing examples from Renaissance Spain and modern America.

Notice that these examples often involve negative emotional reactions. It is sad but true that there seem to be more instances of negative than positive emotional conditioning, surely because there are so many untoward events that befall all of us (Figure 7–8).

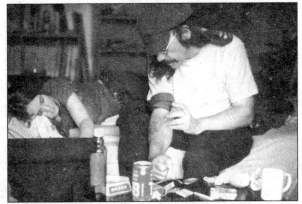

FIGURE 7–8 CONDITIONED DRUG REACTIONS. The injection of a drug is an unconditioned stimulus for lowered blood pressure, increased respiration, and other compensatory reactions. When a drug is regularly injected in the same environment, that environment becomes a conditioned stimulus, evoking these compensatory reactions. When a customary high dose is used in novel surroundings, these compensatory responses are not activated. The body's conditioned countermeasures are not called forth, and the physiological effects of the drug are stronger than usual, increasing the chances of a fatality (Siegel, 1983).

It should be emphasized that positive feelings also can be acquired through classical conditioning. A student reported how she became fond of a cream-colored jeep in this way. Owned by her first boyfriend, it was associated with tasty dinners, hugging, fresh air, and a multitude of other good times. Seeing that car arriving and stopping at her house, she said, was enough to elicit a very definite feeling of excitement, of butterflies in the stomach. During that intense period of being in love, she experienced the same emotional reaction at the sight of any cream-colored jeep she happened to see in the street (Figure 7–9).

Through conditioning, even mildly aversive stimuli can evoke a positive response. Your author once entered an animal psychology laboratory and encountered what he considered to be the usual foul odor of animal research labs. His young daughter exclaimed, "Oh, I *love* that smell." Then she added, "It reminds me of Snoopy." Odors commonly become conditioned stimuli, and Snoopy had provided her with cuddliness and warmth in earlier days. Snoopy was her pet white rat.

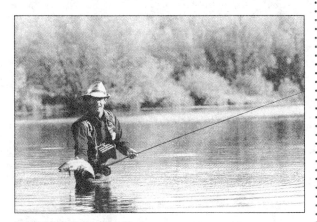

FIGURE 7–9 CLASSICAL CONDITIONING IN ADVERTISING.
Advertisers aim to develop positive emotional responses to their products. To achieve this goal, they use classical conditioning, associating the product—such as fishing gear, clothes, or a vacation tour—with a beautiful person, delicious food, peaceful nature scene, or all of these stimuli, thereby eliciting a positive emotional reaction.

Why do we love our mothers, according to Ivan Pavlov? The answer was partly in front of our baby faces. Mother was paired with milk, warmth, cuddliness, and support from our very first days. For most of us, this early pairing of mother with all sorts of comforts lasts quite a long time, augmented or diminished by events in subsequent years.

How do you make people fall in love with you, according to Pavlov? The answer is—by pairing yourself with appropriate stimuli. When you are with your target person, try to avoid smog, flat tires, and food poisoning, and certainly stay away from the income tax. Pair yourself with laughter, good food, warmth, and pleasant music. And if you have an opportunity, pair yourself with appropriate stimulation of free nerve endings in various parts of the body of your target person. Afterward, he or she may begin to tremble a bit and declare, "I'm in love with you." You'll know that this response is partly a conditioned emotional reaction—love, Pavlovian style.

• RESPONDENT AND OPERANT BEHAVIOR •

A careful distinction must be made at this point. We shall turn shortly to another form of conditioning, called operant conditioning, and therefore we must recognize another form of behavior, operant behavior. It differs significantly from respondent behavior, just discussed in the context of classical conditioning.

RESPONDENT BEHAVIOR

The cats licked their chops at the sound of the scraping benches; punished monks felt a bit anxious when confronted with the kitchen floor. Pavlov studied the acquisition of these emotional and physiological reactions through classical conditioning. He was interested in behavior automatically *elicited* by a stimulus. This behavior is called **respondent behavior** because it occurs as an automatic response to a specific stimulus. The individual responds involuntarily, without intending to do so.

In animals and human beings, we note responses that are inborn and puppetlike, called reflexes. A *reflex* is a relatively simple, involuntary reaction to some stimulus, typically involving a specific part of the body. A depressor applied to the back of the tongue produces the gagging reflex. A tap on the knee causes the patellar reflex, or knee jerk. The chill of winter made the brethren at the monastery shiver. All of these are respondent behaviors, inborn responses to specific stimuli.

The influence of classical conditioning is not restricted to these rather narrow, overt reactions, however. Other respondent behaviors are more subtle: The palms perspire; the pupils dilate; breathing becomes heavier. Still others are more diffuse, such as feelings of fear, hunger, love, and other emotions. A major part of everyday life, they are influenced not only by conditioning but also by cognitive processes, considered later.

The point to be appreciated here is that respondent behaviors, however broad or narrow, are "extracted," so to speak, by some specific stimulus in the environment. Goose bumps elicited by cold are an inborn reflex. Goose bumps elicited by the sight of a stone floor or the sound of an old school song are a conditioned response, acquired through classical conditioning. Regardless of how they originate and the stimulus by which they are elicited, respondent behaviors tend to be physiological and emotional, involving the smooth muscles and glands, as in perspiring, feeling nauseous, feeling elated, and so forth.

∾

OPERANT BEHAVIOR

How do we cope with these emotional reactions? What do we do about them? Poor Brother Mendo finally began his lengthy stay on the kitchen floor,

and he felt immediate discomfort. How would he cope with his distress?

Our coping behavior apparently emerges under circumstances quite different from those accompanying respondent behavior. This behavior is called **operant behavior** because the organism responds in a voluntary manner, operating on its environment, producing a certain outcome. This behavior is not elicited automatically by some stimulus; it is *emitted* voluntarily by the individual. Operant behavior was of special interest to B. F. Skinner, an active and eminent figure in psychology for 60 years (Lattal, 1992).

The forms of operant behaviors are endless. They include virtually all voluntary efforts at adjustment. A punished monk attempts to escape from the kitchen floor; scavenger cats want to satisfy their hunger. These responses usually involve the skeletal muscles, as the individual deals with the situation by praying, running, reading, writing, hiding, speaking, and so forth. These behaviors generally have an effect on the environment and, unlike respondent behavior, the individual is free to emit or not to emit them. Behavior of this sort is sometimes called a *free operant.* It is also known as *instrumental behavior,* for it is instrumental in achieving a certain outcome.

Operant behaviors are learned chiefly through their consequences. The individual does whatever works best in a given situation, at least at the moment. Sometimes this activity is intentional. Sometimes it occurs without full awareness. In both cases, the behavior may become a habit, depending on the effect it produces in the environment.

In summary, there are two broad classes of behavior, respondent and operant, and they differ in the degree to which they are under the individual's control. Respondent behaviors are essentially involuntary, concerning feelings and reflexive physiology. They are elicited by the environment. Operant behaviors are more voluntary, emitted by the individual as he or she deals with some event in the environment.

• OPERANT CONDITIONING •

With this discussion of two kinds of behavior, we turn for a moment from the scavenger cats in the monastery to experimental cats in a psychologist's "puzzle box" at the turn of this century. Here we begin to consider operant conditioning.

The problem for these experimental cats, studied by an American psychologist named E. L. Thorndike, was to escape from the box and reach a nearby dish of food. Each food-deprived animal, tested individually, engaged in various random behaviors in the box, such as walking, scratching, pawing, stretching, and so forth, and eventually it pulled on a latch in the prescribed manner. Then the door opened; the cat escaped; and it consumed the food. On subsequent trials it pushed the latch correctly earlier and earlier.

The same result occurred when the cat was required to pull on a loop, bump a pole, or produce some other specific response to gain its release. The animal at first responded in various ways but eventually, immediately after it was placed in the box, it repeated the behavior it had emitted just prior to its escape. Thus the cat's behavior was molded by the environment. Such behaviors are said to follow the **reinforcement principle,** formerly called the *law of effect:* An organism tends to repeat those behaviors that bring about satisfaction, and it tends to discard those that bring about dissatisfaction or annoyance (Thorndike, 1898, 1911).

Later, B. F. Skinner began to study this process in detail, using rats and pigeons in laboratory experiments. He became a highly visible figure in the field of psychology, especially in studies of this form of learning, which he called operant conditioning (Iversen, 1992). Expressed simply, in **operant conditioning** behavior is determined by its consequences; an organism operates on its environment, and the probability of a given response depends on its prior consequences.

PROCESS OF OPERANT CONDITIONING

There are two basic differences between Pavlov's classical conditioning and Skinner's operant conditioning. The behavior is involuntary in classical conditioning, and the focus is on the meaning of a stimulus. The behavior is voluntary in operant conditioning, and the concern is with the consequences of the behavior (Table 7–2). This distinction between meanings and consequences will be considered again, in detail, later.

	CLASSICAL CONDITIONING	OPERANT CONDITIONING
Type of behavior	Involuntary responses; reflexes, glandular reactions.	Voluntary responses; reactions of the skeletal muscles.
Learning outcome	A formerly neutral stimulus signals a forthcoming event.	An operant response produces certain consequences, solving a problem.
Typical example	The scraping of benches elicited salivation in the cats.	The cats ran to find fallen food, thereby obtaining a meal.

TABLE 7–2 COMPARISON OF CLASSICAL AND OPERANT CONDITIONING. There are similarities and differences in these processes. Only the principal differences are indicated here.

The basic idea in operant conditioning is that behavior is determined *by its consequences.* We engage in operant behavior, and it has certain consequences. Behavior that produces positive consequences tends to be repeated.

Brother Mendo, in the early stages of his long confinement, alleviated his pain a bit by humming little tunes to himself. This behavior made him feel better, and so he continued to sing softly to himself. The monastery cats also emitted behaviors that produced positive consequences. At the proper moment, they scampered from their warm hearth to snatch a scrap of food dropped from the tables. Even an infrequent morsel was enough to keep them at this task.

In addition, operant behavior is sustained by eliminating negative consequences. A cook in any kitchen, after burning himself, adopts a different procedure. If he invariably is not burned using the new procedure, he is likely to repeat it. In the same way, a person trying to operate a keyboard, ride a bicycle, or solve some other problem also adopts behavior which gains positive outcomes or wards off negative outcomes. Operant behaviors are supported by their consequences.

CONDITIONING PROCEDURES. In the laboratory, the experimental animal typically is placed in a *Skinner box,* more technically referred to as an *operant chamber,* which contains a lever and a device for dispensing food or water. There is no research interest in lever pressing per se but, as in Pavlov's work with salivation, this behavior is convenient for studying the conditioning process.

A food-deprived rat is free to move within the confined area, and eventually it presses the lever that triggers the food-delivery mechanism, producing a food pellet. After gaining this outcome, the subject continues its apparently random activity, but sooner or later it presses the lever again, obtaining another pellet. As time passes, the lever is pressed more and more frequently; finally, the rat, like the cats in the box, consistently operates the lever to obtain a favorable outcome, in this case food pellets (Figure 7–10).

The central concept here is **reinforcement,** which is any outcome following a response that increases the probability of a recurrence of that response. Whenever a person operates on the environment and obtains food, a smile, or a pat on the back, or avoids a spanking, a parking fine, or an illness, the probability increases that the individual will operate on its environment in this same way in the future. People sometimes speak of reward and punishment in these contexts, but these terms also have popular meanings and generally are not used in studies of conditioning processes.

To be more specific, in **positive reinforcement** the *appearance* of food, an *A* in school, or some comparable event increases the probability that a response will be repeated. Negative reinforcement, in contrast, involves the removal of an object or circumstance. In **negative reinforcement** the *disappearance* of extreme heat, confinement, or some comparable event increases the probability of a repetition of the response. All reinforcement, positive *or* negative, increases the likelihood that the preceding response will be repeated. The difference is this: In positive reinforcement, a satisfier appears; in negative reinforcement, an annoyer disappears.

The term *reward* is less precise, for it does not indicate whether the outcome involves the appearance or disappearance of a particular event. This lack of precision also occurs with punishment. In its popular use, *punishment* might refer to a spanking, which is the appearance of an event, or the loss of an allowance, which is the disappearance of some circumstance. For these reasons, many traditional behaviorists avoid the concept of punishment, as well as the practice of punishment, as noted later. The important point to note here is that negative reinforcement does *not* mean punishment. It is the *removal* of an aversive situation; it is a favorable event, a form of "reward" with many useful appli-

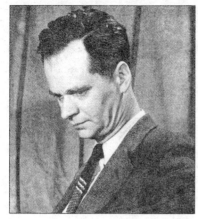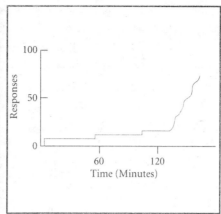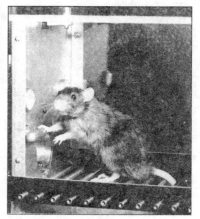

FIGURE 7-10 B. F. SKINNER AND OPERANT CONDITIONING.
When the rat presses the lever in this apparatus, food is delivered. As the graph shows, no lever presses occurred for the first 5 or 10 minutes; then they increased gradually; and after 2 hours they increased sharply.

cations, even in school, for it increases the probability of a certain response (Tauber, 1990; Table 7-3).

To simplify things, the term *reinforcement*, when used without a modifier, refers to a positive reinforcement, and we follow this use throughout these discussions. Remember, all reinforcement increases the probability of behavior.

BASIC TERMS. Other elements of operant conditioning are less specific than those for classical conditioning, primarily because in operant conditioning it is difficult to identify the original stimulus—the stimulus that first evoked the response. In lever pressing it may have been the sight of the lever, smells associated with the box, stimuli within the rat, or some combination

of these factors. The rat did press the lever, however, and this voluntary behavior, an **operant response,** had an effect on the environment. It produced a **reinforcing stimulus,** the food, thereby increasing the probability that this response will be repeated.

Sometimes another stimulus plays a role. Called a **discriminative stimulus,** it indicates when reinforcement is available. When the discriminative stimulus is present, a proper response will be reinforced. This stimulus does *not* automatically elicit the response, as in classical conditioning. Rather, it signals that reinforcement is available—if the response is emitted. In the Skinner box, perhaps food pellets are available only when a light is lit. Very quickly, the rat learns to press the lever when the light appears. Otherwise, it ignores the lever.

	DISPOSITION	
	Presentation	Removal
Positive	*Positive reinforcement.* Example: Receiving praise	*Deprivation.* Example: Losing a privilege
STIMULUS		
Negative	*Punishment.* Example: Receiving a spanking	*Negative reinforcement.* Example: Avoiding criticism

TABLE 7-3 CONSEQUENCES IN OPERANT CONDITIONING. Reinforcement, positive or negative, increases the probability of a response. Punishment and deprivation decrease the probability of a response.

This sequence tends to be repeated until the organism is no longer motivated to seek reinforcement (Figure 7–11).

It is not always possible to identify a discriminative stimulus, but one certainly seems evident in the plight of poor Brother Mendo, for his punishment was worse than yet described. He was required to eat his meals from the kitchen floor in the company of the monastery cats, and Saint Ildefonso forbade any punished monk to touch those fearless creatures. Accustomed to encountering one of the brethren in this predicament, they drove him wild by stealing his choicest morsels. For Brother Mendo, the kitchen floor was humiliating, painful, and frustrating, and it deprived him of his meals.

For the pesky scavenger cats, the operant cycle is readily evident. Brother Mendo's newly filled dish was a discriminative stimulus; stealing that food was their operant response; and having a meal was reinforcement.

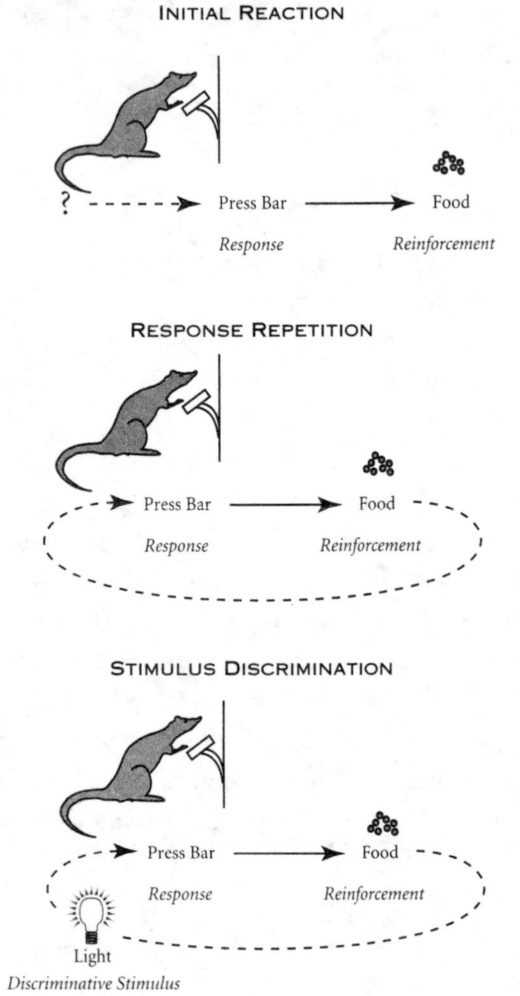

OPERANT CONDITIONING PRINCIPLES

In operant conditioning, the acquisition of a response usually requires several trials, just as in classical conditioning. These two conditioning processes, classical and operant, also share other principles, specifically: stimulus generalization, discrimination, extinction, and spontaneous recovery. They also differ in certain respects.

Insofar as a discriminative stimulus can be identified, **stimulus generalization** occurs when a stimulus *not* used in the original conditioning evokes the response. For example, a rat that has learned to press a lever may press a similar handle or bar, demonstrating stimulus generalization. In **discrimination,** the subject learns to respond only to certain stimuli and not to others. Only the press of the lever is reinforced, not a press of other apparatus; thus, the rat develops discrimination.

These conditioning principles have been observed in numerous organisms. Horses, for example, when observing a circle 6.4 centimeters in size, learned to press a lever with their lips, for which they received food. With slightly smaller or larger circles, they still pressed the lever, displaying stimulus generalization. When the circles were very different in size from the original stimulus, lever pressing diminished, indicating discrimination. Later, some horses were

INITIAL REACTION

? - - - → Press Bar ——→ Food
Response *Reinforcement*

RESPONSE REPETITION

→ Press Bar ——→ Food
Response *Reinforcement*

STIMULUS DISCRIMINATION

→ Press Bar ——→ Food
Response *Reinforcement*
Light
Discriminative Stimulus

FIGURE 7–11 PROCESS OF OPERANT CONDITIONING. The initial stimulus is unknown; the rat presses the lever, an operant response, which produces food, a reinforcing stimulus. This outcome increases the probability that the response will be repeated. Eventually, some discriminitive stimulus, such as a light, may appear, indicating when food is available. The rat learns to press the lever only when the light is on, obtaining food.

trained to respond to the original circle but not to any of the others, for which no reinforcement was offered, and complete discrimination was promptly achieved (Dougherty & Lewis, 1991).

Similarly, **extinction** occurs in operant conditioning, meaning that after several trials without reinforcement, the conditioned response fails to appear. When food no longer follows a lever press, the horse or rat or other organism ceases this behavior (Figure 7–12).

When sufficient time has elapsed since extinction, **spontaneous recovery** may take place, in which a previously extinguished response reappears without further training. This outcome is most likely when the individual has been removed from the original conditioning situation for a considerable period. All of these principles were defined more fully earlier, in the context of classical conditioning.

USE OF REINFORCEMENT. It should be noted in passing that operant conditioning is not limited to the availability of food or water or some other necessity of life, called **primary**

reinforcement because it satisfies some inborn, physiological need. Some animals and most human beings respond for long periods of time to **secondary reinforcement,** which satisfies a learned or acquired need, arising through experience. Money is a good example of a secondary reinforcer. It does not satisfy any physiological need directly, and yet it is a powerful reinforcer. The words "Well done," the letter *A*, and countless other events or symbols constitute secondary reinforcement.

For all of us, the approval of parents, friends, colleagues, and other adults and children is a most important influence on behavior. We do not live by bread alone.

Primary or secondary, the reinforcement in operant conditioning is most efficient when it *immediately* follows the desired response. As a rule, the smaller the interval between response and reinforcement, the faster is the conditioning. Even a delay of a few seconds can retard the conditioning process.

Feeling very chilly, Brother Mendo pulled at the cord on his tunic, tightening the cloth around

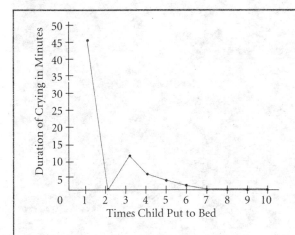

FIGURE 7–12 ELIMINATING AN OPERANT BEHAVIOR. A sick infant required much parental attention early in life. After he regained his health, his parents needed to stay with him at bedtime to prevent temper tantrums. When the parents were instructed to leave the child's bedroom immediately, his crying stopped. Lack of crying at the second bedtime perhaps was due to fatigue (Williams, 1959).

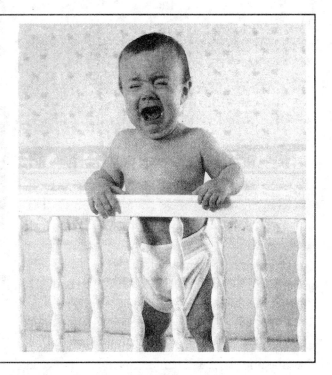

his body. Immediately, he felt a bit warmer. A few minutes later he pulled the cord again, once more obtaining immediate reinforcement.

In addition to immediate reinforcement, there are other considerations in developing an operant response. The first concerns shaping, used for learning complex responses. The second concerns schedules of reinforcement, used for strengthening an already established habit. The third involves a controversial issue, the use of punishment.

METHOD OF SHAPING. In conditioning a rat to press a lever, we can simply wait for this behavior to occur. At some point in its wanderings around the operant chamber the rat probably will press the lever, producing a food pellet. Some minutes, hours, days, or even weeks later, it will press the lever again and receive some more food. Eventually the rat will press the lever regularly, and the response will become well established.

But learning will occur more rapidly if we use a special operant principle. To avoid a long wait for the full response, we provide reinforcement for simpler behaviors that will lead to the full response. Thus, we begin by supplying a food pellet whenever the rat moves even a short distance in the direction of the lever. If we give a few more reinforcers, it will remain in this area, but then we give no more reinforcers until the rat moves still closer to the lever. The animal is thus brought to the wall containing the lever. Then it receives no more reinforcement until it touches the lever, perhaps sniffing it on the first occasion. Next, it must push the lever slightly to receive reinforcement; food is no longer given for merely touching the lever. Later, the rat must push the lever through a larger arc, for only these responses are reinforced. Finally, the rat must make the full response, pressing the lever through its complete arc to obtain a reinforcer.

This approach to learning is called **shaping,** for each successive step is slightly more demanding than the prior step, and reinforcement is contingent on success at that step. The learner gains mastery on a step-by-step basis. These intermediate tasks or steps, accomplished during the process of shaping, are known as **successive approximations.** For example, circus animals have been taught seemingly remarkable feats in this way (Figure 7–13).

Shaping can occur on an accidental basis. A child at dinner asks for the milk in a soft voice. The adults, engaged in conversation, pay no attention. The child asks in a louder voice, and someone passes the milk. As the days go by, the child continues to use this increased volume, but if he is ignored, he asks still more loudly. This behavior, if

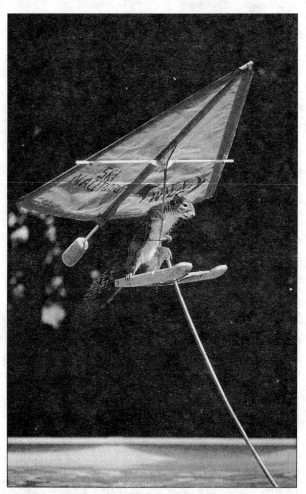

FIGURE 7–13 SHAPING BEHAVIOR.
Many successive approximations were required to reach the final level of skill demonstrated by the airborne, water-skiing squirrel. Notice that the response is compatible with the animal's inborn behavior. Squirrels are accustomed to flying through the air.

reinforced, will continue, but if even this plea goes unattended later, eventually the child uses a very loud voice. As a result of these unintentional successive approximations, he shouts: "Please pass the milk." At that point, an adult may turn and say: "Try to speak more softly! Whoever taught you to speak like that?"

Used intentionally, shaping pervades our approach to the teaching-learning situation, not only in schools and business but also in the home, as the child, for example, learns to read letters, then words, then phrases and sentences, then easy books, and so forth. The steps are known as *successive* approximations to indicate that their sequence must be carefully arranged in order of difficulty. Mastery at each level prepares the learner for the next higher level.

REINFORCEMENT SCHEDULES. Acquisition of any habit is best accomplished by **continuous reinforcement,** or 100% reinforcement, in which each correct instance is reinforced, even in shaping. After the basic pattern is established, however, a different procedure is used to *increase the frequency of the response.* This procedure is known as *intermittent* or **partial reinforcement** because sometimes correct responses are reinforced and sometimes they are not. Under this condition, the response rate increases because more work is required to obtain each reinforcement and because, in some partial schedules, it is never clear when the next reinforcement will become available.

On a **fixed-ratio schedule** (*FR*), the subject is rewarded for only a certain proportion of correct responses. The subject might begin at FR 2, meaning one reinforcement for every two correct responses. After the subject has adapted to this schedule, then it might be changed to FR 3, in which reinforcement is available only after every third correct response. Gradually, over the course of days and weeks, the proportion of reinforcement

can be increased to FR 4, FR 6, FR 9, and so forth up to FR 30 or much more. With these changes, rats and pigeons and countless other animals can be made to perform at very high rates, pressing a bar, pecking a disc, and so forth. Among human beings, piecework in industry illustrates this schedule, especially when a bonus becomes available for pieces produced beyond a certain number. Rental agencies follow this principle more subtly when they offer dividends or reduced rates after each transaction of a certain amount.

To maintain a consistently high rate of responding, variable schedules are used, in which there is no indication when the next reinforcement will occur. On a **variable-ratio schedule** (*VR*), reinforcement is provided on an irregular basis but according to an overall proportion of correct responses. A VR 6 schedule, for example, involves *on the average* one reinforcement for every six responses, but the individual may emit eight responses and receive reinforcement, then three responses and receive reinforcement, and then seven responses before receiving reinforcement. The average is one reinforcement for every six responses, but there is no indication of when the next reinforcement will appear. Gambling establishments operate almost exclusively on this principle. The customer never knows when the next reinforcement will occur, producing a higher rate of response than would occur with a fixed-ratio schedule offering the same overall reinforcement (de Luca & Holborn, 1992).

Reinforcement on a **fixed-interval schedule** (*FI*) is available only after a certain interval of time has passed. Then reinforcement is available for the next correct response. For FI 30″ for example, a reinforcement is available every 30 seconds, and the rat receives it for the first correct response after that interval has passed, regardless of when the last previous reinforcement was obtained. Many organisms learn to discriminate this fixed interval between reinforcements quite accurately. Thus, the response rate increases just before the beginning of each new interval. At the human level, a fixed-interval schedule occurs in a wide variety of contexts, from college to Congress. When an assignment is due every Friday, homework rises to its highest level on Thursday, just before the next opportunity for reinforcement (Figure 7–14).

The **variable-interval schedule** (*VI*) varies around an overall average of time, rather than responses, and irregular intervals are used to achieve this average. On a VI 8′ schedule, reinforcement is available *on the average* of once every eight minutes. Thus, an individual might respond fifteen minutes before receiving reinforcement, then receive a reinforcement for the first response after just 1 minute, then after six minutes, then after ten minutes, and so forth, averaging one reinforcement every eight minutes. Under such conditions, pigeons have pecked for hours at the rate of five pecks per second; some have responded 10,000 times with a very low reinforcement rate (Skinner, 1953). Human beings act in much the same way, although without the pigeon's incredible persistence.

To summarize, we can say that continuous reinforcement is most effective during acquisition, when the response is being learned. The schedules of partial reinforcement are most effective later in generating a high rate of response.

After a schedule of partial reinforcement, especially variable reinforcement, a response is highly resistant to extinction. The reason is that the partial schedule itself contains some *extinction* trials— meaning trials without reinforcement. This resistance to extinction after partial reinforcement is called, not surprisingly, the **partial-reinforcement effect**. After training on a variable schedule, for example, pigeons have responded thousands of times without reinforcement.

USE OF PUNISHMENT. Many psychologists, including Skinner, have spoken widely against the uses of punishment. For humanitarian and practical reasons, they find fault with **punishment,** defined as any outcome following a response that decreases the probability of a recurrence of that response.

Clearly, B. F. Skinner and Saint Ildefonso have very different views on this subject, and yet it would be inappropriate to decide that one is correct, the other wrong. Rather, they stress different

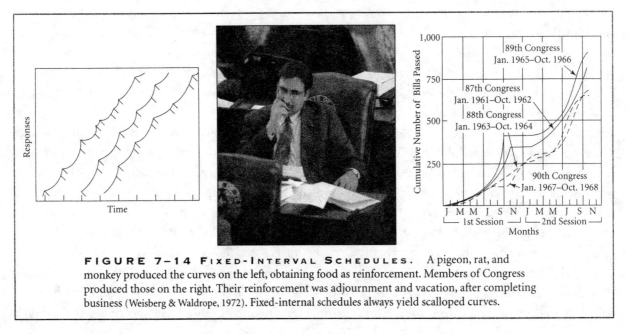

FIGURE 7–14 FIXED-INTERVAL SCHEDULES. A pigeon, rat, and monkey produced the curves on the left, obtaining food as reinforcement. Members of Congress produced those on the right. Their reinforcement was adjournment and vacation, after completing business (Weisberg & Waldrope, 1972). Fixed-internal schedules always yield scalloped curves.

aspects of the outcome. Saint Ildefonso would point out that punishment usually decreases the undesired response, at least for a while. Skinner would state that punishment is only temporarily effective and that the cost of suppressing the response is not worth the negative consequences it often generates.

The humanitarian reasons are obvious. Punishment can be cruel, and it can produce undesirable side effects in the punished individual, animal or human being, including anxiety, lethargy, conflict, illness, hyperactivity, and repetitive behavior. Animals have shown these reactions in experimental situations; clinical observations of severely punished children also provide evidence. Furthermore, punishment can lead to dislike of the punitive agent and the punished activity. These negative attitudes toward the home, school, or parent can remain for long periods, even a lifetime (Mathis & Lampe, 1991).

The punishment administered to Brother Mendo was rather severe, and it left him starving, except for the food that the finicky cats decided not to eat. According to the custom of that day, he might instead have been required to walk around all week with a stick in his mouth—perhaps to remind him not to stick his foot there. (Oh, Brother!) In any case, such punishments probably prompted low self-esteem among the brethren and unfavorable attitudes toward monastery life.

From a practical standpoint, Skinner argued that punishment is not effective in eliminating undesirable behavior; it simply suppresses that behavior. Also, punishment does *not* teach the desired behavior. It does not directly support a correct response. It may even be a stimulus to misbehavior through the attention it gains, relief from guilt feelings, or by serving some other subtle or latent purpose.

One critical factor is the immediacy with which punishment follows the response. Delayed and uncertain punishment, of whatever strength, is less effective than weaker punishment administered earlier (Figure 7–15).

Those who argue for the use of punishment point out that immediate suppression of the undesirable response may be very important, especially in the case of dangerous or threatening behavior.

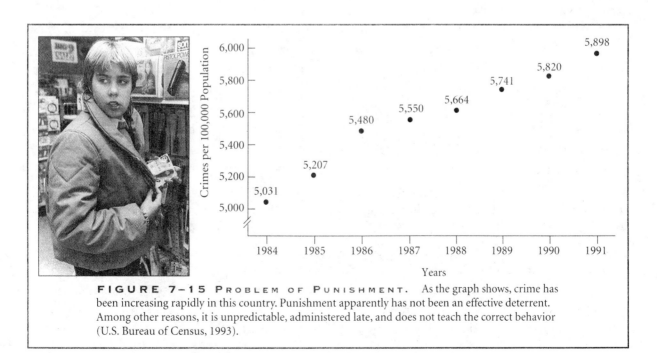

FIGURE 7–15 PROBLEM OF PUNISHMENT. As the graph shows, crime has been increasing rapidly in this country. Punishment apparently has not been an effective deterrent. Among other reasons, it is unpredictable, administered late, and does not teach the correct behavior (U.S. Bureau of Census, 1993).

Certain antisocial actions must be suppressed, even if punishment does not teach the person what to do. At least it indicates what not to do. Furthermore, during the period of suppression, rewards can be used to encourage more desirable behavior. In this context, it should be emphasized again that negative reinforcement is not punishment. Receiving high grades in a course and therefore becoming exempt from the final examination would be an instance of negative reinforcement.

In summary, there are three rules for punishment, if it must be used at all. (1) Administer punishment promptly and consistently. (2) Keep the level of punishment as mild as possible, making it largely informative. (3) Ensure that the correct response is known and available.

INFLUENCE OF OPERANT CONDITIONING

The procedures of operant conditioning are widely used today, knowingly or otherwise, within and outside psychology. Advocates of this approach to psychological issues believe that, if properly applied, it can make an enormous difference in the improvement of the human condition (Skinner, 1961, 1984; Thyer, 1991). In particular, it appears to be important in the theory and practice of shaping behavior of the young (Gewirtz & Peláez-Nogueras, 1992).

OPERANT CONDITIONING AS RECIPROCAL. In many situations, the response of one individual influences the response of the other. This situation is called **reciprocal conditioning,** for each individual's behavior is reinforcing to another. In the dining room, the hungry cats and monks were involved in reciprocal conditioning. The monks intentionally dropped the food, causing the cats to run, and the cats, by running, prompted the monks to drop food. Without fully realizing it, they kept one another dropping food or running to obtain it.

This reciprocity was depicted in a popular cartoon. "Wow! Have I got that guy conditioned," said one rat to another after some Skinnerian experiments. "Every time I push the lever, he gives me food."

In reciprocal conditioning, an individual operates on his or her environment and the environment, which includes the living organisms in it, operates on the individual as well. The parent controls the child, but as any parent knows, the child also controls the parent. A representative government creates and amends laws to control the people, but the people determine what laws the government will make. There are exceptions to this rule—including prisoners, the very elderly, and emotionally disturbed people, who sometimes have little control over their caretakers—but according to B. F. Skinner and others in operant conditioning, it applies in a broad way to most interpersonal relationships.

What is love, according to B. F. Skinner? It is an intricate pattern of reciprocal conditioning—or mutual reinforcement. Each partner supports behavior that the other partner emits. Suppose a man, for example, likes to wear expensive clothing and jewelry, and this style of dressing is admired by his significant other. Her admiration supports his dressing style; his manner of dress elicits her admiring remarks. Mutual reinforcement of desired behaviors—love, Skinnerian style.

LEARNING SKILLS AND SOLVING PROBLEMS. Operant conditioning has been widely used to teach animals tasks and tricks. Monkeys have been trained for assisting the handicapped, horses for crowd control, and dolphins for entertainment (Figure 7–16).

Pigeons have been trained as inspectors in a pill factory, a job for which they are well suited because of their high visual capacity. They identified defective pills with 99% accuracy, using their beaks to knock them off a slowly moving conveyor belt. Their performance was superior to that of human workers in the same role, and special safeguards were set up against possible errors, chiefly by requiring the birds to work in pairs or small groups, thus producing several judgments about the same pill (Verhave, 1966). They were never hired, however, apparently due to the fear of adverse publicity.

In fact, by training the monastery cats, Brother Mendo finally obtained a full meal. One night when Saint Ildefonso and all the other monks were asleep, he left the kitchen, found a big sack, rounded up all of the cats, and put them into the sack. Afterward, he crept out under an arch, found a big stick, and began this training, a procedure to which we shall return shortly.

At the human level, operant conditioning is employed for training in contexts too numerous to describe here, ranging from toilet training to pilot training. Later we shall note its role in personality, therapy, and weight control. In school, it has been used to increase reading skills (Brown, Fuqua, & Otts, 1986). At home, it has been used to eliminate fears and stuttering in children (Glasscock & MacLean, 1900; Onslow, Costa, & Rue, 1990). And it has all sorts of applications in health, ranging from promotion of dental care to use of safety belts (King & Fredericksen, 1984; Sowers-Hoag, Thyer, & Bailey, 1987).

People also employ operant conditioning in *self-management*, using the principles to change their own behavior. Individuals who want to exercise more, eat less, work harder, stop smoking, and so forth establish a set of behavioral objectives for themselves and then arrange a schedule of reinforcement contingent on meeting these objectives. Usually the schedule employs shaping, and therefore the objectives gradually become more demanding, day by day, week by week. The approach here,

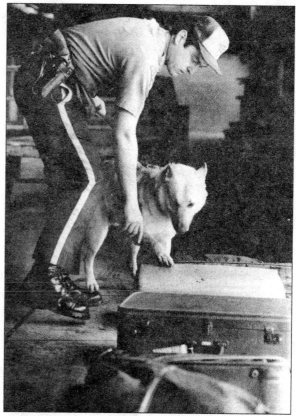

FIGURE 7–16 TRAINED ASSISTANCE BY DOGS. Through operant conditioning, dogs are trained to find drugs, capture suspects, help handicapped people, rescue victims and provide other forms of assistance.

however, is more cognitive self-regulation than it is operant conditioning, for the person is deciding in a purposeful, intended fashion how to change his or her behavior.

The reinforcement in these instances may be a bit of self-indulgence, such as a weekday movie or lunch-hour diversion. As the behavior continues to improve, it should become reinforcing in its own right, for the person is feeling healthier or becoming more productive. The behavior then becomes intrinsically satisfying; there may be no need for additional reinforcement.

CONDITIONING AND SOCIETY. In the novel *Walden Two* (1948), B. F. Skinner advocated careful use of operant conditioning for redesigning societies and improving human life. The issue is highly controversial, for it calls for reshaping human behavior through rearrangement of the environment by social scientists, but these views have found considerable support. One reason is that conditioning processes occur anyway as we interact with each other. Rather than leave them to chance, behaviorists prefer to apply the principles thoughtfully, with certain objectives in mind.

In another book, *Beyond Freedom and Dignity* (1971), B. F. Skinner emphasized that there is a selection process in the environment, and it pertains to behavior as well as to physical structure. Charles Darwin was concerned with the influence of the environment on the physical structure of the species over the millennia—the survival of the fittest organisms. B. F. Skinner was concerned with the influence of the environment on the behavior of the individual over the lifetime of the organism—the survival of reinforced responses. According to Skinner, virtually all of our major problems—overpopulation, energy depletion, pollution, and the nuclear threat—stem from reinforcement of inappropriate behaviors.

The difference between our present society and the one he proposes is that the reinforcement, or control, would be more carefully planned, rather than springing up haphazardly from the self-interests and political successes of many different people. The evolution of our present culture is the result of a massive but prescientific effort to control ourselves, others, and our environment. As Skinner said, we see what humanity under these circumstances has made of itself, but we have not yet discovered what scientific human beings, using a behavioral technology, can make of themselves. "A constantly experimental attitude toward everything—that's all we need" (Skinner, 1948).

For some, B. F. Skinner's view is not subversive or dangerous but rather impractical. Operant conditioning, opponents argue, does not apply to complex human behavior. Skinner's principles, if they are a plausible interpretation of basic habits, are insufficient to account for the broad range of human behavior. In training the cats, for example, Brother Mendo searched for a sack, the cats, and a big stick and then began the training. How do we explain this array of behaviors, comprising a sequence of events? In response, Skinner and his followers have pointed to further operant principles, including the concept of chaining.

CONCEPT OF CHAINING

A moment's reflection shows that human behavior does not occur in separate segments but in a more or less continuous flow, as just suggested. In a baseball game, the batter hits the ball, runs down the baseline, touches first base, and watches the coach for further signals, all in a rapid, integrated sequence. Similarly, the driver of an automobile emits a sequence of intricately interconnected behaviors. These acts cannot occur in a random order. Except for minor variations, only one sequence will achieve the goal. In this sequence, known as **chaining**, any given response in a series is connected to the preceding response and to the subsequent response, each in different ways.

In such a sequence, called a *behavior chain*, each response has two functions. It serves as reinforcement, usually secondary, for the previous response, and it serves as a cue to emit the next response in the chain. Brother Mendo's response of looking for a sack was reinforced when he found it, and it was a cue to look for the cats. Finding each cat was reinforced because then he could put it in the sack, and it was the cue to look for another cat or to creep off to the arch. Arriving under the arch was reinforced because then he could begin to use the stick, and so forth.

Each new condition in such a sequence is termed a *response-produced cue* because it arises from the prior response and also serves as a cue for the next response in the chain. In terms of operant conditioning, such a cue is a discriminative stimulus. These cues are usually visual or auditory, but some are kinesthetic, such as those that arise from turning the key in the ignition of a car, depressing the accelerator, or turning the wheel. The feel of these responses is satisfying because we know that we can move to the next response in the chain.

TWO-FACTOR THEORY

How did Brother Mendo train the monastery cats to leave him in peace? A behavior chain was involved, but clearly there was something else too, which brings us to the question of the relationship between these two types of conditioning, classical and operant. How do they interact, if at all? One answer to this question involves the **two-factor theory** of conditioning, in which signs or signals are learned through the first factor, classical conditioning, and the responses for coping with these signals are acquired through the second factor, operant conditioning.

LEARNING SIGNALS AND SOLUTIONS. In one early experiment using the two-factor theory, guinea pigs were placed individually in a revolving drum. When a buzzer sounded, they received an electric shock. Through classical conditioning, pairing the buzzer and the shock on a number of trials, the buzzer became a conditioned stimulus, and the animals acquired a conditioned response, trembling at the sound of the buzzer. However, each animal in one group could avoid the shock by running at the beginning of the signal;

those in another group always received a shock regardless of their behavior. Eventually the guinea pigs in the first group began to run at the sound of the buzzer. For these subjects, operant conditioning had occurred, as well (Brogden, Lipman, & Culler, 1938).

According to this viewpoint, complex behavior involves a combination of classical and operant conditioning, wherein each form of conditioning makes a different contribution to the total learning situation. In classical conditioning, sometimes called *signal learning*, an organism learns the meaning of stimuli in its environment, at least in terms of positive or negative evaluation. It becomes prepared for what lies ahead (Kohn & Kalat, 1992). Operant conditioning is called *solution learning*, for here the organism learns about consequences— what to do about the desirable and undesirable events in its environment. Both components are involved in many learning situations.

In fact, it was through two-factor conditioning that Brother Mendo solved his problem. His solution, described with wit and wisdom by Lope de Vega, is a fictional part of this narrative and certainly cannot be condoned. The wit is obvious, and the wisdom is found in Lope de Vega's foreknowledge, depicting in light comedy two-factor theory three centuries before Pavlov, Skinner, and others provided scientific evidence.

As Brother Mendo explained: Standing there with the sack and stick on that dark night, first he would cough and then he would

> immediately whale the daylights out of the cats. They whined and shrieked like an infernal pipe organ. I would pause for a while and then repeat the operation—first a cough, and then a thrashing. I finally noticed that even without beating them, the beasts moaned and yelped like the very devil whenever I coughed (qtd. in Bousefield, 1955).

Afterward, he let the cats loose. Then he put away the sack and stick and sat down again.

This training served him well during the rest of his days on the floor. "If an animal approached my food," he pointed out, "all I had to do was cough, and my, how that cat did scat!"

The original training of the cats occurred in a classical framework. Coughing immediately preceded each beating, and eventually it signaled that the painful treatment was about to occur. When the animals heard the cough later, they fled, solving the problem through operant conditioning. They did not literally avoid a beating, but they removed themselves from an anxiety-producing situation, never discovering that the cough was really harmless.

Thus, the cats learned to be afraid through classical conditioning, for the cough was paired with the beating. They learned what to do about their fear through operant conditioning; they ran away.

And here we come to a very different kitchen—this one in twentieth-century America, mentioned at the outset of this chapter, inhabited by the college student named Dolores. One evening her whole family was in the kitchen, busy and harried with preparations for moving from Texas to Virginia. Then her mother became annoyed with her brother and scowled darkly. Immediately Dolores became anxious, just seeing her mother's expression, and suddenly moved to the dishwasher, attempting to fill it even though there were *no* dishes in the sink. Why did she do that?

This puzzling move, she decided later, was a habit. She had been unknowingly conditioned by her mother to do the dishes every time her mother scowled or became distressed (Pinto, 1992).

When Dolores was a child and did something wrong, her mother scowled in exasperation and then spanked her. The scowl was followed by a spanking. Eventually, through classical conditioning, Dolores became anxious simply upon seeing that scowl. Later, through operant condition-

ing, she learned what to do about her anxiety. She washed the dishes whenever her mother scowled. By this behavior, Dolores elicited praise for helping with housework, and at the same time she removed herself as a target for punishment, thereby further diminishing her anxiety (Figure 7–17).

TYPES OF TWO-FACTOR CONDITIONING.
Dolores, the monastery cats, and the guinea pigs in the running wheel all exhibited a specific form of operant conditioning called avoidance conditioning. In **avoidance conditioning** the organism's response does not gain something positive, such as food, but rather prevents something negative, such as a shock, a beating, or a confinement. Another possibility in a negative situation is **escape conditioning**, in which the organism cannot completely avoid the noxious stimulus but instead can terminate the event once it has commenced. Both avoidance and escape are types of *aversive conditioning*, in which the organism eliminates a negative outcome. Thus, they involve negative reinforcement. Two-factor theory also applies when the organism gains a positive outcome, sometimes called *appetitive conditioning* because the organism gains something it wants. Here there is positive reinforcement.

For example, Dolores's family had three household cats. She was responsible for feeding them in the cellar, and she noted that they quickly became conditioned. At the sound of the dry food in the box, they mewed and smacked their lips. When the cellar door was open, they ran downstairs. Thus, they learned the signal for food, the rattle in the box, through classical conditioning. Then they learned what to do about it through operant conditioning; they ran into the cellar to obtain their meal.

At the human level, a man begins to like a certain cologne through its association with a loved one. Then he decides to do something about this preference. He purchases a bottle of the fragrance. Again, classical conditioning is a basis for learning

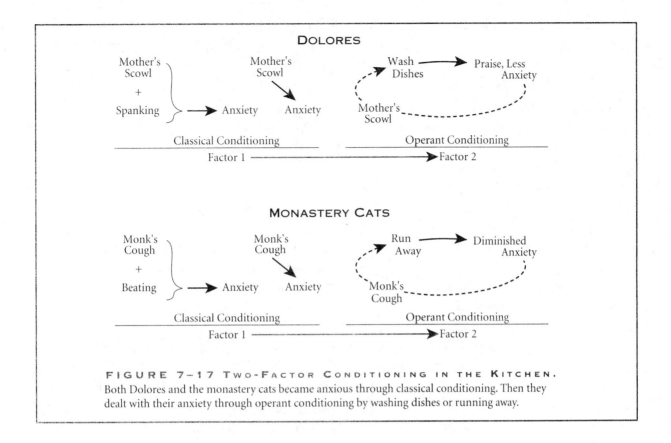

FIGURE 7-17 TWO-FACTOR CONDITIONING IN THE KITCHEN.
Both Dolores and the monastery cats became anxious through classical conditioning. Then they dealt with their anxiety through operant conditioning by washing dishes or running away.

the emotional response—in this case toward a particular odor—and operant conditioning is the basis for learning what to do about it—buying a certain cologne.

RESEARCH CHALLENGES. One purpose of theory is to provide an interpretation of research findings, and in this respect the two-factor approach has proven useful. Both the classical and operant views can be incorporated into a single framework. Two-factor theory presents an overall perspective, and it has suggested that both types of conditioning occur in every such incident.

Another purpose of theory is to stimulate further research on unresolved issues, and here again two-factor theory has been of value, raising the question of whether one or two processes are ultimately involved. For example, biofeedback experiments have suggested that apparently involuntary responses, which are the focus of classical conditioning, can be controlled by operant methods. In biofeedback, electronic devices measure a person's heart rate, brain waves, and so forth, and when this information is made available to the individual, the person often is able to modify his or her heart rate, brain waves, or other bodily processes. This feedback seems to constitute some type of reinforcement in the manner of operant conditioning.

Collectively, such studies suggest that there may be some crossover between the methods and responses in classical and operant conditioning, and some modification of the two-factor theory may be in order. Certain animal studies in avoidance conditioning also restrict application of this theory, for innate behavior sometimes proves resistant to conditioning. However, the two-factor view has maintained a prominent position in learning theory for over 40 years, and at this point there still seem to be two kinds of conditioning. Some version of this theory still appears warranted and useful (Stasiewicz & Maisto, 1993).

OBSERVATIONAL LEARNING

We should also recognize less traditional views of conditioning, including those that incorporate the concept of conditioning into a broader framework. Albert Bandura, in particular, has been influential in developing a perspective that combines elements of conditioning and cognition. The cognitive processes emphasize thinking and memory, which we shall consider shortly in this chapter and extensively in subsequent chapters. At the same time, Bandura's approach offers a practical outlook on the development of certain basic skills.

Imagine teaching a child to tie a shoe solely by operant conditioning. The process could be lengthy indeed, even with shaping. Supplying reinforcement after each correct behavior would be helpful, but the whole learning process could be greatly accelerated by one suggestion: "Watch me!" Then the teacher *shows* the child. In **observational learning,** also known as *social learning theory,* we learn by observing the responses of other people; they demonstrate various behaviors, and we can reproduce those behaviors at a later date. One important premise in this approach is that learning can occur through *observation alone,* without reinforcement. Someone watching another person tie a shoe or train a cat may learn the proper technique simply by observation. Later, when the proper occasion arises, this behavior will be emitted, and then the reinforcement will be obtained (Bandura, 1986, 1989).

PROCESS OF MODELING. In observational learning, the person demonstrating the correct performance is called a *model.* The process of reproducing that performance by watching someone who is competent is known as **modeling.** In this context, we should remark on Dolores's brother in Texas, an indolent adolescent. His behavior offers a good example of modeling.

His job each evening was to collect the three cats from outdoors, sometimes an irksome task, and he noticed Dolores's success with the box of dry food. When she shook it, the animals heard the noise and came running. So he merely modeled his behavior after that of his sister. He opened the back door, shook the box, and the cats came running home. His job was done, even without feeding them.

The brother also discovered some further principles of conditioning. After a while, the cats refused to enter the house when he shook the box. Too many shakings without feedings led to extinction. He also learned about discrimination. The cats continued to behave for his sister. They descended the stairs whenever *she* shook the box (Pinto, 1992).

It is through modeling, claim observational theorists, that children of fearful parents often become fearful, children of critical parents often become critical, and children of confident parents tend to be confident themselves. Even children of aggressive parents are likely to become aggressive, for an adult who punishes aggressive behavior is often demonstrating the very behavior that the child, when away from the punitive model, may imitate.

In one experiment, children three to five years of age were tested for fear of a dog, and then some of them observed a four-year-old child who showed no fear whatsoever. He happily patted the dog, scratched it, and fed it when confined alone with it in a pen. For other children, in a control group, there was no model. They simply observed the dog. After eight sessions under one of these conditions, all children again were measured individually for fear of a dog, and the findings were clear. Mere exposure to the animal made little difference. Instead, the children who observed the fearless model showed a markedly increased capacity to approach the dog, and when all children were exposed to an unfamiliar dog one month later, essentially the same results were found (Bandura, Grusec, & Menlove, 1967).

TYPES OF MODELS. The most effective models typically display characteristics admired by the observers. Dolores's brother, responsible for collecting the cats, watched his older sister. The children in the previous experiment observed a peer. They perhaps were influenced more by this fearless boy than they would have been by a fearless adult, for adults do many things that children know they should not do. In this case the **peer model,** close to the observer in age and background, probably was more influential then a **mastery model,** who demonstrates the behavior to perfection but is more distant socially (Figure 7–18).

In one instance some children watched a **symbolic model,** a person who is not actually present but appears only on television, on the radio, or in a story. This adult became aggressive and was rewarded, and later the children tended to behave aggressively in the same ways. Other children, in variations of this same film, saw the model being punished or ignored, and they did not adopt the model's aggressive style. But when these children were offered incentives for acting like the person in the movie, they too behaved in these aggressive ways (Bandura, 1965).

On such bases, observational learning makes a distinction between learning and performance. Learning, which is a change in behavior resulting from experience, can occur solely through observation; we learn simply by watching someone else. In these instances we can speak of *no-trial learning,* for the behavior has been acquired even without practice. The individual discovers what to do but does not necessarily emit that behavior. In performance, the individual emits the behavior in question if reinforcement is available.

Observational learning emphasizes physical reactions, but other responses can be learned too, including social behavior and emotional responses. One study showed that severe fear of spiders was most often acquired through observational learn-

ing, followed by conditioning and then cognitive processes (Merckelbach, Arntz, & de Jong, 1991). Even hypnotic suggestibility, which involves a mental set, is sometimes said to develop through modeling (Smyth, 1981). Observational learning occurs in numerous species, ranging from fish and octopuses to birds and mammals (Beulig & Dalezman, 1992; Fiorito & Scotto, 1992; Robert, 1990). Kittens, for example, learn to hunt by watching the mother. Those that have not observed an adult cat stalking prey are distinctly less successful in their early attempts (Sigel, 1992).

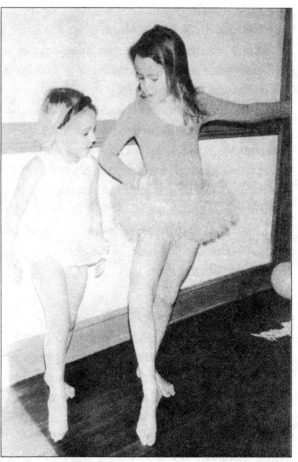

FIGURE 7–18 CHARACTERISTICS OF A MODEL. Typically, the most influential model for children is slightly older and moderately more skillful, as well as emotionally appealing. Thus a sibling may serve as a peer model and also a mastery model, as when a sister or brother is a skilled performer.

LEARNING
AND COGNITION

Human thought is the most outstanding development of psychological evolution. Hence, it is not surprising that many psychologists view memory, thinking, and associated processes, collectively referred to as **cognitive processes,** as playing a vital role in human learning. In fact, one of the strongest criticisms of the conditioning approach is that the contribution of the individual's mental activity is minimized or ignored.

Some cognitive psychologists point out that cognition occurs throughout conditioning phenomena. The conditioned individual develops an *expectancy* based on past experience, and this expectancy determines whether the behavior is repeated or discarded. Expectancy is a mental process, and therefore even in conditioning, the role of cognition must be considered.

In classical conditioning, the individual learns a new signal; in operant conditioning, the individual learns the relationship between a behavior and its consequences (Rescorla, 1992). Brother Mendo understood classical and operant conditioning in this fashion, and he was gratified that the cats had learned so quickly. In less than half an hour under the arch, they had learned the meaning of his cough, and he decided they would remember it if he were ever floored again.

LEARNING SIGNS AND RELATIONS.
Cognitive learning emphasizes understanding, rather than a series of movements. Learned responses are not regarded as conditioned habits but rather as responses to relationships among stimuli. According to the cognitive view, a cat runs down to the cellar to obtain food because it has learned that the cellar and a dark area mean "food" and the upstairs and a light area mean "no food." The cat does not learn a series of specific, rote responses that bring it to the dark area and away from the light area; instead, it learns the significance of the signs.

In a classic experiment on this form of learning, a comparison was made among three groups of hungry rats in a maze. In one group, each subject received food each time it ran the maze, and a steady decrease in error scores was observed. In another group, each subject was given access to the maze without finding food, and there was little improvement in error scores. In a third group, also without food, there was little improvement until the eleventh trial. Then, when food was introduced as reinforcement, performance promptly approximated that of the group that had been rewarded continually. This sudden improvement suggested that the animals had acquired information about the maze that they did not utilize until it became advantageous for them to do so (Tolman & Honzik, 1930). They presumably learned spatial cues while roaming around the maze without reinforcement and then, when food became available, used these cues to find it (Figure 7–19). Such experiments are said to demonstrate **latent learning** because the subject develops a knowledge of the situation that becomes evident only at a later date, when reinforcement is available.

Differences of opinion on the underlying bases of latent learning have a long history, however. Modern experiments that systematically minimize or eliminate visual, auditory, or other cues have suggested that rats employ highly specific associative processes in learning place mazes, rather than forming some overall perceptual representation of the maze (Whishaw, 1991).

Studies of a different sort also support the cognitive perspective. They focus not on learning signs but rather on learning the difference between signs. Let us assume, for example, that the rat has been trained to discriminate between two gray stimuli, responding to the lighter one, which is reinforced with food. After this training, the rat is presented again with this lighter shade of gray, along with a still lighter gray. Which choice does the rat make? Does it choose the original light gray, which is now the darker shade? Or does it choose the new, still lighter gray? In fact, the rat makes its choice on the basis of *comparison* between the stimuli, choosing the still lighter gray in this case. Note that this stimulus is not the specific stimulus that was rewarded previously. Similarly, when the subject is trained to respond to the darker of the two gray stimuli in the original situation, it chooses the darker stimulus when a new pair is presented (Baker & Lawrence, 1951). The outcome in this type of experiment is called **transpositional learning** because the subject makes a comparison, crossing over to the lighter or darker stimulus. It does not maintain a fixed association to the original stimulus.

However, even these results have been interpreted from the conditioning viewpoint, using the concept of stimulus generalization. It is argued that the subject responds to the new *pair* of stimuli in the same way that it responded to the previous pair. The subject selects the lighter, or darker, portion of

each pair in each instance. And it is entirely possible that combinations of conditioning and cognitive components are involved in any such task.

A LEARNING CONTINUUM. Clearly, a number of functions are involved in human learning, regardless of the task to be mastered. The issue, therefore, is not conditioning *or* cognition. Rather, it is the *degree to which* the various processes are involved. Classical conditioning, for example, is not necessarily a low-level, mechanical process. Even in classical conditioning, the organism is an information seeker, alert to relationships among events in understanding the world (Rescorla, 1988). Similarly, cognitive theorists recognize the role of simple habits and reinforcement in most realms of human behavior.

Riding a bicycle, for example, emphasizes the integration of these different forms of learning. It

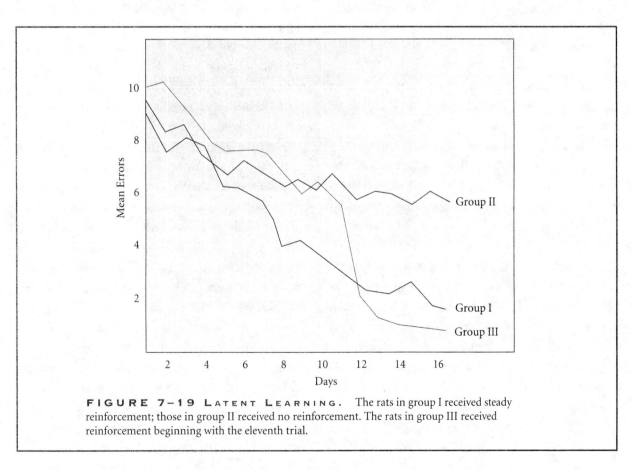

FIGURE 7-19 LATENT LEARNING. The rats in group I received steady reinforcement; those in group II received no reinforcement. The rats in group III received reinforcement beginning with the eleventh trial.

involves motor responses, acquired through conditioning, and also relevant cognitive abilities, such as knowing how to steer, when to brake, what to do to maintain balance, and so forth, all of which become almost automatic after extensive experience (Wierda & Brookhuis, 1991).

Most important in the cognitive tradition is the concept known as insight, sometimes regarded as the highest form of learning in human beings. In **insight,** the solution to a complex problem appears suddenly, not only on the basis of prior experience but also through some new way of perceiving the problem or new combination of earlier experiences. A student suddenly understands how to solve an algebra problem or comprehends the metaphor in a poem. By rearranging or reversing the sequence of letters, for example, you may have suddenly discovered the significance of that earlier sign: SREGNITS. Cognitive psychologists emphasize that insight requires fundamentally new ways of thinking or new combinations of thought, a view that has been prominent for some years, discussed later in the chapter on thought and language.

It thus appears that learning takes place on a continuum of increasing complexity. In this chapter, there is a gradual transition from the simpler forms of learning, emphasized in the conditioning processes, to observational learning, and to the solving of complex problems, of special interest from the cognitive viewpoint. These diverse forms of learning illustrate the multiple bases of behavior.

STUDY OF COGNITIVE PROCESSES.
Looking backward on that evening when she went to the sink with no dishes to be washed, Dolores thought about her behavior, the various factors involved, and developed an explanation with two-factor theory. Similarly, Brother Mendo thought about his problem with the pesky cats, and eventually he developed a scheme for training them. How do we understand these thoughts of Dolores and Brother Mendo in the context of conditioning?

As a rule, traditional behaviorists and other psychologists interested in conditioning do not study thought processes. Instead, they study overt responses, such as Dolores's dishwashing, her mother's scowl, Brother Mendo's coughing, the cats' running, and so forth. No psychologist can study everything, and those concerned with conditioning prefer to limit themselves in this way, utilizing the concepts of reinforcement, shaping, and chaining when referring to complex behavior. If Brother Mendo had previously employed his scheme for training the cats, its reappearance certainly would be explained on the basis of the reinforcement principle.

In recent years, there has been far greater recognition of internal or mental processes, even within the conditioning approach. From this viewpoint, our thoughts do not cause our behavior. They are regarded instead as responses that can be studied in much the same way as overt behavior. They take place inside us, presumably following the same laws as our external responses. The occurrence of each new thought, or response, is thus reinforcement for the preceding one and a cue for the next one. According to this view, Brother Mendo produced internal chains in this fashion, trying one response and then another, each symbolically, until he discovered a procedure for training the monastery cats. Dolores did likewise when she analyzed her behavior in the kitchen.

Some psychologists are content to speculate about thinking in this manner. Others adopt a dualistic approach, as in cognitive-behavioral psychology. They investigate cognitive and conditioning phenomena as separate entities. Still others study mental processes exclusively, which is the domain of cognitive psychology, the subject of the next chapters. Cognitive psychologists are convinced that memory, thought, and language are far too complex to be explained in the behavioristic tradition, and Skinner acknowledged that his view of language was not complete. Thus, psychologists studying these processes often find it convenient to specify these different types of learning (Table 7–4).

TYPE	PROCESS	IN THE KITCHEN
Classical conditioning	A neutral stimulus, after pairing with an unconditioned stimulus, elicits a response.	Dolores became fearful at her mother's scowl; her cats became aroused at the sounds of food.
Operant conditioning	A response is strengthened by satisfying consequences and weakened by annoying consequences.	Dolores washed dishes and escaped her mother's wrath; her cats ran downstairs and obtained food.
Observational learning	Another person's behavior is observed, remembered, and then, depending on its consequences, emitted later.	After watching Dolores, her brother collected the cats simply by shaking the box.
Cognitive learning	A problem is solved by mental processes; overt behavior is not necessarily involved.	Dolores thought about her behavior and then understood her conditioning in the kitchen.

TABLE 7-4 TYPES OF LEARNING

For most behaviorists, however, the emphasis remains on stimulus–response associations. Sometimes the association is between two stimuli, as in classical conditioning; sometimes it is between a response and a reinforcing stimulus, as in operant conditioning. For these reasons, conditioning is also known as *association learning*.

IN PERSPECTIVE. This narrative for conditioning phenomena came from the kitchen. We might ask why, for conditioning can occur anywhere. Of all the places around the the home, however, the kitchen offers the most potential, followed by the bedroom and bathroom. Think of all the opportunities for primary reinforcement in the kitchen: foods, drinks, odors, medications, and hugs and kisses, as well as scalding liquids, sharp knives, broken glass, and electric shocks—to say nothing of the potentially conditioned stimuli and secondary reinforcers: words, tones, gestures, facial expressions, television images, music, and so forth.

The cold, dark kitchen in the seventeenth-century Spanish monastery differed greatly from the bright, modern kitchen in Texas, but the same conditioning processes were at work in both places. Brother Mendo, Dolores, and the various cats were responsive to the reinforcing properties of their environments.

And that concludes our discussion of conditioning in the kitchen. You may remember it through association—with Brother Mendo on the cold floor, Dolores at the dishwasher, and the companionable cats in both kitchens.

CLASSICAL CONDITIONING

I. In the simplest form of learning, called classical conditioning, a previously neutral stimulus develops the capacity to arouse some emotional or physiological response. It does so through association.

2. Some of the important principles of classical conditioning are stimulus generalization, discrimination, extinction, spontaneous recovery, and higher-order conditioning.

3. The most important role of classical conditioning lies in the development of diffuse emotional reactions and certain attitudes.

RESPONDENT AND OPERANT BEHAVIOR

4. Two types of responses are associated with conditioning processes. One type, called respondent behavior, usually involves the smooth muscles and glands; it is particularly amenable to the process of classical conditioning and typically occurs in emotional situations.

5. In operant behavior, the organism is more active, and its responses have more obvious consequences in the environment. These responses typically involve the skeletal muscles, as the organism emits behavior in a voluntary manner.

OPERANT CONDITIONING

6. Habits are acquired through operant conditioning, in which responses are followed by reinforcing stimuli. Primary reinforcement involves the satisfaction of physiological needs. Secondary reinforcement, such as money, a smile, or a high grade, involves the satisfaction of acquired needs.

7. In operant conditioning, an organism's response can be developed by shaping. The response can be increased in frequency by the use of partial reinforcement, including variable and fixed schedules.

8. Operant conditioning procedures are used extensively in childrearing, industry, education, and therapy. According to this view, many of our major social problems stem from lack of scientific control over human behavior, which could be achieved by more carefully planned reinforcements in the environment.

LEARNING COMPLEX RESPONSES

9. In conditioning theory, complex behavior is accounted for partly by chaining, the process of learning a series of related responses. Each response serves as reinforcement for the previous response and also as a cue for the next one.

10. Complex behavior is also accounted for partly by the two-factor theory, in which aspects of classical and operant conditioning are combined.

11. In observational learning, also known as social learning theory, learning can occur by watching a competent person, and the process is called modeling. The learned behavior will not necessarily be emitted, however, until an appropriate moment, usually when reinforcement is available.

12. In the cognitive view, the emphasis is on the organism's knowledge or understanding of the various elements in the learning situation. The cognitive viewpoint is illustrated in latent learning and relationship experiments. Given a complex problem, human beings and other higher organisms arrive at solutions that seem to involve elements of both approaches, conditioning and cognition.

• WORKING WITH PSYCHOLOGY •

⟳ REVIEW OF KEY CONCEPTS ⟳

conditioning
learning
behaviorism

Classical Conditioning
    classical conditioning
    unconditioned stimulus (US)
    unconditioned response (UR)
    conditioned stimulus (CS)
    conditioned response (CR)

simultaneous conditioning
delayed conditioning
trace conditioning
backward conditioning
stimulus generalization
discrimination
extinction
spontaneous recovery
higher-order conditioning
one-trial conditioning

Respondent and Operant Behavior
    respondent behavior
    operant behavior

Operant Conditioning
    reinforcement principle
    operant conditioning
    reinforcement
    positive reinforcement

negative reinforcement
operant response
reinforcing stimulus
discriminative stimulus
stimulus generalization
discrimination
extinction
spontaneous recovery
primary reinforcement
secondary reinforcement
shaping
successive approximations

continuous reinforcement
partial reinforcement
fixed-ratio schedule (FR)
variable-ratio schedule (VR)
fixed-interval schedule (FI)
variable-interval schedule (VI)
partial-reinforcement effect
punishment
reciprocal conditioning

Learning Complex Responses
chaining

two-factor theory
avoidance conditioning
escape conditioning
observational learning
modeling
peer model
mastery model
symbolic model
cognitive processes
latent learning
transpositional learning
insight

❧ CLASS DISCUSSION/CRITICAL THINKING ❧

A NARRATIVE TWIST

Imagine that Brother Enrique, another member of the monastery, committed a misdeed and found himself on the kitchen floor. In an act of friendship, Brother Mendo explained to him the coughing technique. Without training the cats again, would Brother Enrique have found the coughing procedure effective for controlling them? Argue both sides of the case, referring to a specific principle of conditioning in each instance. ❧

TOPICAL QUESTIONS

• *Classical Conditioning.* Using the process of classical conditioning and any stimuli you wish, how might you develop an aversion to drinking or smoking in an adolescent?

• *Respondent and Operant Behavior.* Imagine yourself as an electrician or a construction worker. Identify possible respondent and operant behaviors associated with this work and explain why you categorized them as such.

• *Operant Conditioning.* Using operant conditioning, explain how you would train your grandmother or granddaughter to complain less about your use of the telephone and to exercise regularly.

• *Learning Complex Responses.* Consider a child who has modeled the characteristics of a violent television personality. Discuss television censorship and free speech in this context. Suggest ways to modify television programming to induce more appropriate behavior.

❧ TOPICS OF RELATED INTEREST ❧

Using classical conditioning to reduce fear, often called systematic desensitization, is a mode of therapy (16). Studies in biofeedback (3) show how operant conditioning may be used to control presumably involuntary responses. Observational learning is influential in the development of gender identity (12). Approaches to personality are based on operant conditioning and observational learning (14).

5

MEMORY

BENJAMIN BURTT LIVED A NORMAL CHILDHOOD—
EXCEPT FOR HIS STORY HOUR. EVERY DAY, BEGINNING
WHEN THE BOY WAS 15 MONTHS OLD, HIS FATHER
read aloud to him three short passages from a lengthy drama. Day after day,
his father continued this practice until he had read each passage 90 times
altogether. Then the father changed to another part of the same story, reading three more passages, again 90 times.

Imagine the scene. Harold Burtt, a professor at Ohio State University,
reading aloud while his infant son sat, lay, or squirmed nearby. Still without
mastery of language, Benjamin understood little, said less, and was not permitted toys or other playthings. Running around was not allowed either.
Maybe his father, a college professor, was somewhat accustomed to an inattentive audience.

Every three months the father changed to three new passages, never, of
course, with a word of complaint from his innocent little listener. After all,
the drama his father recited was far too complicated for him to understand.

In fact, it was an adult story of symbolism and human destiny, Sophocles's *Oedipus Tyrannus.* And if that were not enough, the father always read it in the original Greek. For almost two years, the story of King Oedipus unfolded in this way for the unsuspecting child. When the sessions of this unusual story hour finally ended, Benjamin had reached his third birthday. Still learning the syntax and vocabulary of his native English, he had become a somewhat better listener.

The father had selected these passages carefully. They were fairly uniform in difficulty and were written in the same meter and dialogue form, all in iambic hexameter. No choruses were used, and each selection included approximately 20 lines. They were taken from diverse points throughout the play (Burtt, 1932).

What was Professor Burtt's purpose in all of this effort? He wanted to study **memory,** which is the capacity to utilize impressions from previous experience. Specifically, he wanted to discover how early in human life memories could be established. Little Benjamin was an excellent subject because the boy could not engage in extra practice with some-

one else; no other member of the family and no close friend knew Greek. He could test Benjamin's memory later, knowing just which passages had been read to him and at what ages.

The basic message in this chapter, demonstrated in Benjamin's exposure to Greek, is that memory involves three fundamental elements: **encoding,** which is the processing of incoming information; **storage,** the retention of information; and **retrieval,** the recovery of information at some later time. These three elements, which constitute the major topics in the study of memory, are sometimes known as the three *Rs: record, retain,* and *retrieve.* Employing a computer analogy, human memory requires data input, comparable to encoding; saving the information on a disk, comparable to storage; and using the menu to enter old files, comparable to retrieval.

We also approach the Burtts' work with the reader in mind, for the father had a second aim. He wanted to discover how long such memories might last. Today we can add a further question: What can be done to ensure that they last a long time? The outcome of this inquiry should be useful to anyone

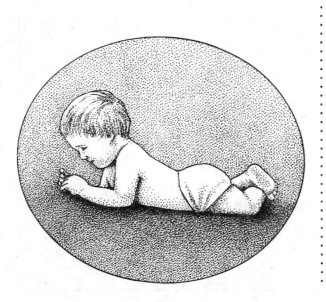

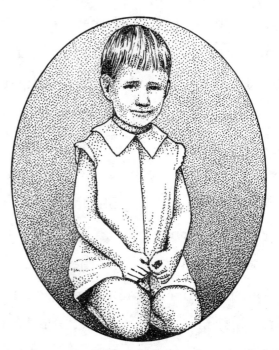

taking courses or trying to pass examinations.

We begin this chapter with the acquisition of memory and then turn to its storage, represented in the memory trace. Afterward, we consider theories of forgetting, which attempt to explain why the trace is sometimes unavailable. Then we conclude with some principles of memorizing.

• ACQUISITION OF MEMORY •

When the first phase of Professor Harold Burtt's project was finally finished, he had read to his son 5,040 Greek syllables. Each one had been repeated 90 times, making 453,600 occasions on which he had recited one Greek syllable or another to the boy, testimony to his perseverance and perhaps his son's malleability (Table 8–1). Harold Burtt, incidentally, showed persistence in other matters as well, from handball to birdwatching. An amateur naturalist, he banded and recorded 164,054 birds. Whatever the endeavor, he was devoted to careful measuring and counting (Thayer & Austin, 1992).

His research with Benjamin reflects a longstanding controversy in the study of memory, one that has recently been rekindled. It concerns the relative values of two different types of investigations: experiments in the laboratory and observations in daily life. The advantage of the laboratory method lies in the opportunities for manipulation and con-

AGE (MONTHS)	PASSAGES FROM SOPHOCLES
15	I, II, III
18	IV, V, VI
21	VII, VIII, IX
24	X, XI, XII
27	XIII, XIV, XV
30	XVI, XVII, XVIII
33	XIX, XX, XXI

TABLE 8–1 BENJAMIN'S SCHEDULE.
The readings continued daily for almost two years. When they were finished, the little boy was just under three years old.

trol. People can be exposed to specific stimuli, and their memories can be precisely tested later (Banaji & Crowder, 1989). The case for naturalistic observation concentrates on the need to understand remembering and forgetting as they occur in daily life. This natural setting more than compensates for the reduced precision (Neisser, 1991). In searching for answers to the perplexing questions of memory, both approaches have proved useful. In fact, both are necessary for steady scientific advancement (Ceci & Bronfenbrenner, 1991).

Harold Burtt's investigation involved both dimensions. It was an experimental study, partly because it controlled the material to which the child was exposed, partly because in the later testing sessions it included some new passages, thereby permitting the precise comparisons essential in the experimental method. At the same time, an adult reading to a child was a naturally occurring event. The setting and even the activity were part of the daily routine for any normal child.

This investigation began 60 years ago, before the widespread use in psychology of the term **information processing,** which refers to the mental operations by which sensory experiences are converted into knowledge. It includes the ways in which we record, retain, and retrieve information; it implies that memory is an active process. Today, it also includes the concept of *parallel distributed processing,* which emphasizes that the brain manages several pieces of different information simultaneously in different brain regions. Most computers today, for example, process information sequentially, one piece after the other. In memory, the human brain not only responds to some eliciting stimulus but, at the same time, attempts to retrieve numerous bits of related information stored in different ways and different places. Human memory, therefore, is an exquisitely intricate and active system of simultaneous information processing.

Within the information processing viewpoint, two broad, complementary approaches to memory have been developed in recent years, one known as stage theory, the other as levels-of-processing theory. While they involve considerable overlap, research on the differences between them demonstrates the ways in which theories become modified, clarified, or rejected. As one view becomes outdated, it provides grounds for its successor. William James described this process in earthy terms: "Science feeds on its own decay" (1890).

We begin with the earlier view, the **stage theory of memory**, which depicts a sequence of three phases qualitatively different from one another: a sensory stage, short-term memory, and long-term memory (Figure 8–1). This three-stage view has been revised, but it forms an essential basis for later discussions (Atkinson & Shiffrin, 1968, 1971).

SENSORY STAGE

At 15 months of age, little Benjamin listened to his father read at a uniform rate, using approximately two seconds per line. Whatever he remembered was acquired through these sounds, for everything we know comes initially through the senses. Immediately after we experience anything, our nervous system contains very briefly an impression of that

information. The term **sensory memory** refers to this momentary residual information within the nervous system, which has not been processed in any significant way.

A convincing demonstration of sensory memory was provided when adult subjects observed three rows of a few letters each for a fraction of a second. Then they were asked to recall them. About half of the letters were recalled in this way, but the investigator believed that virtually all of the letters had been in the subjects' sensory memory. The reason for the poor recall, it was hypothesized, lay in the delay between the disappearance of the letters and the time that elapsed before the subjects could recite all of them.

To test this hypothesis, the subjects were asked to observe briefly on a screen nine letters, appearing in three rows of three letters each. Then, alerted by a special tone that occurred immediately after the stimulation was removed, they were asked to recall one specific row of letters within the block. A high, medium, or low tone requested recall of the top, middle, or bottom row, respectively (Figure 8–2). In these instances the subjects were uniformly successful. They could recall any row of letters in the block, which suggested that after the pattern was withdrawn, the subjects, for a moment, had the

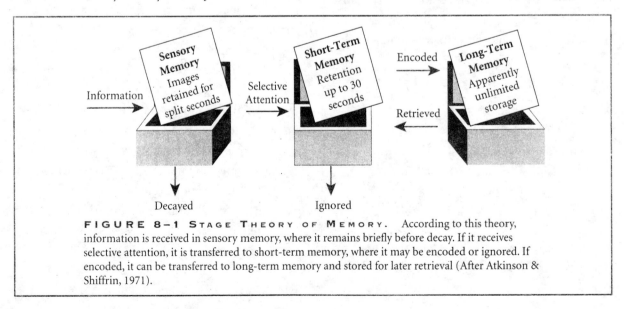

FIGURE 8–1 STAGE THEORY OF MEMORY. According to this theory, information is received in sensory memory, where it remains briefly before decay. If it receives selective attention, it is transferred to short-term memory, where it may be encoded or ignored. If encoded, it can be transferred to long-term memory and stored for later retrieval (After Atkinson & Shiffrin, 1971).

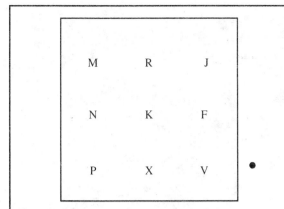

FIGURE 8–2 STUDY OF SENSORY MEMORY. When a low tone was sounded just after disappearance of the letters, it requested recall of the bottom row. The red dot did not appear; it is used here to illustrate the procedure (Sperling, 1960).

whole pattern of nine letters in sensory memory (Sperling, 1960).

In other words, sensory information must be processed immediately if it is to be retained. The speed with which it fades is indicated in these experiments. When the signal for recall was delayed by half a second or less, recall was significantly disrupted. When the delay was a full second, the subjects' success was no greater than it had been earlier, with no tone at all. On this basis, it is generally assumed that unanalyzed information in the visual realm lasts for one second or less. In auditory and other sensory modes, it may have longer or shorter durations.

Have you noticed, for example, that sometimes you can still remember a brief remark even though you were not paying attention a moment earlier? You can process it a split second afterward because the words are still in sensory memory, if not at the next stage, short-term memory. This brief auditory image is known as *echoic memory* because we hear something after the sound has disappeared. In the visual realm, the image is called *iconic memory*, meaning that it is a visual likeness. As might be expected, the stronger the stimulus, the longer the image lasts. The *haptic memory* concerns touch; it is the brief impression still in your nervous system after a fly has left your forehead. Similarly, *kinesthetic memory* refers to memory for certain habitual movements—in the muscles, tendons, and joints. For example, you can still feel a good tennis shot for a moment after the ball has been hit. Presumably, there are such memories for all realms of sensory experience.

❧

SHORT-TERM MEMORY

The sensory image is unprocessed. It appears for a moment, an exact reproduction of the event as revealed by the sense organs, and then it disappears. If any of it is to be useful, it must be handled promptly, passing to another stage. This next stage, **short-term memory** (STM), involves temporary storage, defined in most studies as any interval less than 30 seconds, during which the information is processed or ignored. If ignored, it never becomes a long-term memory. If properly rehearsed, it can go into permanent storage. In either case, short-term memory is a temporary condition.

This early phase is also known as **working memory** because this label emphasizes active memory *processes*, rather than a seemingly static, brief storage. Working memory includes rehearsal of the new information, as well as its manipulation and evaluation (Baddeley, 1990). There is considerable debate about whether short-term memory and working memory refer to the same or different memory functions (Cantor, Engle, & Hamilton, 1991). Whatever the outcome, this research gives further attention to the concept of information processing in memory.

To use a metaphor, short-term memory has been regarded as a receiving platform at the warehouse. It has a limited area, and the workers have a limited time to move some newly acquired material into the warehouse for long-term storage. Something must be done in a hurry, for another shipment will be arriving soon.

LIMITED CAPACITY. The limited capacity of short-term memory was determined when adult learners were asked to memorize various amounts and types of information. It was found that the average person could manage approximately seven separate items. Some people could manage up to nine categories, which seemed to be the effective maximum, and almost all subjects could recall at least five items. The investigator was prompted to speak of the "magical number seven," adding that we should think of it as seven plus or minus two (Miller, 1956).

This limited capacity of short-term memory is both a drawback and an asset. The drawback is obvious, for information that cannot even be received certainly cannot be recalled a few hours, days, or years later. But imagine the difficulties if everything that passed through sensory memory remained in immediate awareness. Yesterday's lecture, today's essay, tonight's news, and the words on this page all would be swirling in our heads at the same time. Our minds would be overloaded with information from our environment, making it more and more difficult to receive and handle incoming information (MacGregor, 1987).

ENCODING: A BASIC PROCESS. To be retained in short-term memory, information must be manipulated or processed properly, as is evident when you ask someone for a telephone number. To be transferred and permanently stored in the vast warehouse of long-term memory, the number requires further processing. This data processing, as indicated earlier, is called *encoding* because it prepares information in a way that makes it likely to be remembered. Encoding is therefore the first component in memory (Figure 8–3).

One encoding process is simple **rehearsal**, in which the information is practiced, covertly or overtly. It is repeated several times, as in saying a telephone number again and again. The aim here is to keep the material available until it can be used, as

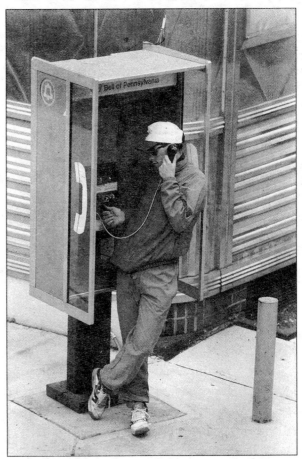

FIGURE 8–3 ENCODING THROUGH REHEARSAL. After dialing for information and obtaining a telephone number, the caller usually cannot afford the slightest diversion. Even a brief remark may disrupt encoding.

in dialing the number, or until it can be stored in some more integrated fashion.

The importance of rehearsal was demonstrated when experimental subjects attempted to remember nonsense syllables for a few seconds. The experimenter showed each subject a three-letter syllable followed by a number. The subject observed the syllable and then, to prevent rehearsal, counted backward by three or four from a randomly selected three-digit number. When asked the syllable three seconds later, the subject remembered it only about half the time. With successively more counting, recall continued to decline, and after 18 seconds, less than 10% of the syllables were recalled (Peterson & Peterson, 1959; Figure 8–4).

In terms of rehearsal, Harold Burtt worked under a handicap with his son. At 15 to 36 months, little Benjamin simply could not rehearse this material himself. To deal with this problem, his father recited each passage 90 times, which constituted prodigious rehearsal for him, although the boy could only sit and listen.

ROLE OF ORGANIZATION. In more complex encoding, there are three basic dimensions, or requirements, one of which is organization. The term *organization* carries its usual meaning, referring to some systematic or functional arrangement. For example, try to remember the following words: *gunners, door, a, floods, can, horrible, by, every.* It may be a difficult task, unless you employ an alphabetical organization—with each word larger than its predecessor.

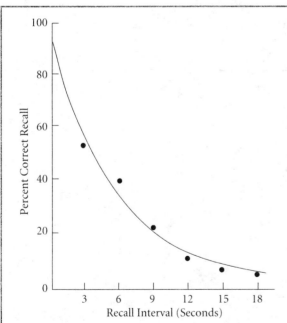

FIGURE 8–4 ROLE OF REHEARSAL. When subjects were prevented from rehearsal, short-term memory showed an almost immediate decline. After just five seconds, there was only about 40% correct recall.

The importance of organization has been demonstrated in experiments comparing free and serial recall. In *free recall* the learner is allowed to reproduce the list in any order; in *serial recall* the items must be remembered in a particular sequence, which requires some organization. When these types of recall are compared using tasks too difficult for success on the first trial, free recall is superior initially. The subject first responds with the last few words on the list, which are still available in short-term memory. Afterward, the subject reports the easiest words, wherever they appear in the list. In learning a complete list of several items, however, the subject almost invariably memorizes it more rapidly when using serial recall, which imposes its own organization (Earhard, 1967; Waugh, 1961). This superiority strongly suggests that memory is powerfully affected by organization, in this case imposed on the material by the sequence.

When there is no organization, the successful learner must develop one. The learner must create a **subjective organization,** a scheme or arrangement for viewing the material developed through personal experience. In memorizing a list of random dates, a woman thinks of them in terms of her eight cousins or the events in a novel. To remember certain facts a man wants to present in an interview, he organizes them around his favorite meal, using the different foods to form a rough framework. Many memory devices are most effective as a means of creating an organization, or order, for recall.

USE OF CHUNKING. Another encoding procedure becomes evident when you try to remember the following string of letters: *O-LDH-ARO-LDA-NDY-OUN-GBE-N.* There are 20 letters, well beyond your short-term memory capacity. If you succeeded, it was undoubtedly because you grouped them in a special way. If you forgot some, try reorganizing them into five words.

Read the immediately preceding sentence just once more, slowly, and then try to repeat it. If you were successful, grouping probably occurred again, despite the fact that the sentence contains not five words but ten, not 20 letters but 50. You probably grouped the elements somewhat like this: If you . . . forgot some, . . . try reorganizing them . . . into five words.

In one study, subjects were asked to sort a deck of cards into categories, with the aim of remembering the single word written on each card. Up to approximately seven, the larger the number of categories used, the better was the recall. Subjects using seven categories were approximately twice as successful as those using only two (Mandler, 1967). The reason: With few piles, there were too many items in each pile to be recalled. With many piles, considerably more than seven, the piles themselves could not be recalled.

This process is called **chunking,** which means combining separate pieces of information into groups, thereby forming fewer but broader categories, or chunks. Sometimes the chunks will be fairly obvious, sometimes not so apparent. With

extensive experience, chunks can be developed containing enormous amounts of information, as demonstrated when chess players viewed a board in the middle of a game. After five or six seconds, the board was emptied and they were asked to replace the pieces. Master chess players often reproduced the entire pattern of 32 pieces; novice players replaced only a half-dozen pieces. As the masters explained later, they could "chunk" the board—but only if it showed a real game in progress, consistent with the knowledge in their permanent memory (de Groot, 1965). With the pieces arranged randomly, chess masters could not remember them any better than beginners (Figure 8–5).

After various karate techniques were presented to 30 practitioners, those who were experts were distinctly superior to the novices in recalling them (Bedon & Howard, 1992). They did so by more successfully combining them into chunks or patterns.

NEED FOR CUING. In addition to organization and chunking, a third procedure for successful encoding involves the use of cues. Perhaps you

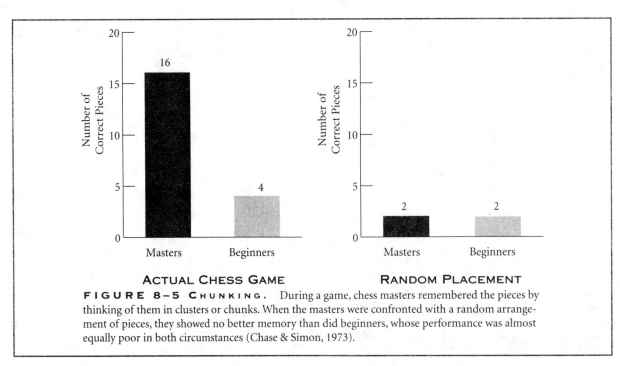

ACTUAL CHESS GAME **RANDOM PLACEMENT**

FIGURE 8–5 CHUNKING. During a game, chess masters remembered the pieces by thinking of them in clusters or chunks. When the masters were confronted with a random arrangement of pieces, they showed no better memory than did beginners, whose performance was almost equally poor in both circumstances (Chase & Simon, 1973).

have taken a test in which you had learned the material but were unable to recall it. There was storage but no retrieval. Specifically, **cuing** is the identification or preparation of some signal, hint, or prompt which can be used to retrieve stored information. Cues can be verbal, visual, auditory, and so forth, ranging from key words to the image of a drawing in a psychology textbook.

In addition to intentional cues, there are spontaneous or unintentional cues, and the closer these are to the original situation, the more likely they are to enhance recall. In **context-dependent memory**, the details of the original setting, where the memory was encoded, can serve as retrieval cues. For example, retrieval may be aided by the presence of the classroom, a friend, or even a lunch box where the material was learned. In **state-dependent memory**, the individual's physical or mental condition may serve as a retrieval cue. If you learned something when you were sad, being in a sad mood may aid that memory. In other words, recall may be enhanced not only by use of the original external cues but also by a return to the original physical or mental state (Bower, 1981).

Not surprisingly, Benjamin was unable to use any such cues. In fact, his encoding of the Greek passages was dubious on all accounts—organization, chunking, and the preparation of cues. These three processes are the chief factors in most memory systems and, as noted at the end of this chapter, they pertain not only to encoding but to storage and retrieval as well.

LONG-TERM MEMORY

Short-term memory involves immediate awareness. The individual is conscious of these memories. The events in long-term memory have been stored, but they do not enter immediate consciousness until the retrieval process begins. In **long-term memory (LTM)** information is retained for *later* use, defined as any interval ranging from 30 or so seconds up to the full life of the organism. It is final storage in the warehouse, not an interim processing stage. It was this aspect of memory that interested Harold Burtt.

Long-term memory differs from short-term memory in another way. It presumably has an unlimited capacity, or at least the limits are not known.

TRANSFER OF INFORMATION. If you listened to a novel list of unrelated words and were asked to recall them shortly thereafter, the outcome would be highly predictable. The first and last words would be most readily recalled. In the **primacy effect,** items at the beginning of a series are better remembered than later ones. In the **recency effect,** items at the end of the list show better recall scores than earlier items. This phenomenon is called the *serial position effect,* meaning that the location of a particular item in a list or passage plays a role in the likelihood that it will be remembered (Figure 8–6).

The serial position effect has several explanations, but two are most relevant to the transfer of information from short-term to long-term memory. First, items at the beginning of the list are

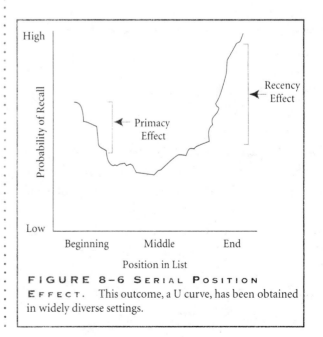

FIGURE 8-6 SERIAL POSITION EFFECT. This outcome, a U curve, has been obtained in widely diverse settings.

most rehearsed. They can be rehearsed until the list grows too long for individual items to be practiced. Second, items at the end of the list are presumably still in short-term memory at the time of recall. In fact, if recall is delayed, the recency effect is sharply diminished (Glanzer & Cunitz, 1966).

The rehearsal process thus plays a role in both instances. This process, incidentally, is sometimes *simple rehearsal*, involving not much more than regular repetition, and sometimes *elaborate rehearsal*, in which the information is processed with special attention to detail and meaning.

The serial position effect also has been obtained with animals. In one study, pigeons, monkeys, and people observed series of four images each. After each series, a test image was presented, and the subjects were trained to indicate whether or not it had appeared in the previous series. In all species, primacy and recency effects were observed. The first and fourth images were recognized with greater accuracy than the others. Furthermore, when the delay between exposure of images was brief, the primacy effect disappeared—apparently for lack of the usual rehearsal of early items. When the delay was lengthy, the recency effect disappeared—apparently because there was no longer any advantage in short-term memory (Wright, Santiago, Sands, Kendrick, & Cook, 1985). This research provides further evidence for the separation between short-term and long-term memory (Squire, Knowlton, & Musen, 1993).

TYPES OF LONG-TERM MEMORY. After decades of research, investigators have decided that long-term memory is not a single element or component. Rather, it consists of several different types, and these multiple kinds of memory appear to be mediated by different brain regions, as is evident in classical conditioning. Memory traces for generalized emotional responses, as in conditioned heart rate and blood pressure, appear to be significantly related to activities in the amygdala. For highly specific conditioned reactions, such as the gagging reflex or eyeblink, another brain area, the cerebellum, plays a critical role (Lavond, Kim, & Thompson, 1993).

One major distinction among the types of long-term memory lies with memory for skills and habits, called *procedural memory*, and memory for facts and events, called *declarative memory*. In **procedural memory,** an individual remembers how to do something, how to perform some act, physical or mental. Procedural memory is involved in making a cup of cocoa, writing a computer program, and playing the trombone.

Most of these memories, especially if complex, are acquired slowly, practiced often, and repeated automatically. If you have learned to use a certain word processor, for example, you perhaps have noticed how much more rapidly and successfully you can do so than when you began, striking the right keys for retrieval, printing, storage, and so forth, often without much thought. There is considerable survival value in procedural memories; they enable us to perform daily habits automatically. And usually our procedural memories are accurate.

We err more often in another type of memory. Called **declarative memory,** it represents a statement of fact; it concerns ideas, dates, definitions, and an endless array of other factual information. The focus is on what, not how. And here two subtypes have been identified. There is, first, **episodic memory,** which involves specific events in the individual's past. There is a time-and-space dimension to episodic memory, directly experienced by the individual. A student says: "I remember that the rain began just as we were entering biology class."

Declarative knowledge of a more general sort, without restriction to time and place, is known as **semantic memory;** it includes mental representation of general ideas and a broad range of information:

the names of animals and plants never encountered directly, their habitats, their organs, their relationships, and countless other pieces of information in biology, for example, and elsewhere. As a rule, we do not remember when such information was acquired. It simply becomes part of our large storehouse of information (Tulving, 1985; Figure 8–7).

Procedural memory is not necessarily better than declarative memory. The outcomes depend on several factors, including prior experience, the number of repetitions, and the effort to remember. Tying shoes and riding a bicycle are well-practiced, well-remembered procedural events. Finding square roots and making Christmas pudding are also procedural memories, rarely practiced and therefore poorly remembered.

Procedural memory, incidentally, often illustrates **implicit memory,** meaning that it can be evoked without conscious effort. A person who has not ridden a bicycle for years simply mounts the vehicle and wheels away—or crashes. In either case, an effort to recall the principles of bicycle riding before attempting the task is of little value. Declarative memory more commonly illustrates **explicit memory,** for it typically involves an intentional, conscious effort to remember. It is formed and utilized with awareness, as when you recite a poem or the basic idea in a book.

STORAGE OF INFORMATION. Are different types of long-term memory stored in different ways? There is considerable speculation on this issue, and three modes of organization have been suggested: schemas and scripts, a conceptual hierarchy, and networks of associations.

Memories of all types are presumed to be stored in a **schema,** which is a general pattern or way of organizing information in a particular culture. For example, when students in England heard a myth told among Native Americans, many elements were foreign to them. When they attempted to recall the myth later, they did so in terms of their own schemas. The tale was organized or adapted to their own patterns of thought. It showed omissions, distortions, and additions reflecting an English way of thinking about things (Bartlett, 1932).

One type of schema often associated with procedural memory is called a **script,** meaning that it depicts a typical sequence of events in a particular setting. It may describe how a specific task is accomplished, or it may indicate more general steps in daily life. College students, for example, have restaurant scripts, dressing scripts, and test-preparation scripts. In the restaurant script there are certain procedures to be followed: obtaining a table, reviewing the menu, ordering a meal, consuming

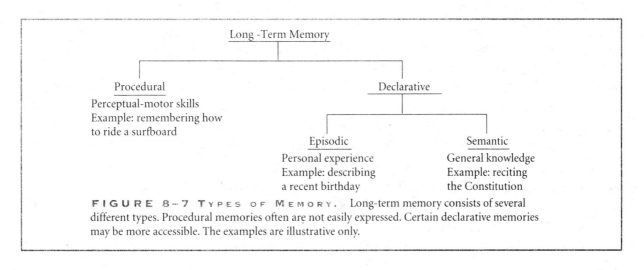

FIGURE 8–7 TYPES OF MEMORY. Long-term memory consists of several different types. Procedural memories often are not easily expressed. Certain declarative memories may be more accessible. The examples are illustrative only.

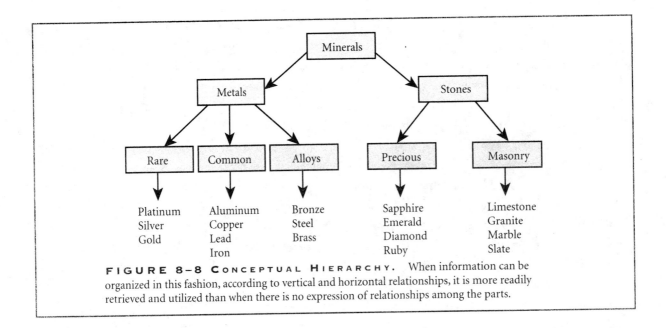

FIGURE 8–8 CONCEPTUAL HIERARCHY. When information can be organized in this fashion, according to vertical and horizontal relationships, it is more readily retrieved and utilized than when there is no expression of relationships among the parts.

the meal, asking for the bill, and so forth. When students were asked to recall procedures for dining in a restaurant, there was high agreement on the script, despite minor variations (Bower, Black, & Turner, 1979).

It is speculated that schemas operate for both input and output of information. Thus, they can be influential while an episodic memory is being constructed, during encoding, and while it is being reconstructed, during retrieval.

Declarative memory, especially, is often considered to be stored according to some hierarchy. In a **conceptual hierarchy,** items with a common property are arranged or classified in a graded order. Our memory of concepts in zoology, for example, includes kingdom, phylum, class, order, and so forth. Similarly, information about government, the church, geology, and other topics is organized this way (Figure 8–8).

In addition, there is considerable speculation about the ways in which semantic memories are reconstructed. The concept of a **network of associations** has been employed here, emphasizing that ideas are connected to each other in patterns,

chains, or pathways, the recall of one idea leading to recall of another, that to another, that to still another, and so forth (Chang, 1986). This viewpoint has a long history, and modern theorists have confirmed it, emphasizing the "spread of activation" from one concept or idea to another. The concept of *red*, for example, is closely associated with the terms for some other colors. It is less closely associated with certain red fruits, such as *cherries* and *apples*. Still other concepts, such as *sunrise* and *sunset*, are even more distantly related (Collins & Loftus, 1975; Figure 8–9).

LEVELS OF PROCESSING

In concluding this discussion of the development of memories, we take a step away from stage theory, which has been valuable in generating research and providing an overall conception of human memory. The stage approach involves considerable hypothesizing, however. Furthermore, the processing of information does not appear to be necessarily sequential. Tracing the flow of information through three stages may fractionate the problem, rather than

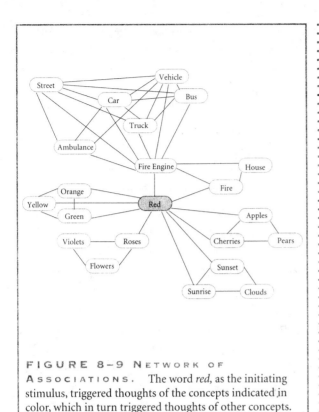

FIGURE 8-9 NETWORK OF ASSOCIATIONS. The word *red*, as the initiating stimulus, triggered thoughts of the concepts indicated in color, which in turn triggered thoughts of other concepts. The shorter lines indicate stronger associations.

give recognition to the presumably interactive and simultaneous processes underlying the memory system as a whole (Atkinson & Shiffrin, 1968, 1971).

A somewhat different view, emerging from stage theory, postulates a *single* memory stage or system. It has arisen because information processing seems to be involved at *all* phases of stage theory. The emphasis, therefore, is on the degree of information processing. According to the **levels-of-processing theory,** information that has been most thoroughly processed, through various cognitive activities on the part of the learner, is most likely to be remembered (Chaik & Lockhart, 1972).

EMPHASIS ON ENCODING. Any modern view of memory, whether or not it postulates stages, gives recognition to encoding, storage, and retrieval. Among levels-of-processing theorists, who

minimize the speculated stages, the emphasis is on the first of these, the encoding process.

In this approach, the short-term memory stage is regarded less as a hypothetical platform and more as a process. If the decision is to store rather than ignore, encoding must commence immediately. According to this view, the extent of encoding determines the level or strength of memory. Information processed only briefly and superficially is not well retained; that which is thoroughly and carefully processed goes into fuller and more permanent storage.

On this basis, the durability of little Benjamin's memory trace was questionable. He heard, perhaps inattentively, passages of a foreign language read aloud by a nearby adult. His father, in contrast, read Sophocles's works himself and probably enjoyed memorizing them, just as he enjoyed recording and remembering the birds in his neighborhood, facts about aviation, and techniques in advertising (Thayer & Austin, 1992). Several cognitive activities undoubtedly went into the formation of all of these memory traces.

DEPTH OF PROCESSING. One danger in the levels-of-processing viewpoint lies in the potential for circular reasoning. Events we remember are those that are fully processed, and when we process events completely, we remember them. It therefore behooves investigators to demonstrate as precisely as possible what is meant by levels of processing and their relationship to encoding.

In one study, subjects were shown a series of words one at a time, each preceded by one of four types of questions. These questions concerned the typeface in which the word appeared, the sound of the word, its category, or its contextual meaning. Believing that the questions constituted a reaction-time test, the subjects answered rapidly for all 36 words, and then an unexpected memory test was administered. It was predicted that memory would be a function of the type of question asked previously, with the question on typeface showing the poorest memory and that on meaning showing the best memory. This result was obtained in several experiments of this sort (Craik & Tulving, 1975).

When the questions merely concerned visual features of the letters, the subjects engaged in shallow processing. Questions about the word's rhyming characteristics prompted an intermediate level of processing. Questions about the word's use in a sentence required the deepest level of processing.

In related experiments, each subject was presented with a series of words and various questions, each question matched to a specific word. Sometimes the question concerned superficial characteristics of the word, such as its length or appearance. How many syllables did it have? Was it written in capital letters? For other words, the questions concerned meaning. Did the word refer to a tool? Was it a synonym for another word? Then the subjects were asked to recall the list of words, a task that they had not anticipated. As predicted, they recalled the words followed by questions about meaning more readily than those followed by superficial questions concerning form and length. Again, it was concluded that depth of processing was a central factor in recall (Parkin, 1984).

CONSTRUCTION AND RECONSTRUCTION. Encoding involves construction, and retrieval also seems to involve construction. It might be argued that both processes involve reconstruction, as well. In any case, the stage approach and the levels-of-processing view are both concerned with the details of these construction processes, although in different ways, and both have asked useful research questions.

In an extended series of studies involving stories and visual figures, reconstructive changes were of three types: simplification, elaboration, and con-ventionalization. In *simplification*, parts of the original story or drawing did not appear in the reproduction. The general features and theme of a scene were retained, but certain details were omitted in telling the story or making the drawing. Certain other details were overemphasized, in the process called *elaboration*, presumably at the expense of the omitted details. A facial feature, mood, or weapon was recalled as larger, more intense, or more prominent than it had been in the original version, especially if it was important to the story. And finally, in *conventionalization*, strange or unfamiliar details were changed into more familiar forms. An unusual object was recalled in a more familiar design (Bartlett, 1932; Figure 8–10).

Reconstruction during the retrieval phase was also demonstrated when subjects watched a videotape of an automobile accident and later were questioned about it. One group was asked about the speed of the cars when they *hit* each other. The other group was asked about the speed of the cars when they *smashed into* each other. Some days afterward, all subjects were asked whether or not there was broken glass at the accident, and the results showed the expected, reconstructive pattern. Among subjects asked earlier what happened when the cars hit each other, 14% recalled broken glass. Among those asked earlier what happened when the cars smashed into each other, 32% recalled broken glass, although there was none at the scene of the accident (Loftus & Palmer, 1974).

Efforts to deal with these numerous facts and theories about the construction of memory have resulted in a **connectionist model** of the mind emphasizing associations among concepts, sensations, and other elements. Describing the workings of the mind in perception and thought, as well as memory, it has been useful in guiding research (Rumelhart, McClelland, & the PDP Research Group, 1986). In general terms, it assumes that the strength of associations among ideas, feelings, or

174

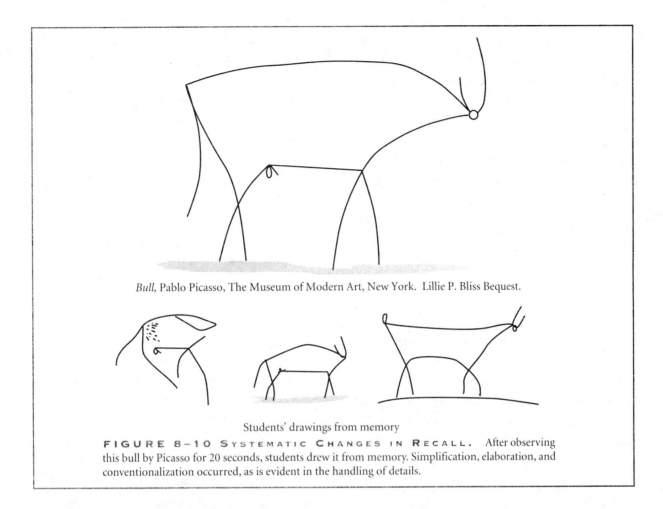

Bull, Pablo Picasso, The Museum of Modern Art, New York. Lillie P. Bliss Bequest.

Students' drawings from memory

FIGURE 8-10 SYSTEMATIC CHANGES IN RECALL. After observing this bull by Picasso for 20 seconds, students drew it from memory. Simplification, elaboration, and conventionalization occurred, as is evident in the handling of details.

memories reflects comparable associations among sets of neurons in the nervous system.

• THE MEMORY TRACE •

Five years after he had read and reread Sophocles's passages, Harold Burtt turned to the next phase in this research. It was time to find out what had transpired in the mind of little Benjamin. Harold remembered the passages. Did Benjamin remember them too?

When storage occurs, it must be based on some change within the individual. Sometimes called a **memory trace** or *engram*, this molecular change is presumed to lie in the nervous system, but we do not yet know with certainty what structures or functions are modified or even whether the concept of a trace is an appropriate description of memory storage (Estes, 1991a). Therefore, some psychologists measure memory indirectly, focusing only on behavior. Others investigate the physiology of memory, focusing on its biochemical bases. One vital concern in memory research is the development of connections between these behavioral and neurological approaches (Hintzman, 1990).

MEASUREMENT OF MEMORY

Psychologists who study memory by examining behavior have developed three methods for measuring memory: recall, recognition, and relearning.

175

METHOD OF RECALL. Harold Burtt began by using the method of recall, which is the most difficult memory task. In **recall,** the person is asked to reproduce a prior experience in any convenient manner, although the instructions may vary somewhat. In *free recall,* there is no significant prompting or cue. A common request is simply: "Tell what you remember" (Figure 8–11). Harold asked Benjamin to relate whatever he could of the original Greek passages, but the boy was completely puzzled. He had no idea that he had ever heard them previously. What did his father mean? What was this all about? Benjamin showed no recall whatsoever, perhaps a disappointing result in view of all the effort by his father.

When various signals or hints are offered, the procedure is called *cued recall.* In the courtroom, a witness might be asked: "Now tell me about the sounds. Do you remember any particular sounds or words?" Cued recall is sometimes called **redintegration,** from *re + integration,* for cues are given to make recall easier. One part is recalled or some prompt is given, and then another part is recalled from this information. Courtroom testimony typically begins with free recall, and when an impasse is reached, cued recall is sometimes used. With eight-year-old Benjamin, even cued recall was of no help.

Especially when remembering visual stimuli, some people give exceptionally accurate testimony without any prompting. This phenomenon, most common in children, is known as **eidetic imagery,** or *photographic memory,* meaning a memory image that possesses the details of a photograph or hallucination. In hallucinations, the person believes the image represents something immediately present in the outer environment. People with eidetic imagery know that they are responding only to an image in the mind.

Sometimes recall is surprisingly accurate and automatic in many people. In **flashbulb memory,** certain details of an emotional experience are recalled with unusual ease and almost perceptual accuracy, as though the event was still in process (Brown & Kulik, 1977). Where were you when you learned of the space capsule *Challenger'*s explosion? Describe the circumstances at the birth of a sibling, death of a pet, or your first kiss. Events of deep personal significance, especially if they occur unexpectedly, often are very well remembered, as if a flash bulb had recorded every detail. The most responsible factors seem to be powerful emotional content and the uniqueness of the event (Sadowski & Quast, 1990).

METHOD OF RECOGNITION. Clearly easier than recall, in a test of **recognition** the previously encountered object or event is merely selected from a series of others not previously encountered. When a witness cannot recall any characteristics of a suspect, a lineup is prepared, and the witness tries to pick the correct person from the group. The information is available. The task is to identify it.

After it was clear that Benjamin had no recall, his father read to him some of the original Greek selections and asked if they seemed familiar. Again, the boy showed no memory whatsoever. Then he

FIGURE 8–11 RECALL TASK. In the space above this caption, draw or write a description of the illustration for the narrative at the beginning of this chapter, depicting the story of Benjamin Burtt and his Greek lessons. This task involves recall.

included some other passages, and still Benjamin showed no recognition.

Despite Benjamin's failure, recognition memory is remarkably successful. People who lament their poor memories are invariably referring to recall, not recognition, for research shows our tremendous capacity for this type of memory. In one instance, students were exposed to approximately 600 randomly selected visual stimuli, called an inspection series. Then some of the stimuli were paired with new stimuli, and the subjects were asked which member of the pair had been seen previously. The median correct recognition score was 88% for sentences, 90% for words, and 99% for pictures (Shepard, 1967). With 10,000 pictures, another researcher concluded that there is no recognizable limit for this type of visual memory (Standing, 1973).

Any recognition task depends heavily on the similarity of the alternatives, however. A teacher or experimenter can make up multiple-choice items that are extremely easy or difficult, depending on the information in the alternatives (Figure 8–12).

Occasionally, we find ourselves in the opposite situation, thinking that we recognize a certain person or place even though we know that cannot be possible. This feeling is referred to as a **déjà vu experience,** defined as an *incorrect* impression that the whole event has been encountered previously (Sno & Linszen, 1990). The French word *déjà* means "already." It *seems* we have already experienced a certain situation, and yet we realize that prior experience is impossible. This feeling arises because some specific part of the new situation—something as subtle as a slight odor, texture, rhythm, or color—is familiar, and then we make the incorrect assumption that the whole scene is familiar.

Sailing into a dozen Mediterranean seaports for the first time years ago, a man believed that he had visited each of them already, although that was impossible. Finally, he decided that this reaction arose because every seaport smelled of fish, seaweed, salt, and gasoline; otherwise, they were quite different. Odors perhaps mask the newness of the rest of a scene, resulting in a déjà vu experience, a view not yet fully confirmed (Sno, Schalken, & de Jonghe, 1992).

Reference to déjà vu is widely made and misused in daily life, as a dramatic way of stating that an event has occurred previously. On seeing the same unusual play twice in a baseball game, Yogi Berra exclaimed, only half-joking, "It's déjà vu all over again!" It was not déjà vu again; it was not even

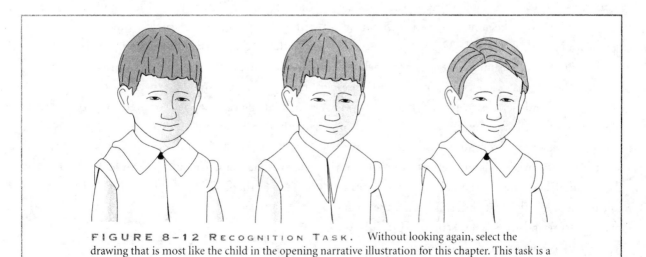

FIGURE 8-12 RECOGNITION TASK. Without looking again, select the drawing that is most like the child in the opening narrative illustration for this chapter. This task is a test of recognition.

déjà vu. It was merely the same play happening twice.

METHOD OF RELEARNING. After Benjamin failed at both recall and recognition, Harold Burtt turned to relearning, the only remaining test of memory. As a method of measuring small amounts of memory, this approach is even more sensitive than recognition. In **relearning,** the individual learns the task again to the original level of success, and the effort required to relearn is compared with the original effort. If relearning is easier, presumably it is because some memory trace remains.

A bright, curious little boy now in elementary school, eight-year-old Benjamin cooperated with his father's request. He listened to his father reading aloud each of ten Greek passages once daily, day after day. The father read at a steady pace, always pausing for 15 seconds after each passage. After 18 days, the father changed to a procedure he called *prompting.* He read very slowly, requesting Benjamin to supply any words he could at the proper point. As these prompting trials continued, the father read less and less, paused more and more, and thereby allowed his son to supply more and more of the missing parts. Their mutual goal was that Benjamin, at some point, would be able to recite each passage in its entirety, from beginning to end, without any help from his father (Burtt, 1932).

Unknown to Benjamin, these passages included seven of the original 21 selections mixed with three new ones. Would he relearn the original selections more easily than the new ones?

This relearning procedure produces a **savings score,** which shows how much effort is saved from the original learning. If the subject demonstrates full memory on the first relearning trial, the memory is perfect and the savings score is 100%. If the number of relearning trials is the same as the original effort, there is no savings. The savings score is zero, and there is no memory. This procedure has been used effectively with a wide variety of subjects, ranging from insects to rhesus monkeys (Minami & Dallenbach, 1946; Swartz, Chen, & Terrace, 1991).

With Benjamin, the relearning procedure involved a deviation from the usual method, for at 15 months of age, when the research began, he certainly could not learn the passages by himself. For this reason, his father read them aloud 90 times each. Then, five years later, when Benjamin "relearned" these passages, his father read them again. We know of these efforts through Professor Burtt's report in a psychology journal, *An Experimental Study of Early Childhood Memory* (1932).

Finally, after more than a year and one-half, Benjamin reached the point of mastery. He had recited each of the passages once, entirely by himself, without error.

With considerable interest, Professor Burtt analyzed the results. He found that Benjamin had needed an average of 317 trials to relearn the original passages. For the new ones, he had required 435 trials. Benjamin thereby gave clear evidence, five years later, of memory for a significant portion of the earlier material. The overall savings score was 27% (Table 8–2).

Each of the seven passages Benjamin relearned came from a different period in his infancy, one of them from age 15 months, another from 18 months, and so forth, up to the last period, beginning at 33 months. Comparison of these results showed what one might expect. The passages presented at the earliest ages required the most relearning, but there were savings even for these passages. Harold Burtt had achieved his first aim. He had shown that human memories could be established as early as the first 15 months of life (Burtt, 1932).

❧

PHYSIOLOGICAL BASES

How do we explain Benjamin's 27% savings score, showing that he remembered material read to him

TYPE OF PASSAGE	TRIALS REQUIRED
Original	
1	382
2	253
3	385
4	379
5	328
6	226
7	265
Average	317
Control	
1	409
2	451
3	445
Average	435

Learning trials for control passages	435
Relearning trials for original passages	−317
Difference	118

$$\frac{435 - 317}{435} = \frac{118}{435} = 27\%$$

TABLE 8-2 RELEARNING AFTER FIVE YEARS. The figures show the average number of trials required for Benjamin to relearn seven original and three comparison passages, resulting in a savings score of 27%.

even before he had mastered language? What happened to Benjamin? What changes occurred in his underlying physiology? Attempts to locate the origins of memory in the nervous system, like the elusive sources of the Nile, have led to considerable speculation.

EVIDENCE IN BIOCHEMISTRY. Early investigations of ribonucleic acid (RNA), which is particularly influential in cell development, have shown the hope and frustration in this work. In these experiments, it was demonstrated that tiny flatworms learned and retained a classically conditioned response (Thompson & McConnell, 1955). Furthermore, when RNA was extracted from the tissues of the trained worms and injected into untrained worms, they learned the response more rapidly (McConnell, 1972). Such research suggested that memory might be transferred through chemistry, and RNA appeared to be *the* memory molecule.

However, there were several limitations in this research, the most important of which has been the difficulty in replicating it. Even the original investigators at times have been unsuccessful, even with larger animals, such as rats and fish. Instead, it appears that other chemical substances may have been involved. Furthermore, it seems that RNA molecules may simply enhance learning in some way, perhaps through protein production, rather than influencing memory per se (Guyette, Chavis, & Shearer, 1980). Quantitative changes in RNA and protein synthesis occur during learning, but there is little evidence that these changes are the fundamental bases of memory (Squire, 1987).

More promising findings have been obtained in recent clinical and experimental studies of neurotransmitter substances. As we saw in the chapter on the biological foundations of behavior, there are transmitters in the synapses for all sorts of human experiences, including sleep, pain, eating, emotion, and memory. For example, patients with Alzheimer's disease, who suffer from pronounced memory loss, show diminished synthesis of acetylcholine, important in cognitive functioning. Several other neurotransmitters, primarily norepinephrine and dopamine, also seem to modulate the development of memory (Morley & Flood, 1990).

The role of transmitter substances was supported when adults learned a 20-word list and a half hour later received either an intravenous infusion of one milligram of physostigmine, a substance that arouses diverse physiological activities, or one milligram of a saline solution, serving as a placebo. Eighteen minutes after the infusion and again 80 minutes afterward, the subjects attempted to recall as many words as possible. In the first recall trial, at 18 minutes, the subjects given physostigmine showed superior memory, and at 80 minutes the difference in favor of physostigmine was even greater (Davis, Mohs, Tinklenberg, Pfefferbaum, Hollister, & Koppell, 1978).

However, physostigmine is an energizer, and a mild dose of caffeine, nicotine, or another stimulant may temporarily increase performance. If we gave little Benjamin a stimulant, even he for a while might do better on something he already knew. It is unlikely that stimulants act only on memory per se, and thus the nature of the synaptic change, chemical or structural, is still uncertain.

One promising area of investigation concerns **long-term potentiation,** which is a sustained, permanent increase in the strength of a synaptic connection. The nerve pathway becomes more readily excitable on a long-term basis. This outcome was demonstrated by stimulating nerve tissue in the brain with a weak electric current and measuring the response. Afterward, when the same neural pathway was stimulated again, it gave a stronger response, and this greater response strength was observed again on later occasions. Highly complex biochemical reactions in the synapses, including protein synthesis, are presumed to be responsible for the increased excitability in long-term potentiation (Lynch & Baudry, 1984).

EVIDENCE IN BRAIN AREAS. For hundreds of years, the role of the brain in human memory has been recognized. But which parts play special roles? One answer to this question is the cerebral cortex, a massive mantle of cells discussed extensively in the chapter on biological foundations of behavior. The most advanced brain structure in an evolutionary sense, it is fundamentally involved in associative thinking and therefore in the retrieval of stored information.

Further studies have pointed to a smaller, subcortical organ, stimulated in studies of long-term potentiation. The **hippocampus** is a curved structure in the temporal lobes of the brain, named for the Latin word for "sea horse," in reference to its shape. Brain injuries from tumor, lack of oxygen, and surgery, as well as controlled studies with animals, cite functions of the hippocampus in memory (Macphail, 1986; Sutherland & McDonald, 1990). It seems to play a central role in *establishing* long-term memories, uniting separate pieces of information into an integrated, whole memory. Later, with the passage of time, this stored memory becomes relatively less dependent on the hippocampus and related structures (Squire & Zola-Morgan, 1991).

In one instance, H. M., a man in his twenties, underwent surgery for epileptic seizures that had beset him since childhood. Before the surgery he was above average in intelligence, as he was afterward, and his memory was normal. But following surgery and a hippocampal lesion, he experienced **anterograde amnesia,** in which no new memories can be established. H. M. could not remember new events in his life, a condition that enormously disrupted his social life. He could make no new friends, for he could not remember having met them. He was a social bore, not recalling what he had just said to anyone (Milner, Corkin, & Teuber, 1968).

Follow-up studies have shown that H. M. can learn *some new motor skills*, such as completing a puzzle or some other simple hand–eye coordination task. He cannot recall having mastered the new task, treating it later as though it were completely new, but he can perform it, even after a lapse of several weeks (Graf, Squire, & Mandler, 1984).

Another form of amnesia, **retrograde amnesia,** also experienced by H. M., involves a loss of memory for old experiences, especially those preceding the traumatic event. The afflicted individual is unable to recall the previous details, such as going to work, reaching the construction site, mounting the framework, reaching for a certain tool, and so forth. A similar form of forgetting may occur more briefly, and in a lesser degree, among people who have received electroconvulsive therapy. In both cases, if memory improves there is a gradual recovery of memory for events closer and closer to the traumatic episode; those immediately preceding it are the last to be remembered, if recovered at all (Figure 8–13).

MULTIPLE BASES OF MEMORY.

It appears that memory cannot be assigned to any particular biochemical element or brain area. The hippocampus may play a special role in the retention of factual information. Memories for procedures—on how to accomplish certain routine tasks—may be stored elsewhere in the brain (Squire, 1987). The site for a particular engram, or memory trace, appears to be partly specific, partly distributed. It may be specific in the sense that certain *sets* of neurons must be activated; it may be distributed in the sense that several brain areas—the hippocampus, cortex, cerebellum, amygdala, and other regions—also play a role (Rosenzweig, 1996).

One fact seems certain: If memory is to occur, some new neural connections must be formed or some old ones must be functionally elaborated.

STRUCTURE OF THE TRACE

In considering the physiological basis of memory, wherever its location, one might ask an equally compelling question: How does the trace work? What is its structure? Two basic hypotheses have been developed about the structure of the memory trace.

REAPPEARANCE HYPOTHESIS.

Spectacular events in brain surgery seem to support the view that memory in some way involves a permanent rearrangement of molecules, just as there is a lasting electromagnetic realignment of particles in a recording tape. This structural alteration, through prior experience, creates a trace that, if properly aroused, will reproduce the event in exact detail, just like the electromagnetic tape. According to this view, Benjamin Burtt would have a full memory of the earlier Greek passages if the proper traces were activated.

Patients' experiences in psychoanalysis, reporting long-forgotten childhood events, add further support to this view, popular for centuries. This outlook, the **reappearance hypothesis,** implies that a full memory will appear whenever the trace is properly retrieved. There is no memory loss; the complete experience is retained, somehow filed away in static fashion, waiting to be aroused. Forgetting is not a failure of storage but rather a failure to retrieve the existing information.

This possibility seemed all the more promising after some midcentury experiments by a well-known Canadian brain surgeon, Wilder Penfield. Patients often remain conscious during such surgery, with only a local anesthetic, for no pain is experienced in the brain itself. With the brain exposed, Penfield stimulated with a needle electrode various regions of the brain of an epileptic person, chiefly to identify possible areas of origin of the

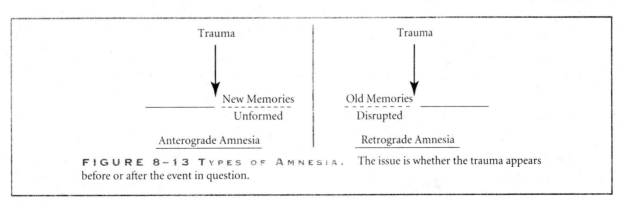

FIGURE 8-13 TYPES OF AMNESIA. The issue is whether the trauma appears before or after the event in question.

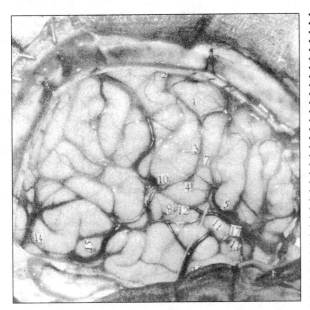

FIGURE 8-14 REAPPEARANCE HYPOTHESIS. Electrical stimulation at point 13 produced descriptions of hearing voices and seeing a circus wagon. The patient was told that the stimulation would be repeated. It was not, and she made no report. Then the same point was stimulated again, eliciting further details about the same voice (Penfield, 1958).

seizures. As he did so, the patient gave detailed reports of immediate experiences, such as seeing lights and hearing sounds. More important, with stimulation in other areas, the patient seemed to be reporting memories: circus wagons in childhood, prior work as a stenographer, and a play seen earlier (Penfield, 1958; Figure 8–14).

RECONSTRUCTION HYPOTHESIS. A contrasting hypothesis states that memories are not fixed images but rather reconstructions. A memory trace is a partial residue from the past, and current memories are built on these remnants. In the **reconstruction hypothesis,** bits and pieces of experience are used to assemble a memory (Neisser, 1967). To recall the Greek lessons, Benjamin would have to reassemble them and fill in the gaps with logic and expectations.

From this perspective, the surgical studies of brain stimulation have been criticized on several grounds. First, they provide no convincing evidence that the patient's report is a memory rather than a fantasy or even a dream. Furthermore, there is no evidence that the report is accurate or even complete. And finally, even if the reports do constitute accurate memories, there is still no evidence that all of our memories are retained permanently (Loftus & Loftus, 1980; Neisser, 1967).

In fact, if every experience remained in permanent storage, totally intact, life could become extremely difficult. Our retrieval system would constantly be overloaded, beset with major thoughts and insignificant matters.

William James advocated the reconstruction view, believing that a permanently existing memory image was highly unlikely. This perspective seems the more probable today, especially according to modern cognitive psychologists. In the levels-of-processing theory and even according to stage theory, memory is regarded as a dynamic process, not a passive experience, a view that has important implications for the ways in which we develop successful memory.

• THEORIES OF FORGETTING •

Around the time of Benjamin's thirteenth birthday, his father gave him a surprise—one the boy was likely to remember. He asked Benjamin to undertake his Greek lessons again. Would Benjamin memorize another ten passages?

So Harold Burtt devoted himself to this second follow-up study. This time, in recognition of Benjamin's greater maturity, he read the ten passages aloud twice daily, again using a rotated sequence. He began with a different passage each day in order to avoid devoting special attention to one passage or another.

Professor Burtt reported that his son's attitude was better than in the earlier tests "because he understood the scientific importance to a greater extent." And certainly Benjamin was a vastly improved learner. In addition, he knew that after he had mastered a certain passage, he would be through with it. On this basis, he required an average of only 149 trials to relearn the original selections. For the new ones, he needed 162 trials. This difference resulted in a savings score of 8%. The memory trace for the original passages was still there, but compared with the earlier savings of 27%, it was unquestionably weaker. Here again Benjamin had no idea which selections he had heard previously and which were new. His father noted all of these findings in a follow-up report, *A Further Study of Early Childhood Memory* (Burtt, 1937; Table 8–3).

This further loss on Benjamin's part brings us to the question of **forgetting**, defined as the inability to recall, to recognize, or to relearn at an improved rate. This condition may be due to storage failure, in which the information was not adequately maintained in the repository, or it may be due to retrieval failure, in which the trace was present but could not be evoked for lack of an appropriate cue. Also, it might have been an encoding failure, in which the information was never fully entered and never became a memory in the first place. Benjamin showed only 8% savings at age 13, partly because at age 3 he had been listening essentially to nonsense syllables, which show a rapid rate of forgetting.

We now turn to several theories that attempt to explain not the rate of forgetting but why memory failures occur at all. These theories of forgetting show once again that psychology is guided by diverse interpretations of its findings.

DECAY THEORY

Benjamin's latest savings score indicated that 92% of the original material had become inaccessible or lost. How did this happen?

According to the **decay theory**, which has much popular appeal, the memory trace deteriorates unless it is used. There is a storage failure, possibly a result of the continuous metabolic action of the cells of the nervous system. The lapse of time, according to this view, may be responsible for forgetting. When you memorize a telephone number and fail to remember it days later, it seems that the memory has just faded away.

Providing clear evidence for decay theory is extremely difficult because the processes postulated in the other theories of forgetting, such as interference and repression, presumably occur at the same time. Thus, the influence of decay alone cannot be readily demonstrated. Some evidence comes from a human adult who lost his sight at the age of two years. When he recovered it years later, he showed no memory of prior visual learning, behaving in the same fashion as someone who was born blind (Hebb, 1966). However, the force of this example is weakened by the fact that children seem to develop and organize their memories differently from adults.

Further claims come from short-term memory experiments, in which much information is lost in just a few seconds. Decay theorists stress that our capacity for processing information is limited and

TYPE OF PASSAGE	TRIALS REQUIRED
Original	
1	142
2	139
3	169
4	151
5	145
6	169
7	127
Average	149
Control	
1	169
2	151
3	166
Average	162

Learning trials for control passages	162
Relearning trials for original passages	−149
Difference	13

$$\frac{162 - 149}{162} = \frac{13}{162} = 8\%$$

TABLE 8–3 RELEARNING AFTER TEN YEARS. The figures show the average number of trials required for Benjamin to relearn seven original and three comparison passages, resulting in a savings score of 8%.

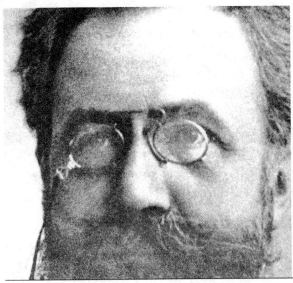

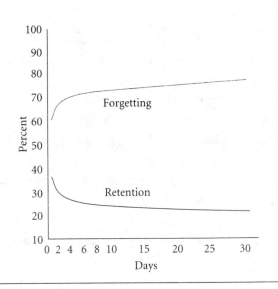

FIGURE 8–15 HERMANN EBBINGHAUS'S MEMORY CURVE.
Despite deficiencies in his work, Ebbinghaus inaugurated the use of quantitative methods in investigating memory. In these curves, obtained by using nonsense syllables, forgetting is the percentage lost; retention is the percentage retained.

that rehearsal prevents decay, chiefly by keeping the material active. When rehearsing stops, decay begins, independently of any outside interference. This theory lacks support, but it is also difficult to demonstrate that there is no deterioration of the memory trace with time.

Hermann Ebbinghaus, a significant figure in early studies of memory, served as his own subject, memorizing over 2,000 nonsense syllables altogether. Devised to provide a large quantity of unfamiliar material for memorization, each syllable was formed by placing a vowel between two consonants. Ebbinghaus memorized each list of several syllables until he could recite it perfectly, and then he tested himself on this material at several later dates. He found that about half of the material was forgotten after just 20 minutes, two-thirds after two days, and almost 80% by the end of the month. Forgetting was rapid at first and then slow (Ebbinghaus, 1913; Figure 8–15).

Later investigators, using many subjects and averaging the results, verified the general slope of the curve that Ebbinghaus found. However, this curve applies only to nonsense material, such as

Ebbinghaus's syllables and little Benjamin's foreign language passages and even here, there is no direct evidence for decay theory.

OBLITERATION OF THE TRACE

Another view that postulates a storage failure focuses on sudden destruction of a trace, presumably in its formative stages, rather than slow deterioration of a well-established trace simply through disuse. According to **obliteration theory,** the trace needs time to become firmly fixed. Certain conditions occurring soon after an experience can eradicate the memory before it becomes permanent.

Various experiments with rats, fish, and other animals have shown the importance of the time factor in obliteration of the memory trace. When rats were given electroconvulsive shocks at several later intervals following the original learning, a test of retention showed that the sooner the shock was administered, the larger was the disruption. When a shock occurred immediately after learning, forgetting was most pervasive (Pinel & Cooper, 1966).

184

This memory disruption apparently occurs by preventing protein synthesis, considered earlier as a possible chemical basis of memory through RNA. In one experiment, goldfish learned to avoid an electric shock by swimming to the darker end of the tank. Immediately after this learning, some of the fish were injected with puromycin, a substance that interferes with protein synthesis. These fish seemed to forget completely what they had just learned. When other fish were injected with puromycin an hour later, memory was unaffected, and injections approximately one half hour after the training resulted in an intermediate memory loss (Agranoff, 1967). As in electroconvulsive shock, the amount of memory loss seems to be closely related to the time of the obliterating stimulus.

In a very different, early experiment, college students, one by one, sat in a lighted room and learned a list of nonsense syllables. Then, to provide a brief rest, some were given simple jokes to read, and afterward they were asked to recall the syllables. For others, the rest period was no joke. Quite unexpectedly, the back of the chair collapsed; an electric shock occurred in the arms of the chair; scrap metal fell from the ceiling; a pistol shot rang out; and the lights went off, producing total darkness. When tested after this commotion, most subjects were in a state of collapse and shock themselves, and they forgot most of the list. One subject could not remember any syllables at all (Harden, 1930).

Take consolation in knowing that you did not participate in that research. According to the code of ethics of the American Psychological Association, it certainly would not be permitted today without the subjects' informed consent, however that might be defined. That investigator scared the nonsense out of those students.

In daily life, people often have amnesia for events immediately preceding or following an emotional upset, but investigators do not know how an emotional trauma interferes with retention. Nor do they fully understand the way in which electroconvulsive shock and lack of protein synthesis disrupt memory. It seems clear, however, that the trace needs time to consolidate or set and that immediate physical *or* emotional shock may disrupt the consolidation process (Squire, 1987).

INTERFERENCE THEORY

Aside from the encoding problem, Benjamin's memory loss might be explained on the basis of interference theory, and his father had been concerned about this possibility. According to **interference theory,** information is lost from memory because it is disturbed or displaced by other information. These disturbances can occur at any time, and therefore the memory problem can be either a storage failure or a retrieval failure (Tulving & Psotka, 1971).

PROACTIVE INTERFERENCE. When memory of earlier learning disrupts the recall of something learned later, the condition is called **proactive interference.** The disruptive events occur *before* the learning in question (Table 8–4).

Children are sometimes remarkable in their accurate recall of a holiday or birthday, often with far more details than the parents. Among the possible explanations, one lies with proactive interference. The child has experienced only a few such occasions before the most recent one. The parents may have been exposed to 40 or more, leaving significant opportunities for interference. When young adults and elderly subjects were compared for facial recognition, a relatively easy task, the results showed a

	LEARNING	LEARNING	RECALL
I	History	Sociology	Sociology
II	—	Sociology	Sociology

TABLE 8–4 PROACTIVE INTERFERENCE. For Group I, learning history disrupted recall of later learning, a sociology assignment.

memory deficit among the elderly, speculated to be the result of proactive interference from previously viewed faces (Flicker, Ferris, Crook, & Bartus, 1989).

Proactive interference is sometimes said to account for certain results obtained by Hermann Ebbinghaus, who found more rapid forgetting than is generally reported today. Since Ebbinghaus learned thousands of nonsense syllables during his experiments, it is quite likely that the earlier learning interfered with the later learning and memory.

RETROACTIVE INTERFERENCE. Another type of interference follows the opposite model. In **retroactive interference,** memories of later experiences disrupt the recall of something learned earlier. The disruptive events occur *after* the learning in question (Table 8–5).

In one instance, college students memorized lists of nonsense syllables and then engaged in various activities or went to sleep. Retention was tested one, two, four, and eight hours later, and it was found that memory was better after any amount of sleep than after a comparable amount of time spent while awake (Jenkins & Dallenbach, 1924; Figure 8–16).

Do these findings pertain to prose, as well as to nonsense syllables? When 391 university students attempted to recall prose passages after exposure to various types of intervening information, retroactive interference occurred just as reliably as it did with nonprose material (Dempster, 1988).

In one early investigation, cockroaches were selected for study because they can be made to remain motionless for long periods of time without the use of drugs or other agents that might disrupt the nervous system. They become completely still when their bodies are in extensive contact with an external object, producing a state of inactivity known as tonic immobility. After three groups of cockroaches learned a simple maze, one group was rendered immobile by inducing them to crawl into a box of tissue paper. A second group was allowed to run freely in their cages. The third group was more active than usual, for these roaches were placed on a moving treadmill. Like pedestrians in a modern airport, they had to keep moving to avoid falling off the treadmill or bumping into a wall. Memory was measured by relearning, and the savings scores clearly favored the motionless group. The normally active subjects performed at an intermediate level. Those trudging on the treadmill needed the most relearning trials. In fact, they showed no memory at all (Minami & Dallenbach, 1946).

These outcomes suggest that forgetting is caused by *what happens* during the passage of time. As we go back and forth on the subway, shuttle about in our cars, and run around town, are we literally losing our minds—or at least our memories? The potentially disruptive influence of such events makes interference theory a recurring issue and decay theory an elusive research topic (Hall, Bernoties, & Schmidt, 1995).

Benjamin's memory loss, if explained on the basis of interference theory, would not be significantly attributed to proactive interference. The original learning, so early in life, left relatively little chance for this type of interference. All sorts of subsequent activities could have disrupted later recall, providing a case for retroactive interference.

Interference theory, incidentally, offers an explanation for the *serial position effect* in long-term memory. If a student memorized Lincoln's Gettysburg Address and then tried to recite it years later, the best remembered parts would be the beginning and ending. Earlier, we noted that rehearsal could account for this outcome when the recall task occurs shortly after learning. But even for

	LEARNING	LEARNING	RECALL
I	Algebra	Chemistry	Algebra
II	Algebra	—	Algebra

TABLE 8–5 RETROACTIVE INTERFERENCE. For Group I, learning chemistry symbols disrupted recall of earlier learning, an algebra assignment.

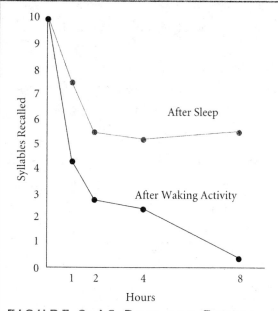

FIGURE 8-16 REST AND RECALL.
Many investigations show that the best preparation for an examination, *after* studying, is a good night's sleep (Jenkins & Dallenbach, 1924).

material learned years ago, the beginning and ending are the favored positions. For the first part of the contents, there can be no proactive interference due to prior material; for the end, there can be no retroactive interference due to subsequent material.

MOTIVATED FORGETTING

Our final view of forgetting, like obliteration theory, does not seem highly relevant in Benjamin's case. It did not emerge through laboratory studies of information processing but rather from Freud's clinical studies of people with adjustment problems. The memory problem is one of retrieval, not storage. In **motivated forgetting,** the full memory trace is presumably available, but the individual does not want to remember. Loss of memory is produced by an unconscious effort to forget, called *repression,* thereby ridding oneself of anxiety, frustration, or some other emotional concern.

Sigmund Freud once came across a name in his medical records and could not recall the patient at all, even though he had treated her for many weeks just six months earlier. Finally, information on his fees brought back all of the facts about the case. The patient was a 14-year-old girl who showed an anxiety reaction that was readily treated, although she still complained of stomach pains. Then, two months later, she suddenly died of sarcoma in the abdomen. Freud was deeply troubled, saddened, and embarrassed by the case, for while the obvious anxiety reaction held his attention, he had over-looked the first signs of the insidious physical ailment (Freud, 1914). Thus, it came to him as no surprise that he was motivated to forget that case.

According to modern psychoanalytic theory, repression can take place not only after the event has occurred but also while it is happening. In other words, repression may become a factor in the initial stages of memory formation, during encoding, and perhaps even in storage. If it takes place while a traumatic event is being encoded, that memory will be particularly inaccessible, for it will be poorly recorded in the first place (Bonanno, 1990).

Many psychologists are not satisfied with the concept of repression. Some point out that forget-ting of negatively toned material may occur simply because there is no effort to remember the experi-ence. Others prefer simpler explanations, especially interference theory.

The role of repression cannot be evaluated in Benjamin's case. The fact that Benjamin could not recall or even recognize the passages, but did show some memory through relearning, indicates that a partial trace remained from the earlier experience. No effort to stimulate that residue evoked a full, intact memory, however, as postulated in motivated forgetting.

• PRINCIPLES OF MEMORIZING •

The reader keeping track of Benjamin's efforts has perhaps surmised that he still had more work to do. His father had read

21 Greek passages in infancy, seven of which were relearned in childhood and seven in adolescence. The remaining seven, with three control passages, would provide one final test in adulthood, at 18 years of age. And they provide an opportunity for comparing the various theories of forgetting (Table 8-6).

This time Benjamin learned more slowly, perhaps because he was tired of this recurring task, every five years, and perhaps because he *was* experiencing some confusion with certain syllables learned earlier. Those from his effort at age 13 at times seemed to disrupt him. And this time, alas, he needed an average of 189 trials for the original passages and 191 for the new ones. The difference was negligible, producing a savings score of 1%. These results left no doubt about what had happened. No significant memory remained at all (Table 8–7).

The effects of the recitations in infancy, definitely manifest at age eight, still evident at age 13, had completely disappeared by age 18. Professor Burtt described this result with professional objectivity in his last report of this work, *An Experimental Study of Early Childhood Memory: Final Report* (1941).

In the last few years, all remaining traces of the stimulation in infancy had disappeared. But why? We have speculated about interference, decay, and even repression, all concerned with storage or retrieval, but something more can be said—about Benjamin's mode of encoding. When the syllables were read to Benjamin in his infancy, he had not mastered his own language, and language can play a vital role in memory. More important, Benjamin had no intention of remembering these syllables.

ROLE OF MOTIVATION

The acquisition of knowledge or a skill without the aim of mastering it is known as *incidental learning*. If you know the name of the city in which this book was published, that information is incidental learning—unless the instructor announced that you must know it for an examination. In contrast, *intentional learning* means that the memory has been acquired with effort, along the lines of the encoding procedures discussed earlier, so completely ignored by Benjamin. The intention to learn is usually vital for long-term storage.

What appears to be forgetting may occur simply because there was no impression, or an inadequate one, in the first place. We fail to remember names, and even passages from rituals recited hundreds of times, because we were inattentive when they were spoken. We do not remember certain details of an exciting event due to concentra-

THEORY	TYPE OF PROBLEM	REASON FOR MEMORY LOSS	EXAMPLE FROM BENJAMIN
Decay	Storage	Gradual deterioration of the trace due to the passage of time	No evidence either way
Obliteration	Storage	Eradication of a newly formed trace before consolidation	No report of this nature by Harold
Interference			
Proactive	Storage or retrieval	Disruption by events before the event in question	Unlikely; Benjamin's lessons took place early in life
Retroactive	Storage or retrieval	Disruption by events after the event in question	A plausible explanation for Benjamin's decreasing memory with increasing age
Motivated forgetting	Retrieval	A memory failure due to repression; the person unconsciously wants to forget	Difficult to evaluate; no clear evidence

TABLE 8–6 THEORIES OF FORGETTING. The decay, obliteration, and interference theories postulate a storage problem. Interference theory also postulates a retrieval problem, as does motivated forgetting.

Type of Passage	Trials Required
Original	
1	202
2	190
3	181
4	220
5	160
6	175
7	193
Average	189
Control	
1	205
2	193
3	175
Average	191
Learning trials for control passages	191
Relearning trials for original passages	−189
Difference	2

$$\frac{191 - 189}{191} = \frac{2}{191} = 1\%$$

TABLE 8–7 RELEARNING AFTER FIFTEEN YEARS. The figures show the average number of trials required for Benjamin to relearn seven original and three comparison passages, resulting in a savings score of 1%.

tion on other details with a higher attention value. Such outcomes do not constitute poor memory, for nothing was learned that might be forgotten later.

The significance of motivation is also evident from the opposite direction, in *overlearning*, which means learning beyond the point at which a task has merely been mastered. The value of this procedure was illustrated when adults learned lists of words beyond one perfect recall. Using half again as many practice trials as were required to reach the first perfect recall was designated 50% overlearning; using twice as many was called 100% overlearning. When these groups were compared with a third group that engaged in no additional practice trials, the results showed a distinct advantage for both amounts of overlearning (Krueger, 1929).

The idea of overlearning is misleading, suggesting that there has been too much practice. A highly motivated learner always passes beyond the point of initial mastery but has not learned the task too well. When college students and their tutors were tested several months after the course was over, the tutors retained more than the students they tutored, presumably because tutoring involved overlearning (Semb, Ellis, & Arauio, 1993).

MEMORY SYSTEMS

If motivation is influential in memory, perhaps sheer practice and determination can make a difference. Years ago, William James decided to answer this question by studying himself. Can memory be improved merely by exercise, just as one strengthens a muscle by exercising it?

James began by memorizing 158 lines from the works of Victor Hugo, applying himself to the task for eight consecutive days. Keeping a careful record of his time, he found that he required an average of 50 seconds to memorize each line. That was the "strength of his memory" before he began his program of memory exercise.

Next, he engaged in intensive memory exercise for 38 days. He attempted to strengthen his memory by memorizing Milton's poetry, spending 20 minutes each day in this effort. Afterward, was his memory stronger? The way to find out was to return to Victor Hugo's poetry. Could he memorize another 158 lines more easily than the earlier ones?

Using the same procedure as before, this time he required 57 seconds per line, just a bit slower than previously. The slightly poorer performance occurred, he said, because he had become "perceptibly fagged." He verified his finding by asking friends to serve as subjects, and they encountered the same result. One's basic memory capacity—or native retentiveness, as James called it—cannot be improved by exercise alone (James, 1890).

However, memory can be improved with **mnemonic devices,** systems designed to aid memory by efficient input and output. The encoding strategies mentioned earlier—organization, chunking, and retrieval cues—are the foundations of most mnemonic devices, which have existed since the time of ancient civilizations (Patten, 1990).

LOCI AND PEG WORDS. One of the more formal mnemonic devices is the **method of loci,** which uses a series of familiar places to aid recall. A locus is a place; loci are places. These places are parts of a well-established route to work, school, or somewhere else, and each item on the list to be remembered is associated with a specific place in this accustomed pathway. That place serves as a cue for recall, and imagery is used in each instance (Figure 8–17). This method illustrates the three basic factors in successful encoding. There is an organization, the accustomed pathway; there is the provision for chunking, accomplished by assigning a group of items at each stopping place; and there is opportunity for cuing, facilitated by creating distinct images at each location (Bower, 1970).

Giving more emphasis to the auditory realm, another approach is not based on a long-standing habit. The framework must be learned, and then it may play an almost irresistible role in recall, as is evident in so many television advertisements. A catchy jingle or simple poem promoting some product becomes unforgettable. In the **peg-word system,** the rhyming words are used as pegs for memorizing the new material. This method is especially useful for serial learning, for each place is numbered and can form a sharp image with the rhyme at that point (Table 8–8).

All mnemonic devices require practice. They do not work by themselves. When students were trained to use chunking, for example, their memory capacities for digits increased enormously. After extensive practice, they reached a level nine or ten times higher than their original level (Chase & Ericsson, 1982).

IN RETROSPECT. Looking backward, Benjamin's failure can be attributed significantly to inadequate encoding, the first element of

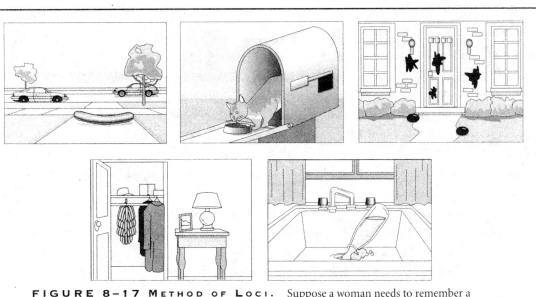

FIGURE 8–17 METHOD OF LOCI. Suppose a woman needs to remember a shopping list of hot dogs, cat food, tomatoes, bananas, and milk. On her habitual route home she encounters several familiar places—walking by the front path, checking the mail box, entering through the front door, hanging a coat in the closet, and going into the kitchen. To remember the shopping list, the person thinks of a large hot dog lying in the front pathway, a hungry cat having its supper in the mail box, tomatoes splattered on the front door, a bunch of bananas hanging in the coat closet, and a milk bottle bubbling its contents into the kitchen sink. To recall these items, she merely procedes mentally down the accustomed route, stopping in the pathway, by the mail box, at the door, and at other places to ask, "What did I put here?"

One is a bun; two is a shoe;
Three is a tree; four is a door;
Five is a hive; six is sticks;
Seven is heaven; eight is a gate;
Nine is wine; ten is a hen.

TABLE 8–8 PEG-WORD SYSTEM.
The verse must be learned first, a relatively easy task
because of its rhyme and rhythm. Then each item
on the list is put in its numbered place. Using the
commuter's shopping list again, a learner might
proceed as follows: one-bun would have a hot dog, a
natural association; two-shoe might have cat food in
the shoe; three-tree would have tomatoes among the
branches, and so forth.

memory. He presumably did not cast the material
into any systematic organization; he apparently did
not use chunking, combining certain pieces of
information into manageable subgroups; and he
surely did not employ cuing, whereby he developed
signals for retrieval of the stored information. Nevertheless, he and his father completed a very
demanding scientific study revealing several important findings.

They showed, in the first place, the value of
using relearning for measuring small amounts of
memory. Compared with recall and recognition,
relearning has the greatest sensitivity for detecting
weak memories. Second, and more important, Professor Burtt accomplished his basic goal. He
demonstrated that human memory can be established in infancy—as early as 15 months of age.
Prior to this experiment, there was little compelling
evidence that experiences at this early point of life
could be retained in any amount. Third, the father

and son together provided support for Ebbinghaus's well-known curves of forgetting, except that
they did so not for a few minutes, a few days, or
one month—but for 15 years.

For these contributions to our understanding
of memory, the Burtts are deserving of special
recognition. It may be quite some time before
another psychologist and partner are willing to
examine memory in the dedicated manner of
Harold and Benjamin. The father recognized his
son, and the hundreds of hours Benjamin donated
from infancy through early adulthood, by adding a
footnote in one report: "To Benjamin P. Burtt, who
served as subject in this rather tedious experiment"
(Burtt, 1932).

By modern standards, the father is doubly
deserving of our gratitude. He also served as a
comparison subject in this research. Benjamin
remained passive throughout the readings, and
part of his forgetting may have been due to
his developing brain structure. But his father
became an active adult learner, reading every passage aloud, pronouncing each syllable slowly
and carefully, 90 times each. Knowing Greek
and the story of Oedipus, he had a context
for remembering these lines, encoding them
within this framework. On these bases, the drama
of King Oedipus became available to him in memory not just through relearning or recognition for
five years or ten years but even through recall into
the very latest decades of his life.

That life was a long one, 101 years.

• SUMMARY •

ACQUISITION OF MEMORY

1. Immediately after we experience something, sensory
memory provides a momentary residual stimulation.
It involves largely unprocessed information, some of

which can be transferred to short-term memory.

2. Short-term memory, the next stage, is also a temporary condition, sometimes known as working
memory. During this period, a limited amount
of information can be processed for permanent
storage in long-term memory. Transfer to long-term
memory requires successful encoding or recoding,

191

which involves: organization, chunking, and the use of cues to aid retrieval.

3. In the third phase, long-term memory apparently has an unlimited capacity and presumably involves different systems of storage for different types of memories—procedural, concerning how to do things, and declarative, concerning factual information.

4. Another approach, sometimes known as levels-of-processing theory, does not involve these hypothesized stages, separate from one another. It states instead that the permanence of a memory depends on the cognitive activities that go into its formation, especially encoding.

THE MEMORY TRACE

5. Memory can be measured by three basic methods: recall, recognition, and relearning. Redintegration is a variation of the method of free recall, for cues or hints are made available.

6. The biochemical nature of the trace is suspected to involve RNA, neurotransmitter substances, and perhaps long-term potentiation, which is a sustained, permanent increase in the strength of a synaptic connection. Several brain areas appear to be involved, especially the hippocampus and cerebral cortex.

7. According to the reappearance hypothesis, the memory trace remains intact in the brain as a structural alteration. In the reconstruction hypothesis, memories are not fixed and filed in the brain but rather reassembled, chiefly on the basis of remnants from past experience.

THEORIES OF FORGETTING

8. In decay theory, forgetting is presumed to involve a storage failure. Through disuse and the passage of time, the trace deteriorates.

9. According to obliteration theory, severe shock destroys the currently forming or newly formed trace before it is firmly established, causing forgetting through a storage failure.

10. There is also evidence that forgetting is produced by what happens over time, apart from some shock immediately after learning. Prior interference is known as proactive interference. Subsequent interference is called retroactive interference.

11. In motivated forgetting, it is hypothesized that unpleasant thoughts are unconsciously excluded from awareness, a process called repression. This problem is a retrieval failure.

PRINCIPLES OF MEMORIZING

12. Motivation is a most important aspect of successful memory. Forgetting may be very rapid when one has no desire to remember; overlearning shows that through extra effort, one can build up resistance to forgetting.

13. For successful encoding, storage, and retrieval, mnemonic devices are useful. The method of loci and the peg-word system illustrate these techniques.

• WORKING WITH PSYCHOLOGY •

❧ REVIEW OF KEY CONCEPTS ❧

memory	*Acquisition of Memory*	short-term memory (STM)
encoding	information processing	working memory
storage	stage theory of memory	rehearsal
retrieval	sensory memory	subjective organization

chunking
cuing
context-dependent memory
state-dependent memory
long-term memory (LTM)
primacy effect
recency effect
procedural memory
declarative memory
episodic memory
semantic memory
implicit memory
explicit memory
schema
script
conceptual hierarchy
network of associations

eory
connectionist model

The Memory Trace
memory trace
recall
redintegration
eidetic imagery
flashbulb memory
recognition
déjà vu experience
relearning
savings score
long-term potentiation
hippocampus
anterograde amnesia
retrograde amnesia

reappearance hypothesis
reconstruction hypothesis

Theories of Forgetting
forgetting
decay theory
obliteration theory
interference theory
proactive interference
retroactive interference
motivated forgetting

Principles of Memorizing
mnemonic devices
method of loci
peg-word system

CLASS DISCUSSION/CRITICAL THINKING

A NARRATIVE TWIST

Assume that Harold Burtt, reciting to his 15-month-old son, had not read *Oedipus Rex* in the original Greek but had read rhyming poetry in English instead. He might have recited Longfellow's *Midnight Ride of Paul Revere*. By using poetry of this sort, would Harold have obtained different results in his study of infant memory? Why or why not? Suggest his reason for using the Sophocles's passages. Which approach seems preferable? Why?

TOPICAL QUESTIONS

• *Acquisition of Memory.* Consider your preparation for an examination on the U.S. Civil War. Indicate in detail the strategies you might use, considering what you know about encoding. In your answer, include the concepts of organization, chunking, and cuing.

• *The Memory Trace.* Suppose your memory is malfunctioning and you are limited to one of its three capacities: recall, recognition, or relearning. Further, suppose you must select a different capacity for different occasions. Which might you choose if you were anticipating a routine day? Going to a high school reunion? Delivering a speech without the use of notes? Explain your reasons.

• *Theories of Forgetting.* Is forgetting a necessary condition for normal human functioning? Speculate on our lives if we could not forget. In this context, suggest a modification in memory capacity that might improve human adjustment.

• *Principles of Memorizing.* Think about a baseball team, a symphony orchestra, or the crew of a ship. Which mnemonic devices might be used to remember the membership in each instance? How would they be employed?

TOPICS OF RELATED INTEREST

Information processing is a central concept in perception (5), as well as in thought and language (9). Neurotransmitter substances, which presumably play an important role in memory, are discussed in the context of the biological bases of behavior (3). Repression, also called motivated forgetting, is the second phase in the three-stage approach in psychoanalysis (14).

6

HOW ORGANISMS EVOLVE

"What but the wolf's tooth whittled so fine
The fleet limbs of the antelope?
What but fear winged the birds, and hunger
Jewelled with such eyes the great goshawk's head?"

ROBINSON JEFFERS in *The Bloody Sire*

A goshawk surveys its surroundings for prey. The exceptionally keen eyes of birds of prey evolved in response to selection pressures that favored those who could spot prey from far above. As Robinson Jeffers poetically suggests, those who could not see well went hungry and produced fewer offspring.

I n Chapter 16 we discussed the history of the theory of evolution and presented some of the evidence that evolution actually happens. But what processes drive evolutionary change? Is natural selection the only cause of evolution? Does evolution always occur all the time in all populations of organisms? In this chapter, we examine evolutionary processes in more detail. As we do, you will see that *evolution is an inevitable consequence of the nature of living things*. It occurs as a direct result of the chemical structure of genes and the interactions between organisms and their environment.

Evolution and the Genetics of Populations

Individual organisms live, reproduce, and die. Individuals, however, do not evolve; populations do. Evolution is the change in gene frequency that occurs in a population over time. Inheritance, therefore, is the link between the lives of individual organisms and the evolution of **populations**, which are all the individuals of a species living in a given area. We will begin our discussion of the processes of evolution by reviewing the principles of genetics as they apply to individuals and then extend those principles to the genetics of populations. You may want to refer to Unit II to refresh your memory on specific points.

Genes, Influenced by the Environment, Determine the Traits of Each Individual

Each cell of every organism contains a repository of genetic information encoded in the DNA of its chromosomes. A gene is a segment of DNA located at a particular place on a chromosome. Its sequence of nucleotides encodes the sequence of amino acids of a protein, usually an enzyme that catalyzes one particular reaction in the cell. Slightly different sequences of nucleotides at a given gene's location, called alleles, generate different forms of the same enzyme. There are usually two or more alleles of a single gene. An individual having alleles of the same type is homozygous, and an individual having alleles of different types is heterozygous. The specific alleles borne on an organism's chromosomes (its genotype), interacting with the environment, determine its physical and behavioral traits (its phenotype).

Let's illustrate these principles with an example that should be familiar to you from Unit II. A pea flower is colored purple because a chemical reaction in its petals converts a colorless molecule to a purple pigment. When we say that a pea plant has the allele for purple flowers, we mean that a particular stretch of DNA on one of its chromosomes contains a sequence of nucleotides that codes for the enzyme catalyzing this reaction. A pea with the allele for white flowers has a different sequence of nucleotides at the corresponding place on one of its chromosomes. The resulting enzyme cannot produce purple pigment. If a pea is homozygous for the white allele, its flowers produce no pigment and are white.

As we will see later, natural selection operates on the phenotype and, in doing so, either favors or selects against the particular genotype that produced it. Thus natural selection alters the gene frequencies within a population.

The Gene Pool Is the Sum of All the Genes Occurring in a Population

A branch of genetics, called **population genetics**, deals with the frequency, distribution, and inheritance of alleles in populations. Because evolution is a change in the genetic makeup of populations over generations, you will need to learn the principles of population genetics to understand the mechanisms of evolution.

In population genetics, the **gene pool** is defined as all the genes that occur in a population. It is made up of all the alleles of all the genes found in all of the individuals. Each particular gene can also be considered to have a gene pool, which consists of all the alleles of that specific gene occurring in a population. For example, in a population of 100 pea plants, the gene pool for flower color would consist of 200 alleles (peas are diploid, so there are two color alleles per plant, multiplied by 100 plants). If we could analyze the genetic composition of every plant in the population, we might find that some have alleles for white flowers, some have alleles for purple flowers, and some have both alleles. If we added up the color alleles of all the plants in the population, we could determine the relative proportions of the different alleles, a number called the **allele frequency**. Let's say that the gene pool for flower color consisted of 140 alleles for purple and 60 alleles for white. The allele frequencies would then be purple, 0.7 (70%), and white, 0.3 (30%).

Evolution Is the Change of Gene Frequencies within a Population

What does all this have to do with evolution? Quite a bit. Suppose a flower-eating cow happens upon a field of purple flowers and, being enamored of purple flowers, eats all of them before they produce seeds. Because the allele for pur-

ple flowers (P) is dominant to the allele for white (p), all the purple alleles in the entire population are in the purple-flowered plants (PP or Pp). If none of these plants reproduce, while the white-flowered plants do reproduce, then the next generation will consist entirely of white-flowered peas (pp). The allele frequency for purple will drop to 0, while the allele frequency for white will rise to 1.0 (100%). As a result of the selective eating habits of the cow, *evolution will have occurred in that field*. The gene pool of the pea population will have changed, and **natural selection**, in the form of foraging by the cow, will have caused the change.

This simple example illustrates four important points about evolution.

1. *Natural selection does not cause genetic changes in individuals.* The alleles for purple or white flower color arose spontaneously, long before the cow ever found the pea field. The cow did not cause white alleles to appear. It merely favored the differential survival of white alleles compared with purple alleles.
2. *Natural selection befalls individuals, but evolution occurs in populations.* Individual pea plants either reproduced or did not, but it was the population as a whole that evolved as its gene frequencies changed.
3. *Evolution is a change in the allele frequencies of a population, owing to differential reproduction among organisms bearing different alleles.* In evolutionary terminology, the **fitness** of an organism is measured by its reproductive success: In our example, the white flowers had greater fitness than the purple flowers, because they produced more viable offspring.
4. *Evolutionary changes are not "good" or "progressive" in any absolute sense.* The white alleles were favored only because of the dietary preferences of this particular cow; in another environment, with other predators, the white allele may well be selected against.

Mutation and the Recombination of Alleles during Sexual Reproduction Provide Sources of Variability

Your observations of the life around you have undoubtedly made you aware that even within a species, most individuals are at least slightly different from one another. The number of different individuals that can be produced from the same set of thousands of genes, considering that most genes come in multiple alleles, is staggering. This variability is produced by genetic recombination and sexual reproduction, which recombine existing alleles. But where did the different genes and alleles come from in the first place? The ultimate source of new genes and new alleles is mutation. Together, these processes provide the raw material for evolution.

Mutations Are the Source of New Genes and Alleles

Cells have efficient mechanisms that protect the integrity of their genes. Enzymes constantly scan the DNA, repairing flaws caused by radiation, chemical damage, or mistakes in copying. Nevertheless, changes in nucleotide sequence can happen. These changes are mutations, and they vary tremendously in their impact. As we explained in Chapter 11, some changes in DNA have virtually no effect on the organism; many, perhaps most, are harmful; and a few may be beneficial or may aid the organism in coping with new or changed environments.

How significant is mutation in altering the gene pool of a population? Mutations are rare, occurring once in 10,000 to 1,000,000 genes per individual in each generation. Therefore, mutation is not a major force in evolution by itself by changing gene frequencies. However, *mutations are the source of new alleles*, new heritable variations upon which other evolutionary processes can work. As such, they are the foundation of evolutionary change. Without mutations there would be no diversity among life forms, and probably no life at all.

As we mentioned earlier, *mutations are not goal-directed*. A mutation does not arise as a result of, nor in anticipation of, environmental necessities (Fig. 17-1). A mutation simply happens and may in turn produce a change in the structure or function of the organism. Whether that

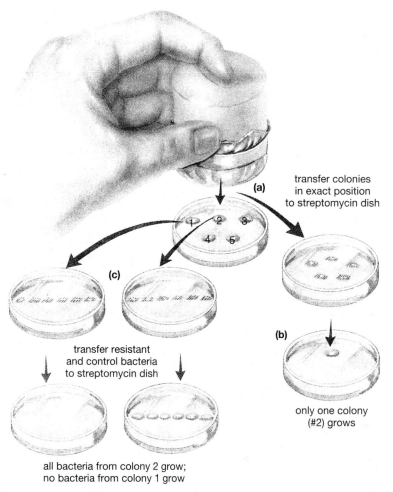

transfer colonies
in exact position
to streptomycin dish

only one colony
(#2) grows

transfer resistant
and control bacteria
to streptomycin dish

all bacteria from colony 2 grow;
no bacteria from colony 1 grow

Figure 17-1 **Mutations occur spontaneously**

Experiment supporting the hypothesis that mutations occur spontaneously and not in response to specific selective pressures. **(a)** Several colonies of bacteria, each the offspring of a single individual and thus having the same genetic makeup, are grown on a solid nutrient medium in a dish. These bacteria have never been exposed to antibiotics. A piece of velvet the exact size of the dish is lightly pressed into the bacterial colonies and then touched to the surface of nutrient medium containing the antibiotic streptomycin in a second dish. Many bacteria from each original colony stick to the velvet and then come off the velvet into the second dish. Thus the exact positions of the "parent" colonies are duplicated in the second dish. **(b)** Only one daughter colony, in position #2, grows on the streptomycin-containing medium in the second dish. If mutations for streptomycin resistance were induced by the presence of streptomycin, then one would predict that any colony transplanted to the streptomycin-containing medium would develop these mutations. If, however, streptomycin resistance is an occasional spontaneous occurrence, then one would predict that the only colony grown on a normal medium that would survive is one that might already have been resistant. These alternatives are tested in **(c)**. Samples of the original colonies 1 and 2 are transferred to streptomycin-containing medium. All bacteria from colony 2 grow, but none from colony 1 grow, suggesting that the bacteria of colony 2 already possessed the mutation for streptomycin resistance prior to exposure and that the presence of streptomycin in the medium did not induce an adaptive mutation for streptomycin resistance.

change is helpful or harmful, now or in the future, depends on environmental conditions over which the organism has little or no control. The mutation provides *potential*; other forces, such as migration and especially natural selection, acting on that potential, may favor the spread of a mutation through the population or eliminate it.

Recombination during Sexual Reproduction Provides New Combinations of Existing Alleles

The production of new combinations of alleles occurs in three ways during sexual reproduction. During meiosis, homologous pairs of chromosomes are separated and parceled randomly into gametes. As a result of this segregation of homologues, each human (having 23 paired chromosomes) can produce 8 million different combinations of chromosomes in his or her gametes. Recombination of alleles on individual chromosomes also occurs regularly as a result of crossing over between pairs of homologous chromosomes, adding to the variability. Then, during fertilization, gametes join in random pairs. Together, these events guarantee that each fertilized egg bears a completely unique combination of alleles, or genotype. Many of these new allele combinations produce measurable differences in behavioral, anatomical, or physiological traits (new phenotypes) that in turn alter the fitness of the individual in a particular environment.

The Equilibrium Population Is a Hypothetical Population in Which Evolution Does Not Occur

It will be easier to understand the forces that cause populations to evolve if we first consider the characteristics of a population that would *not* evolve. In 1908, Godfrey H. Hardy and Wilhelm Weinberg defined an **equilibrium population** as one in which the allele frequencies and the distribution of genotypes remain constant with succeeding generations. In other words, the population remains in **genetic equilibrium** (see "A Closer Look: The Hardy-Weinberg Equilibrium Population"). If allele frequencies do not change, evolution does not occur. A population can remain in equilibrium only if several restrictive conditions are met:

1. *There must be no mutation.*
2. *There must be no **gene flow** between populations;* that is, there must be no net migration of alleles into the population (through immigration) or out of the population (through emigration).
3. *The population must be very large* (theoretically infinite).
4. *All mating must be random,* with no tendency for certain genotypes to mate with specific other genotypes.
5. *There must be no natural selection;* that is, all genotypes must be equally adaptive and reproduce equally well.

Under these conditions, allele frequencies within a population will remain the same indefinitely. If one or more of these conditions are violated, then allele frequencies will change: Evolution will occur.

As you might expect, few if any natural populations are truly in equilibrium. If so, then what is the importance of the Hardy-Weinberg principle? The Hardy-Weinberg conditions are useful starting points for studying the mechanisms of evolution. In the following sections, we will examine each condition, show why it is often violated by natural populations, and illustrate the consequences of its violation. In this way, you can better understand both the inevitability of evolution and the forces that drive evolutionary change.

The Mechanisms of Evolution

As the Hardy-Weinberg conditions predict, there are five major causes of evolutionary change within a population: mutation, migration, small populations, nonrandom mating, and natural selection.

Mutations Are the Ultimate Source of Genetic Variability

A population will remain in genetic equilibrium only if no mutations occur. Although mutations are not common, they are an inevitable result of the imperfections in the way DNA is copied as cells reproduce. When such a copying error occurs in a cell that produces gametes, the mutation may be passed to an offspring and enter the gene pool of a population. Over a sufficiently long time span, genetic change as a result of mutation is a certainty.

Migration Produces Gene Flow between Populations

In biology, the word *migration* has two distinct meanings. In the most familiar context, migration refers to the seasonal movement of many species between summer breeding grounds and winter refuges. In evolutionary biology, however, **migration** *is the flow of genes between populations*. Baboons, for example, live in social groupings called troops. Within each troop, all the females mate with a handful of dominant males. Juvenile males usually leave the troop. If they are lucky, they join and perhaps even become dominant in another troop. Thus the male offspring of one troop carry genes to the gene pools of other troops.

Migration has two significant effects.

1. *Gene flow spreads advantageous alleles throughout the species.* Suppose that a new allele arises in one population and that this new allele benefits the organisms that possess it. Migration can carry this new allele to other populations of the species.
2. *Gene flow helps to maintain all the organisms over a large area as one species.* If migrants constantly carry genes back and forth among populations, then the populations can never develop large differences in allele frequencies. Isolation of populations, with no gene flow

199

to or from other populations of the same species, is a key factor in the origin of new species, as will be discussed in Chapter 18.

Small Populations Are Subject to Random Changes in Allele Frequencies

To remain in genetic equilibrium, a population must be so large that chance events have no impact on its overall genetic makeup. Disaster may befall even the fittest organism. The maple seed that falls into a pond never sprouts; the deer and elk blasted away by the eruption of Mount St. Helens left no descendants. If a population is sufficiently large, chance events are unlikely to alter the overall gene frequency, since they would be expected to interfere equally with the reproduction of organisms of all genotypes. In a small population, however, certain alleles may be carried by only a few organisms. Chance events could reduce or even entirely eliminate such alleles from the population, altering its genetic makeup.

Genetic Drift Is An Example of Random Genetic Change in Small Populations

It is much more likely that chance events will change allele frequencies in a small population than in a large population, by a process called **genetic drift**. Consider, for ex-

ample, two hypothetical populations of haploid ladybugs in which the outer shell is either spotted or solid-colored, controlled by alternate alleles of a single gene. In each population, half the ladybugs are spotted and half are solid-colored (that is, the frequencies of both alleles are 0.5, or 50%), but one population has only four bugs and the other has 1000. Let us assume that each individual that survives to maturity produces two offspring identical to itself. For the population sizes to remain constant, exactly half the individuals must reproduce in each generation. Let us further assume that whether an individual ladybug reproduces is determined entirely by chance.

In the larger population, 500 bugs will be parents to the next generation. Though their survival is random, the odds against all 500 of the reproducing ladybugs being spotted are enormous. In fact, it would be extremely unlikely for even 300 parents to be spotted. In this large population, then, we would not expect a major change in allele frequencies to occur from generation to generation (Fig. 17-2). The effects of chance are minimized by the large population size. In the small population, on the other hand, only two individuals will reproduce. There is a 25% chance that both parents will be spotted (this is the same likelihood as flipping two coins and having both come up heads). If this happens, then the next generation will consist entirely of spotted ladybugs. Within a single generation, it is possible

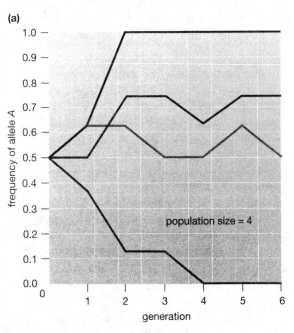

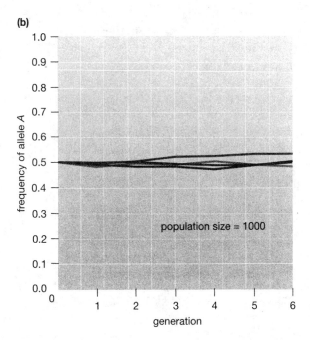

Figure 17-2 Genetic drift

Computer-generated graphs illustrating the effect of population size on genetic drift. In both graphs, the initial population was composed of half *A* and half *a* alleles, and six generations were simulated, with individuals chosen at random to contribute alleles to the next generation. Four simulations were run for each population size, producing the four lines on each graph. **(a)** With a population size of 4, one allele sometimes became "extinct" owing to chance. For example, in the top simulation run, the *a* allele became extinct by the second generation (therefore, the frequency of the *A* allele became 1.0). **(b)** With a population size of 1000, allele frequencies remained relatively constant.

The Hardy-Weinberg Equilibrium Population

The Hardy-Weinberg equilibrium model predicts that, if a large population undergoes no mutation, migration, or natural selection, and if all members of the population mate randomly, then the frequencies of alleles will not change from generation to generation. To see how this can be so, consider our familiar pea plants. Pea seeds can be round (R: dominant) or wrinkled (r: recessive). To determine the genotypes of the offspring of two individuals, for example two heterozygotes, we would draw a Punnett square:

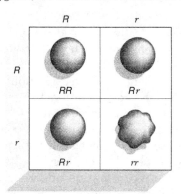

Each parent produces both R and r gametes. The expected offspring are ¼ RR, ½ Rr, ¼ rr. There are two ways to arrive at these frequencies. The first is to add up the offspring in all boxes of the square. Another way of doing it is by probabilities. Each gamete has an equal probability of containing either allele. Therefore we can assign probabilities to the gametes in the Punnett square: R = 0.5, r = 0.5. From the laws of probability, *the probability of two independent events occurring simultaneously is the product of their individual probabilities*. If you flip a coin, the probability of a head is ½. If you flip two coins simultaneously, the probability of two heads is ½ × ½ = ¼. Similarly, we can obtain the probability of obtaining each type of offspring by multiplying the relative proportions of each allele:
We obtain 0.25 RR, 0.5 Rr, and 0.25 rr.

Let us suppose, now, that we have a population of 100 peas, that we collect sperm and egg cells from all of them, and we determine their genotypes. We may find, for example, that there are 60% R alleles and 40% r alleles in the gametes. The proportions of the two alleles R and r are identical to the probability that any given offspring will receive either R or r. We can thus draw a "population Punnett square":

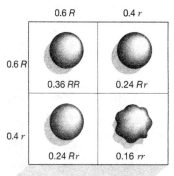

In the "population F_1 generation," we expect the following proportions of genotypes: 0.36 RR, 0.48 Rr, and 0.16 Rr. If the population remains the same size, 100 peas, then we will have 36 RR, 48 Rr, and 16 rr peas. What gametes would this F_1 generation in its turn produce? Under the Hardy-Weinberg conditions, all plants produce equal numbers of gametes, and by the principles of Mendelian genetics, all plants produce equal numbers of gametes with each of the two alleles for seed shape. To keep things simple, let's assume that each plant contributes two gametes, one with each of its two alleles. We therefore collect 72 R alleles from the homozygous dominants, 48 R alleles and 48 r alleles from the heterozygotes, and 32 r alleles from the homozygous recessives, for a total of 120 R and 80 r alleles. The allele frequencies of the gametes from the population F_1 generation, then, are 0.6 R and 0.4 r, just as we started out with. Therefore, the F_2 generation has the same distribution of genotypes as the F_1. If there are no disturbances, this process will go on indefinitely: The population remains in equilibrium.

Rather than going through Punnett squares, there is an easier way of calculating allele and genotype frequencies. The sum of all allele frequencies must equal 1. Let the frequency of the R allele be represented by p, and the frequency of the r allele by q. Then the sum of the frequencies $p + q = 1$. Just as we generated the genotype frequencies in the population Punnett square by multiplying allele frequencies, we can do the same with this equation:

$$(p + q) \times (p + q) = p^2 + pq + qp + q^2 = p^2 + 2pq + q^2 = 1$$

For our particular example, $p = 0.6$ and $q = 0.4$, so the genotypes of the population F_1 generation will be:

$$(0.6)^2 \, RR + 2 \, [(0.6) \times (0.4)] \, Rr + (0.4)^2 \, rr = 0.36 \, RR,$$
$$0.48 \, Rr, \text{ and } 0.16 \, rr$$

This is the same set of frequencies that we calculated with the "population Punnett square."

As these calculations show, in an equilibrium population, allele frequencies and the distribution of genotypes remain constant, generation after generation. In actual experiments, if measurements of allele frequencies in a population show significant changes over time, evolution is occurring in that population.

for the allele for solid-colored shell to completely disappear from the population.

Figure 17-2a illustrates two important points about genetic drift:

1. *Genetic drift tends to reduce genetic variability within a small population.* In extreme cases, all members of a population may become genetically identical (Fig. 17-2a, top line).
2. *Genetic drift tends to increase genetic variability between populations.* Purely as a result of chance, separate populations may evolve extremely different allele frequencies (Fig. 17-2a, top versus bottom lines).

Two special cases of genetic drift, called the population bottleneck and founder effect, further illustrate the enormous consequences that small population size may have on the allele frequencies of a species.

A Population Bottleneck Is an Example of Genetic Drift

In a **population bottleneck**, a species undergoes a drastic reduction in population size, so that only a few individuals contribute genes to the entire future population of the species. As our ladybug example showed, population bottlenecks may cause both *differences in allele frequencies* and *reductions in genetic variability* (Fig. 17-3a). Even if the population then rebounds and the species becomes common, these genetic effects of the bottleneck may remain for hundreds or thousands of generations.

Loss of genetic variability has been documented in the northern elephant seal and the cheetah (Fig. 17-3b). The elephant seal was hunted almost to extinction in the 1800s; by the 1890s only about 20 survived. Because elephant seals breed harem-style, with a single male mating with a stable group of females, one male may have fathered all the offspring at this extreme bottleneck point. The population today has expanded to about 30,000, but biochemical analysis shows that all northern elephant

seals are genetically almost identical. Other species of seals, whose populations have historically always remained large, are much more variable. The rescue of the northern elephant seal from extinction is rightly regarded as a triumph of conservation; however, with very little genetic variation, the elephant seal has much less potential to evolve in response to environmental changes. No matter how many elephant seals there are, the species must be considered to be threatened with extinction. Cheetahs are also genetically uniform, although the reason for the bottleneck is unknown. Consequently, cheetahs too could be gravely threatened by small changes in their environment.

A special case of a population bottleneck is the **founder effect**, which occurs when isolated colonies are founded by a small number of organisms. A flock of birds, for instance, may become lost during migration or may be blown off course by a storm (this is thought to have happened in the case of Darwin's Finches in the Galapagos Islands). Among humans, small groups may migrate for religious or political reasons (Fig. 17-4). Such a small group may have allele frequencies that are very different from the frequencies of the parent population because of chance inclusion of disproportionate numbers of certain alleles in the founders. If the isolation of the founders is maintained for a long period of time, a sizable new population may arise that differs greatly from the original population.

How much does genetic drift contribute to evolution? No one really knows. Only rarely are natural populations extremely small or completely cut off from gene flow from other populations. Populations occasionally do become very small, however, and it may be precisely these small populations that contribute most to major evolutionary changes. As we will see in the next chapter, biologists believe that new species often arise in small populations.

(a)

original population   resulting population

event causing
bottleneck

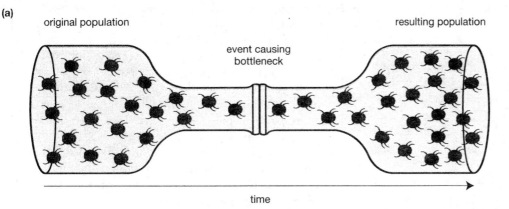

time

(b)

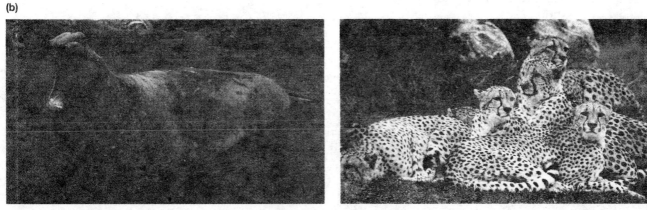

Figure 17-3   **Genetic bottlenecks reduce variability**

(a) If a population is reduced to a very small number of individuals, the gene pool is reduced and a population bottleneck occurs. The recovered population shows reduced genetic and phenotypic variability, because all are offspring of the few organisms that survived the bottleneck. (b) Both the northern elephant seal (left) and the cheetah (right) passed through a population bottleneck in the recent past, resulting in an almost total loss of genetic diversity. As a result, the ability of these populations to adapt to changing environments is very limited.

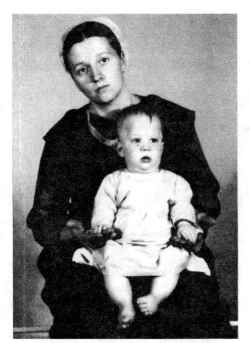

Figure 17-4   **A human example of the founder effect**

An Amish woman with her child, who suffers from a set of genetic defects known as the Ellis-van Creveld syndrome (short arms and legs, extra fingers, occasionally heart defects). Fleeing from religious persecution, about 200 members of the Amish religion migrated from Switzerland to Pennsylvania between 1720 and 1770. Since that time, virtually all the Pennsylvania Amish moved to Lancaster County and have remained reproductively isolated from non-Amish Americans. The population increased to about 8000 by 1964. In that year, geneticist Victor McKusick surveyed the Lancaster County Amish and discovered that they had an allele frequency for Ellis-van Creveld of about 0.07, compared with a frequency of less than 0.001 in the general population. Why? One couple who immigrated in 1744 carried the allele. Inbreeding among the Amish passed the allele along to their descendants: a clear example of a founder effect. In addition, by chance the Ellis-van Creveld carriers had more children than the Amish average, further increasing the allele frequency by genetic drift. The combination of an initially high frequency in the immigrants (1 or 2 out of 200) plus genetic drift has resulted in more cases of Ellis-van Creveld syndrome from Lancaster County than from the entire rest of the world.

Mating within a Population Is Almost Never Random

Organisms seldom mate strictly randomly. For example, most animals have limited mobility and are most likely to mate with nearby members of their species. Further, they may choose to mate with certain individuals of their species rather than with others. The White-crowned Sparrow is a case in point. Although all White-crowned Sparrows sing a fundamentally similar song, each local population has its own song dialect. A female usually chooses a mate that sings the same dialect that her father sang (Fig. 17-5). Among animals, there are three common forms of nonrandom mating: harem breeding, assortative mating, and sexual selection.

In some species, such as elephant seals, baboons, and bighorn sheep, only a few males fertilize all the females. Following some sort of contest, which may involve showing off with loud sounds or flashy colors, making threat-ening gestures, or actual combat, only certain males suc-ceed in gathering a harem and mating (Fig. 17-6).

Many animals mate assortatively—that is, they select mates that are similar to themselves. Humans, for exam-ple, tend to marry members of the opposite sex that are similar in height, race, intelligence, and social status.

Finally, in many mammal and bird species, mate selec-tion is primarily the prerogative of one sex, usually the fe-male. Males display their virtues, such as the bright plumage of a peacock (Fig. 17-7) or the rich territory of a songbird. A female evaluates the males and chooses her mate. This phenomenon, called **sexual selection**, is ex-plored in more detail later in this chapter.

All Genotypes Are Not Equally Adaptive

Genetic equilibrium requires that all genotypes must be equally adaptive—that is, none has any selective advan-tage over the others. It is probably true that some alleles

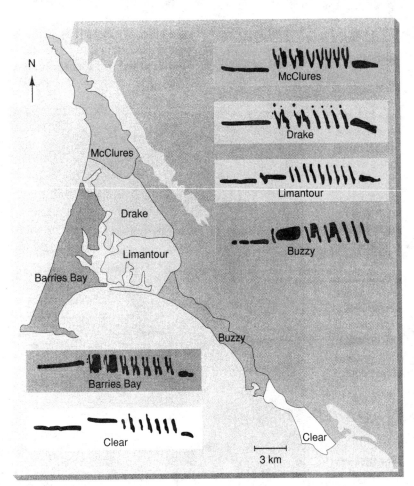

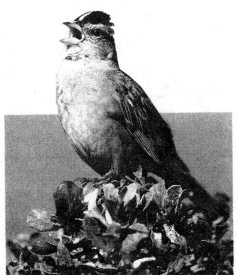

Figure 17-5 **Song-dialect preference illustrates nonrandom mating**

Song dialects among populations of White-crowned Sparrows at Point Reyes National Seashore north of San Francisco. As analysis of the sound patterns shows, the songs are fairly similar, but both birds and human listeners can recognize the different dialects. Male birds of each population learn their local dialect while in the nest and sing it when they mature. Fe-males preferentially mate with males that sing the dialect sung by the females' own fathers—that is, the females' own local dialect.

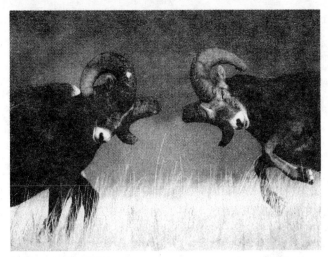

Figure 17-6 **Male competition promotes nonrandom mating**

Sparring contests between males result in extremely nonrandom mating among many animals, including deer, elk, seals, and many monkeys. Here, two male bighorn sheep square off against each other during the fall mating season. Although the horns are potentially deadly weapons, they are used in ritualized ways that minimize the danger of injury to either contestant.

are adaptively neutral, so organisms possessing any of several alleles will be equally likely to survive and reproduce. However, this is clearly not true of all alleles in all environments. Any time an allele confers, in Wallace's words, "some little superiority," natural selection will favor the enhanced reproduction of the individuals possessing it.

Natural selection is not the *only* evolutionary force. As we have seen, mutation provides initial variability in heritable traits. The chance effects of genetic drift may change allele frequencies, even spawning new species. Further, evolutionary biologists are just now beginning to appreciate the power of random catastrophe in shaping the history of life on Earth—mass extinctions that may exterminate flourishing and floundering species alike. Nevertheless, it is natural selection that shapes the evolution of adaptations that humankind has admired for millennia. For this reason, we will examine the mechanisms of natural selection in some detail.

Natural Selection

To most people, the words *natural selection* are synonymous with the phrase *survival of the fittest*. Natural selection evokes images of wolves chasing caribou, of lions snarling angrily in competition over a zebra carcass. Natural selection, however, is not really about *survival* but about *reproduction*. It is certainly true that an organism must survive at least for a while to live long enough to reproduce. In some cases, it may also be true that a longer-lived organism has more chances to reproduce. But no organism lives for-

ever, and the only way that its genes continue into the future is through successful reproduction. When an organism that fails to reproduce dies, its genes die with it. The organism reproduces, lives on, in a sense, through the genes that it has passed on to its offspring. Therefore, although evolutionary biologists often discuss survival, partly because survival is usually easier to measure than reproduction, natural selection is really an issue of **differential reproduction:** Individuals bearing certain alleles leave more offspring (who inherit those alleles) than other individuals with different alleles.

Natural Selection Acts on the Phenotype, Which Reflects the Underlying Genotype

The agents of natural selection cannot directly detect an organism's genotype. Rather, selection acts on phenotypes: the actual structures and behaviors that the organisms in a population display. Genotype and phenotype, however, are related in the following way. If you were to measure the phenotypes of a specific trait in all the individuals in a population, you would find a range of values (Fig. 17-8). This range of phenotypes would arise from differences both in the genotypes of the organisms and in the environments in

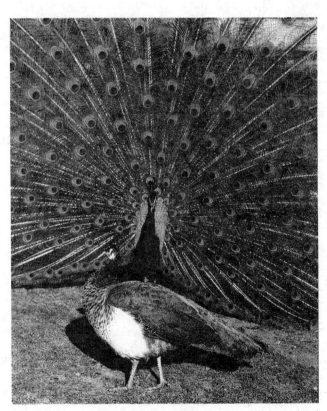

Figure 17-7 **The male peacock's showy tail has evolved through sexual selection**

Many male birds, including peacocks, attract mates by displaying their "wares." The features evolved for female attraction are often irrelevant, or even harmful, to the day-to-day survival of the males.

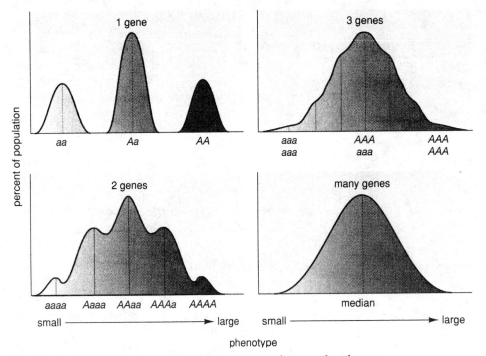

Figure 17-8   **Both genes and environment contribute to the phenotype**

This series of graphs illustrates the distribution of phenotypes that would be expected if one, two, three, or many genes, each with two incompletely dominant alleles (see Chapter 13), contributed to a particular body characteristic (for example, size). The vertical lines represent the precise size expected on the basis of genotype alone. In each case, environmental conditions (for example, amount of available food) create some variation in size, represented by the colored curves. As the number of genes contributing to the characteristic becomes large, the distribution of phenotypes approximates a smooth curve called a normal distribution (lower right-hand graph). The most common value for the phenotype is the middle value, also called the median.

which they live. However, environmental differences influencing phenotypes tend to average out in a large population. Thus, on the whole, genotype reflects phenotype: Most large plants will have genes promoting large size, whereas most small plants will have genes promoting small size. In our discussion of selection, therefore, we will ignore environmental causes of variability.

Natural Selection Can Influence Populations in Three Major Ways

Biologists recognize three major categories of natural selection based on its effect on the population over time (Fig. 17-9):

1. **Directional selection** favors individuals possessing values for a trait at one end of the distribution (representing a range of a particular trait) and selects against both average individuals and individuals at the opposite extreme of the distribution (for example, favors small size, selects against both average and large individuals).
2. **Stabilizing selection** favors individuals possessing an "average" value for a trait and selects against individuals with extreme values.

3. **Disruptive selection** favors individuals possessing relatively extreme values for a trait at the expense of individuals with average values. Disruptive selection favors organisms at both ends of the distribution of the trait (for example, favors both large and small body size).

Directional Selection Shifts Character Traits in a Specific Direction

If environmental conditions change in a consistent way—for example, if the climate becomes colder—then a species may evolve in a consistent direction in response, for example with thicker fur (Fig.17-9a). The evolution of long necks in giraffes was almost certainly due to directional selection: Ancestral giraffes with longer necks obtained more food and therefore reproduced more prolifically than their shorter-necked contemporaries did. Antibiotic resistance in bacteria is another example of directional selection (see Chapter 21).

How fast can directional selection change genotypes? That depends on both the genetic nature of the variability in the population and the strength of selection. The increased frequency of the black form of the peppered moth

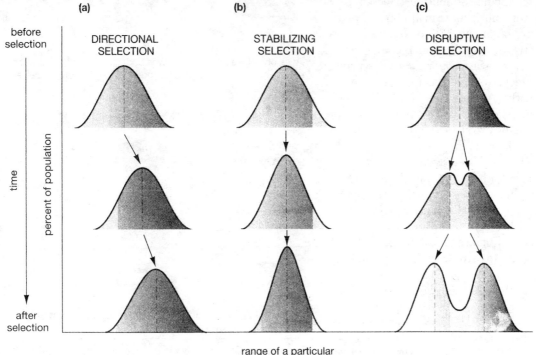

Figure 17-9 Three types of natural selection

A graphical illustration of three types of natural selection, acting on a normal distribution of phenotypes (in these examples, size). In all graphs, the pale areas represent individuals that are selected against—that is, do not reproduce as frequently. **(a)** In directional selection, phenotypes that are either larger or smaller than average (larger illustrated here) are favored. The average phenotype shifts position over the generations. **(b)** In stabilizing selection, the organisms most likely to reproduce are those with phenotypes close to the average for the population. The variability of phenotypes may decline, but the average value remains the same. **(c)** In disruptive selection, phenotypes that are both larger and smaller than average are favored. The population splits into two phenotypic groups.

in Britain during the Industrial Revolution was an extremely rapid case of directional selection (see Chapter 16). In that instance, the color did not vary in a finely graded manner but was either black or pale, controlled by two alleles of a single gene. Predation by birds was also a very strong selective force because pale moths were more visible on increasingly soot-covered tree trunks. Together, these two factors produced a dramatic change in the population in just a few years. If little variability exists in the population, or if the different alleles produce only slightly different phenotypes, then directional selection will drive much slower changes. In some instances, a population may not be able to respond fast enough to the selective forces and may become extinct.

Stabilizing Selection Acts against Individuals Who Deviate Too Far from the Average

Directional selection can't go on forever. Once a species is well adapted to a particular environment, and if the environment doesn't change, then most variations that appear through new mutations or recombination of old alleles will

be harmful. Therefore, the species will often undergo stabilizing selection, which favors the survival and reproduction of "average" individuals (see Fig. 17-9b). Stabilizing selection often occurs when a single trait is under opposing selective pressures from two different sources. Biologist M. K. Hecht, for example, studied lizards of the *Aristelliger* genus. He found that small lizards had a hard time defending territories, but large lizards were more likely to be preyed upon by owls. Therefore, *Aristelliger* lizards were under stabilizing selection favoring an "average" body size.

It is widely assumed, although difficult to prove, that many traits are under stabilizing selection. We have already mentioned several. Although the lengths of legs and necks of giraffes probably originated under directional selection for feeding on leaves high up in trees, they are almost certainly now under stabilizing selection, balancing the demands of eating and drinking. Similarly, female mate choice probably drove the evolution of elaborate sexual displays in many birds, but now increased vulnerability to predation may exert stabilizing selection: If a peacock's tail became so long that he couldn't fly, he would be unlikely to live long enough to woo a female.

Under certain circumstances, stabilizing selection may act not to eliminate variability, but to maintain it. Opposing selective pressures often give rise to **balanced polymorphism**, in which two or more alleles of a gene are maintained in a population because each is favored by a separate selective force. This seems to have occurred with the hemoglobin alleles in native Africans (see Chapter 14). The hemoglobin molecules of people who are homozygous for sickle-cell anemia (having two alleles for defective hemoglobin) clump up into long chains, distorting and weakening their red blood cells. This distortion causes severe anemia and potentially death. Before the advent of modern medicine, people homozygous for sickle-cell anemia were strongly selected against. Heterozygotes, who have one allele for defective hemoglobin and one allele for normal hemoglobin, suffer only mild anemia, though they may be adversely affected during strenuous exercise. Under these circumstances, you might wonder why natural selection has not eliminated the sickle-cell allele. Far from being eliminated, however, the sickle-cell allele is carried by nearly half the people in some areas of Africa. This distribution seems to result from the counterbalancing effects of anemia and malaria, a disease that formerly caused high death rates in equatorial Africa.

Malaria parasites multiply rapidly within the red blood cells of homozygous normal individuals. Before effective medical treatments were discovered, homozygous normals consequently often died of malaria. Heterozygotes, on the other hand, enjoy some protection against malaria. Malaria parasites inside a heterozygote's red blood cells use up oxygen, causing the sickle-cell hemoglobin to clump and the cells to become sickle shaped. Infected, sickled cells are destroyed by the spleen before the parasites can complete their development. Heterozygotes, therefore, have mild anemia but do not succumb to malaria. During the evolution of African populations, heterozygotes survived better than either type of homozygote and reproduced the most. As a result, both the normal hemoglobin allele and the sickle-cell allele have been preserved (Fig. 17-10).

Disruptive Selection Adapts Individuals within a Population to Different Habitats

Disruptive selection (see Fig. 17-9c) may occur when a population occupies an area that provides different types of resources that can be utilized by the species. In this situation, different characteristics best adapt individuals to use each type of resource. For example, an island, such as one of the Galapagos, may have several species of plants, some producing large, hard seeds and others small, soft seeds. Large seeds provide the most food per seed, but they can be cracked and eaten only by birds with large bills. Although large birds can easily eat small seeds, they would probably spend too much energy lugging their large bodies about looking for tiny seeds. If a single species of bird colonized such an island, what would happen? We would expect that larger-bodied, larger-beaked birds would spe-

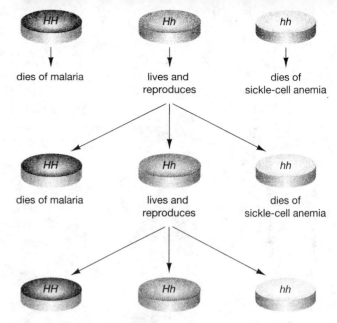

Figure 17-10   **Stabilizing selection can produce balanced polymorphism**

Sometimes two or more alleles, each producing a different phenotype, can be maintained in a population by opposing selection pressures. The alleles for normal (*H*) and sickle-cell (*h*) hemoglobin are maintained by selection against both homozygotes. Heterozygotes (*Hh*) reproduce the most, thereby keeping both alleles present in the population.

cialize on large seeds, while small-bodied, small-beaked birds would specialize on small seeds. Medium-sized birds might not be able to crack open the large seeds and might not get enough energy from small seeds, and so would be selected against. Disruptive selection would favor the survival and reproduction of both large and small, but not medium-sized, birds. Disruptive selection has not been extensively studied, although it has been documented or at least supported by studies of both butterflies and birds.

Natural Selection Takes Several Forms

Natural selection acts by eliminating individuals that do not have the characteristics needed for survival and reproduction in their environment. Characteristics that do help an individual to survive and reproduce in a particular environment are **adaptations**. The process of acquiring these characteristics is also called adaptation because *the end result of natural selection is adaptation to the environment.* An organism's environment can be divided into two components: the abiotic (nonliving) part and the biotic (living) part that consists of other organisms. Adaptations to both biotic and abiotic components occur through natural selection.

The abiotic environment includes physical factors such as climate, availability of water, and minerals in the soil. The abiotic environment provides the "bottom line" requirements that an organism must have to survive and reproduce. However, many of the adaptations that we see in modern organisms have arisen because of interactions with other organisms. As Darwin wrote, "the structure of every organic being is related . . . to that of all other organic beings, with which it comes into competition for food or residence, or from which it has to escape, or on which it preys." A simple example illustrates this concept.

A buffalo grass plant sprouts in a small patch of soil in the eastern Wyoming plains. Its roots must be able to take up enough water and minerals for growth and reproduction, and to that extent it must be adapted to its abiotic environment. Even in the dry prairies of Wyoming, this is a relatively trivial requirement *provided that the plant is alone and protected in its square meter of soil*. In reality, many plants, including other grasses, sagebrush bushes, and annual wildflowers also sprout in that same patch of soil. If our buffalo grass is to survive, it must compete for resources with the other plants. Its long, deep roots and efficient mineral uptake processes have evolved not so much because the plains are dry, but because it must share the dry prairies with other plants. Further, cattle (formerly bison) graze the prairies. Buffalo grass is extremely tough, with silica (glass) compounds reinforcing the blades, an adaptation that discourages grazing. Over millennia, tougher plants were harder to eat and so survived better and reproduced more—another adaptation to the biotic environment.

When two species or two populations of a single species interact extensively, each exerts strong selective pressures on the other. When one evolves a new feature or modifies an old one, the other often evolves new adaptations in response. As the Red Queen told Alice in *Through the Looking Glass*, "Here, you see, it takes all the running you can do to keep in the same place." This constant, mutual feedback between two species is called **coevolution**.

Competition for Scarce Resources Favors the Best-Adapted Individuals

One of the major selective forces in the biotic environment is **competition** with other members of the same species. As Darwin wrote in *On the Origin of Species:* "The struggle almost invariably will be most severe between the individuals of the same species, for they frequent the same districts, require the same food, and are exposed to the same dangers." In other words, no competing organism has such similar requirements for survival as another member of the same species. For example, both Lazuli Buntings and Western Bluebirds are brightly colored in blue, red, and white, and both nest and rear their young in the foothills of the Rocky Mountains in the summer. But they do not compete very much with each other, because they eat different foods: Bluebirds mostly catch insects, while buntings specialize in seeds. Each mosquito picked off by a bluebird makes little difference to a bunting, but makes it harder for other bluebirds to find enough to eat.

Different species may also compete for the same resources, although generally to a lesser extent. As we will discuss more fully in Chapter 46, whether a particular plot of prairie is covered with grass, sagebrush, or trees is at least partly determined by competition among those plants for scarce soil moisture.

During Predation, Both Predator and Prey Act as Agents of Selection

Although we commonly think of predation as one animal preying upon another animal, predation actually includes any situation in which one organism eats another. In some instances, coevolution between predators and prey is a sort of "biological arms race," with each side evolving new adaptations in response to "escalations" by the other. Darwin used the example of wolves and deer: Wolf predation selects against slow or incautious deer, thus leaving faster, more alert deer to reproduce and continue the species. In their turn, alert, swift deer select against slow, clumsy wolves, because such predators cannot acquire enough food.

Symbiosis Produces Adaptations between Species That Live in Intimate Association with One Another

Symbiosis is any relationship in which individuals of different species closely interact for an extended time. Examples of symbiosis are parasitism, in which one species lives

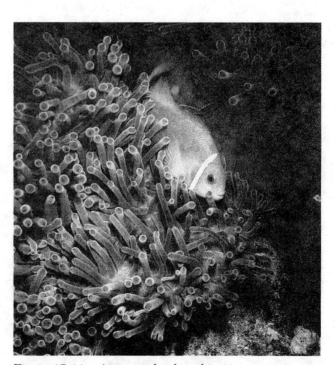

Figure 17-11   An example of symbiosis
Several species of clownfish live in a symbiotic relationship with anemones, each species of fish favoring a particular species of anemone. The fish nestle within the stinging tentacles of the anemone, thus protected from being eaten by other fish. The clownfish evolved specialized skin secretions and behaviors, protecting it from being affected by the anemone. The fish may accidentally drop food onto the anemone once in a while, but the benefits are probably fairly one-sided.

and feeds on a larger species; commensalism, in which one species benefits and the other remains unharmed; and mutualism, in which both species benefit. The different types of symbiosis are described in Chapter 44. From an evolutionary perspective, symbiosis leads to the most intricate coevolutionary adaptations. Although a given predator usually preys on several species and may interact with a particular species only occasionally, partners in symbiosis often live together virtually their entire lives (Fig. 17-11). At least one of the partners, and usually both, must continually adjust to any evolutionary changes developed by the other.

Sexual Selection Sometimes Seems to Oppose Other Forms of Natural Selection

As mentioned earlier, in many species of birds and mammals and even some fish, one of the sexes, usually the female, selects the mate. Males compete for the attention of females through song, elaborate displays, the defense of large territories, or even by building elaborate structures such as that of the bowerbird (see Chapter 42). Choosing a male with a good territory is obviously advantageous, since good territories provide adequate food and shelter to raise young. However, females often also prefer elaborate "fashions" in their mates, such as bright colors and long feathers or fins that may make the male more vulnerable to predation. Why? A popular hypothesis is that structures and colors that do not serve any clear adaptive purpose actually provide the females with an outward sign of the males' fitness. Only vigorous, energetic males can survive when burdened with conspicuous coloration or large tails. Similarly, males sick or under parasitic attack may be dull and frumpy compared with healthy males. Whatever the exact selective mechanisms, it is thought that many of the elaborate structures and behaviors found only in males have evolved through the selective pressure of female mate choice: Only the flashy males transmitted their genes to the next generation.

Darwin was so impressed with these structures that he coined the term *sexual selection* to designate the process of evolution through mate choice. Because conspicuous structures and bizarre behaviors make the males more vulnerable to predators, sexual selection often seems to work in opposition to other forms of natural selection. The trade-off between sexual selection and natural selection through predation has recently been demonstrated through observation and experiment in guppies (small freshwater fish). In streams where predation is a threat, male guppies are inconspicuous, blending with the sandy streambed. But in safer waters, male guppies show more conspicuous colors, apparently as a result of female preference for these markings. University of California biologist John Endler recently transplanted camouflage-colored male guppies from dangerous waters into safe waters. Within a year (about 20 guppy generations) their protected descendants had evolved conspicuous colors. However, nonsexual selective forces may also oppose one another; the height of a giraffe, for example, is a compromise between the advantage of reaching higher leaves for food and the disadvantage of vulnerability while drinking water (Fig. 17-12). In both sexual and nonsexual selection, then, some aspect of the environment (in sexual selection the "opinion" of the opposite sex, which is part of the social environment) influences reproductive success.

(a) 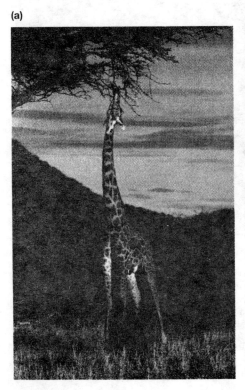 **(b)**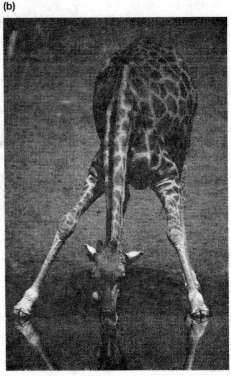

Figure 17-12 **A compromise between opposing selection pressures**

(a) The long neck and legs of a giraffe are a decided advantage in feeding on acacia leaves high up in trees. **(b)** But a giraffe has to get into an extremely awkward and vulnerable position to drink. Feeding and drinking thus place opposing selective pressures on the length of neck and legs.

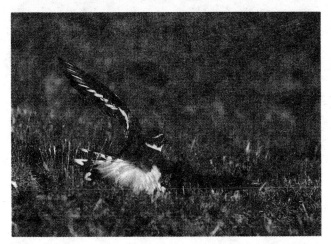

Figure 17-13   Altruism between mother and offspring

A female killdeer lures a predator away from its nest by faking injury. The mother places herself in some small danger (she can always fly away if the predator comes too close) but saves her offspring from much greater danger.

Kin Selection Favors Altruistic Behaviors

Evolution is often portrayed in the popular press as being "red in tooth and claw." This image of bloody and vicious interaction, however, is not the complete picture. Although it is true that competitive and predatory interactions influence the evolution of most species, cooperation and even self-sacrifice can be important selective forces too. **Altruism** refers to any behavior that endangers an individual organism or reduces its reproductive success but benefits other members of its species. Altruistic behaviors are common in the animal kingdom. A mother killdeer flutters just out of reach of a predator, feigning an injured wing and luring the predator away from her nest (Fig. 17-13); female worker bees forego reproduction and devote their lives to raising the offspring of the hive queen (see Chapter 42); and young male baboons scout around the edges of the troop, even though doing so increases their danger from leopards.

You might think that altruism runs counter to natural selection: If altruism is encoded in an organism's genes, those genes are placed at risk every time the altruist performs one of its brave behaviors. But natural selection can indeed select for altruistic genes, if the altruistic individual helps relatives who possess the same alleles. This special case of natural selection is an example of **kin selection** and is explored in "Evolutionary Connections: Kin Selection and the Evolution of Altruism."

Extinction

Natural selection not only produces the fleet limbs of the antelope and the exquisite eyes of the goshawk. It may also lead to the death of all the members of a species, **extinction.** Trilobites, dinosaurs, saber-tooth cats—all are extinct, known

only from fossils. Paleontologists estimate that *at least* 99.9% of all the species that ever existed are now extinct. Why? The actual cause of extinction is probably always environmental change, either in the living or the nonliving parts of the environment. Two characteristics seem to predispose a species to extinction when the environment changes: localized distribution and overspecialization. Three major changes that drive species to extinction are competition among species, novel predators or parasites, and habitat destruction.

Localized Distribution and Extreme Specialization Make Species Vulnerable in Changing Environments

Species vary widely in their range, and hence in their susceptibility to extinction. Some species, such as herring gulls, white-tailed deer, and humans, inhabit entire continents or even the whole Earth, while others, such as the Devil's Hole pupfish (Fig. 17-14), have extremely limited ranges. Obviously, if a species occurs in only a very small area, any disturbance of that area could easily result in extinction. If Devil's Hole dries up from climatic change or well drilling nearby, its pupfish will immediately vanish. Wide-ranging species, on the other hand, usually do not succumb to local environmental catastrophes.

Another factor that may make a species vulnerable to extinction is extreme specialization. Each species evolves a set of genetic adaptations in response to pressures from its particular environment. Sometimes these adaptations limit the organism to a very specialized set of environmental conditions. The Everglades Kite, for example, feeds only on a certain freshwater snail (Fig. 17-15). As the swamps of the

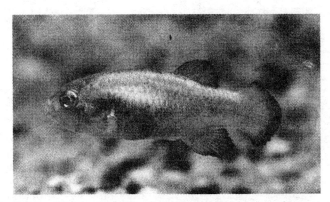

Figure 17-14   Very localized distribution can endanger a species

The Devil's Hole pupfish is found in only one spring-fed water hole in the Nevada desert. During the last glacial period, the southwestern deserts received a great deal of rainfall, forming numerous lakes and rivers. As the rainfall decreased, pupfish populations were isolated in shrinking small springs and streams. Isolated small populations and differing environmental conditions caused the ancestral pupfish species to split up into several very restricted modern species, all of which swim on the brink of extinction.

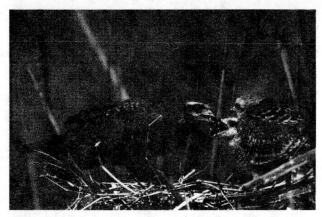

Figure 17-15 **Extreme specialization places species at risk**

The Everglades Kite feeds exclusively on the apple snail, found in swamps of the southeastern United States. Such behavioral specialization renders the kite extremely vulnerable to any environmental change that may exterminate its single species of prey.

American Southeast are drained for farms and developments, the snail population shrinks. If the snail becomes extinct, the kite will surely go extinct along with it.

In the fossil record, such behavioral specialization is hard to recognize. Structural specializations, however, may be just as restrictive. A case in point is giantism. For poorly understood reasons, many animals evolved huge size, including certain amphibians, dinosaurs, and giant mammals, such as mammoths and ground sloths. To support their bulk, these animals must have consumed enormous amounts of food. If environmental conditions deteriorated, those giants may have been unable to find enough food and thus died out. Smaller animals that ate the same food but needed less of it survived.

Interactions with Other Organisms May Drive Species to Extinction

As described earlier, interactions such as competition, predation, and parasitism serve as forces of natural selection. In some cases, these same forces can lead to extinction, rather than adaptation.

Competition for limited resources occurs in all environments. If a species' competitors evolve superior adaptations, and it doesn't evolve fast enough to keep up, it may become extinct. A particularly striking example of extinction through competition occurred in South America 2 to 3 million years ago. For millions of years North and South America were isolated from one another, and each developed a distinctive array of animal life. When the Panamanian land bridge arose, connecting the two continents, massive migrations took place. In general, North American animals displaced their South American counterparts, and many South American species became extinct.

When formerly isolated populations encounter one another, it isn't only competitors that migrate between the

areas—predators and parasites do too. With the exception of humans, who have exterminated hundreds of species, predators probably cause few extinctions. Parasites, on the other hand, can be devastating. In North America, Dutch elm disease and chestnut blight are well-known instances of introduced parasites that almost completely destroyed widespread native species. We cannot tell much about prehistoric parasite invasions, but the extinction of South American animals, mentioned above, might have been at least partly due to diseases carried south by resistant North American migrants.

Habitat Change and Destruction Are the Leading Causes of Extinction

Habitat change, both contemporary and prehistoric is the single greatest cause of extinctions. Presently, habitat destruction due to human activities is proceeding at a frightening pace. Perhaps the most rapid extinction in the history of life will occur over the next 50 years, as tropical forests are cut for timber and to clear land for cattle and crops. As many as half the species presently on Earth may be lost because of tropical deforestation.

Prehistoric habitat alteration usually occurred over a longer time span but nevertheless had serious consequences. Climate changes, in particular, caused many extinctions. Several times, moist, warm climates gave way to drier, colder climates with more variable temperatures. Many plants and animals failed to adapt to the harsh new conditions and became extinct. One cause of climate change is continental drift (Fig. 17-16). As the continents flow about over the surface of Earth, they change latitudes. Much of North America was located around the equator many millions of years ago, an area characterized by consistently warm and wet tropical weather. But drift carried the continent up into temperate and arctic regions. As a result, the tropical weather was replaced by cooler temperatures, less rainfall, and seasonal changes.

An extreme, and very sudden, type of habitat destruction might be caused by catastrophic geological events, such as massive volcanic eruptions. Several prehistoric eruptions, which would make the Mount St. Helens explosion look like a firecracker by comparison, wiped out every living thing for dozens of miles around and probably caused global climatic changes as well.

The fossil record reveals episodes of extensive worldwide extinctions, especially among marine life (Fig. 17-17). Enormous meteorites, several kilometers in diameter, may have hit Earth at these times. If a huge meteorite struck land, it would kick up enormous amounts of dust. The dust might be thick enough, and spread widely enough, to block out most of the sun's rays. Fires started by the impact might be widespread, adding soot to the atmosphere. Many plants would die because they couldn't photosynthesize. Many animals, all of which ultimately depend on plants for food,

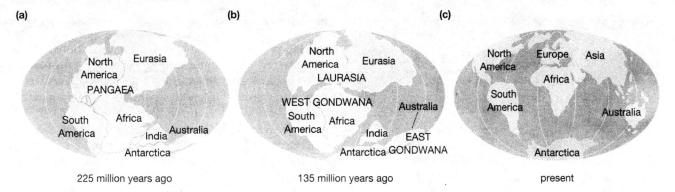

Figure 17-16 **Continental drift has caused climate change**
Although slow, continental drift can cause tremendous environmental changes, as land masses are moved about on the surface of Earth. The solid surfaces of the continents slide about over a viscous, but fluid, lower layer. **(a)** About 225 million years ago, all the continents were fused together into one gigantic land mass, which geologists call Pangaea. **(b)** Gradually Pangaea broke up into Laurasia and West and East Gondwana. **(c)** Further drift eventually resulted in the modern positions of the continents. Continental drift continues today: The Atlantic Ocean, for example, widens by a few centimeters each year.

would also die. Smaller amounts of dust might still block out enough sunlight to cause global cooling, perhaps even triggering an ice age. Widespread extinctions would result.

Did such massive meteorite strikes really occur, and if so, would they cause extinctions? No one knows for sure, but considerable evidence points to meteorites as the causes of at least some major extinctions (Fig. 17-18). Recently, two groups of researchers have suggested that the Chicxulub crater near the Yucatan Peninsula of Mexico was the impact site of the meteorite that might have killed the dinosaurs.

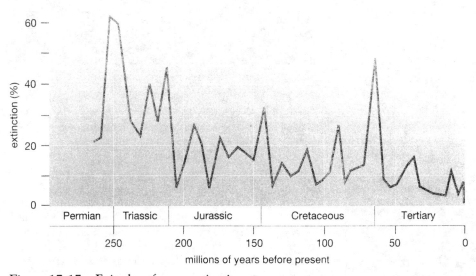

Figure 17-17 **Episodes of mass extinction**
This graph plots the percentage of genera of marine animals that have become extinct during geologic time. The higher the peak, the greater the extent of extinctions. Marine animals were chosen for this study because their fossils are abundant in sedimentary rocks and are easily dated. The large peak of extinctions near the boundary between the Cretaceous and Tertiary periods also approximately coincides with the end of the dinosaurs. Many paleontologists are convinced that the dinosaurs were going downhill for millions of years before this time, so there is hot debate over whether the Cretaceous-Tertiary extinction event (such as a meteorite impact) provided the final blow to the dinosaurs or whether the dinosaurs would have died out at that time anyway.

213

Natural Selection, Genetic Diversity, and Endangered Species

Ever since the Endangered Species Act was passed in 1976, the United States has had an official policy of protecting rare species. In fact, the real goal of the act is not protection but recovery; as one U.S. Fish and Wildlife Service official put it, "the goal is to get species *off* the list." Wildlife biologists try to determine how large a population a species needs to have before it is no longer in danger of extinction from unpredictable events, such as a couple of years of drought or an epidemic of parasites. If a species reaches this critical population size, it is no longer legally "endangered" with extinction.

Does a "large enough" population (which usually is still very small by historical standards) really ensure a species' survival? From our discussion of genetic drift and population bottlenecks, you probably realize that the answer is no. If the population of a species has been reduced to the point where it is placed on the endangered species list, then it probably has lost much of its genetic diversity. As ecologist Thomas Foose aptly put it, loss of habitat and consequent reduction in population size mean that "gene pools are being converted into gene puddles." Even if the species recovers in numbers, its original gene pool has been lost. When the forces of natural selection change at some future time, the species may not have the necessary genetic variability to produce individuals adapted to the new environment, and it may become extinct.

What can be done? The best solution, of course, is to leave enough habitat of diverse types so that species never become endangered in the first place. The human population, however, has grown so large and appropriated so much of Earth's resources that this solution is not possible in many places (Fig. E17-1). For many species, the only so-

lution is to preserve enough habitat so that the remaining population is large enough to retain all or most of the total genetic diversity of the species. If we are to be, as we imagine ourselves, the caretakers of the planet and not merely its ultimate consumers, then protection of other life forms and their genetic heritage will be a continuing responsibility as long as humankind exists.

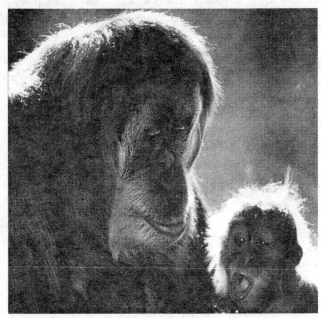

Figure E17-1 **Endangered by habitat destruction**

This orangutan and its young, who live in the tropical rain forests of Borneo, are among the innumerable species whose continued survival is threatened by habitat destruction.

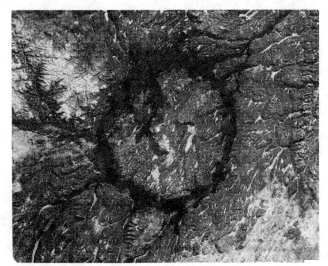

Figure 17-18 **Meteorites may have triggered some mass extinctions**

The Manicouagan crater in Quebec is about 45 miles in diameter. Giant impact craters such as this one often contain a central dome of rock that splashes up after the meteorite has buried itself in the ground, leaving a ring-shaped depression between the outer crater wall and the inner dome. In this satellite photo, water backed up behind a dam fills the crater ring. The Manicouagan meteorite struck a little over 200 million years ago; geologist Paul Olsen suggests that its impact triggered the mass extinction near the Triassic-Jurassic boundary (see Fig. 17-17).

Kin Selection and the Evolution of Altruism

Altruism is any behavior that is potentially harmful to the survival and future reproduction of an individual organism but enhances the reproductive potential of other organisms. Altruism includes worker bees' rearing the offspring of queen bees. Note that altruism does not imply conscious, voluntary decisions to engage in selfless behavior. Rather, most altruistic behaviors have a strong instinctive component; that is, many animals have altruism programmed in their genes.

From an evolutionary viewpoint, how can this be? Surely, if a mutation arose that caused altruistic behavior, and the bearers of that mutation lost their lives or failed to reproduce because of their self-sacrificing behaviors, their "altruistic alleles" would disappear from the population. Maybe, or maybe not. To understand the evolution of altruism, we will need to introduce a new concept: **inclusive fitness**. As formulated by W. D. Hamilton, the inclusive fitness of an allele is the fitness conferred on *all* organisms that have the allele. Therefore, *if an altruist benefits related members of its own species that bear the same altruistic allele, then the altruistic allele may be favored by natural selection.*

To see how altruism might increase the inclusive fitness of an allele, let's consider the Florida Scrub Jay. Year-old jays usually do not mate and reproduce. Instead, these yearlings remain at their parents' nest and help out with next year's brood. Let's assume, for simplicity, that this altruistic behavior is controlled by a single "altruistic" allele and that in the distant past helper jays had the altruistic allele, and nonhelpers had another, "selfish," allele.

At least for one year, altruistic yearlings do not reproduce; some probably die from predation or accidents and never reproduce at all. How, then, can this behavior be adaptive? It all has to do with relatedness and the probability of successful reproduction. First, an animal's offspring inherit 50% of its genes (the other 50% of the offspring's genes come from the other parent). On the average, an animal also shares 50% of its genes with its siblings. Therefore, *a scrub jay is just as related to its siblings as it would be to its own offspring.* The second factor influencing scrub jay reproduction is that ideal habitat for jays is limited. Inexperienced yearling jays would probably have a hard time acquiring a good nest site and would be hard put to feed their offspring. Their best "reproductive bet," then, is to put their energy into helping their parents. Selfish yearling jays that try to nest on their own will probably contribute fewer genes to the next generation than the altruistic yearlings do. This phenomenon, whereby the actions of an individual increase the survival or reproductive success of its relatives, is called kin selection.

As this example suggests, *kin selection can favor the evolution of altruism if the altruistic behavior benefits relatives that bear the same altruistic allele.* In most cases, an animal will not know if another carries the altruism allele, but the animal must at least be able to distinguish relatives from strangers: Relatives stand a good chance of possessing the altruism allele, but you never can tell with strangers. A yearling jay that helped out at the nest of unrelated adult jays would probably waste its time and effort.

Identification of relatives isn't too hard to imagine in the case of jays and their parents. Many biologists objected to other proposed instances of altruistic behaviors, however, arguing that animals cannot evaluate degrees of relatedness. Two findings seem to address this objection. First, many social groups, including wolf packs and baboon troops, are actually family groups. Therefore, an animal would not have to identify relatives in order for its altruistic behaviors to benefit them the most. Second, many animals, including birds, monkeys, tadpoles, bees, and even tunicate larvae, can indeed identify relatives (Fig. 17-19). Given the choice between relatives and strangers, these animals preferentially associate with their relatives, *even if they were separated at birth and have never seen those relatives before.* If animals selectively form related groups, then altruistic behaviors will most likely benefit relatives. Although it is not the only mechanism, kin selection has been a powerful selective force in the evolution of altruism in many species, probably including humans.

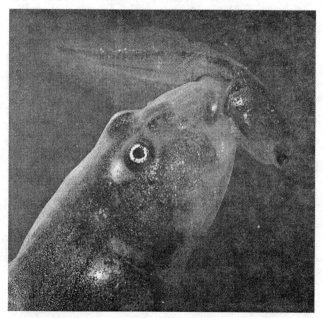

Figure 17-19 **Cannibalistic animals don't eat close relatives**

Spadefoot toad tadpoles, found in transient water holes of the Arizona desert, are cannibalistic. Many of their prey, however, are released unharmed after being tasted briefly. Researchers have discovered that the tadpoles can indeed distinguish, and spit out, their own brothers and sisters, preferring to eat unrelated members of their own species.

Evolution and the Genetics of Populations

The gene pool of a population is the total of all the different alleles of all the genes carried by the members of a population. The sources of genetic variability within a population are mutation, which produces new genes and alleles, and recombination during sexual reproduction. In its broadest sense, evolution is a change in the frequencies of alleles in the gene pool of a population due to enhanced reproduction by individuals bearing certain alleles.

Allele frequencies in a population will remain constant over generations only if the following conditions are met: (1) There must be no mutation; (2) there must be no gene flow, no net migration of alleles into or out of the population; (3) the population must be very large; (4) all mating must be random; (5) all genotypes must reproduce equally well (that is, no natural selection). These conditions are rarely, if ever, met in nature. Understanding why they are not met leads to an understanding of the mechanisms of evolution.

The Mechanisms of Evolution

1. Mutations are random, undirected changes in DNA composition. Although most mutations are neutral or harmful to the organism, some prove advantageous in certain environments. Mutations are rare and do not change allele frequencies very much, but they provide the raw material for evolution.
2. Migration is the flow of genes between populations. If the alleles that migrants carry are different from those in the populations from which they come or to which they migrate, migration will cause changes in allele frequencies.
3. In any population, chance events kill or prevent reproduction by some of the individuals. If the population is small, chance events may eliminate a disproportionate number of individuals bearing a particular allele, thereby greatly changing the allele frequency in the population. This change is termed genetic drift.
4. Many organisms do not mate randomly. If only certain members of a population can mate, then the next generation of organisms in the population will all be offspring of this select group, whose allele frequencies may differ from those of the population as a whole. Population bottleneck and founder effect, two types of genetic drift, illustrate the consequences small populations have on frequency of alleles.
5. The survival and reproduction of organisms are influenced by their phenotype. Because phenotype depends at least partly on genotype, natural selection will tend to favor the reproduction of certain alleles at the expense of others.

Natural Selection

Natural selection is really an issue of differential, or unequal, reproduction. Three types of natural selection are:

1. *Directional selection.* Individuals with characteristics that are different from average in one direction (for example, smaller) are favored both over average individuals and over those that differ from average in the opposite direction.
2. *Stabilizing selection.* Individuals of the "average value" for a characteristic are favored over individuals of extreme values.
3. *Disruptive selection.* Individuals of extreme characteristics are favored over individuals with average values.

Natural selection occurs as a result of the interactions of organisms with both the biotic (living) and abiotic (nonliving) parts of their environments. Within a species, sexual selection and altruism are two types of natural selection. When two or more species interact extensively so as to exert mutual selective pressures on each other for long periods of time, they both evolve in response. Such coevolution can occur as a result of any type of relationship between organisms, including competition, predation, and symbiosis.

Extinction

Two factors that contribute to the likelihood of extinction of a species are localized distribution and overspecialization. Factors that actually cause extinctions include competition among species, novel predators or parasites, and habitat destruction.

✽ KEY TERMS

adaptation	equilibrium population	kin selection
allele frequency	extinction	migration
altruism	fitness	natural selection
balanced polymorphism	founder effect	population
coevolution	gene flow	population bottleneck
competition	gene pool	population genetics
differential reproduction	genetic drift	sexual selection
directional selection	genetic equilibrium	stabilizing selection
disruptive selection	inclusive fitness	symbiosis

Multiple Choice

1. Genetic drift is a _____ process.
   a. random
   b. directed
   c. selection-driven
   d. coevolutionary
   e. uniformitarian

2. Most of the 700 species of fruit flies found in the Hawaiian archipelago are each restricted to a single island. One hypothesis to explain this pattern is that each species diverged after a small number of flies had colonized a new island. This mechanism is called
   a. sexual selection
   b. genetic equilibrium
   c. disruptive selection
   d. the founder effect
   e. assortative mating

3. You are studying leaf size in a natural population of plants. The second season is particularly dry, and the following year you find that the average leaf size in the population is smaller than the year before. But the amount of overall variation is the same, and the population size hasn't changed. Also, you've done experiments that show that small leaves are better adapted to dry conditions. Which of the following has occurred?
   a. genetic drift
   b. directional selection
   c. stabilizing selection
   d. disruptive selection
   e. the founder effect

4. You have bacteria thriving in your gastrointestinal tract. This is an example of
   a. inclusive fitness
   b. balanced polymorphism
   c. symbiosis
   d. kin selection
   e. altruism

5. Lamarckian evolution could occur
   a. if each gene had only one allele
   b. if individuals had different phenotypes
   c. if the genotype was altered by the same environmental changes that altered the phenotype
   d. if the phenotype was altered by the environment
   e. under none of these conditions

6. Of the following possibilities, the best way to estimate the Darwinian fitness of an organism is to measure the
   a. size of its offspring
   b. number of eggs it produces
   c. number of eggs it produces over its lifetime
   d. number of offspring it produces over its lifetime
   e. number of offspring it produces over its lifetime that survive to breed

Review Questions

1. What is a gene pool? How would you determine the allele frequencies in a gene pool?

2. Define an equilibrium population, and outline the conditions that must be met for a population to remain in equilibrium.

3. How does population size affect the likelihood of changes in allele frequencies by chance alone? Can significant changes in allele frequencies (that is, evolution) occur because of genetic drift?

4. If you went out and measured the allele frequencies of a gene and found large differences from the proportions predicted by Hardy-Weinberg equilibrium, would that prove that natural selection is occurring in the population you are studying? Review the conditions that lead to Hardy-Weinberg equilibrium, and explain your answer.

5. People like to say that "you can't prove a negative." Study the experiment in Figure 17-1 again, and comment on what it demonstrates.

6. Describe the three types of natural selection. Which type(s) is (are) most likely to occur in stable environments and which type(s) in rapidly changing environments?

7. What is sexual selection? How is sexual selection similar to and different from other forms of natural selection?

8. Briefly describe competition, predation, symbiosis, and altruism, and give an example of each.

9. Define kin selection and inclusive fitness. Can these concepts help to explain the evolution of altruism?

1. In North America, the average height of human adults has been increasing steadily for decades. Is directional selection occurring? What data would you need to justify your answer?

2. Malaria is rare in North America. In populations of African Americans, what would you predict is happening to the frequency of the hemoglobin allele that leads to sickling in red blood cells? How would you go about determining if your prediction is true?

3. By the 1940s the Whooping Crane population had been reduced to under 50 individuals. Thanks to conservation measures, their numbers are now increasing. But what special evolutionary problems do Whooping Cranes have after passing through a population bottleneck?

4. In many countries, conservationists are trying to design national park systems so that "islands" of natural area (the big parks) are connected by thin "corridors" of undisturbed habitat. The idea is that this arrangement will allow animals and plants to migrate between refuges. Why would such migration be important?

5. Extinctions have occurred throughout the history of life on Earth. Why should we care if humans are causing a mass extinction event now?

6. A preview question for Chapter 18: A species is all the populations of organisms that potentially interbreed with one another but that are reproductively isolated from (cannot interbreed with) other populations. Using the five assumptions of the Hardy-Weinberg equilibrium population as a starting point, what factors do you think would be important in the splitting of a single ancestral species into two modern species?

Allison, A. C. "Sickle Cells and Evolution." *Scientific American*, August 1956. The story of the interaction between sickle-cell anemia and malaria in Africa.

Alvarez, W., and Asaro, F. "An Extraterrestrial Impact," and Courtillot, V. E. "A Volcanic Eruption." *Scientific American*, October 1990. Leading geologists debate the question, What caused the mass extinction of the dinosaurs at the end of the Cretaceous period?

Fellman, B. "To Eat or Not to Eat." *National Wildlife*, February–March 1995. How animals performing altruistic behaviors identify their relatives.

Gould, S. J. "The Evolution of Life on the Earth." *Scientific American*, October 1994. The importance of chance and catastrophe in shaping modern life.

May, R. M. "The Evolution of Ecological Systems." *Scientific American*, September 1979. Coevolution accounts for much of the structure of natural communities of plants and animals.

O'Brien, S. J., Wildt, D. E., and Bush, M. "The Cheetah in Peril." *Scientific American*, May 1986. According to molecular and immunological techniques, a population bottleneck has reduced the genetic variability of the world's cheetahs almost to zero.

Ryan, M. J. "Signals, Species, and Sexual Selection." *American Scientist*, January–February 1990. Ryan explores a variety of experiments on sexual selection, including the genetic basis of male characteristics and female choice.

Stebbins, G. L., and Ayala, F. "The Evolution of Darwinism." *Scientific American*, July 1985. A synthesis of molecular and classical evolutionary methodologies.

N E T W A T C H

On-line resources for this chapter are on the World Wide Web at:
http://www.prenhall.com/~audesirk (click on the table of contents link and then select Chapter 17).

7

THE SOCIAL
BEHAVIOR
OF ANIMALS

> *"The elements of our own behavior are found in all organisms."*
>
> E. G. CONKLIN, 1944

Elaborate instincts: The male satin bowerbird instinctively builds an intricate structure, or bower, that attracts females of the same species.

The Australian satin bowerbird male selects a prime location on the forest floor and picks it clean. Then, after covering the site with coarse grass and twigs, he constructs his elaborate bower, a prop for his courtship dance. Meticulously, he weaves two parallel walls of twigs a foot high and 4 inches thick. Then he chews a twig until its end bristles into a brush and uses it to paint the walls with a mixture of saliva and berry juice. Not satisfied, he decorates the sunny southern end of the avenue between the walls with blue objects: blue berries, blue feathers, even blue bits of glass or plastic. If his bower and treasure trove are sufficiently enticing, a female may come to watch him dance. At the sight of her, he leaps about, showing off each treasure. A successful dance ends with mating. The female then flies off to build a nest and tend her eggs alone.

The satin bowerbird's behavior seems incredibly complex and intelligent—until we look at other bowerbirds. Lauderbach's bowerbird collects only red and pale gray objects. The fawn-breasted bowerbird decorates his bower floor and walls with pale green berries. The great bowerbird favors white treasure piles with pale green borders. Each builds a particular shape of bower unique to its species, decorates it in species-specific colors, and performs a species-specific dance that clearly reveals the overwhelming role of heredity in this elaborate courtship ritual. The females, in turn, respond instinctively only to those bowers built by males of their species. Clearly, communicating his species is an important function of the male bowerbird's elaborate courtship behavior.

Social behavior is a necessity for nearly all animals, since at least minimal social interactions are required for sexual reproduction. Social interactions occur between parent and offspring in those species that nurture their young. In addition, most animals interact competitively in pursuit of resources such as food, living space, or mates. Some species, such as bees and ants, form complex societies based on instinctive social interactions. As we explore in Chapters 43 and 44, social interactions help regulate population size and density and govern some of the community interactions that provide the framework for ecosystem structure. Because many social behaviors are genetically coded, they provide raw material for natural selection, as we will examine more closely at the end of this chapter. All social behavior is based on the ability to communicate, so we start with an exploration of that phenomenon.

Communication

Social behavior is exhibited to some degree by all but the simplest organisms. The basis of all social behavior is communication, and the ultimate outcomes are survival and reproduction. In the context of animal behavior, **communication** is defined as the production of a signal by one organism that causes another to change its behavior in a way beneficial to one or both.

Although animals of different species may communicate (picture a cat, its tail erect and bushy, hissing at a strange dog), most communication occurs between members of the same species. Potential mates must communicate, as must parents and offspring. At the same time, members of the same species compete most directly with one another for food, space, and mates. Communication is often used to resolve such conflicts with minimal damage.

The mechanisms by which animals communicate are astonishingly diverse and use all the senses. In the following sections, we look at communication by visual displays, sound, chemicals, and touch.

Visual Communication Includes Active and Passive Signals

Animals with well-developed eyes, from insects to mammals, use vision to communicate. Visual signals may be **active**, in which a specific movement (such as baring fangs) or posture (lowering head, erecting fur) conveys a message (Fig. 42-1). Alternatively, visual signals may be **passive**, in which case the size, shape, or color of the animal conveys important information, often concerning its sex and reproductive state. For example, when female mandrills become sexually receptive, they develop a large, brightly colored swelling on their buttocks (Fig. 42-2). Active and passive signals may be combined, as illustrated by the lizard in Figure 42-3, the courtship display of the male peacock (see Fig. 42-14a), and the courtship behavior of the three-spined stickleback fish (see Fig. 42-15).

Like all forms of communication, visual signals have both advantages and disadvantages. On the plus side, they are instantaneous and can impart a great deal of information in a short time. The animal can convey the intensity of its response by varying its visual signals (Fig. 42-4). Visual communication is quiet and unlikely to alert distant predators, although the signaler does make itself conspicuous to those nearby. On the negative side, visual signals are usually ineffective in darkness or dense vegetation, though female fireflies signal potential mates using species-specific patterns of flashes. Finally, visual signals are limited to close-range communication.

Communication by Sound Has Many Advantages

The use of sound overcomes many of the shortcomings of visual displays. Like visual displays, sound communication is almost instantaneous. But unlike visual signals, sound can

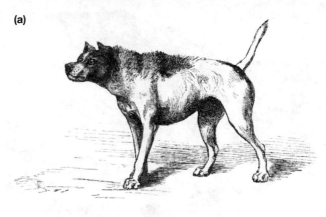

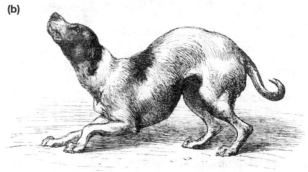

Figure 42-1 Aggressive and submissive displays

These dogs were drawn by Charles Darwin, a perceptive student of animal behavior. **(a)** Upright stance, erect hair, ears, and tail, and a direct stare combine to make the aggressor appear formidable indeed. **(b)** Notice how those displays are reversed in the submissive pose.

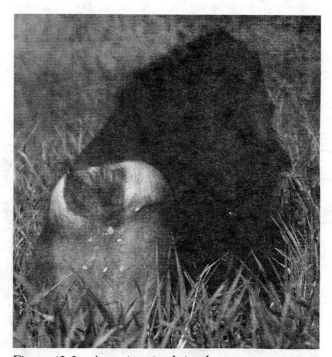

Figure 42-2 A passive visual signal

The female mandrill's colorfully swollen buttocks serve as a passive visual signal that she is fertile and ready to mate.

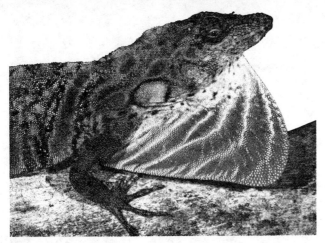

Figure 42-3 **An aggressive display**

The South American *Anolis* lizard raises his head high in the air (an active visual signal), revealing a brilliantly colored throat pouch (a passive visual signal) warning others to keep their distance.

be transmitted through darkness, dense forests, and even water, as the intricate songs of humpback whales testify. If the animal is sufficiently energetic, its call may carry much farther than the eye can see. When the small kangaroo rat drums the Arizona desert floor with its hind feet, the sound can be heard more than 45 meters (150 feet) away. The howls of a wolf pack carry for miles on a still night, and the low, resonant song of the humpback whale can possibly be heard by other whales up to hundreds of miles away.

Auditory signals are similar to visual displays in that they can transmit rapidly changing information almost instantaneously (think of words and of the emotional nuances conveyed by the human voice during a conversation). Changes in motivation may be signaled by a change in the loudness or pitch of the sound. An individual may convey different messages by variations in the pattern, volume, and pitch of the sound produced. Ethologist Thomas Struhsaker studied vervet monkeys in Kenya in the 1960s and found that they produced different calls in response to threats from each of their major predators: snakes, leopards, and eagles. In 1980, other researchers reported that the response of other vervet monkeys to each of these calls is appropriate to the particular predator. The "bark" that warns of a leopard or other four-legged carnivore causes monkeys on the ground to take to trees and those in trees to climb higher. The "rraup" call signaling an eagle or other hunting bird causes monkeys on the ground to look upward and take cover, while monkeys already in trees drop to the shelter of lower, denser branches. The "chutter" call indicates a snake and causes the monkeys to stand up and search the ground for this slower predator.

The use of sound is by no means limited to birds and mammals. Male crickets produce species-specific songs that attract female crickets of the same species (see "Scientific Inquiry: Robot Cricket Finds Her Mate" in Chapter 41). The annoying whine of the female mosquito as she prepares to bite alerts nearby males that she will soon have the blood meal necessary for laying eggs. Male water striders vibrate their legs, sending species-specific patterns of vibrations through the water that attract mates and repel other males (Fig. 42-5). From these rather simple signals to the virtuoso performance of human language, sound is one of the most important forms of communication.

Chemical Communication Uses Pheromones

Chemical substances produced by an individual that influence the behavior of others of its species are called **pheromones.** Chemicals may carry messages over long distances, and, unlike sound, take very little energy to produce. Pheromones may not even be detected by other species, including predators who might be attracted to visual or auditory displays. Like a signpost, a pheromone

(a)

(b)

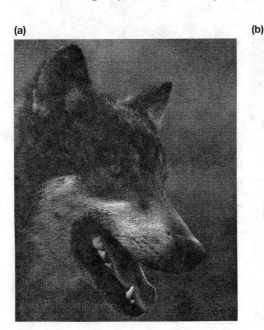
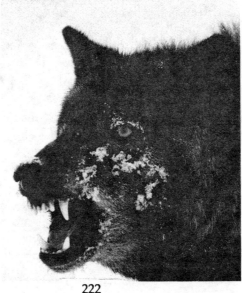

Figure 42-4 **Graded visual signals**

(a) A relaxed, nonaggressive wolf. (b) The wolf signals aggression by lowering the head, ruffling the fur on its neck and along its back, facing the opponent with a direct stare, and exposing its fangs. These signals may vary in intensity, communicating different levels of aggression.

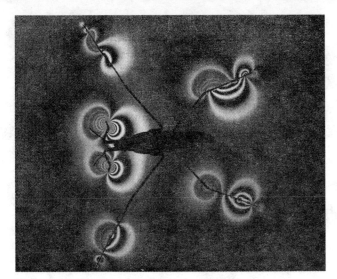

Figure 42-5   Communication by vibration

The light-footed water strider relies on the surface tension of water to support its weight. By vibrating its legs, the water strider sends signals radiating out over the surface of the water. These vibrations advertise the species and sex of the strider to others nearby.

persists over time and can convey a message after the animal has departed. Wolf packs, hunting over areas up to 1000 square kilometers (386 square miles), mark the boundaries of their travels with pheromones in urine that warn other packs of their presence. As anyone who has walked a dog can attest, the domesticated dog reveals its wolf ancestry by staking out its neighborhood with urine that carries a chemical message: "I live in this area."

This type of communication requires that an animal be able to synthesize as well as respond to a different chemical for each message. As a result, in general, fewer messages are communicated with chemicals than with sight or sound. In addition, pheromone signals lack the diversity and gradation of auditory or visual signals. Nonetheless, chemicals powerfully convey a few simple but critical messages.

Pheromones act in one of two ways. **Releaser pheromones** cause an immediate, observable behavior in the animal detecting them. They convey messages such as "this area is mine" or "I am ready to mate now." Foraging ants who discover food lay a trail of pheromones secreted by abdominal glands from the food back to the nest. Its message: "Follow to find food." **Primer pheromones**, in contrast, stimulate a physiological change in the animal detecting them, usually in its reproductive state. The queen honeybee produces a primer pheromone called **queen substance** that is eaten by her hivemates and prevents other females in the hive from becoming sexually mature. The urine of mature males of certain species of mice contains a primer pheromone that influences female reproductive hormones. This pheromone causes the newly mature female to become sexually receptive and fertile for the first time. It will also cause a female mouse newly pregnant by another male to abort her litter and become sexually receptive to the new male. There is indirect evidence (discussed later in the chapter) that primer pheromones may even influence human reproductive cycles.

The sex attractant pheromones of some agricultural pests, such as the Japanese beetle and gypsy moth, have been synthesized. These synthetic pheromones can be used to confuse and disrupt mating or to lure these insects into traps. Pest control using pheromones has major environmental advantages. Pesticides kill beneficial as well as harmful insects and select for resistant insect strains. In contrast, pheromones are specific to one species, and insects resistant to the attraction of their own pheromones would not reproduce.

Communication by Touch Helps Establish Social Bonds

Physical contact between individuals is used in several ways, particularly to establish and maintain social bonds among group members. Primates, including humans, are "contact species" in which a variety of gestures including kissing, nuzzling, patting, petting, and grooming play an important social function (Fig. 42-6a). The greeting ceremony of wolves and dogs involves mutual licking, sniffing, and gentle nipping around the mouth (Fig. 42-6b). The bond between parent and offspring is often cemented by close physical contact, and sexual activity is frequently preceded by ritualized contact (Fig. 42-6c).

Touch can also influence human well-being. Recent research shows that when the limbs of premature human infants are stroked and moved for 45 minutes daily, the infants are more active, responsive, emotionally stable, and gain weight more rapidly than premature infants receiving the standard hospital treatment.

Social Behavior

Many social interactions use a combination of sight, sound, scent, and touch, as illustrated by the waggle dance of the honeybee (described later in this chapter). These complex behaviors play many different roles in the lives of animals. The following sections discuss the forms of communication animals use as they compete for limited resources, reproduce, and cooperate in complex societies.

Competition for Resources Underlies Many Forms of Social Behavior

Aggressive Displays Minimize Injury

One of the most obvious manifestations of competition for resources such as food, space, or mates is **aggression**, or antagonistic behavior, usually between members of the same species. Although the expression "survival of the fittest" evokes images of the strongest animal emerging triumphantly from among the dead bodies of its competitors, in reality most aggressive encounters between members of the same species are rather harmless. Natural selection has favored the evolution of symbolic displays or rituals for resolving conflicts. During fighting, even the victorious an-

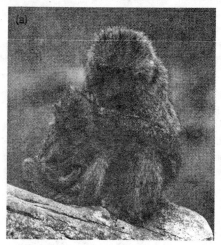
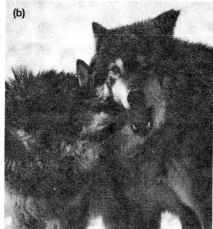
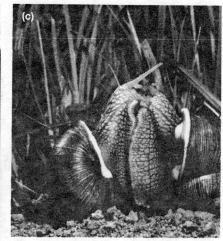

Figure 42-6   Communication by touch

(a) An adult olive baboon grooms a juvenile. Grooming not only reinforces social relationships but also removes debris and parasites from the fur. (b) Wolves from the same pack engage in a greeting ceremony that involves nuzzling and licking. This behavior may indicate submission, as when a subordinate animal licks a dominant one. Wolf pups use muzzle licking to beg for food. (c) Touch is also important in sexual communication. These land snails *(Helix)* engage in courtship behavior that will culminate in mating.

imal may be injured, so serious fighters may not survive to pass on their genes. Aggressive *displays*, in contrast, allow the competitors to assess each other and acknowledge a winner on the basis of its size, strength, and motivation rather than on the wounds it can inflict.

During visual aggressive displays, animals exhibit weapons, such as claws and fangs (Fig. 42-7a), and often behave in ways that make them appear larger (Fig. 42-7b). Competitors may stand upright and erect their fur, feathers, ears, or fins (see Figs. 42-1a, 42-3, and 42-4). The displays may be accompanied by intimidating sounds (growls, croaks, roars, chirps) whose loudness can help decide the winner. Fighting is usually a last resort when displays fail to resolve the dispute.

In addition to visual and vocal displays of strength, many animal species engage in ritualized combat. Deadly weapons may clash harmlessly (Fig. 42-8) or may not be used at all. Frequently these encounters involve shoving rather than slashing. Again, the strength and motivation of the combatants are determined, and the loser slinks away in a submissive posture that minimizes the size of its body (see Fig. 42-1b).

Dominance Hierarchies Reduce Aggressive Interactions

Aggressive interactions use a great deal of energy, may cause injury, and can disrupt other important tasks such as finding food, watching for predators, courting a mate,

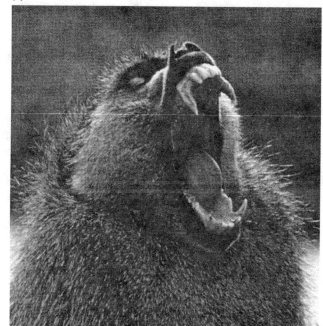

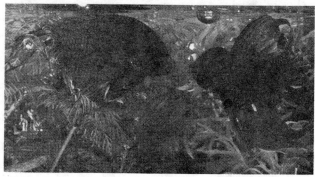

Figure 42-7   Aggressive displays

(a) Threat display of the male baboon. Despite the potentially lethal fangs so prominently displayed, aggressive encounters between baboons rarely cause injury. (b) The aggressive display of the male fighting fish includes elevating the fins and flaring the gill covers, thus making the body appear larger.

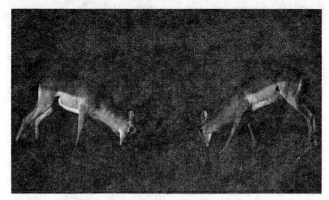

Figure 42-8 **Displays of strength**

Ritualized combat of male impalas, a type of African antelope. The deadly horns, which could stab a predator, clash harmlessly. Eventually one impala, sensing greater vigor in his opponent, will often retreat unharmed.

or raising young. So there are adaptive advantages to resolving conflicts with minimal aggression. In a **dominance hierarchy,** each animal establishes a rank that determines its access to resources. Domestic chickens, after a period of squabbling, sort themselves into a reasonably stable "pecking order." Thereafter, when competition for food occurs, all hens defer to the dominant bird, all but the dominant bird give way to the second, and so on. Conflict is minimized because each bird knows its place. Dominance among male bighorn sheep is reflected in the size of their horns (Fig. 42-9). In wolf packs, one member of each sex is the dominant, or "alpha," individual to whom all others are subordinate. Although aggressive encounters occur frequently while the dominance hierarchy is being established, after each animal learns its place, disputes are minimized. The dominant individuals obtain most access to the resources needed for reproduction, including food, space, and mates.

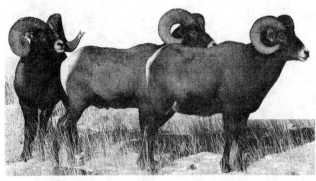

Figure 42-9 **A dominance hierarchy**

The dominance hierarchy of the male bighorn sheep is signaled by the size of the horns; these rams increase in status from right to left. These backward-curving horns, clearly not designed to inflict injury, are used in ritualized combat.

Territoriality Parcels Out Resources

Territoriality is the defense of an area where important resources are located. The defended resources may include places to mate, raise young, feed, or store food. Territorial animals generally restrict most or all of their activities to the defended area and advertise their presence there. Territories may be defended by males, females, a mated pair, or by entire social groups (as in the case of the defense of their nest by social insects). However, territorial behavior is most often seen in adult males, and territories are usually defended against members of the same species, those who compete most directly for the resources being protected. Territories are as diverse as the animals defending them. For example, they can be small depressions in the sand used as nesting sites by cichlid fish (Fig. 42-10), a hole in the sand used as a home by a crab, a tree where a woodpecker stores acorns (Fig. 42-11), or an area of forest providing food for a squirrel.

Acquiring and defending a territory require considerable time and energy, yet territoriality is seen in animals as diverse as worms, arthropods, fish, birds, and mammals. The fact that organisms as unrelated as worms and humans independently evolved similar behavior suggests that territoriality provides some important adaptive advantages. Although the benefits depend on the species and the type of territory it defends, some broad generalizations are possible. First (as with dominance hierarchies), once a territory

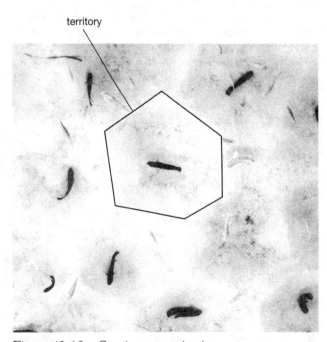

Figure 42-10 **Contiguous territories**

Nesting males of the mouthbrooding cichlid fish (*Oreochromis mossambicus*) guard territories. When space is abundant, these territories are circular. When the population density rises, the territories approach hexagonal shapes because they are so closely packed. A female visits the territories and selects a male, who fertilizes the eggs she releases. She then gathers the eggs in her mouth (where they will develop) and departs.

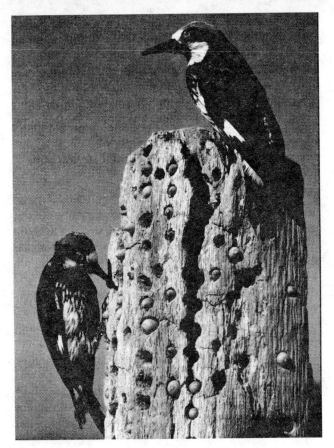

Figure 42-11   A feeding territory

The acorn woodpecker excavates acorn-sized holes in dead trees, stuffing them with green acorns for dining during the lean winter months. He defends the trees vigorously against other acorn-eating birds of other species, such as jays.

is established through aggressive interactions, relative peace prevails as boundaries are recognized and respected. The saying "good fences make good neighbors" also applies to nonhuman territories. One reason for this respect is that an animal is highly motivated to defend its territory and will often defeat larger, stronger animals if they attempt to invade it. Conversely, an animal outside its territory is much less secure and more easily defeated. This principle was demonstrated by Niko Tinbergen's experiment using the stickleback fish, described in Figure 42-12.

Defending reproductive territories is advantageous for certain species. The reproductive success of these animals is enhanced by a high-quality breeding territory, which might have features such as large size, abundant food, and secure nesting areas. Males who successfully defend the most desirable territories have the greatest chance of mating and passing on their genes. For example, experiments have shown that male sticklebacks who defend large territories are more successful in attracting mates than are males who defend small territories. Females who select males with the best territories increase their reproductive success and pass their genetic traits (often including their mate-selection preferences) to their offspring.

Territoriality limits the population size of some species, helping to keep it within the limits set by the available resources. For example, the Scottish red grouse defends feeding and nesting territories. Scientists found that variations in territory size were correlated with the availability of food. In years when food was abundant, territories in the study area were smaller and the number of mating pairs was greater than in lean years.

Territories are advertised through sight, sound, and smell. If the territory is small enough, the owner's mere

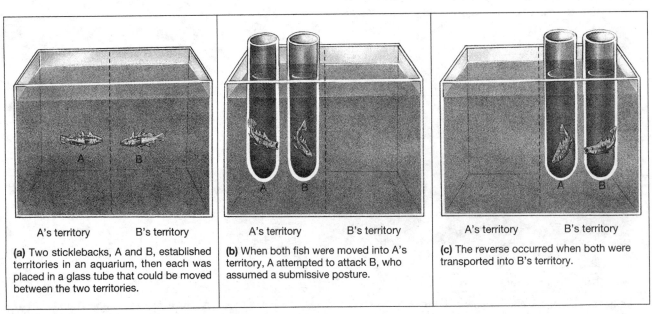

A's territory B's territory	A's territory B's territory	A's territory B's territory
(a) Two sticklebacks, A and B, established territories in an aquarium, then each was placed in a glass tube that could be moved between the two territories.	**(b)** When both fish were moved into A's territory, A attempted to attack B, who assumed a submissive posture.	**(c)** The reverse occurred when both were transported into B's territory.

Figure 42-12   Territory ownership and aggression

Niko Tinbergen's experiment demonstrating the effect of territory ownership on aggressive motivation.

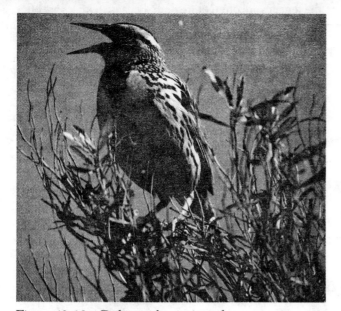

Figure 42-13   Defense of a territory by song

A male meadowlark announces ownership of his territory to all listeners.

presence, reinforced by aggressive displays at intruders, may be a sufficient defense. A mammal that owns a territory but cannot always be present may scent-mark its terrestrial boundaries using pheromones. Male rabbits use pheromones secreted by chin and anal glands to mark their territories. Hamsters rub the areas around their dens with secretions from special glands in their flanks.

Vocal displays are a common form of territorial advertisement. Male sea lions defend a strip of beach by swimming up and down in front of it, calling continuously. Male crickets produce a specific pattern of chirps to warn other males away from their burrows. Birdsong is a striking example of territorial defense. The cheerful melody of the male meadowlark is part of an aggressive display, warning other males to steer clear of his territory (Fig. 42-13). The loudest songbird generally defends the largest territory and is most successful in attracting a mate and driving away intruders. In

ingenious experiments using the wood thrush, ethologist W. Dilger of Cornell University "invaded" the territories of male wood thrushes with a stuffed wood thrush accompanied by a loudspeaker through which he played recordings of the thrush's territorial song. When the volume was turned low, the resident thrushes attacked the stuffed bird, but they retreated rapidly when the volume was raised.

Sexual Reproduction Requires Social Interactions between Mates

Successful reproduction requires that several conditions be met. Animals must identify one another as members of the same species, as members of the opposite sex, and as being sexually receptive. Many animals resist the close approach of another individual; this resistance must be overcome before mating can occur. Some animals, such as frogs and many species of fish, must release eggs and sperm at precisely the same moment for fertilization to occur. The need to fulfill all these requirements has resulted in exceedingly complex, diverse, and fascinating courtship behavior.

Individuals who mate with members of other species, or members of the same sex, waste considerable energy and do not pass on their genes. Thus, animals have evolved elaborate ways to communicate their species and sex, often using vocalizations. The raucous, nighttime chirping that can keep campers awake is probably a chorus of male tree frogs, each singing a species-specific song. Male grasshoppers and crickets advertise species and sex by their calls, as does the female mosquito with her high-pitched whine. Male birds use song to attract a mate as well as defend a territory. For example, the male bellbird uses its deafening call to defend large territories and attract females from great distances. The females fly from one territory to another, alighting near the male in his tree. The male, beak gaping, leans directly over the flinching female and utters an earsplitting note. The female apparently endures this to compare volumes of the various males, choosing the loudest (who would also be the best defender of a territory) as a mate. Males and females of other bird species join

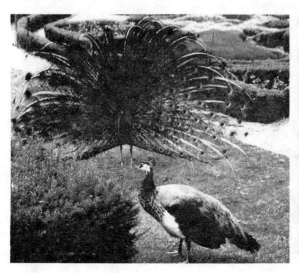
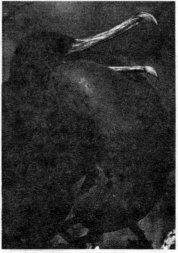

Figure 42-14   Sexual displays

(a) The extravagant tail of the male peacock is displayed during courtship. This oversized tail hampers flight and increases the male's vulnerability to predators. It probably evolved as females consistently selected the flashiest birds as mates, preferring this exaggerated releaser to a more practical tail. (b) The male frigate bird of the Galapagos Islands inflates a scarlet throat pouch to attract passing females.

in elaborate duets that help synchronize reproductive readiness and reinforce the bond between them.

Many species court using visual displays. The firefly, for example, flashes a message identifying its sex and species. Male fence lizards bob their heads in a species-specific rhythm, and females distinguish and prefer the rhythm of their own species. The tail of the male peacock and the scarlet throat of the male frigate bird serve as flashy advertisements of sex and species (Fig. 42-14). In contrast, the females are often quite drab. Because females are often in close association with their young, eye-catching (and predator-attracting) displays could be dangerous.

Species and sex recognition and the synchronization of reproductive behavior often require a complex series of signals, both active and passive, by both sexes. Such signals are beautifully illustrated by the complex underwater "ballet" executed by the male and female three-spined stickleback fish (Fig. 42-15).

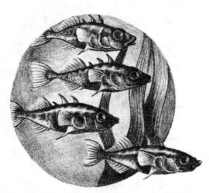

(a) A male, inconspicuously colored, leaves the school of males and females to establish a breeding territory.

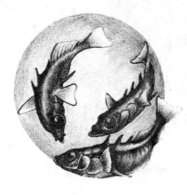

(b) As his belly takes on the red color of the breeding male, he displays aggressively at other red-bellied males, exposing his red underside.

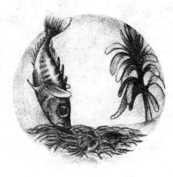

(c) Having established a territory, the male begins nest construction by digging a shallow pit that he will fill with bits of algae cemented together by a sticky secretion from his kidneys.

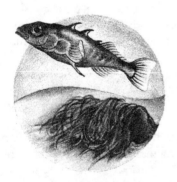

(d) After he tunnels through the nest to make a hole, his back begins to take on the blue courting color that makes him attractive to females.

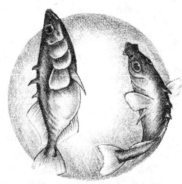

(e) An egg-carrying female displays her enlarged belly to him by assuming a head-up posture. Her swollen belly and his courting colors are passive visual displays.

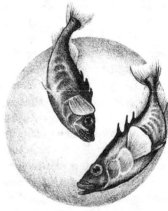

(f) He leads her to the nest using a zigzag dance.

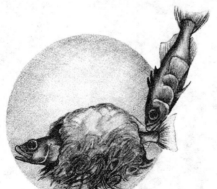

(g) After she enters, he stimulates her to release eggs by prodding at the base of her tail.

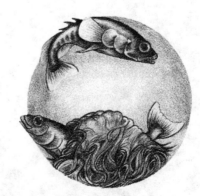

(h) He enters the nest as she leaves and deposits sperm that fertilize the eggs.

Figure 42-15   Courtship of the three-spined stickleback

insect. While she eats, the male mates and runs. The male of another species gains extra time to mate by "gift-wrapping" the insect in a silken web that she must remove before she can eat the gift.

Social Behavior within Animal Societies Requires Cooperative Interactions

Social groupings of animals are conspicuous but by no means universal. Group living has both advantages and disadvantages, and the relative weight of the positive and negative factors varies considerably among different animal species.

On the negative side, social animals may encounter:

1. Increased competition within the group for limited resources
2. Increased risk of infection from contagious diseases
3. Increased risk that offspring will be killed by other members of the group
4. Increased risk of being spotted by predators

For a species to have evolved social behavior, the benefits must have outweighed the costs. Benefits to social animals include:

1. Increased ability to detect, repel, and confuse predators
2. Increased hunting efficiency or increased ability to spot localized food resources
3. Advantages resulting from the potential for division of labor within the group
4. Conservation of energy
5. Increased likelihood of finding mates

The degree to which animals of the same species cooperate varies significantly from one species to the next.

Pheromones can play an important role in reproductive behavior. The sexually receptive female silk moth, for example, sits quietly and releases a chemical message so powerful that it may be detected by males 4 to 5 kilometers (2.5 to 3 miles) away. The exquisitely sensitive and selective receptors on the antennae of the male respond to just a few molecules of the substance, allowing him to travel upwind along a concentration gradient to find the female (Fig. 42-16). Water is an excellent medium for dispersing chemical signals, and fish often use a combination of pheromones and elaborate courtship movements to ensure synchronous release of gametes. Mammals, with their highly developed sense of smell, often rely on pheromones released by the female during her fertile periods to attract males. The irresistible attraction of a female dog in heat to nearby males is one example. The primer pheromone in male mouse urine is another.

Most encounters between individuals of solitary species are competitive and aggressive. During the brief mating season, their reluctance to allow others to approach closely must be overcome for their mate but retained toward others. These conflicting needs introduce an element of tension into sexual encounters that may be overcome by submissive signals. The female Siamese fighting fish appeases the aggressive male with a submissive, head-down posture. Either the male or female of several species of birds defuses aggressive impulses by mimicking juvenile behavior such as begging. Courting male hamsters emit high-pitched cries like baby hamsters, eliciting a maternal response from the female.

Presenting "gifts" seems to inhibit aggression in some species. Finches present their mates with nesting material, terns give fish, and flightless cormorants offer one another gifts of seaweed (Fig. 42-17). The female of one species of fly sometimes devours the male when he makes sexual advances. The males of a closely related species avoid this fate by presenting the female with a gift: a dead

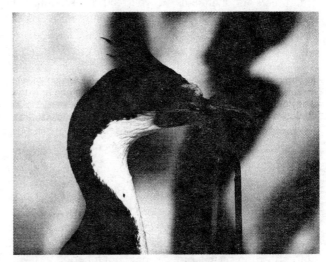

Figure 42-17   Courtship gifts defuse aggression

A flightless cormorant from the Galapagos Islands returns to its nest bearing a "gift" of seaweed for its mate, who will aggressively snatch it away. A bird who fails to bring a gift will be driven away by its mate. The gift appears to allow the nesting bird to take out its aggressive impulses harmlessly.

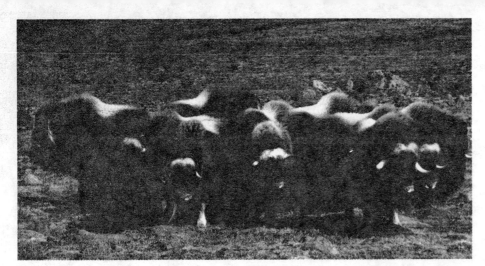

Figure 42-18 Cooperation in loosely organized social groups

A herd of musk oxen functions as a unit when threatened by predators such as wolves. Males form a circle, horns pointed outward, around the females and young.

Some animals, such as the mountain lion, are basically solitary; interactions between adults consist of brief aggressive encounters and mating. Other animals cooperate on the basis of changing needs. For example, the coyote is solitary when food is abundant but hunts in packs in the winter when food becomes scarce. Loose social groupings, such as herds of musk oxen (Fig. 42-18), pods of dolphins, schools of fish, and flocks of birds provide a variety of benefits. For example, the characteristic spacing of fish in schools or the V pattern of geese in flight provides a hydro- or aerodynamic advantage for the individuals, reducing the energy required to swim or fly. Zoologists hypothesize that schooling fish confuse predators—their myriad flashing bodies make it difficult for the predator to focus on and pursue a single individual.

At the far end of the social spectrum are a few highly integrated cooperative societies, found primarily among the insects and mammals. As you read this section, you may notice that some cooperative societies are based on behavior that seems to sacrifice the individual for the good of the group. How could such behavior evolve? In "Evolutionary Connections: Altruism, Kin Selection, and the Selfish Gene," we explore the evolutionary basis for self-sacrificing behaviors that contribute to the success of cooperative societies. In the following section, we present examples of complex societies in insect, fish, and mammal species that vividly illustrate cooperative behavior.

Honeybees Form Complex Insect Societies

The most rigidly organized, most complex societies (humans excepted) are found among the social insects. In these communities, the individual is a mere cog in an intricate, smoothly running machine; it could not function by itself. Social insects are born into one of several castes within the society. These castes are groups of similar individuals genetically programmed to perform a specific function.

Honeybees emerge from their larval stage into one of three major preordained roles (Fig. 42-19). One role is that of queen. Only one queen is tolerated in a hive at

(a)

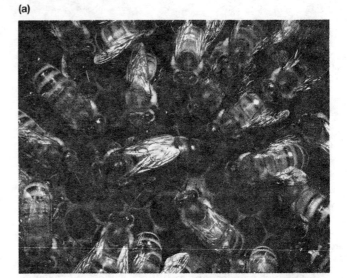

(b)

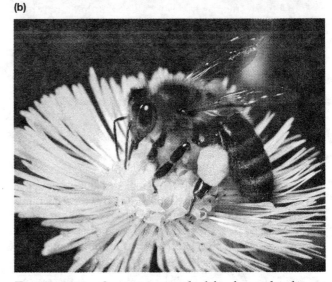

Figure 42-19 Some stages in the life of a worker bee

(a) Workers crowd around the queen (center), feeding her and licking the pheromone called queen substance from her body, which renders them sterile. (b) A forager collects pollen and nectar from a flower. Note the yellow pollen baskets on her legs.

any time. Her functions are to produce eggs (up to 1000 per day for a lifetime of 5 to 10 years) and to regulate the lives of the workers. Male bees, called drones, serve merely as mates for the queen. Lured by her sex pheromones, drones mate with the queen during her first week of life, perhaps as many as 15 times. This relatively brief "orgy" supplies her with sperm that will last a lifetime, enough to fertilize over 3 million eggs. Their sexual chore accomplished, the drones become superfluous and are eventually driven out of the hive or killed.

The hive is run by the third class of bees, sterile female workers. The tasks of the worker are determined by her age and conditions in the colony. The newly emerged worker starts as a waitress, carrying food such as honey and pollen to the queen, other workers, and developing larvae. As she matures, special glands begin wax production, and she becomes a builder, constructing perfectly hexagonal cells of wax where the queen will deposit her eggs and the larvae will develop. She will take a shift as maid, cleaning the hive and removing the dead, and as a guard, protecting the hive against intruders. Her final role in life is that of a forager gathering pollen and nectar, food

for the hive. She will spend nearly half of her 2-month life in this role. Acting as a forager scout, she will seek new and rich sources of nectar and, having found one, will return to the hive and communicate its location to other foragers using the **waggle dance,** an elegant form of symbolic communication (Fig. 42-20). Much of the meaning of the waggle dance was deciphered by Karl von Frisch during 35 years of research beginning in 1915.

Pheromones play a major role in regulating the lives of social insects. Honeybee drones are drawn irresistibly to the queen's sex pheromone (queen substance), which she releases during her mating flights. Back at the hive, she maintains her position as the only fertile female using the same substance (now acting as a primer pheromone). The queen substance is licked off her body and passed among all the workers, rendering them sterile. The queen's presence and health are signaled by her continuing production of queen substance; a decrease in production (which occurs normally in the spring) alters the behavior of the workers. Almost immediately they begin building extra-large "royal cells" and feeding the larvae that develop in them a special glandular secretion known as "royal jelly."

(a)

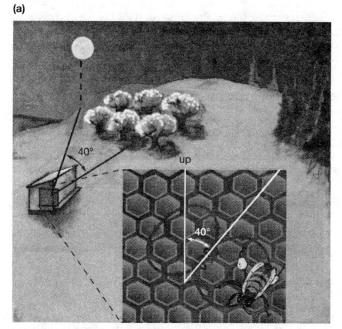

(b)

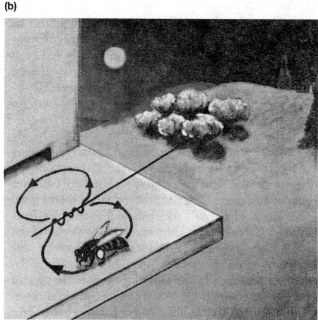

Figure 42-20   Bee language

The waggle dance. A forager, returning from a rich source of nectar, performs a waggle dance that communicates the distance and direction of the food source, as other foragers crowd around her, touching her with their antennae. The bee moves in a straight line while shaking her abdomen back and forth ("waggling") and buzzing her wings. The bee repeats this over and over in the same location, circling back in alternating directions. The richness of the food source is communicated by the vigor of the dance, and how long it continues. The rate at which she circles communicates the distance of the nectar source from the hive; the higher the rate, the closer the food source. The smell of the flowers on her body tells the other foragers what scent to search for. The direction of the food source is communicated by the direction of the waggling portion of the dance. **(a)** If the dance is performed on a wall inside the hive, the angle that the straight run deviates from the vertical represents the angle between the sun and the flowers. **(b)** On a horizontal surface outside, the waggling run is aimed directly toward the flowers.

This unique food alters the development of the growing larvae so that, instead of a worker, a new queen emerges from the royal cell. The old queen will then leave the hive, taking a swarm of workers with her to establish residence elsewhere. If more than one new queen emerges, a battle to the death ensues, with the victorious queen taking over the hive.

Bullhead Catfish Illustrate a Simple Vertebrate Society

Vertebrates possess far more complex nervous systems than insects, and one might therefore expect vertebrate societies to be proportionately more complex. With the exception of human society, however, they are not. Perhaps because the vertebrate brain *is* more complex, vertebrate societies tend to be simpler than those of the social insects such as honeybees, army ants, and termites. Each individual is unique, and this uniqueness is enhanced because vertebrates exhibit more-flexible learned behavior. Although much social behavior has an innate component, vertebrates show a great deal more flexibility (and thus unpredictability) and less of the robotic precision that makes complex insect societies possible.

The social interactions of bullhead catfish, described by John Todd of the Woods Hole Oceanographic Institution in Massachusetts, provide a fascinating illustration of a relatively simple vertebrate in which complex social interactions are based almost entirely on pheromones. Todd observed these nocturnal fish in large aquariums in the laboratory. He discovered that when a group was housed together, territories were staked out, and a dominance hierarchy was established, with the dominant fish defending the largest and best-protected area of the tank. Contests between tankmates consisted of open-mouthed aggressive displays. Once a fish became dominant, its aggressive displays caused the subordinate fish to flee. Actual violence occurred only when a stranger was introduced into a tank with an established hierarchy. In this case, the established group exhibited cooperative behavior. The dominant fish allowed others to take refuge in his protected territory, then fought the intruder (Fig. 42-21). When the newcomer was defeated, the dominant fish chased the others back out of his territory.

Todd discovered that blinding the bullheads did not cause any appreciable change in their social interactions. When their sense of smell was temporarily blocked, however, the fish acted like permanent strangers, interacting aggressively for weeks until their sense of smell returned. Both the status of an individual and a change in status are communicated by scent. If a dominant fish was removed from his tank and later returned, usually both his territory and his status were remembered and respected by his tankmates. But if he was removed and subjected to defeat in the tank of a more aggressive fish, his pheromones were somehow altered. Upon return to his home tank, he was attacked by his former subordinates.

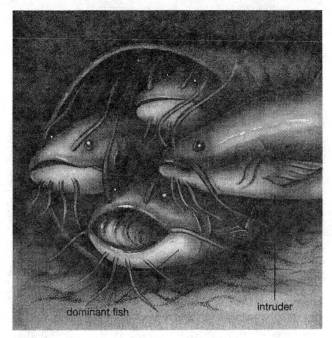

Figure 42-21   Cooperation among bullhead catfish
Three bullhead catfish occupy a section of pipe in a laboratory tank. The dominant fish is usually the exclusive occupant of the pipe, which is part of his territory. When an intruder is introduced into the tank, however, he allows two subordinate fish to seek refuge in the pipe and reacts aggressively to the intruder.

When many newly caught fish are placed in the same tank, bullheads may form a dense and peaceful community lacking territories or dominance hierarchies. Todd established such a community in one tank and placed a pair of aggressive rival fish in an adjacent tank. When water was pumped continuously from the "community tank" into the adjacent tank, the aggressive bullheads too became peaceful, resuming their fighting only when the flow was stopped. Under the crowded conditions of the community tank, an "anti-aggression pheromone" is apparently produced, minimizing conflict.

Naked Mole Rats Form a Complex Vertebrate Society

The most complex nonhuman society among mammals is formed by naked mole rats. These nearly blind, nearly hairless relatives of guinea pigs live in large underground colonies in southern Africa. Colonies ranging from 10 to 300 individuals inhabit a series of tunnels up to 2.5 kilometers (about 1.5 miles) long. The tunnels are interrupted by sleeping, nesting, and food-storage chambers and end in communal latrines. Mole rats eat fleshy roots they encounter while digging. By capturing colonies, permanently marking each individual, and maintaining the colonies in narrow glass-sided chambers (like ant farms), biologists have learned that mole rat societies have much in common with those of social insects such as the honeybee.

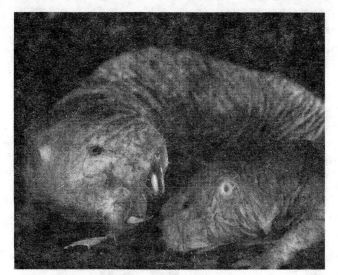

Figure 42-22   **The naked mole rat queen**
Encountering a lazy worker while patrolling the colony's underground tunnels, the queen threatens and shoves it, stimulating the worker to greater efforts.

The colony is dominated by a single reproducing female, the queen, to whom all other members are subordinate (Fig. 42-22). The queen is the largest individual in the colony and maintains her status by aggressive behavior, particularly shoving. The queen prods and shoves lazy workers, stimulating them to become more active. As in honeybee hives, there is a division of labor among the workers, in this case based on size. Small young rats clean the tunnels, gather food, and tunnel. Tunnelers line up head to tail and pass excavated dirt along the completed tunnel to an opening. Just below the opening, a larger mole rat flings the dirt into the air, adding it to a cone-shaped mound. Biologists observing this behavior from the surface dubbed it "volcanoing." In addition to volcanoing, large mole rats defend the colony against predators and members of other colonies.

If another female begins to become fertile, the queen apparently senses changes in the estrogen levels of the subordinate female's urine. The queen then selectively shoves the would-be breeder, causing stress that prevents her rival from ovulating. Large males are more likely to mate with the queen than are small ones, although all adult males are fertile. When the queen dies, a few of the females gain weight and begin shoving one another. Sometimes the aggression escalates and a rival is killed. Finally a single female becomes dominant; her body lengthens and she assumes the queenship and begins to breed. Litters averaging 14 pups are produced about four times a year. During the first month, the queen nurses her pups, and the workers feed the queen. Then the workers begin feeding the pups solid food.

Because the queen produces the pups who grow up to form the colony, all colony members are quite closely related. This genetic relatedness helps explain why behavior has evolved in which workers devote their lives to helping the queen reproduce rather than reproducing

themselves (see "Evolutionary Connections: Altruism, Kin Selection, and the Selfish Gene").

Human Ethology

Some scientists hypothesize that many human tendencies have a genetic basis, and they are attempting to study human ethology. However, human ethology is, and will remain, a less rigorous science than animal ethology. We cannot treat people as we do laboratory animals, nor can we control all the variables that influence our attitudes and actions. Nevertheless, scientists have attempted to isolate the genetic components of human behavior, and in the following sections we review some of these studies and their findings.

Newborn Infants Exhibit Some Innate Behaviors

Much of the behavior of very young infants is likely to have a large innate component, because there has been little time for learning to occur. The rhythmic movement of a baby's head in search of the mother's breast is a human fixed action pattern during the first days after birth. Suckling, which can be observed even in the human fetus, is also innate (Fig. 42-23). Other fixed action patterns seen in newborns or even premature infants include walking movements when the body is supported, and grasping with the hands and feet. Another example is smiling, which may occur soon after birth. Initially, smiling can be re-

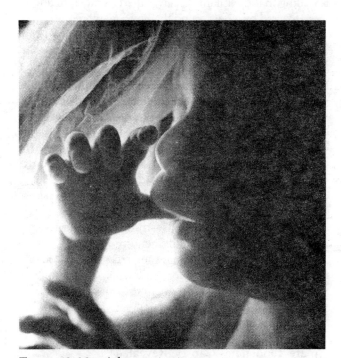

Figure 42-23   **A human instinct**
Thumb sucking is a difficult habit to discourage in young children, because sucking on appropriately sized objects is an instinctive, food-seeking behavior. This fetus sucks its thumb at about 4 1/2 months of development.

leased by almost any object looming over the newborn. Before an infant is 2 months old, supernormal stimulus (see Chapter 41) consisting of two dark, eye-sized spots on a light background will elicit smiling even more successfully than an accurate representation of a human face. As the child matures, learning and further development of the nervous system interact to limit the response to increasingly accurate representations of a face.

Another way to minimize the effects of learning is to observe children who are blind, deaf, or both, and have been unable to learn through sight and sound. Without ever having seen or heard them, these children produce normal smiles and laughter and expressions of frustration and anger.

As discussed in the previous chapter, some animals have a strong innate tendency to learn specific things during certain periods of development, a behavior called imprinting. The human fetus begins responding to sounds during the third trimester of pregnancy and, by 6 weeks after birth, is able to distinguish a variety of consonant sounds, strong evidence that the human brain is programmed to interpret language. Babies are notoriously difficult experimental subjects, and ingenious techniques have been devised to test them. One of the most successful uses the infant's ability to make sucking movements. The baby responds to the presentation of various consonant sounds by sucking on a pacifier containing a force transducer that records the sucking rate. After hearing one sound (such as "ba") repeatedly, the infant becomes bored with it and decreases her sucking rate. A new sound (such as "pa") causes an increase in sucking, revealing that the infant perceives these as different and is more excited by a new sound than by a familiar one.

The sucking-measurement technique has recently been used to demonstrate that newborns in their first 3 days of life can be conditioned to produce certain rhythms of sucking using their mother's voice as reinforcement. Infants clearly preferred their own mothers' voices over other female voices, as indicated by their sucking rhythm (Fig. 42-24). The ability of the infant to learn his or her mother's voice and respond positively to it within days of birth has strong parallels to imprinting and may help initiate bonding with the mother.

The ability of young children to acquire language rapidly and nearly effortlessly is almost certainly an example of developmentally programmed learning. Between ages one and eight, children typically acquire a vocabulary of 28,000 words whose meanings they recognize. If you are currently struggling with a foreign language class, you are probably painfully aware that your critical period for language acquisition is long past.

Innate Tendencies Can Be Revealed by Exaggerating Human Releasers

A behavior probably has an instinctive component if the stimulus that causes it (the releaser) can be exaggerated beyond the bounds of reality and elicit an even stronger re-

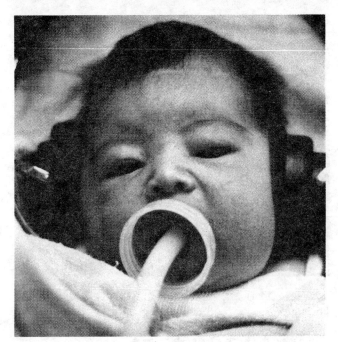

Figure 42-24 **Newborns prefer their mother's voices**

Using a nipple connected to a computer that plays audio tapes, researcher William Fifer of the New York State Psychiatric Institute demonstrated that newborns can be conditioned to suck at specific rates for the privilege of listening to their own mothers' voices through headphones. For example, if the infant sucks faster than normal, her mother's voice is played, if she sucks more slowly, another woman's voice is played. Researchers found that infants easily learned and were willing to work hard at this task just to listen to their own mothers' voices, presumably because they had become used to her voice in the womb. This response may be a human version of imprinting.

sponse. The eye-spots that cause young infants to smile are one example. In turn, the smile of an infant, along with certain characteristic baby features, may release protective feelings in adults. These features include a relatively large head with a domed forehead, chubby cheeks, small nose, short arms and legs, and a small, rounded body. Even 3-year-old children respond to these features with "mothering" behavior. The marketplace has exploited the releasing aspects of these features by exaggerating them in representations of baby animals and people and using their innate appeal to sell dolls, posters, calendars, and cards (Fig. 42-25).

One human signal with an innate, physiological basis is the involuntary enlargement of the pupil of the eye when viewing something pleasant, be it a loved one or a hot fudge sundae. We also react to this signal in others. To test this reaction, researchers showed male subjects identical photographs of smiling women that had been retouched to enlarge or contract the pupils. The subjects overwhelmingly preferred the women with large pupils, although none were consciously aware of the pupil size. We react positively to someone who gazes at us with dilated pupils (although recognition of this fea-

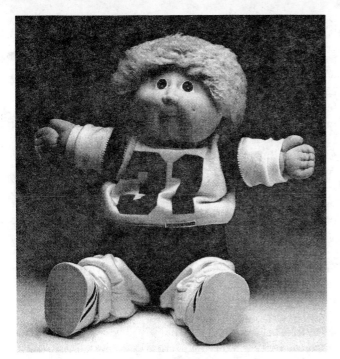

Figure 42-25   **Human releasers**

We instinctively respond to certain features associated with infants and very young children, such as big eyes, small noses, rounded faces, and large heads. These are sometimes exaggerated to produce supernormal stimuli, as in this example.

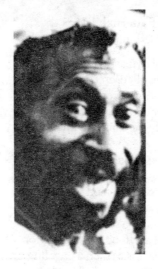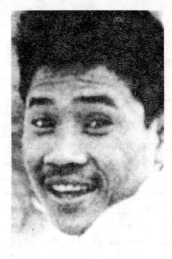

Figure 42-26   **Common gestures**

Gestures that have similar meanings in diverse and isolated cultures may be evidence of a common biological heritage. Here, motion pictures freeze the "eye flash" greeting (in which the eyes are widely opened and the eyebrows rapidly elevated) in a person from New Guinea (left) and Bali (right). Watch for this probably innate response in yourself when you encounter a friend. These photos were taken by I. Eibl-Eibesfeldt, who conducted this research.

ture is subconscious), because it implies interest and attraction. The positive response to enlarged pupils was recognized as long ago as the middle ages, when women sometimes artificially enlarged their pupils with eye-drops containing the drug belladonna (meaning "beautiful woman" in Italian).

Simple Behaviors Shared by Diverse Cultures May Be Innate

Another way to study the instinctive bases of adult human behavior is to compare simple acts performed by people from isolated and diverse cultures. This comparative approach, pioneered by the ethologist I. Eibl-Eibesfeldt, has revealed several gestures that seem to form a universal, and therefore probably innate, human language. Such gestures include a variety of facial expressions for pleasure, rage, and disdain and movements such as the "eye flash" and a hand upraised in greeting (Fig. 42-26).

Do People Respond to Pheromones?

Humans may have unconscious responses to pheromones. Our sense of smell is relatively poor, and the role of odor as a means of human communication is largely unknown. However, an interesting study by Martha McClintock of Harvard provided indirect evidence that primer pheromones may influence female reproductive physiolo-

gy. Using dorm-living college women as subjects, she found that the menstrual cycles of roommates and close friends became significantly more synchronous over a 6-month period. The cycles of women randomly chosen from the dormitory did not. Further, she found that college women who spent time with men frequently had significantly shorter menstrual cycles than those who didn't. Additional support comes from another study in which the timing of the menstrual cycle was altered by placing extract of male underarm sweat on the upper lip of women. Anatomist David Berliner believes he has isolated an odorless human pheromone from skin cells that produces a sense of well-being; he is currently marketing this discovery in the form of a perfume.

In most vertebrates, pheromones are detected by a small pitlike structure inside the nose called the vomeronasal organ (VNO), but the VNO was believed to be nonexistent in humans. In the mid-1980s, researchers finally took a closer look and were able to find a VNO, small but unmistakable, in nearly every human nose they examined. Preliminary studies suggest that certain odorless chemicals cause responses in the sensory cells lining the VNO. In other vertebrates, nerve fibers from the VNO travel to the hypothalamus and amygdala, brain structures important in producing unconscious and emotional responses. While far from conclusive, these findings are tantalizing and call for further investigation of the role of both primer and releaser pheromones in human behavior.

Comparisons of Identical and Fraternal Twins Reveal Genetic Components of Behavior

By studying identical and fraternal twins, investigators can come as close as possible to controlled breeding experiments in humans. Fraternal twins arise from two individual eggs and are no more similar genetically than other siblings. However, they are exactly the same age and share a very similar environment. In contrast, identical twins, arising from a single fertilized egg, have identical genes. The most fascinating twin findings are based on anecdotal observations of identical twins separated soon after birth, reared in different environments, and reunited for the first time as adults. They have been found to share nearly identical taste in jewelry, clothing, humor, food, and names for children and pets. Personal idiosyncrasies such as giggling, nail biting, drinking patterns, hypochondria, and mild phobias may be shared by these unacquainted twins.

More-rigorous studies are also supporting the heritability of many human behavioral traits. These studies have documented a significant genetic component for traits such as activity level, alcoholism, sociability, anxiety, intelligence, dominance, and even political attitudes. On the basis of tests designed to measure many aspects of personality, identical twins are about twice as similar in personality as fraternal twins. Further, identical twins reared apart were found to be as similar in personality as those reared together, indicating that the differences in their environments had little influence on their personality development.

The field of human behavioral genetics is controversial, because it challenges the long-held belief that environment is the most important determinant of human behavior. As discussed in Chapter 41, we now recognize that all behavior has some genetic basis and that complex behavior in nonhuman animals often combines elements of both learned and innate behavior. In the case of our own behavior, the debate over the relative importance of heredity and environment continues and is unlikely ever to be fully resolved. Human ethology is not yet recognized as a rigorous science, and it will always be hampered because we can neither view ourselves with detached objectivity nor treat each other as laboratory animals. In spite of these limitations, there is much to be learned about the interaction of learning and innate tendencies in people.

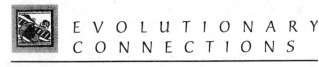

E V O L U T I O N A R Y
C O N N E C T I O N S

Altruism, Kin Selection, and the Selfish Gene

Darwin's concept of the survival of individuals best adapted to their environment and able to leave the largest number of offspring remains the foundation of evolutionary theory. Social animals, however, often behave in ways that appear to endanger the individual, decreasing its chance to survive and reproduce. There are many examples. Worker honeybees and naked mole rats do not reproduce but care for the offspring of the queen. Worker ants die in defense of their nest. Young, mature Florida Scrub Jay males may remain at their parents' nest and help them raise subsequent broods instead of breeding themselves. Young adult jackals may also help their parents raise a new litter. In colonies of Belding ground squirrels, individuals may sacrifice their lives to warn the group of an approaching predator. These behaviors fulfill the biologist's definition of **altruism:** behavior that may decrease the reproductive success of one individual to the benefit of another.

How can such behavior be reconciled with the survival of the fittest? Why aren't the individuals that perform such self-sacrificing deeds rapidly eliminated from the population, taking the genes contributing to this behavior with them? In fact, the laws of natural selection operate in such a way that "selfish" behavior (that is, behavior that increases the chance of perpetuating itself) will always be most successful. So, in some way, altruism must be selfish, but how? A major insight into the selfishness of altruistic behavior is supplied by the theory that natural selection does not operate exclusively on the individual but operates at the level of the gene. From this theoretical viewpoint, individuals are short-lived carriers of genes. Genes, however, may persist for millions of years, passing from one generation to the next. One important way in which genes may be preserved is by individuals' performing innate behavior, even self-sacrificing behavior, that enhances the survival of others carrying the same genes. From this standpoint, genes promote the survival of copies of themselves in other individuals, a concept referred to as the **selfish gene.** This theory was proposed by the ethologist Richard Dawkins (a student of Niko Tinbergen) in his engaging book *The Selfish Gene.*

Statistically, closely related individuals are most likely to carry the same genes. Thus, an individual promotes survival of the types of genes it carries through inherited behaviors that maximize survival not only of that individual, but of its close relatives as well. This concept, called **kin selection,** is also discussed in Chapter 17. Kin selection helps to explain a variety of altruistic behaviors. Male honeybees, for example, are haploid, whereas females are diploid. Female workers share, on the average, 75% of their sisters' genes. If they were to mate and reproduce, they would share only 50% of the genes of their offspring. To maximize survival of their own genes, then, rather than reproducing, they are better off helping their mother (the queen) raise more of their sisters, who share a greater percentage of their genes than would their own offspring. In fact, this is what happens in the honeybee societies described in this chapter. The same is true for naked mole rats, in which colony members share about 80% of their genes.

Alarm calls of Belding ground squirrels (Fig. 42-27) may also be explained by kin selection. Paul Sherman, an

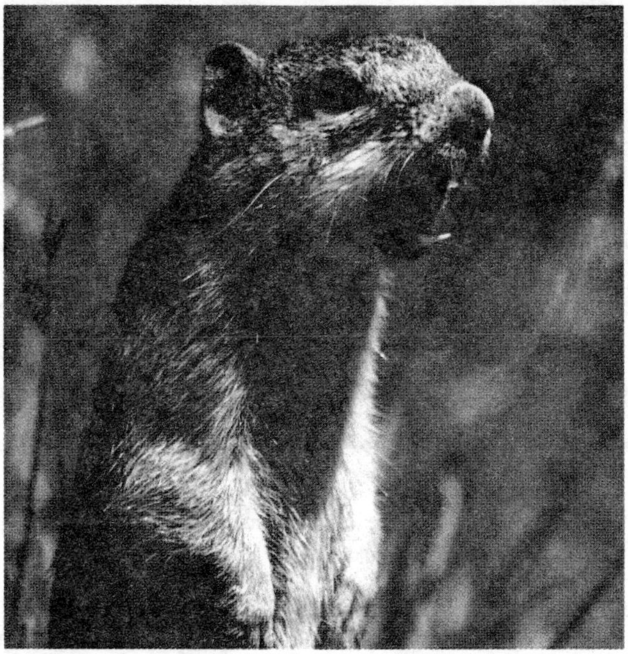

Figure 42-27 **Altruistic behavior**

A Belding ground squirrel sounds an alarm as danger approaches.

evolutionary ecologist at Cornell University, studied colonies of these rodents for several years, marking individuals so that they could be recognized. He observed that the squirrel calling an alarm often drew the attention of the predator and was sometimes killed, but it allowed other members of the colony to seek shelter. In ground squirrel colonies, males leave the burrow in which they were born and establish new burrows some distance away. Females, in contrast, stay close to home. So females in a given area are usually closely related, but males are not. Kin selection theory predicts that females should give more alarm calls than males, because their calls benefit relatives who share more of their genes, justifying the danger. It would also predict that females surrounded by close relatives would call more often than those without close relatives nearby. Sherman's data confirmed both of those predictions, supporting the theory of kin selection.

The concept of kin selection and the selfish gene provides important insights into how self-sacrificing, seemingly nonadaptive behaviors can evolve and persist within a species: Genetically programmed behaviors that sacrifice the individual will be favored by natural selection if they promote the survival of others carrying the same genes. The selfish gene concept helps explain the evolution of altruism.

SUMMARY OF KEY CONCEPTS

Communication

Communication, an action by one animal that alters the behavior of another, is the basis of all social behavior. It allows animals of the same species to interact effectively in their quest for mates, food, shelter, and other resources. Animals communicate through visual signals, sound, chemicals (pheromones), and touch.

Visual communication is quiet and can convey subtle, rapidly changing information. Visual signals may be active (body movements) or passive (body shape and color). Sound communication can also carry a wide range of rapidly changing information and is effective where vision is impossible. Although sound may attract predators, the animal may remain hidden while communicating.

Chemical signals take the form of releaser or primer pheromones. Releaser pheromones cause an immediate, observable behavior in the animal detecting them. Primer pheromones alter the physiological state of the recipient; releaser pheromones influence the recipient's behavior. Pheromones can be detected after the sender has departed, conveying a message over time. Physical contact reinforces social bonds and helps synchronize mating in a variety of animals, from mammals to snails.

Social Behavior

Although competitive interactions are often resolved through aggression, serious injuries are rare. Most aggressive encounters are settled using displays that communicate the motivation, size, and strength of the combatants.

Some species establish dominance hierarchies that minimize aggression and regulate access to resources. On the basis of initial aggressive encounters, each animal acquires a status in which it defers to more dominant individuals and dominates subordinates. When resources are limited, dominant animals obtain the largest share and are more likely to reproduce.

Territoriality, a behavior in which animals defend areas where important resources are located, also allocates resources and minimizes aggressive encounters. In general, territorial boundaries are respected, and the best-adapted individuals defend the richest territories and produce the most offspring.

Successful reproduction requires that animals recognize the species, sex, and sexual receptivity of potential mates. In some cases, they must also overcome a resistance to close approach by another individual. These requirements have resulted in the evolution of sexual displays that use all possible forms of communication.

Social living has both advantages and disadvantages, and species show a wide variation in the degree to which their members cooperate. Some form cooperative societies. The most rigid and highly organized are those of the social insects such as the honeybee, where the members follow rigidly defined roles throughout life. These roles are maintained through both genetic programming and the influence of primer pheromones. Nonhuman vertebrates also form complex, but usually less rigid, societies, such as are found among bullhead catfish. Naked mole rats exhibit the most complex and rigid vertebrate social interactions, resembling insect societies.

Human Ethology

The degree to which human behavior is genetically influenced is highly controversial. Because humans cannot be treated as laboratory animals, and because learning plays a major role in nearly all human behavior, investigators must rely on studies of newborn infants, observation of responses to exaggerated stimuli, comparative cultural studies, correlations between certain behaviors and physiology (which suggest a role for pheromones), and studies of identical and fraternal twins. Evidence is mounting that our genetic heritage plays a role in personality, intelligence, simple universal gestures, our responses to certain stimuli, and our tendency to learn specific things such as language at particular stages of development.

✖ KEY TERMS

active visual signal	kin selection	releaser pheromone
aggression	passive visual signal	selfish gene
altruism	pheromone	territoriality
communication	primer pheromone	waggle dance
dominance hierarchy	queen substance	

✖ THINKING THROUGH THE CONCEPTS

Multiple Choice

1. Which of the following is a function of a territory?
   a. reduction of aggression b. a site in which to nest
   c. a mating area d. a food-storage area
   e. all of the above
2. Which of the following is an advantage of social groupings of animals?
   a. increased ability to detect, repel, or confuse predators
   b. increased hunting efficiency
   c. increased likelihood of finding mates
   d. energy conservation
   e. all of the above
3. Which of the following pairs of communication forms and advantages are NOT accurate?
   a. pheromones, long-lasting
   b. visual displays, instantaneous
   c. sound communication, effective at night
   d. pheromones, convey rapidly changing information
   e. touch, maintains social bonds
4. In an insect society, such as the honeybee society,
   a. the division of labor is based on biologically determined castes
   b. all adult members share labor equally
   c. all adult members have the opportunity to reproduce
   d. reproduction is altered seasonally among the adults
   e. the organization of the society is flexible and adaptable
5. A specific act of altruism will most likely occur between
   a. a male and a female
   b. a female and an unrelated neighbor
   c. a parent and its offspring
   d. two females
   e. two males
6. When a male rat defeats another male and takes over his harem, the new male often kills any current litters. What principle does this behavior represent?
   a. altruism b. kin selection
   c. operant conditioning d. sexual selection
   e. parental investment

Review Questions

1. List four senses through which animals communicate, and give one example of each form of communication. After each, present both advantages and disadvantages of that form of communication.
2. Distinguish between passive and active visual signals, providing an example of each. Which can convey the most rapidly changing information?
3. What are graded visual signals, and what is their purpose?
4. Define and distinguish between primer and releaser pheromones. Give an example of each.
5. A songbird will ignore a squirrel in its territory but act aggressively toward a member of its own species. Explain why.
6. Identify the criteria for successful reproduction. For each, provide an example of how a specific animal satisfies these criteria.
7. Why are most aggressive encounters among members of the same species relatively harmless?
8. Discuss advantages and disadvantages of group living.
9. What type of animal tends to form the most complex societies, and why?
10. Describe one of the experiments that reveal the importance of chemical communication in bullhead catfish. Suggest why visual communication is not highly developed in this species.
11. In what ways do naked mole rat societies resemble those of the honeybee?

APPLYING THE CONCEPTS

1. You raise honeybees but are new at the job. Trying to increase honey production, you introduce several queens into the hive. What is the likely outcome? What different things could you do to increase production?
2. Describe and give an example of a dominance hierarchy. What role does it play in social behavior? Give a human parallel, and describe its role in human society. Are the two roles similar? Why or why not? Now repeat this exercise for territorial behavior, both in humans and in another species of animal.
3. Humans perform many altruistic behaviors, both for their relatives and for unrelated individuals. Discuss possible reasons why people might make sacrifices for unrelated individuals, and whether or not this behavior might be adaptive.
4. Remember "Cabbage Patch" dolls and their enormous popularity? Based on your readings in this chapter, suggest why they were so appealing.
5. You are manager of an airport, where planes are being endangered by large numbers of flying birds, which can be sucked into engines, disabling them. What might you do to discourage birds from nesting and flying near the airport and its planes, without harming the birds?
6. As parents, you decide you would like your child to speak a second language. When, ideally, would you start teaching the child this language, and why?

FOR MORE INFORMATION

Dawkins, R. *The Selfish Gene*, 2nd ed. New York: Oxford University Press, 1989. Exceptionally clear explanation of the evolutionary basis of altruistic behavior, written for laypeople and scientists.

Eisner, T. and Wilson, E. O. *Animal Behavior*. New York: W. H. Freeman and Co., 1975. An outstanding collection of articles on animal behavior collected from *Scientific American*, written in a readable style by some of the field's best researchers.

Goldman, B. "The Essence of Attraction." *Health*, March/April 1994. Describes the discovery and marketing of a potential human pheromone.

Kirchner, W. H., and Towne, W. F. "The Sensory Basis of the Honeybee Dance Language." *Scientific American*, June 1994. Combines a historical look at the work of Karl von Frisch with a modern update on recent research that has almost fully elucidated the mechanisms of honeybee communication during the waggle dance.

Locke, J. L. "Phases in the Child's Development of Language." *American Scientist*, September/October 1994. Learning about speech begins before birth and continues to develop before any intelligible words are produced.

Macdonald, D., and Brown, R. "The Smell of Success." *New Scientist*, May 1985. Describes the amazing diversity of mammalian pheromones.

Radetsky, P. "Silence, Signs, and Wonder." *Discover*, August 1994. Discusses sign language as a means of communication and relates it to brain function.

Seeley, T. D. "The Honey Bee Colony as a Superorganism." *American Scientist*, November–December 1989. The honey bee society exemplifies the concept of kin selection in which the society, rather than the individual, serves as a "vehicle for the survival of genes."

Sherman, P. W., Jarvis, J. U. M., and Braude, S. H. "Naked Mole Rats." *Scientific American*, August 1992. Describes the newly investigated society of the naked mole rat, a vertebrate whose social behavior resembles that of some social insects.

Stevens, J. "The Biology of Violence." *BioScience*, May 1994. Discusses the genetic aspects of violence.

Wilson, E. O. "Empire of the Ants." *Discover*, March 1990. This entertaining article discusses the diversity of ant behavior that has contributed to their enormous success.

Wright, K. "The Sniff of Legend." *Discover*, April 1994. Discusses the discovery of human pheromones and a sixth sense organ that detects them.

NET WATCH

On-line resources for this chapter are on the World Wide Web at:
http://www.prenhall.com/~audesirk (click on the table of contents link and then select Chapter 42).

RELATION OF CUE TO CONSEQUENCE IN AVOIDANCE LEARNING[1]

John Garcia and Robert A. Koelling

An audiovisual stimulus was made contingent upon the rat's licking at the water spout, thus making it analogous with a gustatory stimulus. When the audiovisual stimulus and the gustatory stimulus were paired with electric shock the avoidance reactions transferred to the audiovisual stimulus, but not the gustatory stimulus. Conversely, when both stimuli were paired with toxin or x-ray the avoidance-reactions transferred to the gustatory stimulus, but not the audiovisual stimulus. Apparently stimuli are selected as cues dependent upon the nature of the subsequent reinforcer.

A great deal of evidence stemming from diverse sources suggests an inadequacy in the usual formulations concerning reinforcement. Barnett (1963) has described the "bait-shy" behavior of wild rats which have survived a poisoning attempt. These animals utilizing olfactory and gustatory cues, avoid the poison bait which previously made them ill. However, there is no evidence that they avoid the "place" of the poisoning.

In a recent volume (Haley & Snyder, 1964) several authors have discussed studies in which ionizing radiations were employed as a noxious stimulus to produce avoidance reactions in animals. Ionizing radiation like many poisons produces gastrointestinal disturbances and nausea. Strong aversions are readily established in animals when distinctively flavored fluids are conditionally paired with x-rays. Subsequently, the gustatory stimulus will depress fluid intake without radiation. In contrast, a distinctive environmental complex of auditory, visual, and tactual stimuli does not inhibit drinking even when the compound stimulus is associated with the identical radiation schedule. This differential effect has also been observed following ingestion of a toxin and the injection of a drug (Garcia & Koelling, 1965).

Apparently this differential effectiveness of cues is due either to the nature of the reinforcer, i.e., radiation or toxic effects, or to the peculiar relation which a gustatory stimulus has to the drinking response, i.e., gustatory stimulation occurs if and only if the animal licks the fluid. The environmental cues associated with a distinctive place are not as dependent upon a single response of the organism. Therefore, we made an auditory and visual stimulus dependent upon the animal's licking and water spout. Thus, in four experiments reported here "bright-noisy" water, as well as "tasty" water was conditionally paired with radiation, a toxin, immediate shock, and delayed shock, respectively, as reinforcers. Later the capacity of these response-controlled stimuli to inhibit drinking in the absence of reinforcement was tested.

METHOD

The apparatus was a light and sound shielded box (7 in. x 7 in. x 7 in.) with a drinking spout connected to an electronic drinkometer which counted each touch of the rat's tongue to the spout. "Bright-noisy" water was provided by connecting an incandescent lamp (5 watts) and a clicking relay into this circuit. "Tasty" water was provided by adding flavors to the drinking supply.

Each experimental group consisted of 10 rats (90 day old Sprague-Dawley males) maintained in individual cages without water, but with *Purina Laboratory Chow ad libidum.*

The procedure was: A. One week of habituation to drinking in the apparatus without stimulation. B. Pretests to measure intake of bright-noisy water and tasty water prior to training. C. Acquisition training with: (1) reinforced trials where these stimuli were paired with reinforcement during drinking, (2) nonreinforced trials where rats drank water without stimuli or reinforcement. Training terminated when there was a reliable difference between water intake scores on reinforced and nonreinforced trials. D. Post-tests to measure intake of bright-noisy water and tasty water after training.

In the x-ray study an audiovisual group and a gustatory group were exposed to an identical radiation schedule. In the other studies reinforcement was contingent upon the rat's response. To insure that both the audiovisual and the gustatory stimuli received equivalent reinforcement, they were combined and simultaneously aired with the reinforcer during acquisition training. Therefore, one group serving as its own control and divided into equal subgroups was tested in balanced order with an audiovisual and a gustatory test before and after training with these stimuli combined.

One 20-min. reinforced trial was administered every three days in the x-ray and lithium chloride studies. This prolonged intertrial interval was designed to allow sufficient time for the rats to recover from acute effects of treatment. On each interpolated day the animals received a 20-min. nonreinforced trial. They were post-tested two days after their last reinforced trial. The x-ray groups received a total of three reinforced trials, each with 54 r of filtered 250 kv x-rays delivered in 20 min. Sweet water (1 gm saccharin per liter) was the gustatory stimulus. The lithium chloride group had a total of five reinforced trials with toxic salty water (.12 M lithium chloride). Non-toxic salty water (.12 M sodium chloride) whose rates cannot readily distinguish from the toxic solution was used in the gustatory tests (Nachman, 1963).

The immediate shock study was conducted on a more orthodox avoidance schedule. Tests and trials were 2 min. long. Each day for four consecutive acquisition days, animals were given two nonreinforced and two reinforced trials in an NRRN, RNNR pattern. A shock, the minimal current required to interrupt drinking (0.5 sec. at 0.08–0.20 ma), was delivered through a floor grid 2 sec. after the first lick at the spout.

The delayed shock study was conducted simultaneously with the lithium chloride on the same schedule. Non-toxic salty water was the gustatory stimulus. Shock reinforcement

was delayed during the first trials and gradually increased intensity (.05 to .30 ma) in a schedule designed to produce a drinking pattern during the 20-min. period which resembled that of the corresponding animal drinking toxic salty water.

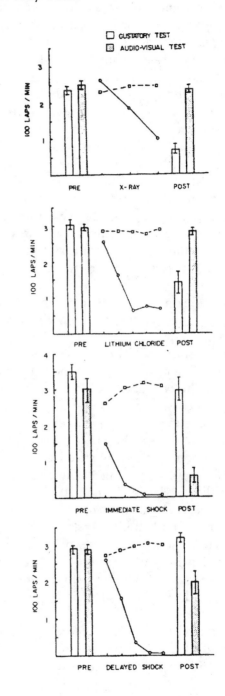

FIGURE 1 The bars indicate water intake (± St. Error) during a gustatory test (a distinctive taste) and an audiovisual test (light and sound contingent upon licking) before and after conditional pairing with the reinforcers indicated. The curves illustrate mean intake during acquisition.

RESULTS AND DISCUSSION

The results indicate that all reinforcers were effective in producing discrimination learning during the acquisition phase (see Figure 1), but obvious differences occurred in the post-test. The avoidance reactions produced by x-rays and lithium chloride are readily transferred to the gustatory stimulus but not to the audio-visual stimulus. The effect is more pronounced in the x-ray study, perhaps due to differences in dose, The x-ray animals received a constant dose, while the lithium chloride rats drank a decreasing amount of the toxic solution during training. Nevertheless, the difference between post-test scores is statistically significant in both experiments (p < 0.01 by ranks test).

Apparently when gustatory stimuli are paired with agents which produce nausea and gastic upset, they acquire secondary reinforcing properties which might be described as "conditioned nausea." Auditory and visual stimulation do not readily acquire similar properties even when they are contingent upon the licking response.

In contrast, the effect of both immediate and delayed shock to the paws is in the opposite direction. The avoidance reactions produced by electric shock to the paws transferred to the audiovisual stimulus but not to the gustatory stimulus. As one might expect the effect of delayed shocks was not as effective as shocks where the reinforcer immediately and consistently followed licking. Again, the difference between post-test intake scores is statistically significant in both studies (p< 0.01 by ranks test). Thus, when shock which produces peripheral pain is the reinforcer, "conditoned fear" properties are more readily acquired by auditory and visual stimuli than by gustatory stimuli.

It seems that given reinforcers are not equally effective for all classes of discriminable stimuli. The cues, which the animal selects from the welter of stimuli in the learning situation, appear to be related to the consequences of the subsequent reinforcer. Two speculations are offered: (1) Common elements in the time-intensity patterns of stimulation may facilitate a cross modal generalization from reinforcer to cue in one case not in another. (2) More likely, natural selection may have favored mechanisms which associate gustatory and olfactory cues with internal discomfort since the chemical receptors sample the materials soon to be incorporated into the internal environment. Krechevsky (1933) postulated such a genetically coded hypothesis to account for the predispositions of rats to respond systematically to specific cues in an insoluble maze. The hypothesis of the sick rat, as for many of us under similar circumstances, would be, "It must have been something I ate."

REFERENCES

Barnett, S. A. *The rate: a study in behavior*. Chicago: Aldine Press, 1963.

Garcia, J., & Koeling, R. A. A comparison of aversions induced by x-rays, toxins, and drugs in the rat. *Radiat. Res.*, in press, 1965.

Haley, T. J., & Snyder, R.S. (Eds.) *The response of the nervous system to ionizing radiation*. Boston: Little, Brown & Co., 1964.

Krechevsky, I. The hereditary nature of 'hypothesis', *J. comp. Psychol.*, 1932, 16, 99–116.

Nachman, M. Learned aversion to the taste of lithium chloride and generalization to other salts. *J. comp. physiol. Psychol.*, 1963, 56, 343–349.

NOTE

1. This research stems from doctoral research carried out at Long Beach V.A. Hospital and supported by NIH No. RH00068. Thanks are extended to Professors B. F. Ritchie, D. Krech and E. R. Dempster, U.C. Berkeley, California.

JOURNAL ARTICLE REVIEW FORM

Name_____ Date _____

Article Name: _____

Article Authors: _____

1. Why did the authors perform this study? (What question(s) did the authors want to answer?)

2. Identify the IV(s) and the DV(s) used in this study (Note: there may be more than one of each).

3. How was the welfare of human subjects or animal subjects safeguarded?

4. What were the major findings of this study?

5. Why were these results significant?

6. What would be a good follow-up to this study? (What study should be done next?)

1. The Kallikak study, similar to many studies that have attempted to settle the nature-nurture question, produce results that:
   a. clearly support the greater influence of heredity
   b. clearly support the greater influence of environment
   c. could be used to support either hereditary or environmental influence
   d. demonstrate that neither heredity nor environment have much to do with human characteristics

2. In classical conditioning, what is "learned" is an association between:
   a. a neutral stimulus and an unconditioned stimulus
   b. a conditioned stimulus and a conditioned response
   c. an conditioned response and a unconditioned response
   d. an unconditioned stimulus and an unconditioned response

3. The true test by Pavlov that his dog had been conditioned to salivate to the ringing of a bell was:
   a. to sound the bell when no meat was presented
   b. to present the meat before ringing the bell
   c. to present the meat after ringing the bell
   d. to present the meat at exactly the same time the bell was rung

4. The best example of the following of an operant response is:
   a. a baby crying when the pediatrician gives it an injection
   b. a dog salivating to a conditioned stimulus
   c. a puppy running about the yard for no apparent reason
   d. shivering when walking in a cold wind

5. "Schedules of Reinforcement" really is referring to:
   a. amount of reward the animal receives
   b. rewarding some, but not all, responses
   c. the pattern in which rewards are freely delivered
   d. secondary reinforcement

6. A fundamental principle of rewards is that the smaller the reward given for a well-learned response:
   a. the less likely the animal will continue to respond
   b. the more likely the animal will continue to respond
   c. frustration will ultimately interfere with responding
   d. the more easily the animal is distracted

7. In reality, the "short" of short term memories is:
   a. a few seconds
   b. a few minutes
   c. a few hours
   d a few months

8. In an institution, patients are given brightly-colored plastic chips whenever they perform a desired behavior. Later they can exchange their chips for items such as candy, note paper, or a magazine. This is known as a(n) _____.
   a. reinforcement exchange   c. behavior contract
   b. token economy   d. management code

9. Cognitive psychologists suggest the primary reason for forgetting is:
   a. decay   d. repression
   b. interference   e. changes in memory over time
   c. encoding mistakes

10. Darwin believed the environment:
    a. played little or no part in evolution
    b. was important only when there was no genetic basis for a characteristic
    c. defined which traits would are adaptive
    d. none of the above
11. Mr. Schneider has four children at home and is a single parent. He is tired and stressed because he works three part-time jobs to keep food on the table for his children. In evolutionary terms, Mr. Schneider is behaving with:
    a. selfishness.
    b. maladaptation.
    c. altruism.
    d. spite.
12. The "winners" in the game of evolution are those individuals who:
    a. survive to adulthood
    b. survive to adulthood and mate
    c. survive to adulthood, mate, and produce offspring
    d. can successfully modify their environments to ensure plenty of food, safe living quarters, etc.
13. Sexual dimorphism is when males and females of a species:
    a. clearly look different
    b. act very differently
    c. have very different roles in rearing young
    d. all of the above
14. Because they must invest a fairly long period of time caring for their offspring before and after the offspring are born, reproductive strategy for a females would include

    _____.
    a. as many matings as possible, competition for males, and conservative behaviors
    b. as many offspring as possible, selectivity in mate choice, and risk-taking
    c. few offspring, competition for males, and risk-taking
    d. few offspring, selectivity in mate choice, and conservative behavior and values
15. Likely the most profound insight by Darwin for describing evolution was:
    a. reproductive fitness
    b. natural selection
    c. adaptations
    d. only the strong survive

PART THREE: BEHAVIORAL DEVELOPMENT

We all pass through phases during development from fetus to adulthood and each stage leaves its indelible imprint. That is the substance of the initial chapter in Part Three that provides an overview of the field of "Developmental Psychology." The next chapters, on Reproduction and the Endocrine System, revert to the beginning stages for a more detailed look at development or, as biologists say, "ontogeny." A special topic emerging from those chapters is the notable influence hormones during early fetal life have on later behaviors that are as central to each of us as any other—whether we identify ourselves as male or female. That those same early hormonal influences may determine our sexual orientation as an adult is one of the more provocative ideas in the behavioral sciences today. The I.Q. chapter serves two primary functions. One is to look at the development of intelligent behaviors and other characteristics (extroversion, aggressiveness and so forth) that determine individual differences among people. Second, the I.Q. chapter describes the logic of test construction for the measurement of these characteristics, as well as describing the pitfalls confronted by psychologists who attempt to measure such uniquely human characteristics. Part Three concludes as the other parts of the text, with a Classic Reading and a practice test.

∾ ∾ ∾ ∾ ∾ ∾

8

HUMAN
DEVELOPMENT

THE PLAINS OF IOWA WERE SPARED THE BATTLES OF OUR CIVIL WAR, BUT A CLUSTER OF BUILDINGS REMAINED AS A MONUMENT TO THAT GREAT STRUGgle. By the 1930s, the hospital and barracks were housing instead a small army of children, residents of the Iowa Soldiers' Orphans' Home. Neglected or rejected by their next of kin, they were wards of the state.

The Home from the outside had a deserted look because the children were rarely allowed outdoors for unrestricted play. Instead, they spent most of the time inside, a procedure that facilitated their care. The infants lived together in the nursery, little girls in one dormitory, little boys in another, the older girls in a cottage, and so forth. These confinements further simplified the management of these bereaved little citizens.

C.D., a baby of 13 months, lay inert most of the time. She did not even try to pull herself into an upright position in her crib. She showed no interest in playthings and uttered few spontaneous sounds. Her little neighbor, B.D., three months older, also ignored the few toys in the nursery, and she too lay mute or cried, without babbling. In short, both babies appeared to be retarded.

Neither infant came from a promising background. The mother in both cases was reportedly retarded, and there was no information on the father. Examinations by a psychologist, pediatrician, and nurses made dire predictions. "C.D. will be unable to make her way outside the care and protection offered by an institution." For B.D., the prognosis was equally unfavorable (Skeels & Dye, 1939).

Indeed, for these children, life's prospects were dim. If they could leave, where would they go?

At this time, the Iowa Board of Control of State Institutions had just introduced new psychological services. For this purpose, the Board appointed to its first position Harold M. Skeels, who was recently finished with his clinical training. Skeels' work at this orphanage tells a remarkable story, for it includes much of the life span and shows how these little girls led psychologists to a new view of human development.

The study of **human development** concerns the ways in which people change as they grow older. It emphasizes the patterns that occur for most people throughout the life span. In this chapter, after a brief consideration of developmental issues and hereditary influences at conception, we progress to each of the major life stages—the prenatal phase and infancy, childhood and adolescence, adulthood and old age. The chapter concludes with a comment on individual differences.

In approaching these stages, William Shakespeare's celebrated description is helpful. It begins:

At first the infant,
Mewling and puking in the nurse's arms.
And then the whining school-boy, with his satchel
And shining morning face, creeping like snail
Unwillingly to school. And then the lover,
Sighing like a furnace, with a woeful ballad
Made to his mistress' eyebrow. . . .
—As You Like It, 2:7

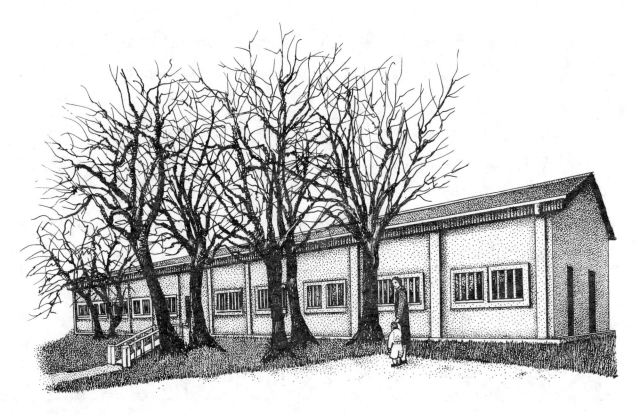

These words illustrate an important procedural question: Should our discussion proceed chronologically, from infancy to childhood, then adolescence, and so forth, as Shakespeare suggests? Or should it proceed topically, focusing on physical, cognitive, and then social development, the chief topics in human development today? Grounds for the latter approach are also evident in Shakespeare's words: The infant, mewling and puking, demonstrates physical development; the whining schoolboy, creeping like a snail to school, is en route to further cognitive development; and the lover, sighing unto his mistress' eyebrow, certainly displays social and emotional development. In fact, all three areas of development occur at *all* chronological stages (Table 12–1).

Both approaches are used here. The chronological approach forms the basic structure, as revealed in the chapter outline, which begins with conception and continues through old age. Within each chronological stage, the discussion proceeds essentially from physical to cognitive and then to social development.

• DEVELOPMENTAL ISSUES •

At the outset, however, certain developmental issues deserve our attention. Emerging in many areas of human development, they have precipitated considerable research and theory in the field.

The first issue concerns the **critical period,** a brief interval in the life span during which the individual is unusually responsive to certain forms of stimulation. The question here is not whether such periods exist but rather for which areas of development, and when, and how long, and with what outcomes? It is quite clear, for example, that ingestion of certain drugs during a woman's first weeks of pregnancy can damage the brain and heart of the unborn child. For the use of drugs, these early weeks are a critical period. Ingestion of the same drugs at the end of the pregnancy will have a lesser effect (Overholser, 1990).

In contrast, the importance of cognitive and social stimulation for the infant is widely debated, prompted in part by the story of the orphans in Iowa. If an environment is negative, does it create irreversible cognitive damage? Research in language acquisition suggests that there may be a critical period for this task, after which language cannot be readily or normally mastered (Curtiss, 1977; Itard, 1807).

Many experts consider adolescence a critical period in human development, especially for sexual stimulation. The individual may become almost irreversibly attached to some other person or event, even by chance. According to some, the roots of impotence, cross-dressing, and sexual fixations have been traced to this period (Money, 1986). For others, the significance of adolescence is overestimated. The instability is not as universal and the period not as critical as popular accounts suggest (Galambos, 1992). In any case, the question of critical periods extends from conception through the adolescent years.

A second issue, with a long history in psychology, concerns the roles of heredity and environ-

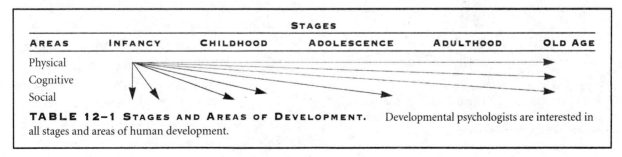

TABLE 12–1 STAGES AND AREAS OF DEVELOPMENT. Developmental psychologists are interested in all stages and areas of human development.

ment in human development. Called the **heredity–environment issue,** it arises over the relative contributions of each set of factors, inborn and acquired, in the different spheres of human development. Years ago, when C.D. and B.D. were living in the orphanage, the usual answer cited heredity, and these children seemed to be retarded on that basis. Today we recognize that both factors are always present and contribute in complex ways to human development (Figure 12–1). Also known as the *nature–nurture issue,* this controversy has been lengthy and vigorous (Mealey, 1990; Rushton, 1991).

Nature has provided some help in assessing these influences. Pairs of **identical twins,** who develop from a single fertilized ovum and therefore have exactly the same heredity, sometimes have been adopted into different homes. In a collection of extensive searches in Europe and North America, such twins were brought together and compared. They were found to be much more alike in physical characteristics and appearance than were comparable pairs of **fraternal twins,** who share no more inheritance than other brothers and sisters. In height, the identical twins showed a close resemblance (Erlenmeyer-Kimling & Jarvik, 1963). In intelligence there was an average difference in IQ of about 8 points, but an important factor here is

whether the twins had received comparable schooling. Differences in educational opportunity can produce significant differences in intelligence (Anastasi, 1988). Finally, in personality traits, the separately reared identical twins were sometimes similar and sometimes as different as fraternal twins (Gottesman, 1963; Newman, Freeman, & Holzinger, 1937).

These findings permit some generalizations about the relative influence of heredity and environment, provided that we ignore extreme circumstances. Environmental factors influence physical appearance, but they are comparatively more influential in cognitive and social development, in which one's parents, friends, and cultural milieu play decisive roles. The opposite statement might be made for heredity. Under normal conditions, heredity is highly influential in physique and less influential but certainly still important in cognitive and social development.

One ongoing study, known as the *Minnesota Twin Study,* has involved 402 sets of twins, identical and fraternal, reared together or apart. The debate continues, for recent results suggested that about 50% of personality diversity is attributable to genetic factors, an estimate considerably higher than that expected by many psychologists (Tellegen, Lykken, Bouchard, Wilcox, Segal, & Rich, 1988).

Through such investigations, it has become apparent that the heredity–environment debate is not an either-or issue. The result of any given inherited potential inevitably depends on the environment and vice versa, a condition known as the **interaction principle.** The current concern is with the relationships between these two sets of factors, an interplay of forces that can be extremely complex and intermixed (Magnusson & Törestad, 1993; Scarr, Weinberg, & Levine, 1986).

The interaction principle has been most clearly demonstrated in laboratory manipulations with animals. In one instance, newborn rats selectively bred for brightness or dullness were maintained for

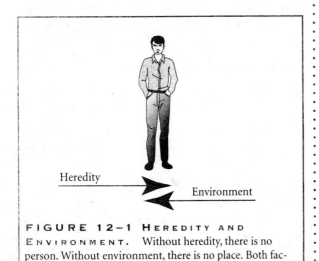

FIGURE 12–1 HEREDITY AND ENVIRONMENT. Without heredity, there is no person. Without environment, there is no place. Both factors must be taken into account.

forty days in one of three environments: restricted, neutral, or enriched. Later, they were tested for learning ability. It was found that the bright and dull groups differed by fewer than nine points when they came from either the restricted or enriched environment. However, there was a difference of 47 points between the bright and dull groups from the neutral environment. Heredity had a marked influence in that setting but not in the others (Cooper & Zubek, 1958; Figure 12–2).

This same principle applies to other species. In the production of beef, Galloway cattle fare better than Aberdeen Angus in poor grazing areas, but Angus produce more beef in good grazing areas (Haldane, 1946). Whether the Galloway or Aberdeen Angus cattle have the more favorable heredity for beef production depends on the area in which they are grazing—that is, on the environment. Among African cichlids, heredity enables a male fish to defeat the others in combat. It thereby gains ascendancy in its enviroment. Then, *after* it attains the dominant position in this particular setting, it shows rapid growth of brain cells and gonads. In other words, the environment then influences its physical development. (Davis & Fernald, 1990). Once again, heredity and environment are intricately connected in a feedback system in which they influence one another.

Similarly, a human being does not inherit a specific behavioral trait but rather a tendency or predisposition that becomes manifest in one way in one situation, differently in another, and perhaps remains latent in a third. Except in highly unusual instances, neither heredity nor environment is omnipotent (Plomin & Rende, 1991).

• AT CONCEPTION •

Like the rest of us, the development of the Iowa orphans was influenced by both heredity and environment, inevitably in interaction. On the hereditary side, they and we began life in a very small way, as a single cell. The fertilized cell, resulting from the union of the father's sperm and the mother's egg, is but half the size of the dot over this *i*, and yet *all* the inborn influences on our physical, mental, and even social development are set at this miraculous moment of conception.

DETERMINERS OF HEREDITY

Within the fertilized cell, complex organizations of chemical materials called **chromosomes** carry the information about an individual's inheritance. They received this name because they were first seen by scientists as colored strands. Microscopic studies have shown that there are 46 chromosomes in every human cell, and on the basis of size and form, they can be arranged into 23 pairs.

One pair consists of the sex chromosomes, and one member of this pair, *X* or *Y*, results in the development of a male or female. The male receives an *X* from the mother and a *Y* from the father, resulting in *XY*. The female receives an *X* from each parent. Therefore, the orphan girls, like all girls, had

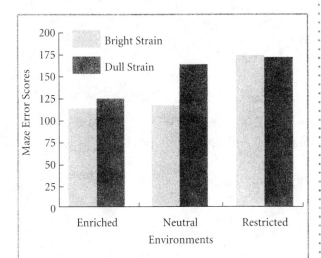

FIGURE 12–2 INTERACTION EFFECT. Maze learning by rats showed the influences of heredity only in a neutral environment. They were obscured by environmental influences in the highly restricted and enriched conditions (Pettigrew, 1964).

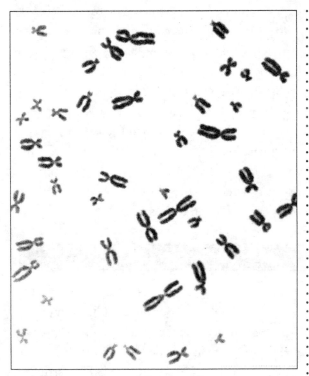

FIGURE 12–3 HUMAN CHROMOSOMES.
Chromosomes are not located in pairs, side by side. Rather, each chromosome can be matched to another according to size and structure.

an *XX* combination (Figure 12–3).

Within the chromosomes are the fundamental determiners of heredity, called **genes,** which contain the basic hereditary blueprint, specifically directing the development of most physical characteristics and certain behavioral traits. The numbers of genes is still a matter of guesswork, with estimates varying from 1,000 to 100,000 per chromosome. In a series of continuing studies, it has been discovered that *deoxyribonucleic acid* (DNA) is the basic genetic substance of all kinds of living organisms, including human beings. All genes are comprised of DNA molecules. The structure of this molecule has been established and it is possible to study genes at the molecular level.

Whenever a cell divides, its chromosomes and their thousands of genes are duplicated. As the cells multiply, the complete genetic code is passed on to each of the resulting cells, giving all cells except the reproductive cells an identical inheritance.

Beginning at puberty, the reproductive cells, the **sperm** cells in the male and the **ova,** or egg cells, in the female, undergo a division different from that just described. As they split and become duplicated, they receive *only one member of each pair* of chromosomes. Ova receive half of the female's chromosomes; sperm receive half of the male's chromosomes. Different ova produced by the same individual receive different chromosomes, and the same is true for sperm.

Thus, there are millions of possible combinations of chromosomes among the reproductive cells of any one female. There are also millions of possible combinations in the male. Taken together, the potentially different inheritances for any given individual, with chromosomes from the male *and* female, rise into the billions. They become even higher when, during the cell division process, chromosomes occasionally split apart, and a segment of one chromosome is exchanged with a segment of another split chromosome.

❧

GENETIC PROCESSES

By inheriting pairs of chromosomes, human beings also inherit pairs of genes, again one member of each pair from each parent. These genes may be dominant or recessive for any given trait. A **dominant gene** takes precedence over the other member of the pair. It is expressed when two members of a gene pair are alike *or* different. A **recessive gene,** in contrast, is influential only when it is paired with another recessive gene of the same type. Otherwise, it has no influence.

These conditions are readily illustrated in the determination of eye color. For example, one of the orphan children had brown eyes and, because genes come in pairs, let us refer to these genes as *BB.* The capital *B* is used because the gene for brown eyes is dominant. Another child might have had *Bb;* if so, she also would have had brown eyes because of the dominant *B.* The lowercase *b* denotes the gene for blue eyes, a recessive gene. It will not exhibit any effect unless it appears with another recessive gene for this trait.

If someone with *BB* marries someone with *bb*, all of the offspring will be brown-eyed, *Bb*, receiving one gene from each parent. But if both parents are *Bb*, in a sufficiently large sample three-fourths will be brown-eyed, as *BB* or *Bb*, and only one-fourth blue-eyed, as *bb* (Figure XII.1, Color).

Today it is understood that few human characteristics are controlled by a single-gene pair. One exception is Huntington's chorea, an inherited nervous condition with involuntary twitching and convulsions, as well as mental deterioration. In this case the *H* or abnormal gene is dominant, and the *h* for the normal condition is recessive. A union of *Hh* parents would produce the same distribution seen for *Bb* parents, and the offspring would have a 75% chance of manifesting the disease, but fortunately this dominant gene is rare.

POLYGENIC TRAITS. Most human characteristics show countless differences. Therefore they are thought to be influenced by multiple pairs of genes with *no* dominance. Whenever any characteristic appears in varying degrees or forms, such as physique or intelligence, it is known as a **polygenic trait,** meaning that it has been influenced by multiple pairs of genes.

Human subjects cannot be bred in accordance with scientific research. Thus, investigators often use animals to study the ways in which multiple pairs of genes seem to operate. In one instance 142 rats were tested for their capacity to learn a maze. The differences were remarkable. For example, one rat made only 5 errors and another made 214 before learning the maze. Those rats making few errors were designated bright, and those making many errors were designated dull. Keeping the environment constant, the investigator then mated the brightest rats in each generation with one another. He also mated the dullest rats in each generation

with one another. At first, in the early generations, there was not much difference between the offspring in the two groups, suggesting that maze learning is not controlled by a single dominant gene. If a single gene had been dominant, a more pronounced difference in learning would have appeared in the first generations. Instead, seven generations were required before two distinct types of rats—maze-bright and maze-dull—were produced by this process of selective breeding (Tryon, 1940; Figure XII.2).

The genetic backgrounds of human beings cannot be manipulated in this manner, but sometimes hereditary influences appear overwhelming anyway. For example, there seemed little doubt about the inheritance of the two little girls at the orphanage. Weak and frail, clearly slow in development, C.D. and B.D. spent their days rocking and whining, although no organic problem could be identified.

By chance, when Harold Skeels went to the orphanage to offer psychological services in 1932, he observed them on one of his early visits. At 13 and 16 months of age, they should have been in the dormitories with the other children. Skeels could not help but notice their physical and mental retardation. They behaved more like the newborn babies in the cribs, making almost no effort to play with anything or anyone. He called them "pitiful little creatures" (Skeels & Dye, 1939).

BEHAVIORAL GENETICS. At both the animal and human levels, a field of study called **behavioral genetics** aims to discover the hereditary foundations of the ways organisms respond in their environment. This research is often misunderstood, for it has the capacity to demonstrate not only genetic but also environmental influences on behavior, depending on the design of the research (Plomin & Neiderhiser, 1992; Rose, 1995).

In behavioral genetics, an individual's full genetic makeup can only be assumed. Thus, the sets of genes assumed to underlie any given trait are referred to as the **genotype.** For blue eyes, the genotype is *bb*, referring to the postulated genetic structure. The observable trait, blue eyes, is the **phenotype,** derived from the stem *pheno*, meaning "showing" or "displaying." The phenotype is blue eyes; the genotype is *bb.*

With animals, research may begin with the phenotype, or performance, as just illustrated with maze learning among rats. Those that were most successful were mated with one another, as were those least successful. For research beginning instead with the genotype, males and females from the *same* litter are mated over and over for many generations, producing a *pure* strain, meaning that the animals have essentially the same genetic background. Then, when two or more different inbred strains are exposed to the same environment, any difference in behavior between them can be attributed to the difference in genetic makeup.

At the human level, the obvious control for genetic makeup involves members of pairs of identical twins. In later chapters, on intelligence and adjustment disorders, we shall consider the merits of such studies.

• PRENATAL PHASE AND INFANCY •

One principle of development applies even before birth. Called **differentiation,** it states that human development proceeds from simple to complex and from the general to the specific. In biology, this process refers to the steady development of many specialized organs, emerging out of an originally undifferentiated mass of tissue. In psychology, it indicates that our behavior becomes increasingly specific and complex as we progress from infancy to adulthood. Our use of the hands, acquisition of language, expression of feelings, and virtually all other human capacities develop in this way, from a generalized response to highly specific reactions.

EARLY NEURAL GROWTH

Expressed as stages, the prenatal changes appear in three periods. The period of the fertilized ovum, or **zygote,** lasts for about ten days after conception, characterized by rapid cell division. The period of the **embryo,** from the second week to the end of the second month, is marked by the beginning of the heartbeat at three weeks and by some developing sensory and motor mechanisms, such as the eyes, hands, and feet. And finally, beginning at the third month and extending until birth, the period of the **fetus** shows all sorts of dramatic developments, including the bulk of neuronal development, between 10 and 20 weeks, and the first sensitivity to stimulation, which occurs in the head region (Figure XII.3).

Researchers in neurology study malformations in the nervous system during these periods, arising from many sources. Collectively, these sources are called **teratogens,** meaning environmental or chemical factors that disrupt normal development, producing birth defects. In a pregnant woman, the disease known as *rubella*, a form of measles, is a teratogen. It can cause retardation and deafness in the offspring. Alcohol consumption can cause growth deficiencies and mental retardation, a condition known as *fetal alcohol syndrome* (Overholser, 1990). Even maternal malnutrition has detrimental effects, producing babies more susceptible to diseases. Teratogens, moreover, are most influential during embryonic and early fetal development, rather than just before birth. These first weeks are therefore a critical period.

No significant teratogens occurred in the prenatal life of the two orphan girls, as far as we know. No birth injuries or glandular dysfunctions were observed. Their retardation could not be explained on these bases.

The transition from the human womb to our immeasurably complex outside world has been called the *birth trauma.* The newborn is suddenly confronted with diverse social and nonsocial stimuli. Its sensory and motor immaturity and the absence of relevant past experience render it relatively unresponsive at first, making the transition easier.

At birth, the individual begins *infancy*, a term derived from Latin, referring to the first one or two years of postnatal human life. Literally, it means "unable to speak."

At this point the infant's brain is only about one-fourth of its adult size, but it soon increases enormously in complexity and interconnections. Six months later, the brain achieves half of its full size.

Initially, the areas below the brain's surface, or cortex, control most of the infant's reactions. These subcortical structures are most important in automatic responses, such as breathing and reflexes. The grasping reflex of the newborn infant is well known. When stimulated in the palm, the infant involuntarily makes a fist, grasping the stimulating object. About a month after birth, this reflex disappears, and then it returns three or four months later. It is speculated that this dormant interval, which occurs in other reflexes as well, allows time for development of the neural structures underlying voluntary responses.

SENSORIMOTOR DEVELOPMENT

At the Orphans' Home, all newborn babies lived in the nursery, sleeping in individual cribs without toys or mobiles. Instead, they gazed at protective coverings on the sides of the cribs. Later, they were moved to small dormitories, where two caretakers cleaned, fed, and clothed them.

In newborn babies, it is not possible to identify physical, cognitive, and social developments as distinct from one another because differentiation has not proceeded to this point. These functions have not yet emerged as separate entities. Hence, rather than speaking of physical development, the focus in the prior discussion was on the development of the nervous system, which underlies *all* behavior and

experience. Similarly, in the following discussion we are concerned with sensory and motor development, for the infant's capacities have not yet developed to the point where we can speak easily of cognition—apart from sensory and motor ability. In fact, to measure the cognitive ability of C.D. and B.D., we would measure vision, hearing, general activity, and so forth, for these are the means by which an infant eventually becomes intelligent about its environment.

When psychologist Harold Skeels assessed the mental development of these two orphans, C.D. demonstrated an IQ of 46 and B.D. an IQ of 35. It seemed that B.D., under optimal circumstances, might have performed up to 10 points higher. At these young ages, further evidence was needed, and therefore a second test was used. It yielded essentially the same results.

The girls performed so poorly that foster placement could not be anticipated. With the orphanage at Davenport already overcrowded, adoption unlikely, and the prognosis dismal, Skeels recommended early transfer to an institution for mentally retarded people, where they were destined anyway. Two months later, this transfer was made to the institution at Woodward. These tearful little creatures, 15 and 18 months of age, were sent off to new lives (Skeels & Dye, 1939). Their runny noses, poor muscle tone, and lack of responsiveness would be someone else's problem.

SENSORY DEVELOPMENT IN EARLY INFANCY. The infant's visual world is largely colorless, at least initially, but color vision improves rapidly during the first month. By six months of age, the infant's capacity approaches the adult level. There is currently no satisfactory explanation for the young infant's color deficiency, but it may be related to an overall insensitivity to differences in light intensity (Brown, 1990).

In one series of studies, 43 infants ranging in age from two days to six months were tested in a special apparatus. It consisted of a large frame for holding visual stimuli over the infant's bed, a series of stimuli, and a peephole through which the investigator could observe the direction and length of fixation of the infant's gaze. Each infant was exposed to various patterned and unpatterned stimuli up to eight times. The results showed considerably more visual attention to the patterned surface than to plain but colored ones and most attention to an outline of a human face. This finding indicates that the visual world of even the very young infant is not entirely formless (Fantz, 1961).

Hearing also appears quickly after birth. The newborn is responsive only to loud noises, but soon pitch, quality, and other aspects of sound are discriminated. Sensitivity to temperature and other stimuli, and the capacities for taste and smell, although present in the fetus, continue to increase in the following weeks.

MOTOR DEVELOPMENT IN INFANCY. During the prenatal and early postnatal years, there is a universal tendency in vertebrates to develop faster at the head than at the tail. The head of a human fetus has reached a greater proportion of its ultimate size than the lower body parts, and the same condition holds for a young child. Since the direction of the head is referred to as *cephalic* and the direction of the tail as *caudal*, this head-to-tail growth is known as **cephalocaudal development.** Similarly, structures close to the center of the body develop faster than those at the extremes. A comparison of the body parts shows that early in life the trunk grows more; later, the arms and legs grow more. This center-to-extremities growth is known as **proximodistal development,** meaning from near to far. In summary, in our early years we grow downward from the top, outward from the center.

The most obvious postnatal developments pertain to the muscles. The baby learns to control the head before the legs, illustrating the cephalocaudal sequence. The baby moves the arms as a whole before gaining effective control of the hands and fingers, demonstrating proximodistal development.

As its muscles grow, and especially as neural development continues, the normal infant progresses to successive stages in *locomotion,* which is the capacity to move oneself from place to place. In the first year, this progression goes from lying to sitting to standing and finally to walking with assistance. These stages are essentially predictable, and ages have been identified at which they often occur, although there are distinct variations in the rates at which even normal children reach them.

At the time they were recommended for transfer, C.D. and B.D. were well behind the usual rate of development. C.D., 13 months of age, made no attempts to sit or stand unaided. B.D., at 16 months, was unable to walk, even with assistance. In normal development, the younger baby would have been crawling up and down stairs; the older one would have been standing and walking alone (Figure 12–4).

Compared with later development, these early physical changes take place with remarkable speed. The only comparable period of physical development—less dramatic but remarkable in its own way—is the adolescent growth spurt.

SOCIAL-EMOTIONAL DEVELOPMENT

Six months after the transfer of the two little girls, Harold Skeels's responsibilities were expanded beyond the orphanage to include two state institutions for the mentally retarded. One day while visiting the wards at Woodward, he noticed "two outstanding little girls." They were healthy, playful children, toddling about like most others of their age. He hardly recognized them as the hopelessly retarded pair transferred to the institution a half year earlier. In disbelief, he tested them again and found that they were approaching the lower level of normal development. After another 12 months, he

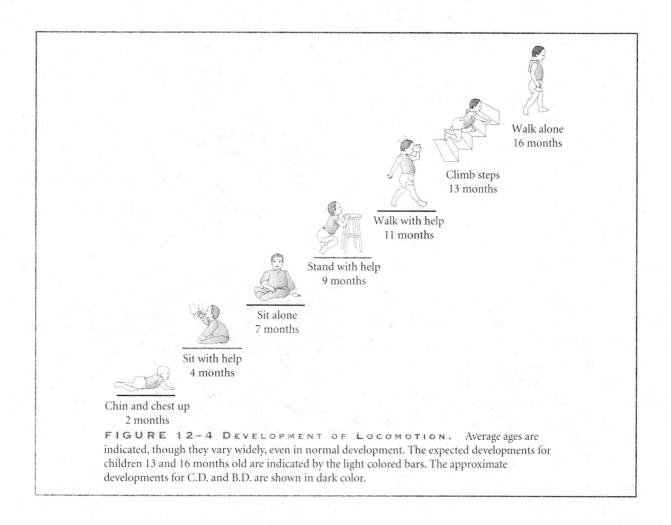

Walk alone
16 months

Climb steps
13 months

Walk with help
11 months

Stand with help
9 months

Sit alone
7 months

Sit with help
4 months

Chin and chest up
2 months

FIGURE 12–4 DEVELOPMENT OF LOCOMOTION. Average ages are indicated, though they vary widely, even in normal development. The expected developments for children 13 and 16 months old are indicated by the light colored bars. The approximate developments for C.D. and B.D. are shown in dark color.

tested them once more, obtaining still higher results, within the normal range. Finally, when the little girls were 40 and 43 months of age, Skeels obtained IQs of 95 and 93, respectively, just slightly below average (Skeels & Dye, 1939).

These physical and cognitive developments were truly remarkable, but the girls also showed noticeable social development. They seemed happier and more stable emotionally. Skeptical of the tests and of the permanence of these improvements, Skeels suggested no change in their lives. The children would stay in the institution, and he would return later to check their progress (Skeels & Dye, 1939).

The principle of differentiation, just as it holds for physical and cognitive development, also applies to social development. There is no identifiable social responsiveness in newborn infants, as clearly distinct from emotional, sensory, or motor behavior. The baby looks for its mother and perhaps reaches for her. Later it smiles, cries in anger, coos, and learns to express affection. Only gradually does the behavior of the newborn become differentiated into the many different social and emotional reactions of the child and adult.

IMPRINTING AND ATTACHMENT. In the early decades of this century, the role of early experience in human development was not understood as we know it today. It had been described by poets and philosophers, and Alexander Pope had written: "Just as the twig is bent, the tree's inclin'd" (*Moral*

Essays, I, 1734). However, it had not yet come under careful scrutiny by scientists, who were just beginning studies of social behavior in animals.

Under normal circumstances, for example, newborn ducklings and goslings follow their mother soon after hatching, perhaps because they are stimulated initially by her movements or vocalizations. This learned attachment of young animals to members of their own species is called **imprinting,** and it is acquired during a certain *optimal* time for learning. This period varies for different species. In geese, it is up to 16 hours after birth. Afterward, readiness to learn to follow declines rapidly. The young bird is so ready during these early moments—a critical period—that this behavior can be elicited by almost any perceptible object that moves, living or inanimate. Furthermore, once this attachment has been established, it is essentially irreversible (Lorenz, 1958; Figure 12–5).

Most researchers refuse to speculate regarding any fixed interval for human social responsiveness. The first 3 days after birth, for example, may be sufficient for initiating in the human infant a special responsiveness to the mother's voice (DeCasper & Fifer, 1980). Within 30 weeks, infants acquire the concept of a human face (Cohen & Strauss, 1979). Some investigators therefore speak of a *sensitive period,* implying its importance but not its irreversibility.

Through their regular interactions, an intense and enduring emotional relationship often develops between an infant and its human caretaker, called **attachment.** It begins by three months of age, perhaps earlier, when the baby takes special note of the caretaker and develops a special affection for that particular person. By six months, this attachment becomes an important source of security as the child begins to investigate the world around it. Any disruption in this relationship produces stress and even depression in either or both individuals.

The observations of imprinting in animals

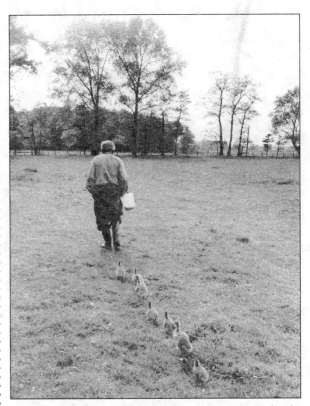

FIGURE 12–5 IMPRINTING. Immediately after birth of these goslings, Konrad Lorenz waddled and quacked his way around a meadow for two hours, occasionally glancing back at the piping little creatures marching obediently behind him. Lorenz was the first moving object in their lives, and they developed a learned attachment to him, called imprinting, shown here in later days.

foretold in a rough manner the later scientific interest in attachment among human beings, but the findings are hardly comparable. Imprinting in animals is essentially predictable, remarkably firm, and not highly variable from one individual to another. Attachment is a more elusive concept, not yet supported by substantial evidence or clearly distinguished among the many different terms for early human social support (Newcomb, 1990).

EMERGING EMOTIONAL REACTIONS. Investigations of early emotional development have fostered a wide array of techniques. In one instance, infants were systematically stimulated by toys, parents, and food. A panel of judges, not informed of the circumstances, identified the infant's reaction only on the basis of its facial expression. The results indicated that the expression of interest is present shortly after birth, along with the startle pattern and distress. These are followed by a true social smile at about one to two months, then anger at three to four months, fear at six months, and so forth (Izard, Huebner, Risser, & Dougherty, 1980). As in earlier studies, negative emotional reactions generally were identified earlier than positive expressions.

At six or seven months, the infant becomes afraid with unfamiliar people, a condition called **stranger anxiety.** The baby cries, turns away, hides, or clings to the parent. These responses typically disappear sometime after the first year. Around this same period, occasionally lasting for many months, a related concern arises. In **separation anxiety,** the child shows great distress on being away from the parent. Both types of anxiety appear to be significantly influenced by biological factors in maturation, for they are common in many cultures.

Among theoretical explanations for these anxieties, the Darwinian view postulates that the various emotions have survival value or at least had this capacity in earlier evolutionary history. The negative emotions, in particular, are viewed in this way: Fear stimulates flight from predators; anger prompts retaliation; and the startle pattern provides a reflex withdrawal from an unexpected stimulus. Smiling and crying also have survival value, eliciting the attention of adults.

CARETAKER–CHILD INTERACTION. When Harold Skeels reexamined the two orphan girls again and again, they showed unmistakable development, eventually reaching the normal range. There seemed little doubt that the original evaluations had given a reasonably accurate assessment of their functioning at the orphanage, and yet each successive examination showed more normal development. What had happened?

Attention had happened—good old tender, loving care. In the institution for the mentally retarded, each child had been placed separately on a ward for older girls and women ranging in age from 18 to 50 years old. One of these women spontaneously became the adoptive mother of each child. The others served as adoring aunts. Equally important, the ward attendants became attracted to C.D. and B.D., the only preschool children in the area. The setting was abundant in affection and interesting stimulation for them, although most of their caretakers had no more mental ability than a nine-year-old child (Skeels & Dye, 1939).

Back at the orphanage, these children would have lived in an overcrowded, underfurnished dormitory. With only one or two caretakers for every 12 to 18 children, sustained contacts with adults for these boys and girls were rare, limited chiefly to physical care.

The difference between life at the orphanage and life at the institution for the mentally retarded lay not in the satisfactions of biological needs, which were approximately equal in the two institutions. One difference was the availability of toys and other equipment. More important was the difference in **caretaker–child interaction,** which refers to attention and responsiveness to a child on the part of adults, including diverse opportunities for play and support. It was in the context of these games and related experiences with women and older girls that the two younger ones showed such marked changes, including improved emotional development.

The two little girls of course differed from one another, and many differences in infant behavior cannot be attributed to environmental influences (Kagan, Snidman, Julia-Sellers, & Johnson, 1991). One task of the caretaker is to recognize early the baby's temperament and to respond accordingly.

At some point during the second year, normal babies use words in combinations. This cognitive-motor development represents the beginning of speech and therefore the transition from infancy to childhood.

The stage of childhood lasts about ten to twelve years, until adolescence, which is defined differently in different cultures and even for the two sexes. In the United States, the stage of adolescence today it is often considered to span the years 11 to 18 in girls and 13 to 20 in boys. Especially in adolescence, the three areas of development—physical, cognitive, and social—occur at very different rates in different people, meaning that some developments may not be complete until the twenties. Both childhood and adolescence are considered in three phases: early, middle, and late.

The two orphans, C.D. and B.D., were in early childhood when they received the abundant attention and affection from the retarded girls and women. After slightly more than two years, Skeels decided that they were behaving in an essentially normal manner. It was unlikely that life with retarded people would meet their future developmental needs, and so the girls were returned to the orphanage to await adoption. This adoptive placement occurred a year later, when they were about four years old.

This totally unexpected development, especially in such an unlikely place as an institution for the mentally handicapped, so impressed Harold Skeels that he made another radical proposal. A whole group of orphans should be transferred to live with the mentally retarded. Little could be lost, he pointed out, because those who did not attain normal development would simply remain where they were destined anyway. Naturally, the Board of Control of State Institutions responded to this plan with grave misgivings, fearing damage to the children and to the reputation of their institutions.

A compromise was reached. To escape the stigma of being committed as mentally retarded at an earlier age than usual, the children would be considered house guests at the institution, their names remaining on the orphanage roster. Each child would be placed singly on a ward, or in some cases in pairs, and there would be periodic reevaluations. All of these arrangements were described in Skeels's report on this procedure, *A Study of the Effects of Differential Stimulation on Mentally Retarded Children* (Skeels & Dye, 1939).

Under this plan, 11 children were transferred to the state institution at Glenwood, making a total of 13 who went earlier than usual to live with the mentally retarded. Their average age was 19 months, and reevaluation was scheduled to take place within two years.

PHYSICAL DEVELOPMENT

Human **physical development** involves the growth of all structures of the body. These structures underlie all behavior and experience; therefore, physical, cognitive, and social development are interrelated.

PHYSICAL CHANGES IN CHILDHOOD. Biological inheritance manifests itself not only in physical characteristics but also in a certain sequence of physical development. When this sequence is universal among all normal members of a given species and depends almost solely on biological factors, it is called **maturation.** This shared unfolding of structure and behavior, which takes place almost automatically and inevitably, suggests a common inheritance among the group members. Even among retarded and precocious individuals, the *sequence is the same* as it is for normal or average individuals. It simply occurs at a different rate.

Maturational influences also appear in the

changes in body proportions. In length, the ratio of the head to the total body at birth is 1:4. By age six years, it becomes 1:6. After twelve years, it remains approximately 1:8. A similar change occurs in the ratio of the head to the limbs. The newborn infant can hardly reach the top of its head, for its arms, legs, and head are almost the same length. These proportions change steadily until, at adolescence, the limbs are more than twice the length of the head (Figure 12–6).

Increases in physical size continue until approximately the eighteenth year, and they can be considered in stages. During infancy, they are more rapid than at any other time in life. In early childhood, ages two through five, the rate decreases but remains rapid. Then the years of middle and late childhood, from five to eleven or so, bring a marked change. Growth is so slow that it sometimes seems there is none at all.

ADOLESCENT GROWTH SPURT. The second spurt of physical growth in the human life cycle marks the stage of **adolescence,** a time when girls and boys reach reproductive capacity and also experience marked intellectual and emotional changes. Some of the physical changes are obvious, such as the increasingly feminine and masculine proportions in physique and the rapid increases in height and weight in both sexes, but they are not synchronized among or within adolescents. Girls generally mature earlier than boys, some much sooner than their friends of both sexes. Others are late. Boys, too, mature at very different rates, as do the separate body parts. The chin, nose, neck, and feet may grow early and rapidly, leaving many adolescent boys gawky and awkward—out of step with themselves, as well as with their peers.

The most significant of these changes are less obvious, arising from hormonal secretions beginning at about the tenth year. A marked rise in the production of **estrogens,** the female sex hormone, is partly responsible for the girl's changing figure and increasing interest in the opposite sex. The secretion of **androgens,** the male hormone, begins a bit later, stimulating the male sex characteristics. The beginning of reproductive capacity, called **puberty,** occurs with the onset of menstruation in girls, sometime after age 11, and the presence of sperm cells in boys, approximately one or two years later.

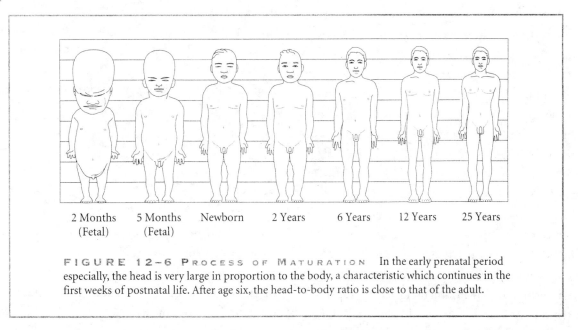

| 2 Months (Fetal) | 5 Months (Fetal) | Newborn | 2 Years | 6 Years | 12 Years | 25 Years |

FIGURE 12–6 PROCESS OF MATURATION   In the early prenatal period especially, the head is very large in proportion to the body, a characteristic which continues in the first weeks of postnatal life. After age six, the head-to-body ratio is close to that of the adult.

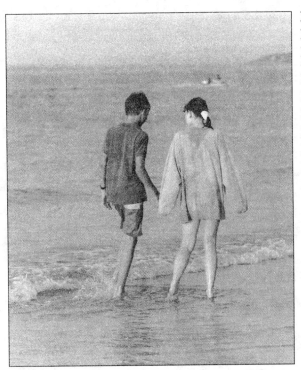

FIGURE 12–7 ADOLESCENCE AS A CRITICAL PERIOD. One major task is the acceptance of sexual impulses and their integration into the personality.

Two generations ago the average British girl reached puberty at 15, and centuries earlier she reached it at 16 or later. This trend toward earlier onset of menstruation has been found throughout developed parts of the world. A most likely contributor is improved nutrition throughout the growth period. Comparisons of well-nourished and poorly nourished populations support this idea, showing a sharp difference in the median age at first menstruation (Tanner, 1971). Still another possibility is the increased stimulation and stress in developed countries, brought about by the automobile, telephones, television, and other complexities of modern urban life (Adams, 1981). The adolescent spurt is a universal inheritance, but the time of its occurrence depends partly on the interplay of environmental factors, especially nutrition and social changes (Hamburg & Takanishi, 1989).

PROBLEMS OF ADOLESCENT SEXUALITY. Attracted to sexual experience by earlier puberty and sexually oriented mass media, adolescents are engaging in intercourse at younger and younger ages. This activity, unless guided by principles of safe sex, involves two dangers: sexually transmitted disease and unwanted pregnancy. The chief concern in both cases is prevention (Turkington, 1992; Figure 12–7).

Instances of AIDS among teenagers have been increasing precipitously, and the other hazard, adolescent pregnancy, can become an enormous handicap for adolescent girls—and boys too. And yet, among teenagers who are sexually active, less than one-third employ contraceptives regularly; approximately one million girls become pregnant each year (Dryfoos, 1990).

On these bases, the need for sex education seems paramount. But who should offer it? How should it be presented? What should it contain? With these questions largely unanswered, teenage pregnancy in this country is markedly higher than in other industrialized countries, such as Sweden, where sex education is part of the school curriculum. Teenage sexual activity is approximately the same in both places, and therefore the responsible factor seems to be effective sex education (Figure 12–8). Surveys of adolescents in this country and abroad have shown that even without extensive sex education in school, instruction from parents is extremely limited, reported by only 14% in some cases (Finkel & Finkel, 1983; Mayekiso & Twaise, 1993).

COGNITIVE DEVELOPMENT

As the child matures, its mental capacities become more prominent and varied, and these changes are known as **cognitive development**. The term *cognition* means knowing or understanding; it includes not only intelligence but also such complementary or component processes as perceiving, recognizing,

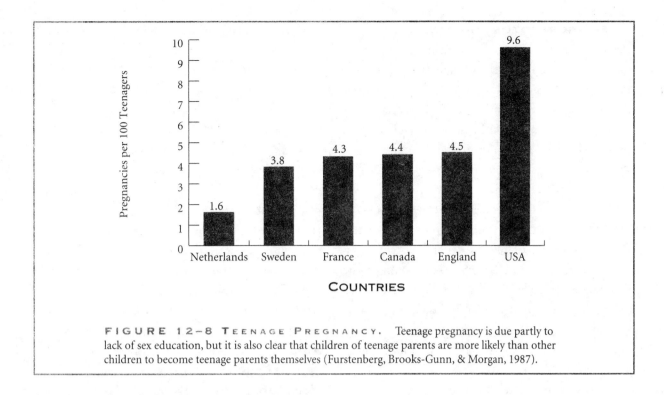

FIGURE 12–8 TEENAGE PREGNANCY. Teenage pregnancy is due partly to lack of sex education, but it is also clear that children of teenage parents are more likely than other children to become teenage parents themselves (Furstenberg, Brooks-Gunn, & Morgan, 1987).

recalling, and interpreting information, as well as all forms of reasoning.

One of the foremost figures in this area has been a Swiss psychologist, Jean Piaget. Early in his resarch, he turned to a difficult question: What is the nature of knowledge? In search of answers, he decided to talk with children, who are in the early stages of acquiring it.

Through his studies on thought, morality, and language in the child, Piaget made an enduring contribution to developmental psychology, fostering experiments unrivaled in the history of the field (Beilin, 1992). Eventually, he came to the view that the child's thinking is not just a simpler version of adult thought. It is *qualitatively* different, based on a different understanding of reality, one that slowly changes according to maturation and experience as the child actively develops new mental processes.

Two processes underlie these changes, according to Piaget. The first, **assimilation,** is the process of fitting new information into our current understanding of the world. Encountering a new event,

we use an old way of interacting with it. The child's first footwear includes stockings and booties; through assimilation, the child learns that shoes, slippers, and similar objects also go on the feet. However, when young children begin dressing themselves, they often put their shoes on the wrong feet. When corrected, or through experience, the child learns that shoes, unlike stockings and booties, are shaped to fit a specific foot. This response, **accommodation,** is the process of altering our current understanding, or cognitive structure, to make it more consistent with the new experience. In accommodation, we modify our old way of thinking to fit the new facts.

Adults behave similarly, for example, when they learn computer programs. They approach a program on the basis of what they already know and then modify their knowledge appropriately. This process is cyclical, moving from assimilation to accommodation, back to assimilation, and so forth, whether the problem is understanding how clothes fit or how computer programs work.

SENSORIMOTOR PERIOD. The first of Piaget's four stages occurs from birth to approximately 18 to 24 months of age, at which time infants do not think in the sense that older children do. This stage of cognitive development is called the **sensorimotor period** because the child merely senses things and acts on them.

At this stage, infants do not seem to conceive of objects as having any permanent, independent existence apart from their own experience with them. They do not carry around in their heads the symbols or images of objects. Or at least they show no awareness of an object when not looking at it, handling it, or otherwise acting on it. When Piaget dangled a rattle in front of his daughter's face, Jacqueline wriggled with delight. But when he hid it under a blanket as she watched, she immediately lost interest.

A few months later, Jacqueline behaved differently, as did her cousin Gerard when his ball rolled under an armchair. He retrieved it with difficulty, and later, when it rolled under the sofa, he looked there, too. When he could not find it, he crossed the room and explored under the armchair, where the ball was previously found. Gerard had acquired **object permanence,** which is the understanding that an object continues to exist even when it is not directly available to the senses (Piaget, 1954).

This understanding of object permanence is one of the accomplishments that mark the end of the sensorimotor period, a step that is enormously important because it permits children to represent objects to themselves. They need not act on something for it to exist in their minds. They have memories. They can carry images of rattles, balls, and other things in their heads, which is perhaps the beginning of thinking.

It was during the sensorimotor period that the two orphans, C.D. and B.D., were transferred to live with retarded people. This early action took place essentially by chance. However, the subsequent transfer of 11 more children was intentionally arranged to coincide with the end of the sensorimotor period, as we know it today, a time at which mental developments are rapid and dramatic.

PREOPERATIONAL THOUGHT. In this new stage, called the **preoperational period,** children can represent things to themselves, but they still do not readily understand the use of symbols, cannot perform logical manipulations with information, and cannot readily change the direction of their thinking. Children are preoperational throughout most of the preschool and early school years, from age 18 or 24 months to age six or seven years (Piaget & Inhelder, 1969).

One prominent characteristic of preoperational thought is its egocentrism. In **cognitive egocentrism,** for example, children do not realize that their thoughts are not necessarily shared by other people. Asked what happened at school, one child said, without further explanation, "Tommy did it." In **perceptual egocentrism,** children do not realize that their perceptions are not necessarily shared by other people. A three-year-old girl, playing hide-and-seek, shut her eyes and said, "Ha, ha! Can't see me!" (Clinchy, 1975).

In a test of perceptual egocentrism, each child was seated at a table that held a model of three mountains. Seated at this same table but in a different chair was a doll, and the child's task was to select from a series of pictures the one that represented the way the mountains looked from the doll's viewpoint. The child could walk around and observe the model from any position at the table but had to return to his or her own seat to select the picture. Preschoolers had little success with this task. Not understanding how the operation of changing location gave a different view, they consistently selected the picture that matched the mountains as seen from their own vantage point (Piaget & Inhelder, 1967).

Another characteristic of preoperational thought is evident when an object is changed in some way. The child is impressed with how it appears, rather than with less striking characteristics, such as how it was made. The aim in the **conservation task** is to discover whether a child recognizes that certain basic properties of something remain constant when only its appearance is changed.

Among many forms of the conservation task, one involves two identically shaped, tall jars containing equal amounts of liquid. After the child asserts that the contents are equal, the contents of one jar are poured into a third jar, which is low and wide. The amount of liquid has not changed; it is conserved. But the preoperational child, attending to the height of the tall column of liquid, typically maintains that there is more liquid in that tall, thin beaker than in the short, wide one. This thought is called *preoperational* because the child reasons in terms of the dominant perceptual experience rather than the logical operations involved (Figure 12–9).

CONCRETE OPERATIONS. Around age six, the child begins to master conservation problems. One six-year-old girl and an experimenter dropped marbles, one by one, into different beakers. The child's fell into a short, wide beaker and the experimenter's into a tall, thin one. The child, who could count to 30, counted the marbles as they dropped, and at first she maintained that she and the experimenter had the same number.

"How do you know?" she was asked. "Because I counted 'em. You've got ten and I've got ten." As the column of marbles mounted more impressively in the tall beaker, she began to hesitate. Finally, even though she counted 20 in each, she decided that the experimenter had more. Then she became confused: "You've got more, 'cause they're spread out more. No . . . I don't know" (Clinchy, 1975). This confusion is a sign of cognitive growth because the child considers other factors besides the dominant perceptual features.

During the stage of concrete operations, which lasts until age 11 or perhaps longer, the child becomes capable of reversing the procedure. One examiner made two straight clay "worms" of equal length and then formed the child's into a curly worm, testing the conservation of length. When asked if they were still the same length, the child said: "Acourse. If you pull my worm straight, he'll look like yours. They were both the same to start" (Clinchy, 1975). This capacity to use logic to solve problems when the physical objects are directly available is called **concrete operations.**

At the close of this stage, the individual can solve problems requiring classification, ordering, and sequencing, but only in specific situations, with the materials present. The child can arrange a series of sticks from tallest to shortest without making errors. The child can think of a given stick as both shorter than the preceding one and longer than the

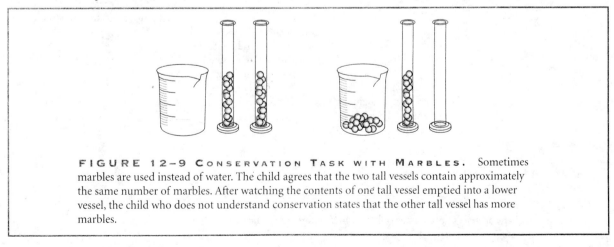

FIGURE 12–9 CONSERVATION TASK WITH MARBLES. Sometimes marbles are used instead of water. The child agrees that the two tall vessels contain approximately the same number of marbles. After watching the contents of one tall vessel emptied into a lower vessel, the child who does not understand conservation states that the other tall vessel has more marbles.

next one. Children at this stage have mastered the operations required in solving such problems, which is why we speak of concrete operations (Piaget, 1950).

FORMAL OPERATIONS. Suppose, however, that we asked the child to solve for the first time the lily-pad problem. A frog sits on the only lily pad on a pond. The pad reproduces itself, doubling every 24 hours; the next day there are two pads, the following day four, and so fourth. At the end of a month, the pond is covered completely. At what point in the month will the frog find the pond half covered?

In thinking about this problem, regardless of the solution, the adult uses **formal operations,** which is the capacity for reasoning apart from concrete situations. It is abstract reasoning, Piaget's final level of cognitive development. Around age 11 or older, the average child, entering adolescence, begins to engage in this type of thinking, although at a less sophisticated level than most adults. The adolescent well into formal operations may think of different approaches to the lily-pad problem and then realize that it is most readily solved by working backward from the end of the month, rather than forward from the beginning. If the pads double each day, then the pond must be half covered on the next-to-last day of the month.

In the previous stage, the child was able to classify, enumerate, and place objects and events in time and space, but in formal operations the child can *imagine* the possibilities inherent in a problem. Probably the most important feature of formal operations is that reality is seen as just one aspect of what might be. The adolescent generates hypotheses and tests them to find which one seems most valid and can even leave reality altogether, reasoning entirely in abstract terms. Not all adolescents and adults do so, however. Many never leave concrete operations (Figure 12–10).

The capacity for formal operations means that the cognitive world of the adolescent and adult is very different from that of the child, who lives largely a here-and-now existence. Adolescents, in particular, begin to imagine other worlds, especially ideal ones. They imagine worlds with better governments, better economic systems, better schools, better health care and even—ah, yes—better parents. Some of these things are not hard for any of us to imagine. Then they make comparisons with their current circumstances and often rebel or change their lifestyles. As formal operations develop, adolescents move beyond conventional standards of morality toward the construction of their own moral principles (Elkind, 1967).

It has been hypothesized, incidentally, that this

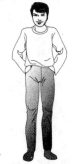

Formal operations, 11–
Logical, abstract reasoning; developing and testing hypotheses

Concrete operations, 7–11
Conservation and logical reasoning with concrete objects and events

Preoperational, 2–7
Perceptual and cognitive egocentrism; lack of conservation

Sensorimotor, 0–2
Lack of object permanence; response only to immediate environment

FIGURE 12–10 STAGES OF COGNITIVE DEVELOPMENT.
The ages are approximate; only the chief features are indicated.

mental growth contributes to certain fallacies adolescents may have about themselves. Self-conscious about their new and uncontrollable physical and psychological developments, they may imagine that they are under special scrutiny by others. This *imaginary audience*, it is speculated, partly accounts for teenagers' extreme concern about looking alike, thereby increasing peer support and diminishing the chances of being noticed. In the *personal fable,* the adolescent decides that his or her surprising new thoughts are unique. No one else has had them. The adolescent may think: "My parents never understood love the way I do." "No disaster will happen to me." Only gradually do they realize that their newly discovered mental abilities are shared by their mother and father, who at one time also questioned *their* parents' childrearing, business, religion, and other practices (Elkind, 1967, 1984).

A clear illustration of formal operations is apparent in Harold Skeels's work. He made an extraordinary proposal: to transfer mentally retarded children to a ward for mentally retarded girls and women in order to make the children normal. At face value, the proposal was preposterous. However, Skeels had reasoned from the preliminary findings with C.D. and B.D. He imagined a similar outcome—or rather hoped "that possibly 50 percent of the cases might show at least some improvement" (Skeels & Dye, 1939).

CRITIQUE OF PIAGETIAN THEORY.
One process underlies many of the changes in all stages, according to Piaget. It is *overcoming* egocentrism, which in this instance does not refer to personal interests or selfishness. Rather, **egocentrism** means that the individual's view of the world is self-centered. The individual assumes that the only understanding of the world is the one he or she possesses. Experience plays a vital role in enabling the individual to diminish egocentrism as the child discovers that objects exist even when not immediately present, that other people have thoughts different from his or her own, that there are agreed-upon systems for ordering and classifying things, and that the reality one experiences is just one of many possibilities. Needless to say, even adults never completely overcome this egocentrism.

How does the child make these advances? Piaget pointed to assimilation and accommodation, but his work is largely a description of what the child can and cannot do. There is a large difference in thought, for example, between a child in the preoperational stage and a child in concrete operations, but how does the child move to successive stages? How do these changes occur? How does the child overcome egocentrism? These questions remain to be answered. Several factors, external and internal, presumably influence the child's performance and hence, to a lesser degree, placement at a particular stage.

According to critics, differences in children's constructions of reality are influenced not only by differences in the various tasks they can perform but also by differences in information processing. In focusing on stages, which are somewhat arbitrary classifications, Piaget underestimated the *continuity* in cognitive development, which becomes manifest especially in the study of individual children (Niaz, 1991). Piaget's contribution to our understanding of children's thoughts has been enormous, yet its influence in the context of our advancing knowledge is regularly debated (Beilin, 1992; Halford, 1990).

INFORMATION PROCESSING VIEWPOINT.
Foremost among the other approaches to cognitive development is the **information processing viewpoint**, which emphasizes *how* the individual obtains and utilizes information, focusing on the mental operations by which the child converts sensory experience into knowledge. Perception, memory, and thinking are the basic concerns in the information processing approach. More inferential than Piaget's original work, this approach is also more directly concerned with the operations that

go on inside the "black box," a metaphor referring to the fact that mental functions cannot be observed directly. They take place inside the skull and can only be inferred.

In the information processing viewpoint, the idea of task specificity is important. It means that the performance on a particular problem or task pertains only to *that* task. The results are not generalizable; they cannot be applied beyond the immediate, specific situation.

The most widely cited Piagetian tasks are the conservation experiments, and follow-up studies show that the outcomes are often task specific. A child at age six or so may successfully manage conservation of liquid or solids, with water or marbles transferred from one container to another, but may be unable to solve a problem in conservation of length, in which a piece of string laid out straight is judged to be longer than one of equal length rolled into a ball. The solution to the conservation problem depends not only on the child's age, or stage, but also on the type of conservation task involved (Figure 12–11).

Similarly, the three-mountain problem allegedly shows the child's inability to put herself perceptually in someone else's place, but this same child may perform successfully on a simpler test of perceptual egocentrism, hiding a doll from the experimenter while viewing it herself. This less complex task is still a test of perceptual egocentrism (Flavell, Shipstead, & Croft, 1978).

The steady unfolding of the child's intellect is not an automatic process, as Piaget himself pointed out. It requires appropriate stimulation. The child becomes a little scientist or explorer, seizing opportunities to twist and pull, pick and drop, poke and rub, shake and break, trying to understand our world. In this context, Piagetians speak of "growledge"—meaning that children somehow grow their knowledge. However, the ways in which they achieve this development remain largely unknown, for studies in information processing and neural science are still far apart. To understand these processes, a bridge between these two fields will be necessary (Simon, 1990).

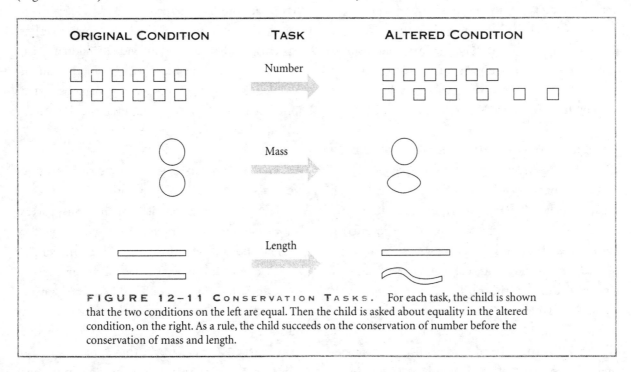

FIGURE 12–11 CONSERVATION TASKS. For each task, the child is shown that the two conditions on the left are equal. Then the child is asked about equality in the altered condition, on the right. As a rule, the child succeeds on the conservation of number before the conservation of mass and length.

MORAL DEVELOPMENT

As children develop increased responsiveness to the environment, they begin to learn how society works—what is right, wrong, expected, and so forth. Gradually they learn the rules of their social group and the world at large, a process called **moral development**.

KOHLBERG'S APPROACH TO MORAL REASONING. The concept of moral development includes two basic dimensions: moral reasoning and moral behavior. Human beings need to learn what is appropriate, and then they need to guide their behavior in these ways. In this respect, moral development occupies a position midway between cognitive and social development.

One of the earliest modern theories of moral reasoning was presented by an American psychologist, Lawrence Kohlberg, who viewed moral development from a cognitive perspective. His work provided evidence for six levels of moral reasoning, occurring in pairs. Therefore three basic levels were identified: preconventional, conventional, and postconventional.

In **preconventional morality,** characteristic of children ages four or five through ten, the basis for a moral judgment is the *physical consequences* of an act. Children of these ages judge misbehavior by the amount of damage someone does or by the amount of punishment that the person receives.

Two boys at the orphanage had a fight, but only one, with telltale bruises on his face, was caught and punished. In the preconventional view, the boy who was never punished was not such a bad child.

Around age ten, the approximate time for reaching **conventional morality,** there is a broader social concern, an effort to *maintain the social order,* but only in a stereotypical "good child" manner.

The laws are still fixed, and conformity is the goal; the aim is to avoid disapproval.

Even if one boy in the fight is being severely beaten, the bystander who does not intervene is a good child—according to conventional morality. The moral aim is to be a good boy or good girl, and not entering the fight achieves this goal. It gains the approval of authority.

The major difference between the second and third levels lies in the awareness of independent moral principles. Recognizing that there is an almost inevitable conflict of interests within a large group, the person at the level of **postconventional morality** understands the relativism of personal values and standards. According to Kohlberg, only a minority of the population reach this stage which, if entered at all, begins no earlier than age 13. At this level, there is a concern for human rights in the broadest sense and respect for the dignity of *people as individual human beings* (Kohlberg, 1969).

A bystander at the fight may decide to ring the fire alarm, not because there is a fire but because he or she feels that all physical hostility is immoral and wants the fire department to intervene. The law or rule of not ringing a false alarm is disobeyed because fighting violates a personal moral principle. This individual—according to postconventional morality—is responding to his or her own conscience.

MORAL BEHAVIOR. The other issue is moral behavior, and the question here concerns the correlation between ways of thinking and ways of behaving. Does the child who shows high moral reasoning also display high moral behavior?

In one early study, children were assessed for honesty in a wide variety of situations, ranging from recreational activity to school work. For example, they tried to identify some interesting objects. Then they were asked to go alone to the next room to return them, but a special observer could detect whether they kept any of these objects. After many tests of this sort, the most pronounced finding was that stealing, lying, or any other form of dishonesty occurred unpredictably from one situation and one child to another (Hartshorne & May, 1928). Some years later, these findings were reexamined, chiefly because they gave so little support for any persistent traits. Again, however, the evidence for moral behavior in young children was not impressive (Rushton, Brainerd, & Pressley, 1983; Rushton, Jackson, & Paunonen, 1981).

Moral reasoning is a necessary but not sufficient condition for moral behavior. The task of teaching moral reasoning and moral behavior in diverse situations lies before us, especially in the home and school. One problem in American society today, many contend, is a decline in moral instruction (Bok, 1988).

CRITIQUE OF KOHLBERG'S THEORY. The first effort to demonstrate empirically and in detail that morality can be viewed in stages, Kohlberg's theory is a pioneering effort. There is some doubt, however, about its applicability across cultures. The upper levels do not appear in certain societies, and they are found only on rare occasions in others. Further, it has been argued that Kohlberg's theory contains a political bias; it offers implicit support for people who believe in principles that may conflict with established laws. They should reach the upper levels of postconventional morality more readily than those who adhere to laws approved by the governing bodies.

A limitation of a different sort arises because Kohlberg's work was based essentially on studies of boys. These all-male samples reflected an assumption that gender differences may exist, and yet the morality of girls, as a separate issue, has not been investigated extensively. Using boys, Kohlberg's view of morality focuses on respecting others' rights. It stresses justice. Carol Gilligan has pointed out that girls develop moral reasoning along different lines.

Their focus is on developing personal relationships, caring for others, and becoming attached to them. It stresses care. Gilligan's approach states that the issues of intimacy, nurturance, and affiliation should be reflected in any view of morality (Gilligan, 1982). The difference in these views is sometimes known as the *justice–care debate*, reflecting the emphasis in each instance. Various theoretical and practical proposals have been made to resolve these differences (Brown & Tappan, 1991; Puka, 1991).

SOCIAL DEVELOPMENT

Morality had been an issue back at the orphanage in Iowa. Harold Skeels had prematurely transferred 13 children to the wards for mentally retarded women. According to what he had learned from C.D. and B.D., that transfer was morally defensible. Then, rather suddenly, he came to an important realization. The tests administered to those children before their transfer also had been administered routinely to *all* children who stayed at the orphanage. He could conduct an empirical study, comparing the scores of children who were transferred with those of children who stayed at the orphanage. And he could do so without any concerns about morality or any resistance from the Board of Control. He would simply look at the old records.

Examining the orphanage files, Skeels identified 12 *non*transferred children who might serve as a comparison group. One of the boys in this group suffered from mild deafness, but otherwise the transferred and comparison groups were similar in age, and their average time with the retarded women or at the orphanage spanned about two years.

Skeels's purpose was to detect any differences in scores that had occurred during that time. And his findings were remarkable. The transferred group had achieved an average gain in IQ of 28 points. Among the comparison group, there was an average loss of 26 points. The mean IQ of the transferred children was close to normal, and the comparison

	TRANSFERRED GROUP				COMPARISON GROUP		
CASE	FIRST IQ	LAST IQ	CHANGE	CASE	FIRST IQ	LAST IQ	CHANGE
1	89	113	+24	1	91	62	−29
2	57	77	+20	2	92	56	−36
3	85	107	+22	3	71	56	−15
4	73	100	+27	4	96	54	−42
5	46	95	+49	5	99	54	−45
6	77	100	+23	6	87	67	−20
7	65	104	+39	7	81	83	+2
8	35	93	+58	8	103	60	−43
9	61	80	+19	9	98	61	−37
10	72	79	+ 7	10	89	71	−18
11	75	82	+ 7	11	50	42	−8
12	65	82	+17	12	83	60	−23
13	36	81	+45				
Average	64	92	+28	Average	87	61	−26

TABLE 12–2 CHANGES IN IQ OF SKEELS'S CHILDREN. C.D. is case 5, and B.D. is case 8. Their gains were the largest among all the transferred children.

group had fallen into the retarded range (Skeels & Dye, 1939; Table 12–2).

This positive outcome for the transferred children, according to Harold Skeels, was due to the stimulation and caretaker–child interaction they had received in the institution for the mentally retarded. In contrast, the overworked matrons at the orphanage made their young charges stand up, sit down, and do most other things in unison. There was little time for interactions and activities with other children or adults, thereby fostering **social development,** a person's growing capacity for successful relations with other people.

GENDER IDENTITY. Social development is often closely linked to gender identity; they can have considerable significance for one another. The term **gender identity** means that people recognize themselves as belonging to one sex or the other; they have confidence in themselves as male or female. This outcome is prompted by adult expectations, social stereotypes, and the more subtle ways in which the sexes are treated differently.

The concepts of male and female are among the earliest that young children acquire. Formed in a rudimentary sense in the first two years, they play a crucial role in further development, even into adulthood and the workplace (Ely, 1995).

Long-term studies show a decrease in traditional sex roles for men and women, but the change is substantially greater for women (McBroom, 1987). In this regard, gender theory approaches the study of sex roles from either of two directions. Some investigators maximize the differences by contrasting the sexes; others minimize them by stressing the equality or similarity between the sexes (Hare-Mustin & Marecek, 1988). Still others, especially psychoanalysts, raise fundamental questions about the function of gender identity in people's lives. For personal adjustment, the capacity to tolerate ambiguity in gender categories may be as important as achieving a single sex-appropriate view of oneself (Goldner, 1991).

PSYCHOSOCIAL STAGES: CHILDHOOD. At various points in this book, the works of stage theorists are noted: Freud, concerned with sexual development; Piaget, with emphasis on cognitive development; and Kohlberg, who investigated moral development. Each examined development in the early years rather than across the life span.

Erik Erikson, a psychoanalyst who acknowledged a debt to Sigmund Freud, has been responsible for much of the current interest in the entire life cycle, and he decided that human development occurs in eight stages. These are called **psychosocial stages** because many aspects of psychological and social functioning are interrelated and show consistent changes during the life cycle. At each stage, the focus is on a specific crisis in our relationships with other people (Erikson, 1963). The ways in which these crises are managed play a major role in the individual's capacity to respond successfully to personal and social problems at later stages. In childhood, these successive stages are four in number: trust, autonomy, initiative, and industry.

The newborn's first awareness is of physical needs, most obviously the need for nourishment. If the caretaker fulfills these needs consistently, the infant develops trust. In this crisis of **trust versus mistrust,** the infant acquires a sense of reliance on and confidence in its environment or, through early deprivation of these needs, it becomes unresponsive and distrustful. It was just after this stage that Skeels's transferred group was sent from the orphanage to live with the retarded women and girls. Developmental psychologists would point out that the chances for a positive outcome would have been decidedly diminished if the transfer had occurred later.

By the second year of life, the muscular and nervous systems have developed markedly. The child is no longer content to sit and watch, but judgment develops more slowly. The caretaker's decisions about how much freedom to allow are therefore very important in the crisis of **autonomy versus doubt,** from which the child emerges with a sense of independence or with feelings of fear and dependence.

Once a sense of independence has been established, the child wants to try out various possibilities. It is during this crisis of **initiative versus guilt,** from age three to six years, that the child's willingness to try new things is facilitated or inhibited. If the caretaker responds to the child's creative effort in attempting to paint the bathroom, for example, rather than to the resulting mess, the crisis tends to be resolved in a favorable direction.

From six to twelve years the child develops a greater attention span, needs less sleep, and gains rapidly in strength. Therefore, he or she can expend much more effort in acquiring skills. Eager to learn real skills, rather than pretend to have them, the child reaches a new stage. In this crisis, **industry versus inferiority,** the fortunate child is guided to tasks that are appropriate for him or her at the given moment, developing a sense of accomplishment, rather than feelings of failure (Figure 12–12).

THE IDENTITY CRISIS. Adolescence means growing up, which often includes the well-known adolescent–parent conflict. The adolescent at times demands considerable freedom, borrowing the car and staying out late. At other times, the adolescent shows sustained dependence, needing assistance with school or personal relationships. In nonindustrialized countries, the adolescent rebellion is moderate or nonexistent. The apparent reason is that

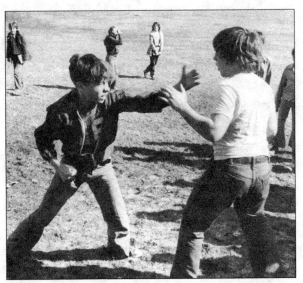

FIGURE 12–12 SOCIAL DEVELOPMENT THROUGH PLAY. Children's play includes constructive, imaginary, and rough-and-tumble activities, all influential in social development.

entrance into an agricultural or hunting-and-gathering society is far easier than finding a place in a highly developed culture. Young people in our country need a temporary place for themselves while they search for a more permanent place in the larger social context (Elkind, 1984; Galambos, 1992).

In the crisis of **identity versus role diffusion,** the adolescent gradually develops a sense of self as a consistent and unique person or instead begins to experience a fragmented, disconnected, and unclear sense of self. Through Erikson's work, the period of adolescence is regarded as involving an **identity crisis,** a search for self-understanding marked by emotional upheaval and difficulties in establishing a consistent personality. However, uncertainty about attitudes, values, ethics, career opportunities, and religious beliefs appears at later stages too.

• ADULTHOOD AND OLD AGE •

With the full life cycle in mind, Harold Skeels one day began a highly improbable task. Almost a quarter of a century after his original work, he set out to find all 25 of his former subjects, 13 from the transferred group and 12 from the comparison group. What had become of the little girls and boys who lived for a while with the mentally retarded women? What about those who stayed at the orphanage? Now about 30 years old, where were all of these people? What places had they taken for themselves in society?

Some of them still lived in Iowa, not far from the orphanage site, but others had moved to the farthest corners of the country, including Florida and California, and efforts to contact them were time-consuming and frustrating. Once located, each subject was interviewed, along with the adoptive parents whenever possible, and these findings were presented in another report, *Adult Status of Children with Contrasting Early Life Experiences: A Follow-up Study* (Skeels, 1966).

Among the 12 people in the comparison group, four were still institutionalized, and one had died in an institution. The state had cared for these people for a combined total of 273 years. In the transferred group, *none* of the 13 members was institutionalized, and the state had cared for them for only 72 years. The maintenance costs for the comparison group were five times greater than those for the transferred group.

An equally impressive difference appeared in the work records for both groups. All members of the transferred group worked inside or outside the home. Only half of the comparison group were so employed, sometimes intermittently. The transferred group also appeared to be in better physical health. In all respects, that group had become more firmly established in adulthood.

The stage of adulthood, the longest in human life, has been least studied in psychology. For many years it was thought that adulthood contained no significant developmental changes, but now it is regarded as a period with numerous important transitions—from the intermittent dependency of late adolescence to the intermittent or total dependency of old age. It is basically divided into three stages: young adulthood, from the twenties to 45 or so; middle adulthood, from 45 to 65; and old age, from 65 onward.

PHYSICAL CHANGES

One reason that adulthood was ignored in earlier research is that the physical changes are slower and less obvious than those that occur during childhood and adolescence. Moreover, after the twenties, the basic process is decline.

From this perspective, two generalizations should be kept in mind, for they summarize the findings on physical decline and aging. First, it is not readily apparent whether diminished physical functions are due to aging or to disease. It has been very difficult to demonstrate that decreased ability is a natural result of aging per se. Second, differences in physical ability among individuals of the same age are generally less pronounced at midlife than in the later years. The elderly show wider variations than do younger adults (Jones, 1987).

PHYSICAL DECLINE IN ADULTHOOD. Maximum physical growth occurs around ages 18 to 20. Certainly by age 30, power, agility, and endurance are at their peaks and, except in highly trained athletes, the decline has commenced. Skeels's subjects were around this age when he commenced his follow-up studies.

Athletes who continue to improve their performance later do so chiefly by increasing their knowledge about competitive situations and by restricting themselves to certain roles, such as the designated hitter in baseball or the field goal kicker in football, or by restricting themselves to certain sports, such as golf, in which strength and endurance are not prime factors. Even for the average person, the environment plays a role in physical condition, always in the context of a given heredity. Men and women in their sixties, through careful programs of exercise, rest, nutrition, and avoidance of stress, can maintain a better physical condition than those in their thirties who ignore these factors.

By the late forties and fifties, as muscle strength and capacity more clearly decline, there is an increase in body weight, a decrease in hair on the head—especially in men—and the appearance of wrinkles in the skin. Body fat tends to accumulate in the trunk and to decrease on the limbs, and therefore physical appearance sometimes changes without any marked change in weight. The need for assistance in daily routines, such as seeing and chewing, becomes evident in the use of eyeglasses and dental crowns.

PHYSICAL CONDITION OF THE ELDERLY. As the late years in the full life cycle are approached, hearing aids, canes, and pill boxes accompany the crowns and eyeglasses. Old age, indeed, is not for sissies. Posture, stature, and locomotion also change noticeably. The bent or stooped look occurs through alterations in bone structure, a decrease in muscle mass, and loss of elasticity in the tendons and ligaments. Elderly people *have* shrunk. They are stiffer and shorter than they were in earlier years, even if they can stand up straight.

These exterior changes reflect changes in the interior, not only in the heart and lungs but also in the brain. After midlife, the brain begins to decrease in volume at the rate of one or two percent each decade, chiefly through the slow loss of neurons in physical deterioration (Miller, Alston, & Corsellis, 1980). This rate of change is less than that elsewhere in the body and by itself represents no significant loss of mental ability. Redundancy in the nervous system apparently prevents any appreciable decline in abilities, and it is clear that certain brain areas can take over functions of other areas. It has also been suggested that the brain may prune some synapses to achieve its proper adult organization. In other words, efficient networks for performing certain tasks may require a reduction in the potential for performing others (Greenough & Juraska, 1979).

With our increasingly older population, experts in this field now have begun to speak of the young-old, referring to people in the first decade after retirement, and the old-old, who range upward from 75. Again, individual differences are important. Many old-old function better than young-old.

∾

COGNITIVE ABILITIES

When physical and cognitive development in adulthood are compared, one difference is readily apparent. Unlike physical development, there is no inevitable decline in cognitive ability beginning in early adulthood. In fact, there may be no decline until middle adulthood or much later, depending to a significant degree on the type and extent of mental activity in the adult's life. In other words, exercise, rest, and nutrition may help slow the inevitable physical decline beginning in the late twenties, keeping the body in its best possible physical condition, but various mental activities during these same years may even increase cognitive ability.

The difference in mental ability between the two groups in Harold Skeels's research remains essentially unknown in adulthood, despite the large difference in childhood and the different employment histories. Out of respect for these adults, Skeels did not administer mental tests. However, he did obtain information on their educational levels, finding that the transferred group was far superior here, too (Table 12–3).

COGNITIVE DEVELOPMENT IN ADULT-HOOD. While progressing in a career and certain hobbies, a person's activities often demand more and more attention to mental tasks, and with this practice and experience, mental capacity typically increases. As indicated in the next chapter on intelligence, there may be a gradual improvement in

TRANSFERRED GROUP		COMPARISON GROUP	
CASE	GRADE	CASE	GRADE
1	11	1	2
2	5	2	2
3	15	3	4
4	15	4	3
5	10	5	0
6	12	6	13
7	12	7	8
8	12	8	2
9	6	9	3
10	14	10	6
11	16	11	2
12	12	12	3
13	13		
Average	12	Average	4

TABLE 12–3 LEVEL OF EDUCATION OF SKEELS'S ADULTS. Only two of the transferred children failed to attend high school. Only one of the comparison children reached that level.

intellectual ability even into the sixth and seventh decades of life. A key factor, perhaps *the* key factor, is the extent to which the individual engages in stimulating and challenging mental activity.

In this regard, we can speak of **metacognition,** meaning the extent to which an individual understands his or her own cognitive processes. Metacognition is knowing what one knows, thinking about one's own thinking. To improve our thinking, we need to become aware of how our thinking works, evaluating its successes and failures, regulating it according to the problem. Without conscious effort, many adults commonly develop increased metacognition over the years (Powell & Whitlaw, 1994). The process of teaching people to think about their thinking may hold special promise in education.

COGNITION IN THE ELDERLY. The most obvious change among the old-old, and even in many young-old, is a *decline in speed* in mental functions, including perception, recall, problem solving, and other forms of information processing. Like physical movement, mental activity becomes slower through changes in the nervous system. There is abundant evidence for diminished speed in almost every cognitive task in which speed has been measured (Light, 1991; Birren & Fisher, 1995).

There is also a *decline in learning,* but if learning is defined as the rate of acquiring new information, the underlying problem is still the speed of processing new information. This decline also may arise through decreasing confidence, lack of exposure to contemporary educational opportunities, and a diminished attention span (Botwinick, 1984).

The *memory problems* of the elderly are legion, and apparently they arise in two general ways, apart from the possible changes in neurophysiology. First, perception may be part of the problem. With decreased sensory abilities, elderly people do not obtain new information in an efficient, well-organized fashion. Second, these problems should be understood not as storage problems but as problems in retrieval, for laboratory studies have shown that the elderly perform quite differently on tests of recognition and recall. When young adults and the elderly are compared on recognition of well-learned material, their scores are almost equal; when compared on recall, the elderly do more poorly (Mitrushina & Satz, 1989; Poon, 1985).

Failing memory is especially evident in **Alzheimer's disease,** a progressive brain disorder in the later years characterized not only by forgetting but also by disorientation, slowness of speech, and general apathy. A fatal disease, Alzheimer's eventually results in total mental and emotional deterioration. In this respect, the caregiver becomes a patient too, experiencing the consequences of coping with an important problem that has no immediate solution (Ehrlich & White, 1991; Parks & Pilisuk, 1991).

In normal health, verbal abilities are often maintained or even improved until well past the middle of life. People engaged in scholarly tasks, working at jobs that require special attention to words, or simply practicing language skills, show no diminution in verbal ability in the sixth and seventh decades or later (Schaie & Willis, 1986; Figure 12–13). They approach new problems with a vast background, and this wisdom or experience may compensate for deficits in speed and perceptual-motor abilities.

∾

SOCIAL RELATIONS

Since the middle of this century, the highly complex social environment of the adult has received increasing research attention, and several points of transition have been identified. These developmental tasks do not occur with the regularity of childhood changes, but they occur for most adults: joining the labor force, getting married, becoming a parent, raising an adolescent, reaching mid-career in

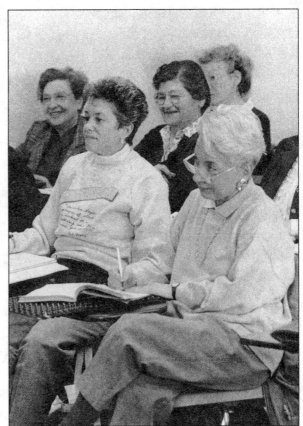

FIGURE 12–13 MAINTAINING COGNITIVE ABILITY. Mental challenges play a vital role in maintaining intellectual ability in the later decades, just as they are essential to mental development in the earlier years.

work, adjusting to life without dependent children, and so forth.

SOCIAL CONCERNS: ADULTHOOD. For young adults, an enormous challenge is posed by *career planning*, which means preparing a satisfying and productive vocational path. A major part of the identity crisis, this problem is complicated by the fact that careers planned today may not even exist in another decade. Moreover, our changing physical, intellectual, and social makeup require constant career adjustment and readjustment during our working lives.

The aim in career planning is to make optimal use of one's talents, but ultimately the career must be a compromise between what one would like to do and what reality offers. In the future, with constant and rapid change in the workplace, the diagnosis and treatment of work-related problems may become a major specialty in psychology (Handy, 1990; Lowman, 1993).

Around the forties or later, men and women often experience a tension or lack of fulfillment in their lives, called the **midlife crisis** or midlife transition. These years may reveal that certain things cannot be accomplished in life, that there can be no new start, and that the end is approaching (Levison, Darrow, Klein, Levinson, & McKee, 1978). In this respect, the midlife crisis—which is *highly* variable in age and intensity, if it appears at all—marks a transition from young adulthood to middle adulthood.

The responsibilities of young adulthood, according to Erik Erikson, can create tensions and frustrations. They are therefore accompanied by an attempt to develop an intimate relationship, physical or psychological, with someone else. If this crisis of **intimacy versus isolation** is adequately resolved, the adult feels personal support in the culture; otherwise he or she feels alienated. But a commitment to someone else, especially in the context of childrearing, requires abandoning one's own goals to some degree, something that is not readily undertaken. Hence Erikson emphasizes that true intimacy is not possible without first achieving identity and gaining confidence in oneself.

If intimacy is reflected in marriage, then the results of Skeels's follow-up study were again dramatic. Of the 13 transferred children, 11 were married. Of the 12 comparison children, only two had married, and one of these marriages ended in divorce. Intimacy is not requisite for matrimony and certainly is not absent among unmarried people, but the very large difference in this traditional measure of becoming partners suggests an overall difference in interpersonal relationships between the two groups (Skeels, 1966).

Erikson has pointed out that the demands of intimacy are often in conflict with those of work. In fact, Sigmund Freud defined mental health in adults as the capacity to love and to work. It is noteworthy, therefore, that all of Skeels's transferred group were employed in some way, while only half of the comparison group were employed. Hence, by both criteria, love and work, the transferred group had found a much firmer place in the community, supporting family members as well as themselves (Table 12–4).

In middle adulthood, Erikson continued, there may be a broadening concern, beyond intimacy. In this crisis, called **generativity versus stagnation,**

TRANSFERRED GROUP		COMPARISON GROUP	
CASE	OCCUPATION	CASE	OCCUPATION
1	Staff sargeant	1	Institutional inmate
2	Housewife	2	Dishwasher
3	Housewife	3	Deceased
4	Nursing instructor	4	Dishwasher
5	Housewife	5	Institutional inmate
6	Waitress	6	Compositor/typesetter
7	Housewife	7	Institutional inmate
8	Housewife	8	Dishwasher
9	Domestic service	9	Floater
10	Real estate sales	10	Cafeteria worker
11	Vocational counselor	11	Gardener's assistant
12	Gift shop sales	12	Institutional inmate
13	Housewife		

TABLE 12–4 TYPE OF OCCUPATION OF SKEELS'S ADULTS.   These differences in occupation also were reflected in the spouses. The occupations of the spouses of the transferred group ranged from dental technician to flight engineer to advertising copywriter. The one spouse in the comparison group was employed in the home.

there is an expansion of one's interests to include the next generation, or else there is a rather restrained and exclusive focus on one's personal goals. The concern in generativity is not just bearing children, for the biological parent is not necessarily interested in future generations. The positive solution to this crisis is manifested in working, teaching, and caring for the young, in nurturing the products and ideas of the culture, and in a more general "belief in the species." This response reflects a desire to leave something of benefit to humanity rather than an exclusive concern with one's own well-being.

SOCIAL CONCERNS: OLD AGE.

If the criterion for entering old age is the generally accepted retirement age of 65, then every day more than 4,000 people in the United States enter this life stage. For many adults, a central part of the self-concept is the vocational self, regardless of the type of work in which one is engaged. Thus, retirement from a formal work setting is a most important transition among the elderly.

According to Erikson, in the final life crisis, **integrity versus despair,** a person finds meaning in memories or instead looks back on life with dissatisfaction. Integrity implies emotional integration; it means accepting one's life as one's own responsibility. It is based not so much on what has happened as on how one feels about it. If a person has found meaning in certain goals, or even in suffering, then the crisis has been satisfactorily resolved. If not, the person experiences dissatisfaction, and the prospect of death brings despair.

With their infirmities, the elderly remind us of the young. As they become more and more limited, the earlier issues of industry, initiative, autonomy, and even trust arise again. With fewer and fewer friends and sometimes no family, loneliness is the critical psychological problem, often managed by maintaining a sense of humor about one's predicament.

CRITIQUE OF ERIKSON'S THEORY.

For many critics, Erikson's later stages seem vague, and there is a reason. The biological changes in adulthood are not nearly as sudden and marked as those in childhood and adolescence, and they are not accompanied by such obvious behavioral changes as the child's first steps, the adolescent's first shave, and the young mother's first lactation. As a result, Erikson's stages for adulthood become more philosophical, less biological. His theory has been criticized for these reasons: What are the operational definitions of intimacy, generativity, and integrity? And what is the evidence that people in adulthood behave in these ways? There is a need for greater precision in these later stages (Hamachek, 1990).

Other critics, on the grounds that self-knowledge can be achieved only after intimacy with someone else, maintain that the stage of intimacy should appear before that of identity. Still others argue that the order may be one way for men and the other way for women. These arguments suggest that these two developmental tasks influence one another, continue throughout adulthood, and are closely related. In fact, advanced stages of identity formation have been found to be associated with increased levels of intimacy formation (Kacergius & Adams, 1980).

In adulthood, the points of change instead seem to be determined more by social factors, especially socioeconomic status. Among people in the lower class, the prime of life is considered to be the late twenties and early thirties, and middle age begins at 40; people in the upper middle class regard 40 as the prime of life and 50 as the onset of middle age (Neugarten, 1968). Education, financial resources, and occupational status all create more opportunities for upper-class and middle-class people and therefore prolong the midlife stages (Hopson & Scally, 1980).

In the context of these criticisms, Erikson's theory has made three special contributions. The first major developmental theory to emphasize the full life span, it has called attention to the phases or periods in adulthood. Second, it has focused on social development, as distinct from other areas of development. Third, it has emphasized the adolescent identity crisis, an expression now so popularized that it is used throughout the adult life cycle. It is particularly relevant in our highly technical, rapidly changing society, one in which lifestyles and career paths may be disrupted without notice (Figure 12–14).

DEATH AND DYING. The subject of death, long taboo or ignored in Western research, has been studied in investigations with terminally ill patients, suggesting that dying also can be viewed in stages.

Five in number, these include: denial, in which the individual, responding to the shock, feels that a mistake has been made; anger, when the patient, accepting the evidence, feels unfairly treated; bargaining, a relatively short period during which the individual promises better behavior in exchange for a longer life; then depression, involving a feeling of hopelessness and grief at the separation from loved ones; and finally acceptance, if there is sufficient time, wherein the person is neither depressed nor angry but resigned to the final outcome of the life cycle (Kübler-Ross, 1969).

The response to this conception has been mixed and sometimes strongly disputed. While it concerns an important and neglected issue in

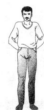
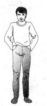

ELDERLY
Integrity vs. despair
Fulfillment in life

MIDDLE ADULTHOOD
Generativity vs. stagnation
Future generations

YOUNG ADULTHOOD
Intimacy vs. isolation
Personal and career commitments

ADOLESCENCE
Identity vs. role diffusion
Sense of self

LATE CHILDHOOD, 6–12
Industry vs. inferiority
Competence, ability

MIDDLE CHILDHOOD, 3–6
Initiative vs. guilt
Effort, willingness

EARLY CHILDHOOD, 1–3
Autonomy vs. doubt
Self-control

INFANCY, 0–1
Trust vs. mistrust
Dependence on others

FIGURE 12–14 PSYCHOSOCIAL STAGES. This sequence shows an expanding social context. Concerns at any stage may reappear later (Erickson, 1963).

American psychology, there is a need for further empirical support, precise definitions, and an overall theoretical structure. It does not apply when death is sudden, and it appears more relevant to cases of early, prolonged illness than to dying at a much later age.

With increasing research interest, there is now emphasis on *healthy death*, which is not a self-contradictory expression. Death, an inevitable conclusion to the developmental process, can be approached in ways that are appropriate and meaningful, resulting in healthy attitudes among the dying person, the family, and the support person (Smith & Maher, 1991). The prospects for a healthy death are most likely following a purposeful, healthy life.

Whether one accepts these psychological stages of death or Erikson's stages of life, there is no doubt that human beings are always in the process of developing. In one way or another, the life of every human being is shaped and reshaped every day.

• INDIVIDUAL DIFFERENCES •

Developmental psychologists sometimes study the ways in which people are alike, as illustrated in the stage theories of Erikson, Freud, Kohlberg, and Piaget. And sometimes they focus on the ways in which they differ, called the psychology of individual differences.

All of the adults in Skeels's comparison group differed from one another, but one person was special. He had achieved an education not only the highest in his group but also equal to or higher than that of all but four members of the transferred group. Through his work in printing, he had earned higher wages than the rest of the comparison group combined. Perhaps this surprising outcome was due in part to his disability, for he was the boy with the mild hearing loss. After leaving the orphanage, he went to a school for the deaf, where he received considerable individual attention. This personal support and careful instruction could have been a significant factor in his later favorable development.

The printer's position in the comparison group prompts us to recognize differences among us. The concept of **individual differences** states that all of us are unique; each of us deviates in one way or another from the average and from all other people in physical, cognitive, social, and other characteristics. Even identical twins are not exactly alike. The aim, in concluding this chapter, is to remind the reader about such variations. Psychologists study them to understand more fully and accurately the complexities of human behavior and experience, thereby according to all individuals greater respect and human dignity (Betz & Fitzgerald, 1993).

When compared with the people in his group, as well as with those in the transferred group, the printer's success also illustrates the interaction principle. It shows that a particular heredity can interact with a particular environment, producing unexpected results.

In addition, the success of the printer demonstrates possible shortcomings in Harold Skeels's research. No investigator can take into account all potentially relevant factors, and in this instance all children were first tested at approximately 18 months of age, when the scores are unreliable predictors of adult intelligence. The capacity of the printer, and indeed of all the subjects in these relatively small samples, might have been quite different from that indicated at the early age. Moreover, the rate of adoption for the transferred children was higher than that of the orphanage children. It could have influenced later adult status considerably. But of course adoption, in turn, was significantly influenced by the earlier gains.

Ideally, the Skeels research should be repeated with larger groups of subjects, more precise measures of early development, and greater control over adoption procedures. But unless we lose sight of what has been learned already, such studies

284

should never take place. Orphanages like those of the 1930s are now prohibited by state law. Infants and young children awaiting adoption today, in hospitals and elsewhere, usually receive considerable individual attention, largely through the efforts of temporary foster families.

This approach to adoption, and indeed our modern view of effective day care for all children, owes much of its origin to two frail, runny-nosed, little orphans. They led Harold Skeels to a group of loving, retarded women.

• SUMMARY •

DEVELOPMENTAL ISSUES

1. The study of human development concerns changes that take place throughout the life span, and certain fundamental issues have arisen. One of these concerns the nature and duration of critical periods, during which the individual is unusually responsive to certain forms of stimulation. The heredity–environment issue concerns the contribution of each factor in human development. Today it is recognized that both heredity and environment are always present and always in interaction.

AT CONCEPTION

2. At conception, our biological inheritance is determined by 23 pairs of chromosomes or, more specifically, by the almost countless genes within the chromosomes. The genes contain the basic hereditary blueprint; they direct the development of many physical characteristics and behavioral traits.

3. Most human traits seem to depend on an interaction of multiple pairs of genes. Through controlled studies of animals, using genotypical and phenotypical perspectives, as well as studies of identical twins, the field of behavioral genetics attempts to discover the hereditary and environmental foundations of behavior.

PRENATAL PHASE AND INFANCY

4. The first three months of prenatal life are particularly susceptible to the influence of teratogens,

meaning factors that disrupt normal development, producing birth defects. Neural development continues after birth, at which time the brain is only about one-fourth of its adult size.

5. The principle of differentiation indicates that development proceeds from the simple to the complex, from general reactions to highly specific responses, and it is evident in both sensory and motor development. The normal human infant, for example, progresses from lying to sitting to standing and to walking on a predictable basis.

6. The phenomena of imprinting and critical periods in animals suggest that the timing of early experiences can be influential in human development as well. These so-called sensitive periods in human beings are not as sharply defined as those in animals, but they can play an influential role in learning and social development.

CHILDHOOD AND ADOLESCENCE

7. When developmental responses appear in a given sequence at about the same age in all members of a species, they are said to be due to maturation, as in cephalocaudal and proximodistal development. In postnatal life, human beings show very rapid physical development for the first two years. A second period of rapid physical development occurs during adolescence, when hormonal secretions produce physiological changes having wide repercussions.

8. Stages of cognitive development have been identified by Jean Piaget. In the sensorimotor stage, the child is simply acting on and experiencing the environment. In the preoperational stage, the child slowly overcomes certain aspects of egocentrism,

perceiving the world from others' viewpoints. As concrete operations are achieved, the child becomes capable of solving concrete problems. Formal operations, not necessarily achieved by all adolescents or adults, involve the capacity for solving abstract problems.

9. The development of morality is studied in two dimensions, moral reasoning and moral behavior. One view of moral reasoning postulates three basic stages: preconventional morality, conventional morality, and postconventional morality. Correlations between moral reasoning and moral behavior have not been substantial.

10. According to Erikson's life span theory of psychological stages, human development involves a series of eight crises, four of which occur in childhood: trust, autonomy, initiative, and industry. The psychosocial crisis during adolescence is that of establishing a personal identity, which means developing a sense of self as a consistent yet unique person.

∽

ADULTHOOD AND OLD AGE

11. Maximum physical growth and ability are achieved by the late twenties, after which a slow but steady decrease begins in strength, quickness, and size. Throughout young adulthood and middle adulthood, the rate of change depends partly on environmental circumstances. The elderly can vary sharply in physical ability, a condition partly responsible for references to the young-old and old-old.

12. There is no inevitable decline in cognitive ability in young and middle adulthood and sometimes even into the early years of old age. There may even be steady improvements, depending significantly on the type and extent of intellectual activity in the individual's adult life. Among the elderly, the inevitable decline is most obvious in the speed of mental functions.

13. Healthy adults, according to Erikson, can find satisfaction in relations with others. The psychosocial crises in adulthood involve intimacy, which occurs with another person, and generativity, which concerns future generations. Elderly people are confronted with the eighth and last psychosocial crisis, achieving integrity, which means developing a sense of meaning in one's life.

∽

INDIVIDUAL DIFFERENCES

14. The concept of individual differences states that everyone is unique. We all differ from one another in physical, cognitive, and social dimensions.

• WORKING WITH PSYCHOLOGY •

∽ REVIEW OF KEY CONCEPTS ∽

human development

Developmental Issues
critical period
heredity–environment issue
identical twins
fraternal twins
interaction principle

At Conception
chromosomes
genes

sperm
ova
dominant gene
recessive gene
polygenic trait
behavioral genetics
genotype
phenotype

Prenatal Phase and Infancy
differentiation
zygote
embryo

fetus
teratogens
cephalocaudal development
proximodistal development
imprinting
attachment
stranger anxiety
separation anxiety
caretaker–child interaction

Childhood and Adolescence
physical development
maturation

adolescence
estrogens
androgens
puberty
cognitive development
assimilation
accommodation
sensorimotor period
object permanence
preoperational period
cognitive egocentrism
perceptual egocentrism
conservation task
concrete operations
formal operations

egocentrism
information processing
  viewpoint
moral development
preconventional morality
conventional morality
postconventional morality
social development
gender identity
psychosocial stages
trust versus mistrust
autonomy versus doubt
initiative versus guilt
industry versus inferiority

identity versus role
  diffusion
identity crisis

Adulthood and Old Age
metacognition
Alzheimer's disease
midlife crisis
intimacy versus isolation
generativity versus stagnation
integrity versus despair

Individual Differences
individual differences

∾ CLASS DISCUSSION/CRITICAL THINKING ∾

A NARRATIVE TWIST

Assume that the transferred orphans in Skeels's study had been sent to live with women in prison, rather than with mentally retarded women. Would this circumstance have produced for the children outcomes different from those obtained with the retarded women? What might have been the chief differences, if any? From the opposite perspective, would the presence of the children have influenced the prisoners? If so, how? If not, why not? Explain your views. ∾

TOPICAL QUESTIONS

• *Developmental Issues.* Suppose you are allowed to study human development from only one perspective, either chronological for just one area of development throughout the life span *or* topical for all three areas at just one stage of life. Which approach would you choose? Why? Describe the specific chronological stages or topics to which you would give most emphasis.

• *At Conception.* Is it possible that a grandparent may make no contribution to the genetic inheritance of his or her grandchild? Explain the reason for your answer, referring to the matter of chance in the assortment of chromosomes within the sperm and ovum and in the association of a particular sperm and ovum at fertilization.

• *Prenatal Phase and Infancy.* The concept of imprinting is typically applied to the attachment of offspring to the mother shortly after birth. To what extent might this concept be applied to teenage lovers in middle adolescence? Discuss the question of readiness. Point out the defects and limitations in this speculation.

• *Childhood and Adolescence.* Is the development of morality primarily a problem in cognitive psychology or social psychology? Pick one side and develop an argument. Then defend the other side of the argument.

• *Adulthood and Old Age.* In which decade of adulthood—the thirties, forties, fifties, or sixties—will you be most gratified with your life? Give specific reasons for your choice and indicate the reasons why you do not choose the other decades.

• *Individual Differences.* Consider the question of individual differences at the various life stages. Are they larger in infancy, childhood, adolescence, middle adulthood, or old age? Defend your answer.

∾ TOPICS OF RELATED INTEREST ∾

Freud's views of sexual development constitute a stage theory (14). The nature–nurture issue reappears in the context of intelligence (13). Individual differences are relevant to discussions of intelligence (13), personality (14), and variability in statistics (18).

9

ANIMAL
REPRODUCTION

*A mother koala with her young reaches for eucalyptus leaves.
Most young mammals require considerable parental care,
feeding, and protection before they are able to face the
world alone.*

The word *reproduction* may bring to mind images of romantic courtship and cute cuddly babies. From an evolutionary perspective, however, romance and the universal appeal of babies are frills that have evolved only because they further the real evolutionary goal: to pass on one's genes to another generation. From this viewpoint, an animal's life can be divided into three stages. First, it is born or hatched from an egg and grows to sexual maturity. Second, it gathers the resources needed to reproduce, which may include stores of food, impressive strength or weaponry, or a territory. Finally, it finds a mate (if necessary) and reproduces, which may include caring for its offspring until they can fend for themselves. The marvelous adaptations that we have discussed in the previous chapters, such as sophisticated sensory equipment or complex digestive systems, have evolved through millennia of mutation and natural selection because they have allowed survival and successful reproduction. Reproduction is the key to the continued existence of the species.

Reproductive Strategies

Animals reproduce either sexually or asexually. As you learned in Chapter 12, in **sexual reproduction** an animal produces haploid gametes through meiosis. Two gametes, usually from separate parents, fuse to form a diploid offspring. Because an offspring receives genes from two parents, it is genetically different from both of them. In most forms of **asexual reproduction,** on the other hand, a single animal produces offspring through repeated mitosis of cells in some part of its body. Therefore, the offspring are genetically identical to the parent.

We humans reproduce sexually, and we tend to regard sexual reproduction as the normal, best way to do it. From a biological standpoint, by bringing together genes from two different parental organisms, sexual reproduction allows for new gene combinations that may enhance the survival and reproduction of the offspring. Nevertheless, asexual reproduction is more efficient, because there is no need to find a mate, court, and fend off rivals, and there is no waste of sperm and eggs that never unite to form an offspring. Not surprisingly, most animals reproduce asexually, at least some of the time.

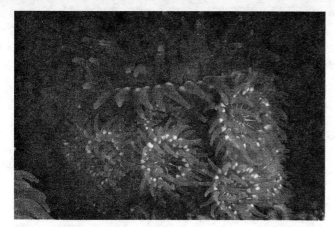

Figure 39-1 Budding

The offspring of some cnidarians, such as the anemone shown here, grow as buds that appear as miniature adults sprouting from the body of the parent. When sufficiently developed, the buds break off and assume independent existence.

Let's begin, then, with a brief survey of asexual reproduction among animals before moving on to sexual reproduction.

Asexual Reproduction Does Not Involve the Fusion of Sperm and Egg

Budding Produces a Miniature Version of the Adult

Many sponges and cnidarians, such as *Hydra* and some anemones, reproduce by **budding** (Fig. 39-1). A miniature version of the animal (a **bud**) grows directly on the body of the adult, drawing nourishment from its parent. When it has grown large enough, the bud breaks off and becomes independent.

Regeneration Produces a New Individual from Parts of Another

Regeneration from body fragments is a potential form of reproduction in some animals such as sea stars (Fig. 39-2a). If sea stars are cut up, fragments that contain part of the center part of the body can regrow the rest of the star. (Oyster "ranchers," attempting to rid their oyster beds of predatory sea stars, used to catch sea stars, hack them to pieces, and throw the parts back into the sea. Much to their dismay, this method merely resulted in more sea stars than ever, as the fragments regenerated entire animals.) A few brittle stars routinely reproduce in a similar fashion; they split apart and each half regenerates a complete animal. Despite these asexual capabilities, sea stars usually reproduce sexually, casting huge numbers of sperm and eggs into the sea.

During Fission, an Animal Divides, Producing Two New Individuals

Some animals reproduce by **fission.** A few corals can divide lengthwise to produce two smaller but complete individuals. Some flatworms and annelids divide across the middle and regenerate the missing parts (Fig. 39-2b). Of course, the "tail half" of the animal must regenerate the head, including the brain!

During Parthenogenesis Eggs Develop without Fertilization

The females of some animal species can reproduce by a process known as **parthenogenesis,** in which haploid egg cells develop into adults without being fertilized. Parthenogenetically produced offspring of some species remain haploid. Male honey bees, for example, are haploid, developing from unfertilized eggs; their diploid sisters develop from fertilized eggs. On the other hand, some fish, amphibians, and reptiles regain the diploid number of chromosomes in parthenogenetically produced offspring by duplicating all the chromosomes either before or after meiosis. The resulting offspring are all females.

Some species of fish, including relatives of the mollies and platies found in tropical fish stores, and some lizards, such as the whiptail, have done away with males completely. Their populations consist entirely of parthenogenetically reproducing females. Still other animals, such as the aphid, can reproduce either sexually or parthenogenetically, depending on environmental factors such as the season of the year or the availability of food (Fig. 39-3).

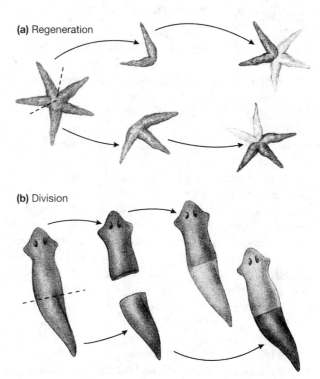

(a) Regeneration

(b) Division

Figure 39-2 Other modes of asexual reproduction

(a) Many sea stars can regenerate new individuals from fragments if the fragment includes part of the center of the body. **(b)** Certain flatworms divide across the middle. At first, each offspring is missing half the adult body, but these are regrown from cells near the broken edge.

Figure 39-3 **A female aphid gives live birth**

In spring and early summer, when food is abundant, aphid females reproduce parthenogenetically. In fact, the development of the reproductive tract proceeds so rapidly that females are born pregnant! In fall, reproduction becomes sexual, as the females mate with males. Aphids have thus evolved the ability to exploit the advantages of asexual reproduction (rapid population growth during times of abundant food, no energy spent in seeking a mate, no wasted gametes) and sexual reproduction (genetic recombination).

Sexual Reproduction Requires the Union of Sperm and Egg

In animals, sexual reproduction occurs when a haploid sperm fertilizes a haploid egg, generating a diploid offspring. In most animal species, an individual is either male or female. These species are termed **dioecious** (Greek for "two houses"). The sexes are defined by the type of gamete that each produces. Females produce **eggs,** which are large, nonmotile cells containing substantial food reserves. Males produce small, motile **sperm** that have almost no cytoplasm and hence no food reserves.

In **monoecious** ("one house") species, such as earthworms and many snails, single individuals produce both sperm and eggs. Such individuals are commonly called **hermaphrodites** (after Hermaphroditos, a male Greek god whose body was merged with that of a female water nymph, producing a being half male and half female). Although most hermaphrodites exchange sperm with other individuals if they have the opportunity (retaining the advantages of genetic exchange), some hermaphrodites can fertilize their eggs with their own sperm if necessary. These animals, including tapeworms and many pond snails, are relatively immobile and may find themselves isolated from other members of their species. Obviously, the ability to fertilize oneself is advantageous under these circumstances.

For dioecious species and for hermaphrodites that cannot self-fertilize, successful reproduction requires that sperm and eggs from different animals be brought together for fertilization. The union of sperm and egg is accomplished in a variety of ways, depending on the mobility of the animals and on whether they breed in water or on land.

External Fertilization Occurs outside the Parent Bodies

In **external fertilization,** the union of the sperm and egg takes place outside the bodies of both parents. Usually, parents release sperm and eggs into water, through which the sperm swim to reach an egg. This procedure, called **spawning,** obviously is restricted to animals that breed in water. Because sperm and egg are relatively short lived, spawning animals must synchronize their reproductive behaviors, both *temporally* (male and female spawn at the same time) and *spatially* (male and female spawn in the same place). Animals employ a combination of environmental cues, chemical signals called pheromones, and behaviors to synchronize spawning.

Most spawning animals rely on environmental cues to some extent. Breeding usually occurs only during certain seasons of the year, but more precise synchrony is required to coordinate the actual release of sperm and egg. Grunion, fish that inhabit coastal waters off southern California, time their unusual reproductive rituals by the season, time of day, and phase of the moon (Fig. 39-4a). On fall nights during the highest tides (which occur during a full moon), grunion swim up onto sandy beaches. Writhing masses of males and females release their gametes into the wet sand and then swim back out to sea on the next wave. Many corals of Australia's Great Barrier Reef also synchronize spawning by the phase of the moon. On the fourth or fifth night after the full moons of November and December, all the corals of a particular species on an entire reef release a blizzard of sperm and eggs into the water (Fig. 39-4b).

Other animals communicate their sexual readiness to one another by releasing pheromones into the water. A **pheromone** is a chemical released from the body of one animal that affects the behavior of a second animal. Pheromones synchronize spawning of many immobile or sluggish invertebrates, such as mussels and sea stars. Usually, when a female is ready to spawn, she releases eggs and a pheromone into the water. Nearby males, detecting the mating pheromone, quickly release millions of sperm. The sperm themselves are lured by a chemical attractant released by the eggs in some, if not most, animals. Such "egg pheromones," which have been detected in animals as diverse as sea stars and humans, help ensure fertilization.

Synchronized timing alone does not guarantee efficient reproduction. Corals, sea stars, and mussels all waste enormous quantities of sperm and eggs because they are released too far apart. In species of mobile animals both temporal *and* spatial synchrony can be ensured by mating behaviors. Most fish, for example, have some sort of courtship ritual in which the male and female come very close together and release their gametes in the same place and at the same time (Fig. 39-5). Frogs carry this ritual one step further, by assuming a characteristic mating pose called **amplexus** (Fig. 39-6). At the edges of ponds and lakes, the male frog mounts the female and prods her in the side. This prod-

(a)

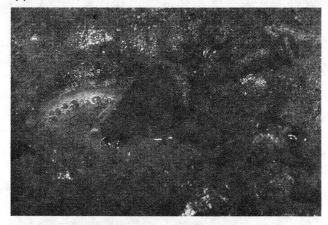

(b)

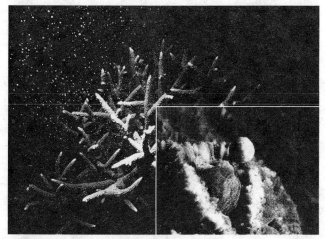

Figure 39-4 **Environmental cues may synchronize spawning**

(a) At the highest tides of fall, grunion swarm ashore on the few undeveloped beaches left in southern California. The fish burrow slightly into the sand and release sperm and eggs. The eggs hatch in the warm sand and develop over the following 2 weeks. When the next-highest tide comes, the young fish wash out of the sand back into the ocean. (b) Along the Great Barrier Reef of Australia, thousands of corals spawn simultaneously, creating this "blizzard" effect. The inset photo shows a package of sperm and eggs erupting from a spawning hermaphroditic coral. Spawning in these corals is linked to the phase of the moon.

ding stimulates her to release eggs, which he immediately fertilizes by releasing a cloud of sperm above them.

Internal Fertilization Occurs within the Female Body

In **internal fertilization,** sperm are taken into the body of the female, where fertilization occurs. This method has two advantages over external fertilization, especially in terrestrial environments. First, sperm require a direct fluid path to reach the eggs, which, on land, can be guaranteed only inside the body of the female. Second, even in aquatic environments, internal fertilization increases the likelihood that most eggs will be fertilized, because the sperm are confined in a small space with the eggs, rather than being left to thrash about in a large volume of water.

Internal fertilization usually occurs by **copulation,** in which the penis of the male is inserted into the body of the female, where it releases sperm (Fig. 39-7). In a variation of internal fertilization, males of some species package their sperm in a container called a **spermatophore** (Greek for "sperm carrier"). Males of some species of mites and scorpions simply drop the spermatophore on the ground. If a female finds the spermatophore, she fertilizes herself by inserting it into her reproductive cavity. The male squid picks up his spermatophore with a tentacle and inserts it into the female. In both cases, the sperm are then liberated inside the female's reproductive tract.

Simply depositing sperm into the body of the female does not guarantee fertilization. Fertilization can occur only if an egg is mature and released into the female reproductive tract during the limited time when sperm are present. Most mammals copulate only at certain seasons of the year or when the female signals readiness to mate. The season or signal often coincides with **ovulation,** or release of the egg cell from the ovary. Copulation itself triggers ovulation in a few animals, such as rabbits. An alternative strategy, employed by many female snails and

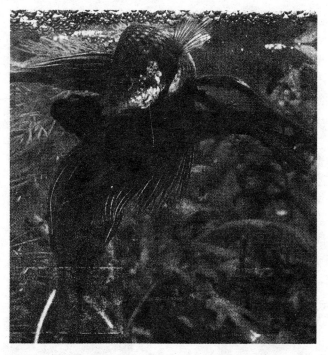

Figure 39-5 **Courtship rituals synchronize release of sperm and eggs**

Violent courtship rituals among Siamese fighting fish (*Betta splendens*) ensure fertilization of the female's eggs, as male and female curl about one another, releasing sperm and eggs together. The male retrieves the eggs as they fall, spits them into his bubble nest (seen here as bubbles floating on the surface above him), and cares for the offspring during their first few weeks of life.

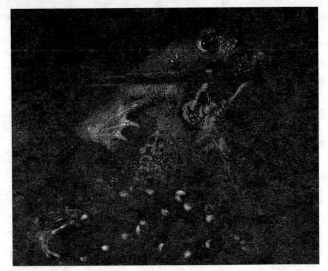

Figure 39-6 Golden toads in amplexus
The smaller male rides atop the female and stimulates her to release eggs. Because the large eggs of frogs and toads are surrounded by a transparent coat of jelly, they are ideal subjects for observing and studying embryonic development.

insects, is to store sperm for days, weeks, or even months, thus assuring a supply of sperm whenever eggs are ready.

Mammalian Reproduction

Male and female sexes of mammals are separate. Mammals reproduce sexually, uniting sperm and eggs through internal fertilization. Many mammals reproduce only during certain seasons of the year and consequently produce sperm and eggs only at that time. Human reproduction is similar to that of other mammals, but it is not restricted by season. Men produce sperm more or less continuously, and women ovulate about once a month. Our discussion will focus on human reproduction.

The Male Reproductive Tract Includes the Testes and Accessory Structures

The male reproductive tract consists of the paired **gonads** (organs that produce sex cells), the **testes** (singular, **testis**) where sperm are produced, and accessory structures that store the sperm, produce secretions that activate and nourish them, and finally conduct them to the inside of the female reproductive tract (Fig. 39-8 and Table 39-1).

The Testes Are the Site of Sperm Production

The testes produce both sperm and male sex hormones. The testes are located in the **scrotum,** a pouch that hangs outside the main body cavity. This location keeps the testes about 4° C cooler than the core of the body and provides the optimal temperature for sperm development. (Tight jeans may look sexy, but they push the scrotum up against the

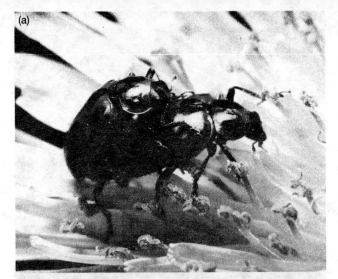

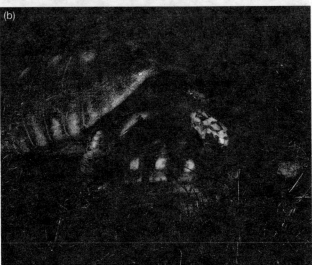

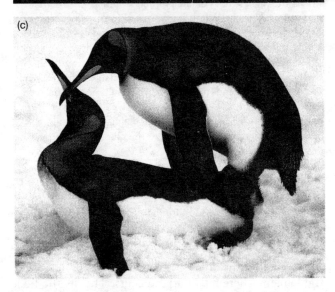

Figure 39-7 Internal fertilization is essential for reproduction on land

(a) Ladybugs mate on a dandelion flower. (b) South American tortoises must cope with confining shells. (c) King penguins mate comfortably in the snow.

294

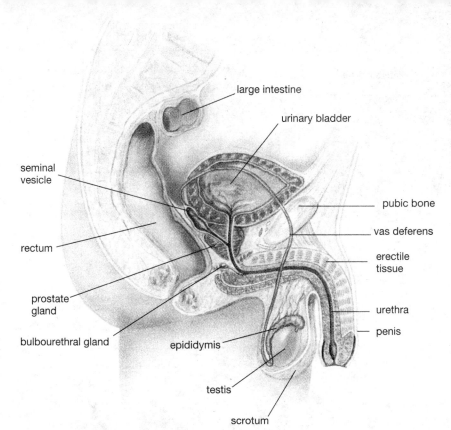

Figure 39-8 **The human male reproductive tract**

The male gonads, the testes, hang beneath the abdominal cavity in the scrotum. Sperm pass from the seminiferous tubules of a testis to the epididymis, and from there through the vas deferens and urethra to the tip of the penis. Along the way, fluids are added from three sets of glands: the seminal vesicles, the bulbourethral glands, and the prostate gland.

TABLE 39-1 ❖ *Structures and Functions of the Human Male Reproductive Tract*

Structure	Type of Organ	Function
Testis	Gonad	Produces sperm and testosterone
Epididymis and vas deferens	Ducts	Store sperm; conduct sperm from testes to penis
Urethra	Duct	Conducts semen from vas deferens and urine from urinary bladder to the tip of the penis
Penis	External "appendage"	Deposits sperm in female reproductive tract
Seminal vesicles	Glands	Secrete fluids that contain fructose (energy source) and prostaglandins (possibly cause "upward" contractions of vagina, uterus, and oviducts, assisting sperm transport to oviducts); fluids may wash sperm out of ducts of male reproductive tract into vagina
Prostate	Gland	Secretes fluids that are basic (neutralize acidity of vagina) and contain factors that enhance sperm motility
Bulbourethral glands	Glands	Secrete mucus (may lubricate penis in vagina)

body, raising the temperature of the testes. Some researchers think that wearing tight pants may reduce sperm counts and decrease fertility. This is not, however, a reliable means of birth control!) Coiled, hollow **seminiferous tubules,** in which sperm are produced, nearly fill each testis (Fig. 39-9a). In the spaces between the tubules are the **interstitial cells,** which synthesize the male hormone testosterone.

Just inside the wall of each seminiferous tubule lie the diploid cells, or **spermatogonia** (singular, **spermatogoni-**

um), from which all the sperm eventually will arise, and the much larger **Sertoli cells** (Fig. 39-9b, c). Each time a spermatogonium divides, it can take one of two developmental paths. First, it may undergo mitosis. Mitosis ensures that the male has a steady supply of new spermatogonia throughout his life. Second, it may undergo **spermatogenesis**—that is, the production of sperm by the process of meiosis followed by differentiation (Fig. 39-9d). Spermatogenesis begins with growth and differentiation

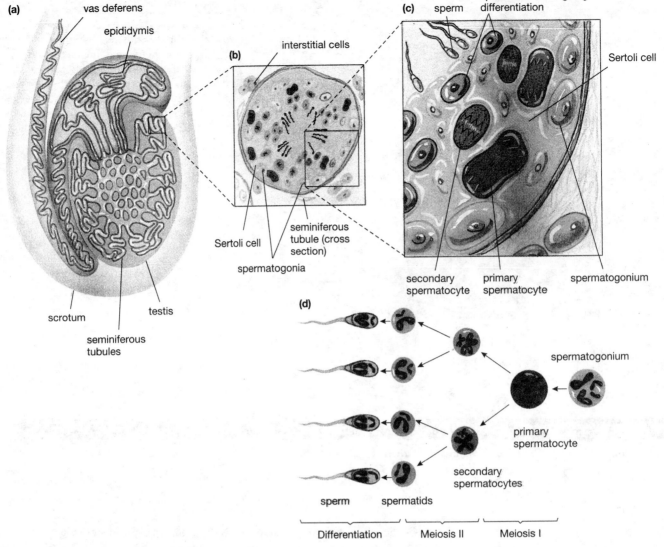

(a)
vas deferens
epididymis
interstitial cells
(b)
scrotum
testis
seminiferous tubules
Sertoli cell
seminiferous tubule (cross section)
spermatogonia

(c) sperm
spermatids undergoing differentiation
Sertoli cell
secondary spermatocyte
primary spermatocyte
spermatogonium

(d)
spermatogonium
primary spermatocyte
secondary spermatocytes
sperm
spermatids
Differentiation
Meiosis II
Meiosis I

Figure 39-9   **The development of sperm cells**

(a) A lengthwise section of the testis, showing the location of the seminiferous tubules, epididymis, and vas deferens. (b) A cross section of a seminiferous tubule. The walls of the seminiferous tubules are lined with Sertoli cells and spermatogonia protruding into the central cavity (lumen) of the tubule. (c) As spermatogonia undergo meiosis, the daughter cells move inward, embedded in infoldings of the Sertoli cells. There they differentiate into sperm, drawing upon the Sertoli cells for nourishment. Mature sperm are finally freed into the lumen of the tubules for transport to the penis. Testosterone is produced by the interstitial cells found in the spaces between tubules. (d) Spermatogenesis is accomplished by meiotic divisions that produce haploid sperm (compare with the actual locations shown in part [c]). Although four chromosomes are shown for clarity, in humans the diploid number is 46 and the haploid number is 23.

of spermatogonia into **primary spermatocytes.** These are large diploid cells that will develop into sperm. The primary spermatocytes then undergo meiosis (see Chapter 12). At the end of meiosis I, each primary spermatocyte gives rise to two haploid **secondary spermatocytes.** Each secondary spermatocyte divides again during meiosis II to produce two **spermatids,** for a total of four spermatids per primary spermatocyte. Spermatids undergo radical rearrangements of their cellular components as they differentiate into sperm.

Sertoli cells regulate the process of spermatogenesis and nourish the developing sperm. The spermatogonia, spermatocytes, and spermatids are embedded in infoldings of the Sertoli cells. As spermatogenesis proceeds, they migrate up from the outermost edge of the seminiferous tubule to the central cavity of the tubule (Fig. 39-9c). The mature sperm, several hundred million a day, are finally liberated into the lumen.

A human sperm (Fig. 39-10) is unlike any other cell of the body. Most of the cytoplasm disappears, leaving a hap-

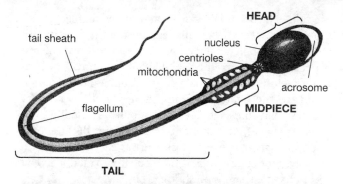

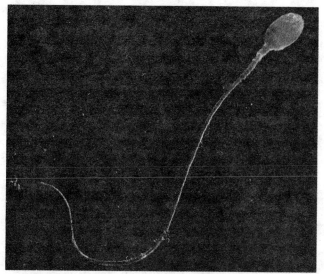

Figure 39-10   A human sperm cell

A mature sperm is a stripped-down cell equipped with only the essentials: a haploid nucleus containing the male genetic contribution to the future zygote, a lysosome (called the acrosome) containing enzymes that will digest the barriers surrounding the egg, mitochondria for energy production, and a tail (actually a long flagellum) for locomotion. The photo is a false-color electron micrograph of a human sperm.

loid nucleus nearly filling the head. Atop the nucleus lies a specialized lysosome, called the **acrosome.** The acrosome contains enzymes that will be needed to dissolve protective layers around the egg, enabling the sperm to enter and fertilize it. Behind the head is the midpiece, which is packed with mitochondria that provide the energy needed to move the tail that protrudes out the back. Whiplike movements of the tail, which is really a long flagellum, propel the sperm along inside the female reproductive tract.

At puberty, the time of rapid growth and sexual maturation, the hypothalamus releases **gonadotropin-releasing hormone (GnRH),** which stimulates the anterior pituitary to produce **luteinizing hormone (LH)** and **follicle-stimulating hormone (FSH).** Spermatogenesis begins as a result of the interplay of LH and FSH and **testosterone** secreted by the testes (Fig. 39-11). Luteinizing hormone stimulates the interstitial cells to produce testosterone. The combination of testosterone and FSH stimulates the Sertoli cells and spermatogonia, causing spermatogenesis.

Testosterone also stimulates the development of secondary sexual characteristics (such as the growth of facial hair in males and breast development in females), maintains sexual drive, and is required for successful intercourse (a term we will use for human copulation). Sperm, however, are not involved in these functions. Therefore, if one could suppress FSH release (blocking spermatogenesis) but not LH release (thereby allowing continued testosterone production), a man would be infertile but not impotent. Efforts are under way to develop a drug to do just that, as a form of male birth control.

Accessory Structures Produce Semen and Conduct the Sperm outside the Body

The seminiferous tubules merge to form a single convoluted tube, the **epididymis** (see Fig. 39-9). The epididymis becomes the **vas deferens,** which leaves the scrotum and enters the abdominal cavity. Most of the hundreds of millions of sperm produced each day are stored in the vas deferens and epididymis. The vas deferens joins the **urethra,** leading from the bladder to the tip of the penis. This final common path is shared, at different times, of course, by sperm (during ejaculation) and urine (during urination).

The fluid ejaculated from the penis, called **semen,** consists of sperm mixed with secretions from three glands that empty into the vas deferens or urethra: the **seminal vesicles,**

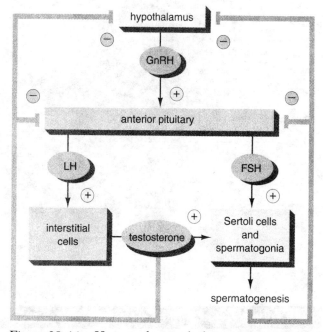

Figure 39-11   Hormonal control of spermatogenesis

Gonadotropin-releasing hormone (GnRH) from the hypothalamus stimulates the anterior pituitary to release LH and FSH. LH stimulates the interstitial cells to produce testosterone. Testosterone and FSH stimulate the Sertoli cells and the spermatogonia, causing spermatogenesis. Testosterone and chemicals produced during spermatogenesis inhibit further release of FSH and LH, forming a negative feedback loop that keeps the rate of spermatogenesis and the concentration of testosterone in the blood nearly constant. + stimulates; − inhibits.

the **prostate gland,** and the **bulbourethral glands.** The secretions activate swimming by the sperm, provide energy for swimming, and neutralize the acidic fluids of the vagina that normally inhibit bacterial growth (see Table 39-1).

The Female Reproductive Tract Includes Ovaries and Accessory Structures

The female reproductive tract is almost entirely contained within the abdominal cavity (Fig. 39-12 and Table 39-2). It consists of paired gonads, the **ovaries** (Fig. 39-13a), and accessory structures that accept sperm, conduct the sperm to the egg, and nourish the developing embryo.

The Ovaries Are the Site of Egg Production

The human female produces precursor egg cells, or **oogonia** (singular, **oogonium**), while still a fetus in her mother's womb, beginning the process of **oogenesis,** the formation of egg cells. The oogonia divide by mitosis and then grow into **primary oocytes.** No oogonia remain after the third month of fetal development, and no new ones form during the rest of her life. Still during the fetal stage, all the primary oocytes begin meiosis but then halt during prophase of meiosis I. At birth, the ovaries contain about 2 million primary oocytes; many die each day, until at puberty (usually 11 to 14 years of age) only about 400,000 remain. Because only a few oocytes resume meiosis during each month of a woman's reproductive span (from puberty to menopause at age 45 to 55), there is no shortage of oocytes.

Surrounding each oocyte is a layer of much smaller cells that both nourish the developing oocyte and secrete female sex hormones. Together, the oocyte and these accessory cells make up a **follicle** (Fig. 39-13b). Approximately once a month during a woman's reproductive years, she undergoes a menstrual cycle, which is described below. During the menstrual cycle, pituitary hormones stimulate

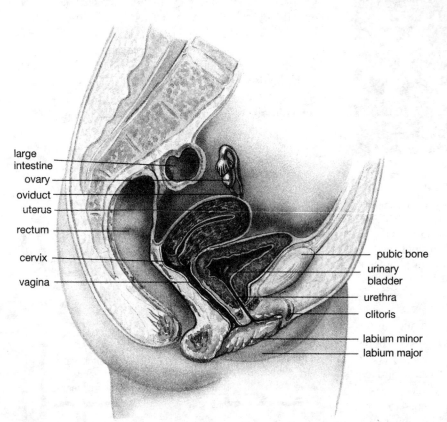

Figure 39-12 **The human female reproductive tract**

Eggs are produced in the ovaries and swept by cilia into the oviduct. A male deposits sperm in the vagina, from which they move up through the cervix and uterus into the oviduct. Sperm and egg usually meet in the oviduct, where fertilization occurs. The fertilized egg attaches to the lining of the uterus, where the embryo develops.

TABLE 39-2 ⁚⁚ *Structures and Functions of the Human Female Reproductive Tract*

Structure	Type of Organ	Function
Ovary	Gonad	Produces eggs, estrogen, and progesterone
Fimbria	Mouth of duct	Cilia sweep egg into oviduct
Oviduct	Duct	Conducts egg to uterus; site of fertilization
Uterus	Muscular chamber	Site of development of fetus
Cervix	Connective tissue ring	Closes off lower end of uterus, supports fetus, and prevents foreign material from entering uterus
Vagina	Large "duct"	Receptacle for semen; birth canal

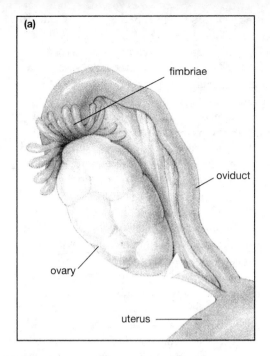

(a)

fimbriae

oviduct

ovary

uterus

(b)

ruptured
follicle

corpus luteum

degenerating
corpus luteum

④ ovulated
secondary
oocyte
(egg)

ovary

③ mature
follicle
with
secondary
oocyte

②

developing
follicles

① primary follicle
containing primary
oocyte

(c)

egg

polar body

polar body

polar body

polar body

secondary
oocyte (egg)

primary
oocyte

oogonium

polar body

Meiosis II
(after fertilization)

Meiosis I

Figure 39-13 Oogenesis in the human female

(a) External view of the ovary and oviduct. **(b)** The development of follicles in an ovary, portrayed in a time sequence going clockwise from the lower right. ① A primary oocyte begins development within a follicle. ②, ③ The follicle grows, providing both hormones and nourishment for the enlarging oocyte. ④ At ovulation, the secondary oocyte, or egg, bursts through the ovary wall, surrounded by some follicle cells (now called the corona radiata). The remaining follicle cells develop into the corpus luteum, which secretes hormones. If fertilization does not occur, the corpus luteum breaks down after a few days. **(c)** The cellular stages of oogenesis. The oogonium enlarges to form the primary oocyte. At meiosis I, almost all the cytoplasm is included in one daughter cell, the secondary oocyte. The other daughter cell is a small polar body that contains chromosomes but little cytoplasm. At meiosis II, almost all the cytoplasm of the secondary oocyte is included in the egg, and a second small polar body discards the remaining "extra" chromosomes. The first polar body sometimes also undergoes the second meiotic division. In humans, meiosis II does not occur unless the egg is fertilized.

development of a dozen or more follicles, although usually only one completely matures. At this time, the primary oocyte completes the first meiotic division (which was halted during development) to become a single **secondary oocyte** and a **polar body,** which is little more than a discarded set of chromosomes (Fig. 39-13c). Meanwhile, the

small accessory cells of the follicle multiply and secrete **estrogen.** As it matures, the follicle grows, eventually erupting through the surface of the ovary and releasing the secondary oocyte (Fig. 39-14). The second meiotic division occurs, not in the ovary, but in the oviduct (the tube leading out of the ovary), and then only if the sec-

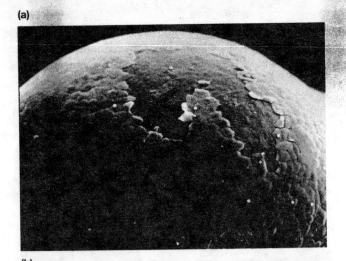

(a)

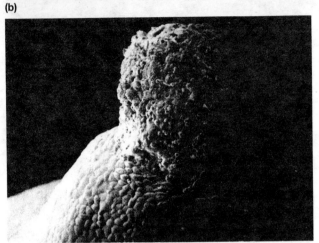

(b)

Figure 39-14 **A follicle erupts from the ovary**

The mature follicle grows so large, and is filled with so much fluid that it moves to the surface of the ovary **(a)** and literally bursts through the ovary wall like a miniature volcano **(b)**. It then releases the secondary oocyte into the oviduct.

ondary oocyte is fertilized. For convenience, we will refer to the ovulated secondary oocyte as the "egg."

Some of the follicle cells accompany the egg, but most remain behind in the ovary. These cells enlarge and become glandular, forming the **corpus luteum,** which secretes both estrogen and a second hormone, **progesterone.** If fertilization does not occur, the corpus luteum breaks down a few days later.

Accessory Structures Include the Oviducts, Uterus, and Vagina

Each ovary is adjacent to, but not continuous with, an **oviduct** (sometimes called the **fallopian tube** in humans; see Fig. 39-13a). The open end of the oviduct is fringed with ciliated "fingers" called **fimbriae** that nearly surround the ovary. The cilia create a current that sweeps the egg into the mouth of the oviduct. Fertilization usually occurs in the oviduct, and the **zygote,** as the fertilized egg is now called, is swept down the oviduct by beating cilia and released into the pear-shaped **uterus,** or womb. Here it will develop for the next 9 months. The wall of the uterus has two layers that correspond to its dual functions of nourishment and childbirth. The inner lining, or **endometrium,** is richly supplied with blood vessels. (This lining will form the mother's contribution to the **placenta,** the structure that transfers oxygen, carbon dioxide, nutrients, and wastes between fetus and mother; see Chapter 40.) The outer muscular wall of the uterus, the **myometrium,** contracts strongly during delivery, expelling the infant out into the world.

Developing follicles secrete estrogen, which stimulates the uterine lining to grow an extensive network of blood vessels and nutrient-producing glands. After ovulation, estrogen and progesterone released by the corpus luteum promote continued growth of the endometrium. Thus, if an egg is fertilized, it encounters a rich environment for growth. If the egg is not fertilized, however, the corpus luteum disintegrates, estrogen and progesterone levels fall, and the overgrown endometrium disintegrates as well. The uterus contracts, squeezing out the excess endometrial tissue (and sometimes causing menstrual cramps in the process). The resulting flow of tissue and blood is called **menstruation** (from the Latin *mensis*, meaning "month").

The outer end of the uterus is nearly closed off by a ring of connective tissue, the **cervix.** The cervix holds the developing baby in the uterus, expanding only at the onset of labor to permit passage of the child. Beyond the cervix lies the **vagina,** which opens to the outside of the body. The vagina serves both as the receptacle for the penis during intercourse and as the birth canal.

The Menstrual Cycle Is Controlled by Complex Hormonal Interactions

The human male produces sperm continuously, thereby increasing the number of potential offspring that a man can father. In contrast, it is fruitless for a woman to ovulate unless her reproductive tract is properly prepared for pregnancy. The human female reproductive system goes through a complex **menstrual cycle,** in which hormonal interactions among the hypothalamus, pituitary gland, and ovary coordinate ovulation with the preparation of the uterus to receive and nourish the fertilized egg.

You may recall from Chapter 35 that hormone release by the anterior pituitary gland is controlled by neurosecretory cells in the hypothalamus. Some of these neurosecretory cells produce gonadotropin-releasing hormone (GnRH), which stimulates endocrine cells in the anterior pituitary to release FSH and LH. A key to understanding the menstrual cycle is that these neurosecretory cells spontaneously release GnRH all the time, unless actively prevented from doing so by other hormones, notably progesterone. We will begin our discussion of the menstrual cycle with the spontaneous release of GnRH.

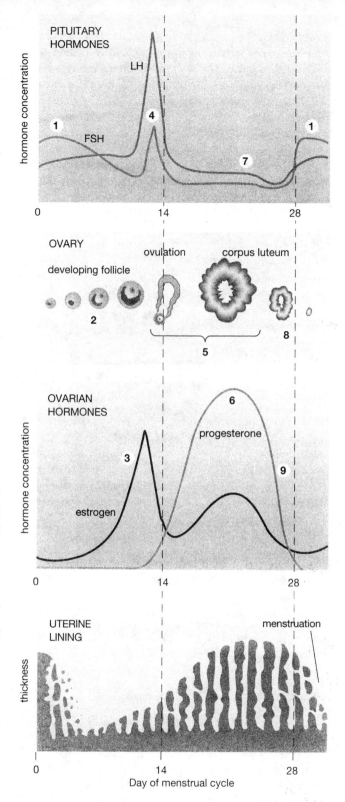

PITUITARY HORMONES

hormone concentration

1 LH 4 FSH 7 1

0   14   28

OVARY

ovulation   corpus luteum

developing follicle

2   5   8

OVARIAN HORMONES

hormone concentration

6

progesterone

3   9

estrogen

0   14   28

UTERINE LINING

menstruation

thickness

0   14   28

Day of menstrual cycle

Figure 39-15   **Hormonal control of the menstrual cycle**

The menstrual cycle is generated by interactions among the hormones of the hypothalamus, anterior pituitary gland, and ovaries. The hormonal changes in turn drive cyclic changes in the uterine lining. The numbers on the graphs refer to the hormonal interactions discussed in the text. They zigzag back and forth among pituitary hormones, ovarian structures, and ovarian hormones, as each of these exerts effects on the others.

Gonadotropin-releasing hormone stimulates the anterior pituitary to release FSH and LH (step 1 in Fig. 39-15). FSH and LH circulate in the bloodstream and initiate the development of several follicles within the ovaries. The follicle cells surrounding the developing oocyte are stimulated by FSH and LH to secrete estrogen. Under the combined influences of FSH, LH, and estrogen, the follicles grow during the next two weeks (step 2). Simultaneously, the primary oocyte within each follicle enlarges, storing both food and regulatory substances (mostly proteins and messenger RNA) that will be needed by the fertilized egg during early development (see Chapter 40). For reasons that are not completely understood, only one, or rarely two, follicles complete development each month.

As the maturing follicle enlarges, it secretes ever greater amounts of estrogen (step 3). This estrogen has three effects. First, it promotes the continued development of the follicle itself and the primary oocyte contained within it. Second, it stimulates growth of the endometrium of the uterus. Third, high levels of estrogen stimulate both the hypothalamus and pituitary, resulting in a surge of LH and FSH at about the twelfth day of the cycle (step 4).

The function of the peak in FSH concentration is still a subject of investigation, but the surge of LH has three important consequences: (1) It triggers the resumption of meiosis I in the oocyte, resulting in the formation of the secondary oocyte and the first polar body; (2) it causes the final explosive growth of the follicle, culminating in ovulation (step 5); and (3) it transforms the remnants of the follicle that remain in the ovary into the corpus luteum.

The corpus luteum secretes both estrogen and progesterone (step 6). The combination of these hormones inhibits the hypothalamus and pituitary, shutting down the release of FSH and LH (step 7), thereby preventing the development of any more follicles. Simultaneously, estrogen and progesterone stimulate further growth of the endometrium, which eventually becomes about 5 millimeters thick. (Note that the effects of progesterone and estrogen depend on the target organ. Progesterone *stimulates* the endometrium but *inhibits* hormone release from the hypothalamus and pituitary.)

In menstrual cycles in which pregnancy does not occur, the corpus luteum disintegrates about 1 week after ovulation. The corpus luteum survives only while it is stimulated by LH (or by a similar hormone released by the developing embryo, described below). However, because progesterone secreted by the corpus luteum shuts off the LH secretion that sustained it, the corpus luteum essentially "self-destructs" around the twenty-first day of the cycle (step 8). With the corpus luteum gone, estrogen and progesterone levels plummet (step 9). Deprived of stimulation by estrogen and progesterone, the endometrium of the uterus also dies, and its blood and tissue are shed, forming the menstrual flow beginning about the twenty-seventh or twenty-eighth day of the cycle. Simultaneously, the reduced progesterone level no longer inhibits the hypothalamus and pituitary, and the spontaneous release of

GnRH from the hypothalamus resumes. Release of GnRH in turn stimulates release of FSH and LH (step 1), which initiates development of a new set of follicles, starting the cycle over again.

During pregnancy, the embryo itself prevents these changes from occurring. Shortly after the ball of cells formed by the dividing fertilized egg embed themselves in the endometrium, they start secreting an LH-like hormone called **chorionic gonadotropin (CG)**. This hormone travels in the bloodstream to the ovary, where it prevents breakdown of the corpus luteum. The corpus luteum continues to secrete estrogen and progesterone, and the uterine lining continues to grow, nourishing the embryo. So much CG is released by the embryo that it is excreted by the mother in her urine; in fact, most pregnancy tests use the presence of CG in a woman's urine to determine pregnancy.

Although negative feedback regulates the levels of most hormones, the hormones of the menstrual cycle are regulated by both positive and negative feedback. During the first half of the cycle, FSH and LH stimulate estrogen production by the follicles. High levels of estrogen then *stimulate* the midcycle surge of FSH and LH release (positive feedback). During the second half of the cycle, estrogen and progesterone together *inhibit* the release of FSH and LH (negative feedback). The early positive feedback causes hormone concentrations to reach high levels, and the later negative feedback shuts the system down again unless pregnancy intervenes.

Copulation Allows Internal Fertilization

As terrestrial mammals, humans use internal fertilization to deposit the sperm in the moist environment of the female reproductive tract. To do this, the penis is inserted into the vagina, where sperm are released during ejaculation. The sperm swim upward in the female reproductive tract, from the vagina through the opening of the cervix into the uterus, and on up into the oviducts. If the female has ovulated within the past day or so, the sperm will meet an egg in one of the oviducts. Only one sperm can succeed in fertilizing it, starting the development of a new human being.

During Copulation, Sperm Are Deposited inside the Female Vagina

The male role in copulation begins with erection of the penis. Before erection, the penis is relaxed (flaccid), because the arterioles supplying it are constricted, allowing little blood flow (Fig. 39-16a). Under the dual influences of psychological and physical stimulation, the arterioles dilate and blood flows into spaces in the tissue within the penis. As these tissues swell, they squeeze off the veins that drain the penis (Fig. 39-16b). Pressure builds up, causing an erection. After the penis is inserted into the vagina, movements further stimulate touch receptors on the penis, triggering ejaculation. Ejaculation occurs when muscles en-

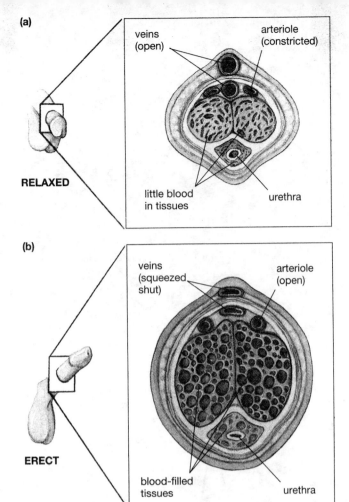

Figure 39-16   Changes in blood flow within the penis cause erection

(a) Normally, smooth muscles encircling the arterioles leading into the penis are contracted, limiting blood flow. (b) During sexual excitement, these muscles relax, and blood flows into spaces within the penis. The swelling penis squeezes off the veins leaving the penis, thereby increasing the pressure produced by fluids within the penis and causing it to become elongated and firm.

circling the epididymis, vas deferens, and urethra contract, forcing semen out of the penis and into the vagina. On average, 3 or 4 milliliters of semen, containing 300 to 400 million sperm, is ejaculated. Male orgasm causes both ejaculation and a feeling of intense pleasure and release.

Similar changes occur in the female. Sexual excitement causes increased blood flow to the vagina and external parts of the reproductive tract, including the labia and clitoris (see Fig. 39-12). The clitoris, which is derived from the same embryological tissue as the penis, becomes erect. Stimulation by the penis of the male often, but not always, results in female orgasm, a series of rhythmic contractions of the vagina and uterus accompanied by sensations of pleasure and release. Female orgasm is not necessary for fertilization.

The intimate contact involved in copulation creates a situation where disease organisms can readily be transmitted. Since the "sexual revolution," which began in the 1960s, many people have had multiple sexual partners, and the incidence of sexually transmitted diseases has greatly increased (see "Health Watch: Sexually Transmitted Diseases").

During Fertilization, the Sperm and Egg Nuclei Unite

Neither sperm nor egg lives very long. An egg may remain viable for a day, and sperm, under ideal conditions, may live for two. Therefore, fertilization can succeed only if copulation occurs within a couple of days before or after ovulation. You will recall that the egg leaves the ovary surrounded by follicle cells (Fig. 39-17a). These cells, now called the **corona radiata,** form a barrier between the sperm and the egg. A second barrier, the jellylike **zona pellucida** ("clear area"), lies between the corona radiata and the egg. Recent research suggests that the human egg releases a chemical attractant that lures the sperm toward it.

In the oviduct, hundreds of sperm reach the egg and encircle the corona radiata, each sperm releasing enzymes from its acrosome (Fig. 39-17b). These enzymes weaken both the corona radiata and the zona pellucida, allowing the sperm to wriggle through to the egg. If there aren't enough sperm, not enough enzymes are released, and none of the sperm will reach the egg. This may be the selective pressure for the ejaculation of so many sperm. Perhaps 1 in 100,000 reach the oviduct, and 1 in 20 of those find the egg, so only a few hundred of the 300 million sperm that were ejaculated join the attack on the barriers surrounding the egg.

When the first sperm finally contacts the surface of the egg, the cell membranes of egg and sperm fuse, and the sperm head is drawn into the cytoplasm of the egg. As the sperm enters, it triggers two vital changes in the egg. First, vesicles near the surface of the egg release chemicals into the zona pellucida, reinforcing it and preventing further sperm from entering the egg. Second, the egg undergoes its second meiotic division, producing a haploid gamete at last. Fertilization occurs as the haploid nuclei of sperm and egg fuse, forming a diploid nucleus that contains all the genes of a new human being.

Human males who have fewer than 20 million sperm per milliliter of semen (about one-fifth the normal amount) usually cannot fertilize a woman during intercourse because too few sperm reach the egg. If the sperm are otherwise normal, such men can father children by artificial insemination, in which a large quantity of their semen is injected directly into the oviduct. In other cases, a blocked oviduct may prevent sperm from reaching the egg. Today, some couples seek high-technology help in the form of *in vitro* fertilization (see "Scientific Inquiry: *In Vitro* Fertilization").

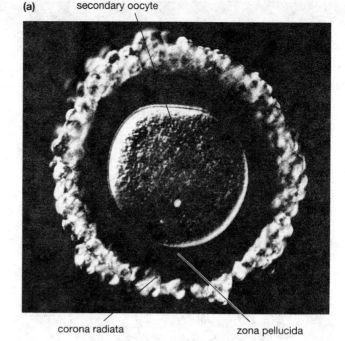

Figure 39-17 **The secondary oocyte and fertilization**

(a) A human secondary oocyte shortly after ovulation. Sperm must digest their way through the small follicular cells of the corona radiata and the clear zona pellucida to reach the oocyte itself. (b) Sperm surround the oocyte, attacking its defensive barriers.

During Pregnancy, the Developing Embryo Grows within the Uterus

The zygote begins to divide while being carried by cilia down the oviduct to the uterus, a process that takes about 4 days (Fig. 39-18). By about 1 week after fertilization, the zygote has developed into a hollow ball of cells, the **blastocyst** (Fig. 39-18b). A thickened region of the blasto-

In Vitro Fertilization

Louise Brown, the first "test-tube baby," was born in England in 1978. Since that well-publicized event, more than 200 centers for *in vitro* fertilization (IVF) have been established in the United States; these have produced over 26,000 healthy babies. The demand for IVF is fueled by an epidemic of infertility. Twenty years ago one out of every six American couples was unable to conceive after trying for 1 year or more; that rate has now tripled. One reason for the increase in infertility is that modern couples often delay childbearing, and fertility declines with age. A second reason is a higher incidence of sexually transmitted diseases such as chlamydia and gonorrhea that can scar and block the oviducts or sperm ducts. Both blocked ducts and low sperm counts can be overcome with IVF, because oocytes are removed directly from the ovaries, and their meeting with sperm is guaranteed within the confines of a small glass dish (*in vitro* means "in glass" in Latin). The popularity of IVF, which costs around $6000 per attempt, is a testimony to the strong biological drive to have children. With an average success rate of 14%, a typical conception via IVF costs over $40,000.

Although the technique is simple in concept, the procedure is complex and delicate. First, the woman is given daily injections of drugs or hormones or both to stimulate multiple ovulation. Using blood tests and ultrasound imaging of the ovaries, doctors determine when the time is ripe for ovulation. Then the woman is injected with human chorionic gonadotropin, which begins the process of expelling the oocytes from the follicles. Just before the oocytes are ejected, surgeons insert a thin fiber-optic viewing device through a small abdominal incision to locate the mature follicles. Next, they insert a long, hollow needle into each ripe follicle and suck out the follicular cells and fluid, which are examined under a microscope. With luck, an oocyte is present (Fig. E39-1). Usually, at least four oocytes are harvested and incubated in a glass dish to which freshly collected sperm are then added. In 48 hours, about two-thirds of the oocytes will have been fertilized and have reached the eight-cell stage. A few of these early embryos (usually two to four) are sucked into a tube and expelled very gently into the uterus. Transplanting multiple embryos increases the success rate for implantation, but at the same time it increases the probability for multiple births, which carry considerably higher risks than single births.

Recently, IVF has become a weapon in the fight to save endangered species. The National Zoo in Washington, D.C., has been working since 1984 to adapt IVF technology to help endangered species reproduce. They have developed a mobile IVF laboratory that can travel to zoos where endangered species are housed. A tremendous advantage of IVF is that it will allow sperm from a male of an endangered species to be transported between continents, if necessary, to fertilize an appropriate female. This method eliminates the danger and trauma of transporting the animals themselves. IVF also overcomes the very real probability that, once together, the animals will refuse to mate. In April 1990, the first "test-tube tiger" was born (Fig. E39-2). Only 200 individuals of this rare Siberian subspecies remain in the wild. Use of IVF increases the chances that we may save this and other precious forms of life on Earth.

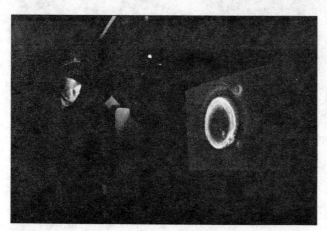

Figure E39-1 Examining the harvested egg
The microscopic egg cell is found in the follicular fluid, and its image is projected onto a screen for examination.

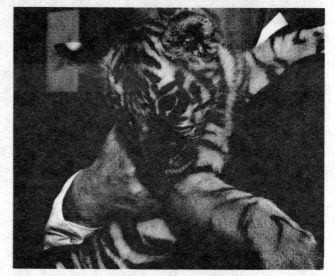

Figure E39-2 The world's first test-tube tiger
Born in 1990, this test-tube tiger is the first successful use of IVF in the fight to save endangered species.

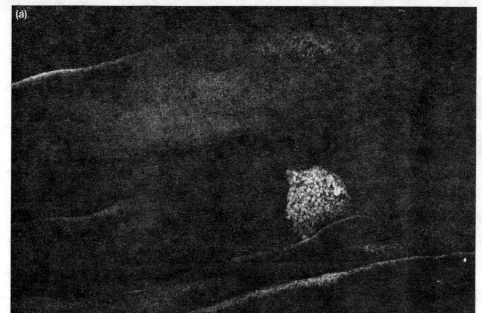

Figure 39-18   **The journey of the egg**

(a) The egg, surrounded by the corona radiata, travels down the oviduct toward the uterus. It emits chemicals that attract sperm, increasing its chances of being fertilized. (b) The egg is fertilized in the oviduct and slowly travels down to the uterus. Along the way, the zygote divides a few times, until a hollow blastocyst is formed. The inner cell mass will form the embryo, while the surrounding cells will adhere to the uterine endometrium, burrow in, and begin forming the placenta.

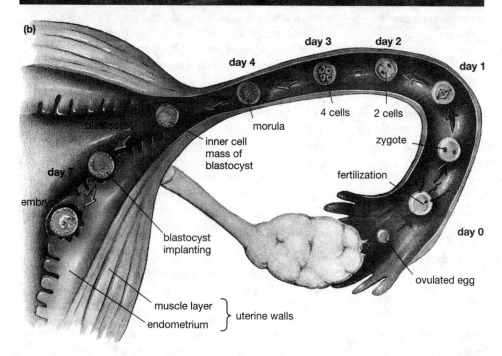

day 3
day 2
day 4
day 1
4 cells
2 cells
morula
blastocyst
inner cell mass of blastocyst
zygote
day 7
fertilization
embryo
blastocyst implanting
day 0
muscle layer
endometrium
} uterine walls
ovulated egg

---

cyst, called the **inner cell mass,** will become the embryo itself, while the sticky outer ball will adhere to the uterus and burrow into the endometrium, a process called **implantation.** Blood from ruptured uterine vessels plus glycogen secreted by glands in the endometrium nourish the growing embryo.

Obtaining nutrients directly from the nearby cells of the endometrium suffices only for the first week or two of embryonic growth. During this time, the placenta, composed of interlocking tissues of the embryo and the endometrium, begins to form. Through the placenta, the embryo will receive nutrients and oxygen and dispose of wastes into the maternal circulation. The details of embryonic development are presented in Chapter 40.

Milk Secretion, or Lactation, Is Stimulated by Pregnancy

As the fetus grows, nourished by nutrients diffusing through the placenta, changes are occurring in the mother's breasts that prepare her to continue nourishing her child after it is born. The breast contains milk glands arranged in a circle around the nipple, each with a duct leading to the nipple. Although the breasts begin enlarging at puberty under the influence of estrogen, their glandular structure does not fully develop until pregnancy occurs (Fig. 39-19). Then, large quantities of estrogen and progesterone (acting together with several other hormones) stimulate the milk glands to grow, branch, and de-

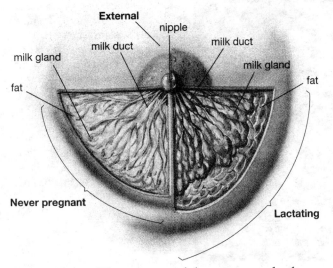

External

nipple

milk duct   milk duct

milk gland   milk gland

fat   fat

Never pregnant

Lactating

Figure 39-19   **The structure of the mammary glands**

During pregnancy, both fatty tissue and the milk-secreting glands and ducts increase in size.

During the first few days after birth, the milk glands secrete a thin, yellowish fluid called **colostrum.** Colostrum is high in protein and contains antibodies that are absorbed directly through the infant's intestine and help protect the newborn against some diseases. Colostrum is gradually replaced by mature milk, which is higher in fat and milk sugar (lactose) and lower in protein.

Reproduction Culminates in Labor and Delivery

Near the end of the ninth month, give or take a few weeks, the process of birth normally begins (Fig. 39-20). Birth is the result of a complex interplay between uterine stretching caused by the growing fetus and fetal and maternal hormones that finally trigger **labor** (contractions of the uterus that result in the birth).

Unlike skeletal muscles, uterine muscles can contract spontaneously, and these contractions are enhanced by stretching. As the baby grows, it stretches the uterine muscles, which contract occasionally weeks before delivery. Recent research suggests that the final trigger for labor is provided by the fetus. The near-term fetus produces steroid hormones that cause increased estrogen and prostaglandin production by the placenta and uterus. These hormones make the uterus even more likely to contract. When the combination of hormones and stretching activate the uterus beyond some critical point, strong contractions begin, signaling the onset of labor. As the contractions proceed, the baby's head pushes against the cervix, making it expand in diameter (dilate). Stretch receptors in the walls of the cervix send signals to the hypothalamus, triggering oxytocin release. Under the dual stimulation of prostaglandin and oxytocin, the uterus contracts even more strongly. This positive feedback cycle is finally halted when the baby emerges. After a brief rest, uterine contractions resume, causing the uterus to shrink remarkably. During these contractions, the placenta is

velop the capacity to secrete milk. The actual secretion of milk is promoted by the pituitary hormone prolactin (see Chapter 35). The level of prolactin rises steadily from about the fifth week of pregnancy until birth.

Immediately after birth, estrogen and progesterone levels plummet, and prolactin, which stimulates milk secretion, takes over. Suckling stimulates nerve endings in the nipples. These signal the hypothalamus, which in turn triggers an extra surge of prolactin and oxytocin from the pituitary. Oxytocin causes muscles surrounding the milk glands to contract, ejecting the milk into the ducts leading to the nipples (see Chapter 35).

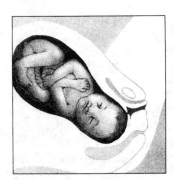

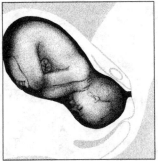

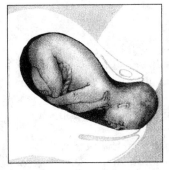

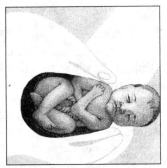

(a) The baby is oriented head downward, facing the mother's side. The cervix is beginning to thin (efface) and expand in diameter (dilate).

(b) The cervix is completely dilated to 10 centimeters (almost 4 inches) and the baby's head has entered the vagina, or birth canal. The baby has rotated to face the mother's back.

(c) The baby's head is emerging (crowning).

(d) The baby has rotated to the side once again as the shoulders emerge.

Figure 39-20   **Delivery**

sheared off from the uterus and is expelled through the vagina as the "afterbirth."

Further release of prostaglandins in the umbilical cord causes the muscles surrounding fetal blood vessels in the umbilical cord to contract, shutting off blood flow. (Tying off the cord is standard practice but is not usually necessary; if it were, other mammals would not survive birth!) Although he or she is still intimately dependent on the parents for survival, a new human being has been born.

On Limiting Fertility

Successful reproduction is essential if any species, including our own, is to endure. During most of human evolution, child mortality was high. Therefore, natural selection favored people who tended to produce many children. With a few tragic exceptions, people today enjoy low infant mortality and a life span triple that of ancient times. Although people today no longer need to have many children to ensure that a few survive to adulthood, we still have reproductive drives appropriate to prehistoric times. As a result, every 4 days a million new people are added to our increasingly overcrowded planet, and controlling human births has become a critical environmental issue. On the individual level, limiting reproduction allows people to plan their families and generally provide the best opportunities for themselves and their children.

Historically, limiting fertility has not been easy. In the past, some cultures have tried such inventive, if bizarre, techniques as swallowing froth from the mouth of a camel or placing crocodile dung in the vagina. Even 50 years ago there were no reliable methods of birth control. Since the 1970s, however, several effective techniques have been developed for **contraception**, or preventing pregnancy. Their mechanisms are described below, and their reliability and some possible side effects are summarized in Table 39-3. Of course, the choice of a contraceptive should be made only in consultation with a physician who can provide more complete information.

Permanent Contraception Can Be Achieved through Sterilization

The most effective, and, in the long run, most effortless method of contraception is **sterilization,** in which the pathways through which sperm or egg must travel are interrupted. In men, the vas deferens leading from each testis may be severed in an operation called a **vasectomy** (Fig. 39-21a). Sperm are still produced, but they cannot reach the penis during ejaculation. The surgery is performed under a local anesthetic, and vasectomy has no known physical side effects on health or sexual performance. The slightly more complex operation of **tubal ligation** renders a woman infertile by cutting her oviducts (Fig. 39-21b).

About 37% of women of childbearing age in the United States have chosen this form of birth control. Ovulation still occurs, but sperm cannot travel to the egg, nor can the egg reach the uterus. Sterilization is generally permanent. Sometimes, however, in a delicate and expensive operation, a surgeon can reconnect the vas deferens or oviducts.

There Are Three Major Approaches to Temporary Contraception

Temporary contraception techniques fall into three general categories: preventing ovulation, preventing sperm and egg from meeting when ovulation does occur, and preventing implantation of a fertilized egg in the uterus.

Synthetic Hormones Can Prevent Ovulation

As you learned earlier in this chapter, during a normal menstrual cycle, ovulation is triggered by a midcycle surge of LH. An obvious way to prevent ovulation is to suppress LH release by providing a continuing supply of estrogen and progesterone. Estrogen and progesterone (usually in synthetic form) are the components of **birth control pills.** "The Pill" is an extremely effective form of birth control, but it must be taken daily, usually for 21 days each menstrual period.

Two new long-term contraceptives, Norplant and Depo-Provera, have been approved for use in the United States since 1990. Both contain synthetic hormones resembling progesterone that prevent ovulation. Norplant consists of six slim, 1.3-inch long silicone rubber rods inserted under the skin of the upper arm. The rods provide gradual, steady diffusion of hormone into the bloodstream for 5 years. In extensive tests, Norplant has proved slightly more effective than the birth control pill. Women using Norplant usually become fertile within months after the capsule is removed. Depo-Provera is injected once every 3 months.

Abstinence and Barrier Methods Prevent Sperm from Reaching the Egg

Abstaining from sexual intercourse is the only completely effective means (other than sterilization) of preventing sperm and egg from meeting. Abstinence also has the advantage of complete safety from possible contraceptive side effects and from sexually transmitted diseases.

There are several effective barrier methods that prevent the encounter of sperm and egg. One is the **diaphragm,** a rubber cap that fits snugly over the cervix, preventing sperm from entering the uterus. In conjunction with a **spermicide,** diaphragms are very effective and have no serious known side effects. Alternatively, a **condom** may be worn over the penis, preventing sperm from being deposited in the vagina. A female condom is now available that completely lines the vagina. Diaphragms and condoms must be applied shortly before intercourse, often at a time when the participants would rather be

TABLE 39-3 ▓ *Birth Control Techniques*[a]

	What Is It?	*How Does It Work?*
NO! (negative response)	Saying NO! is deciding not to be sexually active until you're ready to take on that heavy a commitment.	Say NO! as often as necessary to get your point across. Wear a button that says "NO!" Guaranteed stopper: "If you really loved me, you wouldn't ask."
Natural Family Planning	Combination of cervical mucus (Billings) and basal body temperature (BBT) methods to determine fertile period when you can get pregnant. Billings: based on recognizing changes in mucus discharge that occur just BEFORE ovulation; BBT: based on body temperature changes just AFTER ovulation.	You must learn from a professional nurse practitioner or doctor how to predict your fertile period, using changes in cervical mucus and body temperature.
Condom (for men) Condom (for women)	For men: Thin rubber or latex (latex is strongest) disposable sheath (usually lubricated with non-oxynol-9) worn over penis during sex. Never use Vaseline as a lubricant. ("Natural" condoms don't protect against STDs.) For women: Soft, loose-fitting prelubricated polyurethane pouch with two rings: one inserted deep in vagina, the other, when in place, remains just outside the vagina.	For both: Placed correctly, catches sperm so they can't enter vagina. Also shields you from exposure to AIDS or other STDs. Protects your partner too.
Foam (spermicides)	Sperm-killing foam inserted into vagina before having sex. Choose foam that contains non-oxynol-9 for best protection against pregnancy and STDs.	Inserted deep into vagina with plastic applicator, forms chemical barrier over uterine entrance. Sperm die when they hit foam.
The Sponge[c]	Soft disposable polyurethane sponge filled with one gram of sperm-killing non-oxynol-9 that is activated by moistening sponge with water. Can be put in vagina hours before having sex, is effective immediately, and offers contraceptive protection for up to 24 hours. Some clinics say it's number 1 choice for young lovers.	Sponge moistened with water is placed far back in vagina up to 18 hours before having sex. Sponge fits around cervix, keeps sperm from entering uterus. Traps sperm, killing them on contact.
Diaphragm/ Cervical Cap	The diaphragm and cervical cap are birth control devices that fit over the cervix and prevent pregnancy by preventing sperm from entering uterus. Both must be individually fitted by a medical professional. Both are made of rubber-like materials. Cap is half the size of diaphragm, and can be left in place twice as long.	Place one teaspoonful of spermicide containing non-oxynol-9 inside the dome and another around the edge of diaphragm or cap. Spermicide seals barrier and kills sperm.
The Pill	A pill made of a combination of synthetic hormones almost like those produced by the ovaries. Take at the same time every day whether or not you have sex. It's the day-by-day action of the pills that protects you from pregnancy.	Prevents ovary from releasing an egg. With no egg present for a sperm to fertilize, a woman cannot become pregnant. Caution: Use a back-up method plus the pill in first couple months of use.
IUD (intrauterine device)	Small plastic device treated with copper or hormones. Nylon thread attached for easy checking. Fitted by medical professional.	Prevents egg from being implanted in uterine wall. Copper IUD is replaced every 6 years; hormonal IUD, every year.
Norplant	New! Long-lasting! Doctor inserts 6 tiny flexible progestogen-filled capsules under skin of upper arm to provide protection up to 5 years. Fertility returns when Norplant is removed.	Progestogen is released in steady low doses, preventing pregnancy by blocking ovulations.
Depo-Provera (injectable)	An injectable form of contraception (given as a shot) that protects you from pregnancy for a full 3 months. Contains a chemical similar to the hormone (progesterone) that ovaries produce during the second half of the menstrual cycle.	Depo-Provera works by preventing egg cells from ripening. If an egg is not released from your ovaries during a menstrual cycle, it can't be fertilized by sperm, so you can't get pregnant. But you have to be very sure to get a shot every 3 months—no more, no less.

[a]Modified with permission from *"No!" and Other Methods of Birth Control*, Private Line, P.O. Box 31, Kenilworth, Illinois 60043.

[b]All of these birth control methods (except Norplant and to a lesser extent, Depo-Provera) take effort on your part. Nothing works if you leave it in the dresser drawer!

[c]The company manufacturing the sponge stopped distributing it in 1995 for business reasons. The sponge may or may not be available when you read this. Ask at your drugstore.

Does It Have Any Side Effects?	Are There Any Dangers?	How Reliable Is It?[b]
Only positive ones. If you're not loaded down with a relationship you can't handle, you'll have time to make a life for *yourself* and you won't have to worry about getting pregnant or getting a sexually transmitted disease (STD) such as chlamydia, genital warts, herpes, or AIDS.	Only that people who put pressure on you might make fun of you or drop you cold. But if they do, ask yourself what they really want from you—love and friendship, or sex?	100% effective.
No—but it doesn't offer any protection against sexually transmitted diseases (STDs).	You could become pregnant unless you avoid sex during your fertile period. Some women have trouble identifying mucus changes.	10 to 15 women out of 100 become pregnant in a given year using the Billings or BTT methods. The calendar method alone is not a reliable form of birth control.
For both: Next to not having sex, condoms or pouch used along with spermicidal foam containing non-oxynol-9 are the best available way to protect you against AIDS and other STDs—or pregnancy. (One or both of you could be allergic to spermicidal foam or lubricant.)	NO. AIDS is no joke. Condoms could save your life. Use one every time you have sex even if your partner is on the pill, has an IUD, is wearing a diaphragm—or has had a vasectomy. For women: A pouch, properly used, provides even better protection than a condom against STDs.	2 to 10 women out of 100 become pregnant in a given year when the man uses a condom correctly every time. The time period for clinical testing of the pouch has been too short for accurate statistics. The manufacturer reports that 2 to 3 women out of 100 become pregnant in a given year when the woman uses a condom every time as directed.
Occasionally the foam you're using may cause a mild vaginal irritation, cause bladder or yeast infection, or irritate your partner. Usually a change to a different brand solves the problem, but be sure the foam you use contains non-oxynol-9. If necessary, change to a birth control method that doesn't require a spermicide.	No, except your partner should use a condom when you use foam to give you the best protection, next to not having sex, against STDs and pregnancy. Just remember that protection is not 100% guaranteed.	4 to 29 women out of 100 become pregnant in a given year when using foam alone.
You don't have to worry about hormonal side effects. In clinical trials small number of women tested discontinued using because of itching, irritation, rash or allergic reactions.	Manufacturer's instructions stress use for ONLY 24-hour period. Should NOT be used during menstrual period. Slight danger of toxic shock syndrome (TSS). Sponge does not stop flow of vaginal secretions.	8 to 10 women out of 100 become pregnant in a given year when using the sponge as directed.
None unless the spermicide you're using causes bladder or yeast infection. If it does, change to another brand.	Slight danger of toxic shock syndrome (TSS). Should be used for birth control only, not to control vaginal secretions. Be sure you have inserted it correctly. Don't forget the spermicidal foam or jelly.	5 to 10 women out of 100 in a given year become pregnant when using a diaphragm or cap consistently and correctly. (If you gain or lose weight, your diaphragm may no longer fit correctly and should be checked by a medical professional.)
Positive: regular periods, less anemia, less cramping, less benign breast disease. May inhibit some forms of cancer. Negative: (normally disappear within 3 months) may include nausea, spotting, missed periods, headaches, mood changes, dark skin areas. Major but rare: blood clots, high blood pressure, gallbladder disease, heart attacks, liver tumors.	Some women should not take the pill because of other health problems. A health professional will choose the best pill for you. Read carefully all material in pill package. Follow doctor's advice. Smoking increases the chance of blood clots or stroke, even in young people on the pill.	1 woman out of 300 becomes pregnant in a given year when using the pill correctly. Always check with your doctor about possible interactions between the pill and any other medications you are taking.
Possible cramps and heavy menstrual flow caused by the body's effort to push out IUD. Expect heavy menstrual periods the first few months.	Risk of pelvic inflammatory disease (PID) or tubal pregnancy. Tell doctor if you have fever or stomach pain.	1 to 5 women out of 100 in a given year become pregnant while using an IUD.
Irregular menstrual cycle for first 6 months with longer periods, spotting between periods or skipped periods. Possible headaches, weight gain.	The method is too new for accurate statistics. Counseling to understand method is extremely important. If pregnancy does occur, have Norplant removed at once.	1 woman out of 300 becomes pregnant in a given year when using Norplant for the first 2 years. After 2 years, less protection for overweight women.
Irregular menstrual bleeding at first, then little or no menstruation, weight gain, but not much. Possibly headache, nervousness, abdominal pain, dizziness, fatigue. Check with doctor if you experience any unusual symptoms.	Important that injection be given during first 5 days of menstrual period to avoid possibility of receiving the shot during a pregnancy—which could result in ectopic pregnancy. If you should get pregnant, see your doctor immediately.	1 woman out of 300 in a given year becomes pregnant while receiving Depo-Provera injections as prescribed.

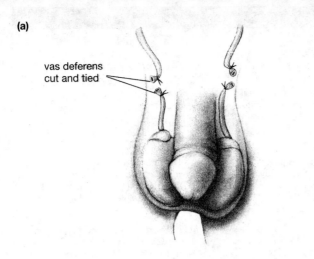

vas deferens
cut and tied

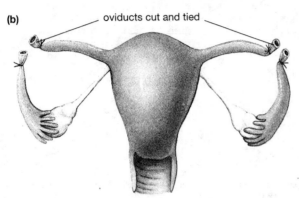

oviducts cut and tied

Figure 39-21   Sterilization

Sterilization is the most effective form of birth control, but it is not dependably reversible. **(a)** In the male, the vas deferens is reached through a small slit in the scrotum. It is cut and each end is tied off. **(b)** In the female, the oviduct is reached through an abdominal incision. It is cut, and each end is tied off.

thinking about something else. Furthermore, if the diaphragm or condom happens to have even a small hole, sperm may still enter the uterus and fertilize the egg. (It seems a cruel irony that a man ejaculating 50 million sperm will often be infertile, but if just a few drops of semen escape past a diaphragm or condom, pregnancy might result.)

Other, less effective, procedures include using spermicides alone, **withdrawal** (removal of the penis from the vagina just before ejaculation), and **douching** (washing sperm out of the vagina before, it is hoped, they have had a chance to enter the uterus). Spermicides have some contraceptive effect, but withdrawal and douching are essentially useless. A final method of preventing fertilization is the **rhythm method:** abstinence from intercourse during the ovulatory period of the menstrual cycle. In practice, rhythm usually has a high failure rate, because of lack of discipline on the part of the users or inaccuracies in determining the menstrual cycle, which varies somewhat from month to month. Because a slight rise in body temperature and changes in the discharge of mucus from the cervix can be used to predict ovulation, the rhythm method can be made more effective if these indicators are monitored and sexual activity is regulated accordingly.

Intrauterine Devices Prevent Implantation

Even if an egg is fertilized, pregnancy will not occur unless the blastocyst implants in the uterus. The **intrauterine device (IUD)** is a small copper or plastic loop, squiggle, or shield that is inserted into the uterus and remains there until removed by a physician. Highly effective (if it stays in place), the IUD seems to work by irritating the uterine lining so that it cannot receive the embryo. A second method of preventing implantation is the "morning after" pill, which contains a massive dose of estrogen. For some women, preventing implantation has the major drawback that it is, in effect, an extremely early abortion.

Abortion Removes the Embryo from the Uterus

When contraception fails, pregnancy may be terminated by **abortion.** Abortion commonly involves dilating the cervix and removing the embryo and placenta by suction. The compound RU-486, taken as a pill, is now routinely used in France to terminate pregnancy up to about a month after conception and may be available in the United States by 1996. This substance binds to progesterone receptors and blocks the actions of progesterone, which are essential to the maintenance of pregnancy.

Because abortions are usually surgical procedures, they are potentially more dangerous to a woman's health than the contraceptive techniques described above. Although science can describe fetal development during pregnancy, it cannot provide judgments about when a fetus becomes a "person," or about the relative merits of fetal versus maternal rights. Therefore, abortion remains controversial.

Additional Contraceptive Methods Are under Development

Further advances in contraception are under development. For example, a vaginal ring that continuously releases synthetic progesterone has been tested in several countries but is not yet on the market. A pill that prevents ovulation by blocking receptors for gonadotropin-releasing hormone is in the testing stage. There are also once-a-month contraceptive pills under development, most of which prevent the uterus from becoming fully prepared for implantation. Another possibility is a contraceptive vaccine that would remain effective for one to several years. One such vaccine induces antibodies against human chorionic gonadotropin, which is essential for the implantation of the embryo in the uterus. Another in-

Sexually Transmitted Diseases

Sexually transmitted diseases (STDs), caused by viruses, bacteria, protists, or arthropods that infect the sexual organs and reproductive tract, are a serious and growing health problem worldwide. The World Health Organization estimates that there are 250 million new cases of STD each year. As the name implies, these diseases are transmitted either exclusively or primarily through sexual contact. Here we discuss some of the more common of these diseases.

Bacterial Infections

Gonorrhea, an infection of the genital and urinary tract, is one of the most common of *all* infectious diseases in the United States, estimated to infect at least 2 million people each year. The causative bacterium, which cannot survive outside the body, is transmitted almost exclusively by intimate contact. It penetrates the membranes lining the urethra, anus, cervix, uterus, oviducts, and throat. In males, inflammation of the urethra results in a discharge of pus from the penis and painful urination. About 10% of infected males and 50% of infected females have symptoms that are mild or absent and do not seek treatment. They become carriers who can readily spread the disease. Gonorrhea can lead to infertility by blocking the oviducts with scar tissue. Treatment by penicillin was formerly highly successful, but penicillin-resistant strains now require use of other antibiotics. Infants born to infected mothers may acquire the bacterium during delivery. The bacterium attacks the eyes of newborns and was once a major cause of blindness. Today, most newborns are immediately given antibiotic eyedrops to kill the bacterium.

Syphilis is a far more dangerous, though less prevalent, disease than gonorrhea. It is caused by a spiral-shaped bacterium that enters the mucous membranes of the genitals, lips, anus, or breasts. Like gonorrhea, it is readily killed by exposure to air and is spread only by intimate contact. Syphilis begins with a sore at the site of infection. Syphilis may be cured with antibiotics, but if untreated, syphilis bacteria spread through the body, multiplying and damaging many organs, including the skin, kidneys, heart, and brain, sometimes with fatal results. About 4 out of every 1000 newborns in the United States have been infected with syphilis before birth. The skin, teeth, bones, liver, and central nervous system of such infants may be damaged.

Chlamydia causes inflammation of the urethra in males and the urethra and cervix in females, but in many cases there are no obvious symptoms, so the infection goes untreated and is spread. Like the gonorrhea bacterium, *Chlamydia* can infect and sometimes block the oviducts, resulting in sterility. Chlamydial infection can cause eye inflammations in infants born to infected mothers.

Viral Infections

Acquired immunodeficiency syndrome, or **AIDS,** is caused by the HIV virus. Because the virus does not survive exposure to air, it is spread primarily by sexual activity and by contaminated blood and needles. The HIV virus attacks the immune system, leaving the victim vulnerable to a variety of infections, which almost invariably prove fatal. Children born to mothers with AIDS sometimes become infected before or during birth. There is no cure, although certain drugs, such as AZT, can prolong life. AIDS is discussed in detail in Chapter 34.

Genital herpes reached epidemic proportions during the 1970s and continues to spread to more than a million new victims yearly. It causes painful blisters on the genitals and surrounding skin and is transmitted primarily when blisters are present. The herpes virus never leaves the body but resides in certain nerve cells, emerging unpredictably, possibly in response to stress. The first outbreak is the most serious; subsequent outbreaks produce fewer blisters and may be quite infrequent. The drug acyclovir, which inhibits viral DNA replication, may reduce the severity of outbreaks. Pregnant women with an active case of genital herpes may transmit the virus to the developing child, causing severe mental or physical disability or stillbirth. Herpes may also be transmitted from mother to infant if the infant contacts blisters as it is born.

Protists and Arthropod Infections

Trichomoniasis is caused by *Trichomonas*, a flagellated protist that colonizes the mucous membranes lining the urinary tract and genitals of both males and females. The symptoms are a discharge caused by inflammation in response to the parasite. The protist is spread by intercourse but can also be acquired through contaminated clothing and toilet articles. Lengthy untreated infections can result in sterility.

Crab lice, also called pubic lice, are microscopic arachnids that live and lay their eggs in pubic hair. Their mouthparts are adapted for penetrating the skin and sucking blood and body fluids, a process that causes severe itching. "Crabs" are not only irritating; they may also spread infectious diseases. They can be controlled through careful hygiene and chemical treatments.

duces the formation of antibodies to a protein called SP-10 that is unique to sperm.

You may have noticed that most of the contraceptive techniques are directed at the woman, not the man. It is much easier to interfere with ovulation than with sperm formation. A woman ovulates only once a month, and ovulation itself does not influence a woman's sexual drives. In contrast, testosterone is essential both for sperm for-mation and sexual performance; early "male pills" caused not only infertility but also impotence. Nevertheless, there is a major research effort under way to develop male con-traceptives equivalent to The Pill. A promising contra-ceptive is a daily dose of testosterone and a modified form of gonadotropin-releasing hormone, which together seem to block sperm production without affecting sexual per-formance. Clinical trials are now under way.

✖ SUMMARY OF KEY CONCEPTS

Reproductive Strategies

Animals reproduce either sexually or asexually. Sexual re-production involves the union of haploid gametes, usual-ly from two separate parents, and produces an offspring that is genetically different from either parent. In asexu-al reproduction, offspring are usually genetically identical to the parent. Asexual reproduction may occur by bud-ding, regeneration, fission, or parthenogenesis.

Among animals that engage in sexual reproduction, the female produces large, nonmotile eggs, and the male produces small, motile sperm. Animals may be either monoecious (a single animal produces both sperm and eggs) or dioecious (a single animal produces one type of gamete). The union of sperm and egg, called fertiliza-tion, may occur outside the bodies of the animals (ex-ternal fertilization) or inside the body of the female (in-ternal fertilization). External fertilization must occur in water so that the sperm can swim to meet the egg. Most internal fertilization is through copulation, in which the male deposits sperm directly into the female reproductive tract.

Mammalian Reproduction

The human male reproductive tract consists of paired testes that produce sperm and testosterone and acces-sory structures that conduct the sperm to the female's reproductive tract and secrete fluids that activate swim-ming by the sperm and provide energy. In human males, spermatogenesis and testosterone production are stim-ulated by FSH and LH, secreted by the anterior pitu-itary. Spermatogenesis and testosterone production are nearly continuous, beginning at puberty and lasting until death.

The human female reproductive tract consists of paired ovaries that produce eggs as well as the hormones estrogen and progesterone, and accessory structures that conduct sperm to the egg and receive and nourish the embryo during prenatal development. In human fe-males, oogenesis, hormone production, and develop-ment of the lining of the uterus vary in a monthly men-strual cycle. The cycle is controlled by hormones from the hypothalamus (gonadotropin-releasing), anterior pituitary (FSH and LH), and ovaries (estrogen and progesterone).

During copulation, the male inserts his penis into the female's vagina and ejaculates semen. The sperm move through the vagina and uterus into the oviduct, where fertilization usually takes place. The unfertilized egg is surrounded by two barriers, the corona radiata and the zona pellucida. Enzymes released from the acro-somes at the tips of sperm digest these layers, permitting sperm to reach the egg. Only one sperm enters the egg and fertilizes it.

The fertilized egg undergoes a few cell divisions in the oviduct and then implants in the uterine lining. Implan-tation and subsequent release of chorionic gonadotropin by the embryo maintain the integrity of the corpus luteum and the endometrium during early pregnancy, preventing further menstrual cycles.

During pregnancy, milk glands in the mother's breasts enlarge under the influence of estrogen, progesterone, and other hormones. After birth, milk secretion is triggered by prolactin and oxytocin, whose release is triggered by suckling.

After about 9 months, uterine contractions are trig-gered by a complex interplay of uterine stretch and prostaglandin and oxytocin release. As a result, the uterus expels the baby and then the placenta.

On Limiting Fertility

Permanent contraception can be achieved by steril-ization: severing the vas deferens in males (vasecto-my) or the oviducts in females (tubal ligation). Tem-porary contraception techniques include those that prevent ovulation: birth control pills, Norplant, and Depo-Provera. Barrier methods prevent sperm and egg from meeting. These include the diaphragm, the con-traceptive sponge, and the condom, accompanied by spermicide. Spermicide alone is less effective. With-drawal and douching are poor techniques. The rhythm method involves sexual abstinence around the time of ovulation. Intrauterine devices prevent implantation of the blastocyst. Abortion causes the expulsion of the developing embryo.

abortion	follicle	prostate gland
acquired immunodeficiency syndrome (AIDS)	follicle-stimulating hormone (FSH)	regeneration
		rhythm method
acrosome	genital herpes	scrotum
amplexus	gonad	secondary oocyte
asexual reproduction	gonadotropin-releasing hormone (GnRH)	secondary spermatocyte
birth control pill		semen
blastocyst	gonorrhea	seminal vesicle
bud	hermaphrodite	seminiferous tubule
budding	implantation	Sertoli cell
bulbourethral gland	inner cell mass	sexual reproduction
cervix	internal fertilization	spawning
chlamydia	interstitial cell	sperm
chorionic gonadotropin (CG)	intrauterine device (IUD)	spermatid
colostrum	labor	spermatogenesis
condom	luteinizing hormone (LH)	spermatogonium
contraception	menstrual cycle	spermatophore
copulation	menstruation	spermicide
corona radiata	monoecious	sterilization
corpus luteum	myometrium	syphilis
crab lice	oogenesis	testis
diaphragm	oogonium	testosterone
dioecious	ovary	trichomoniasis
douching	oviduct	tubal ligation
egg	ovulation	urethra
endometrium	parthenogenesis	uterus
epididymis	pheromone	vagina
estrogen	placenta	vas deferens
external fertilization	polar body	vasectomy
fallopian tube	primary oocyte	withdrawal
fimbria	primary spermatocyte	zona pellucida
fission	progesterone	zygote

✳ THINKING THROUGH THE CONCEPTS

Multiple Choice

1. Budding, regeneration, and splitting apart are processes used by
   a. dioecious species
   b. hermaphroditic organisms
   c. organisms requiring new gene combinations for each generation
   d. sexually reproducing species
   e. asexually reproducing species

2. All of the following are barrier contraceptive devices EXCEPT
   a. IUD
   b. contraceptive sponge
   c. caps that fit over the cervix
   d. diaphragm
   e. male condom

3. In humans, spermatogenesis yields _____ sperm for each diploid germ cell, and oogenesis yields _____ secondary oocyte(s) for each germ cell.
   a. one, four   b. two, one
   c. one, two   d. four, one
   e. four, two

4. Which structure adds the *final* secretions to semen as it moves out of the human reproductive tract?
   a. epididymis
   b. bulbourethral gland
   c. seminal vesicle
   d. prostate gland
   e. interstitial cells

5. During fetal development, oogonia in human females halt meiosis at
   a. the secondary oocyte stage
   b. the polar body stage
   c. metaphase of meiosis II
   d. telophase of meiosis II
   e. prophase of meiosis I

6. The primary hormone that inhibits GnRH is
   a. FSH
   b. LH
   c. progesterone
   d. estrogen
   e. a hypothalamic releasing factor

Review Questions

1. List the advantages and disadvantages of asexual reproduction, sexual reproduction, external fertilization, and internal fertilization, including an example of an animal showing each type.
2. Compare the structures of the egg and sperm. What structural modifications are found in sperm to facilitate movement, energy use, and digestion?
3. What is the role of the corpus luteum in a menstrual cycle? In early pregnancy? What determines its survival after ovulation?
4. Construct a chart of common sexually transmitted diseases. List the disease's name, the cause (organism), symptoms, and treatment.
5. List the structures, in order, through which a sperm passes on its way from the seminiferous tubules of the testis to the oviduct of the female.
6. Name the three accessory glands of the male reproductive tract. What are the functions of the secretions they produce?
7. Diagram the menstrual cycle and describe the interactions among hormones produced by the pituitary gland and ovaries that produce the cycle.
8. Describe the changes in the breast that prepare a mother to nurse her child. How do hormones influence these changes and stimulate milk production?
9. Describe the events that lead to the expulsion of the baby and placenta from the uterus. Explain why this is an example of positive feedback.

APPLYING THE CONCEPTS

1. Identify and discuss some of the ethical issues involved in *in vitro* fertilization.
2. Discuss the most effective or appropriate method of birth control for each of the following couples: Couple A has intercourse three times a week but does not ever want to have children; Couple B has intercourse only once a month, and may want to have children someday; and couple C has intercourse three times a week and wants to have children someday.
3. Female condoms were recently introduced in the United States. What advantages and disadvantages can you think of for this form of birth control?
4. Pelvic endometriosis is a relatively common disease of women in which bits of the endometrial lining find their way onto abdominal organs and respond in typical ways to hormones during a menstrual month. When the uterine lining bleeds during menstruation, so do these implants. Common treatments are oral contraceptives, Danazol (a compound that inhibits gonadotropins), and synthetic GnRH analogues that are paradoxically powerful inhibitors of FSH and LH. How does each of these compounds provide relief?
5. Would contraceptive drugs that block cell receptors for FSH be useful in males and/or females? Explain. What side effects would such drugs have?
6. Think of all the choices a couple have to obtain a child, including: *in vitro* fertilization using the couple's eggs and sperm, *in vitro* fertilization using a donor's sperm or egg, and insemination of a surrogate mother with sperm from the couple's husband. Think of some more. Now describe what ethical issues these various options present?

FOR MORE INFORMATION

Crews, D. "Animal Sexuality." *Scientific American*, January 1994. Explores the wide range of mechanisms that control male and female sexual development among different types of animals.

Eberhard, W. G. "Runaway Sexual Selection." *Natural History*, December 1987. Interesting article on the evolution of male genitalia.

Riddle, J. M., and Estes, J. W. "Oral Contraceptives in Ancient and Medieval Times." *American Scientist*, May–June 1992. How did women control their fertility before modern medicine stepped in?

Ulmann, A., Teutsch, G., and Philibert, D. "RU-486." *Scientific American*, June 1990. Describes the abortion pill now widely used in France and other applications for this drug.

Wassarman, P. W. "Fertilization in Mammals." *Scientific American*, December 1988. Describes the events leading to the penetration of the egg by the sperm, with emphasis on the role and composition of the zona pellucida.

Wright, K. "The Sniff of Legend." *Discover*, April 1994. This article explores human pheromones, sex attractants, and a sixth sense organ in the nose.

NET WATCH

On-line resources for this chapter are on the World Wide Web at:
http://www.prenhall.com/~audesirk (click on the table of contents link and then select Chapter 39).

10

CHEMICAL CONTROL OF THE ANIMAL BODY: THE ENDOCRINE SYSTEM

*The changes that occur throughout the life cycles of all animals
are under the control of hormones. One of the more dramatic
events during the life cycle of certain insects is metamorphosis,
illustrated here by an Indonesian birdwing butterfly emerging
from the pupal case it formed as a caterpillar.*

With the evolution of complex multicellular organisms came the need to coordinate the activities of cells in different parts of the body. Cell-to-cell communication is crucial to the control of movement, growth, reproduction, and the maintenance of homeostasis. Many different mechanisms have evolved by which cells within organisms communicate among themselves. One method is by direct contact. Molecules protruding from the surface membrane identify cells as belonging to an individual of a particular species, as parts of a unique individual organism, and as specific cell types, such as skin or liver. Surface contacts are important in the development of embryos, in which cells migrate around one another to arrive at their proper destination. Direct contact also plays a key role in defense against disease organisms, in which immune cells recognize invading foreign cells by their surface molecules (see Chapter 34).

Cells can also communicate with one another over distances. Cells of the nervous system convey electrical signals over long or short distances, then transmit these signals to other cells by releasing chemicals into the immediate vicinity of the nerve cell ending (Chapter 36). Cells of the **endocrine system**, in contrast, release chemicals into the bloodstream, where they are carried throughout the body and may have wide-ranging effects. These chemicals, or hormones, and the glands and organs that release them, are the subject of this chapter.

Animal Hormone Structure and Function

A **hormone** is a chemical secreted by cells in one part of the body that is transported in the bloodstream to other parts of the body, where it affects particular target cells. Hormones are released by the cells of major endocrine glands and endocrine organs located throughout the body (Fig. 35-1). There are four classes of chemicals used as hormones in the animal kingdom, illustrated in Table 35-1.

Peptide Hormones Include Both Short and Longer Chains of Amino Acids

Most hormones are chains of amino acids ranging from a few to over a hundred amino acids in length. Technically, short amino acid chains are called peptides, whereas longer chains are called proteins. For convenience, however, all hormones composed of amino acid chains are described as **peptide hormones.** Insulin, antidiuretic hormone, all the hormones of the hypothalamus and the anterior and posterior pituitary, as well as many other hormones are peptide hormones.

Some Hormones Consist of Modified Single Amino Acids

A few hormones are modified amino acids. The amino acid tyrosine forms the basis for the hormones epinephrine (also called adrenaline), norepinephrine (also called noradrenaline), and the thyroid hormone thyroxine.

Steroid Hormones Resemble Cholesterol in Structure

Steroid hormones, also called **steroids**, all have a chemical structure resembling cholesterol, from which most of them are synthesized. Steroid hormones are secreted by the ovaries and placenta (estrogen and progesterone), the testes (testosterone), and the adrenal cortex (aldosterone).

Prostaglandins Are Modified Fatty Acids

Nearly every type of cell in the body has been found to produce **prostaglandins**. These substances consist of two fatty acid carbon chains attached to a five-carbon ring.

Hormones Function by Binding to Specific Receptors on Target Cells

Because nearly all cells have a blood supply, once hormones enter the bloodstream, they reach nearly every cell of the body. But in order to exert their precise control, hormones must act only on certain **target cells**. Hormone specificity is determined by receptors on target cells; if a cell lacks a specific receptor for a hormone, the hormone will not affect the cell. In addition, the same hormone may have several different effects depending on the nature of the target cell it contacts. Receptors for hormones are found in two general locations on target cells: on the cell membrane and inside the cell, usually within the nucleus (Fig. 35-2).

Some Hormones Bind to Surface Receptors

Most peptide hormones, as well as epinephrine and norepinephrine, are water soluble but not lipid soluble. Hence, these hormones cannot cross the phospholipid cell membranes. Instead they react with protein receptors protrud-

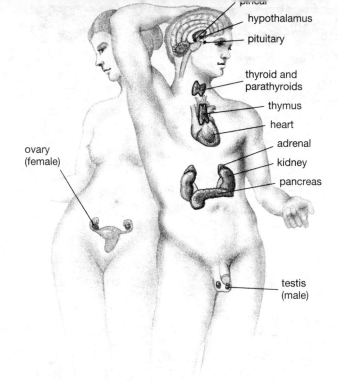

Figure 35-1   Major mammalian endocrine glands

The major mammalian endocrine glands discussed in the text are the hypothalamus-pituitary complex, the thyroid and parathyroid glands, the pancreas, the sex organs (ovaries in females, testes in males), and the adrenal glands. Other organs that secrete hormones include the pineal gland, thymus, kidneys, heart, and digestive tract.

ing from the outside surface of target cell membranes (see Chapter 6). In general, hormones that bind to surface receptors trigger rapid, short-term responses. Some receptors, such as those for norepinephrine, are directly linked to channels that are opened in response to the binding of the hormone. For example, epinephrine binding to receptors on heart muscle cells causes calcium channels to open, allowing more calcium to flow into the muscle cells, which in turn increases the strength of contraction of the heart.

More frequently, a **second messenger** system is used. In second messenger systems, when the hormone binds to the receptor, the shape of the receptor is altered, triggering a series of biochemical reactions that alter the activity of the cell (Fig. 35-2a). In many cases, the binding of the hormone to the receptor activates an enzyme. When activated, the enzyme catalyzes the conversion of ATP to **cyclic AMP** (see Chapter 3), a nucleotide that regulates many cellular activities. Cyclic AMP is often called a second messenger, because it transfers the signal from the first messenger, the hormone, to molecules within the cell. The formation of cyclic AMP initiates a series of reactions inside the cell. Each of these reactions involves an increasing number of molecules, amplifying the original signal. The end result varies with the

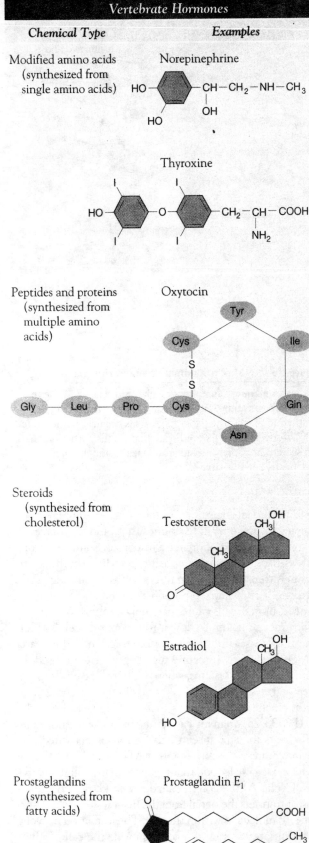

TABLE 35-1 ❊ *The Chemical Diversity of Vertebrate Hormones*

Chemical Type	Examples
Modified amino acids (synthesized from single amino acids)	Norepinephrine
	Thyroxine
Peptides and proteins (synthesized from multiple amino acids)	Oxytocin
Steroids (synthesized from cholesterol)	Testosterone
	Estradiol
Prostaglandins (synthesized from fatty acids)	Prostaglandin E_1

target cell. For example, channels may be opened in the cell membrane, or substances may be synthesized or secreted.

Another second messenger that may be activated by hormones is **calmodulin**. The binding of certain hormones to their receptors triggers the opening of calcium channels, allowing an influx of calcium into the cell. Calmodulin is a protein in the cytoplasm that binds calcium ions, changing shape as a result. The altered shape of the calcium-calmodulin complex allows it to activate enzymes, acting in a manner similar to cyclic AMP.

Other Hormones Bind to Intracellular Receptors

Steroid hormones and thyroid hormones are lipid soluble and are therefore able to diffuse into the cell membrane and bind to receptors inside the cell (Fig. 35-2b). Both steroid and thyroid hormones alter the activity of genes. It may take from minutes to days for these hormones to exert their full effects. Thyroid and most steroid hormones bind to protein receptors in the nucleus. The receptor-hormone complex binds to DNA and initiates the transcription of messenger RNA from specific genes. The messenger RNA then moves into the cytoplasm and directs the synthesis of new proteins, for example, enzymes involved in cell growth and metabolic activity.

Hormones Are Regulated by Feedback Mechanisms

Animals usually regulate the release of hormones through negative feedback (see Chapter 29). During negative feedback, the secretion of a hormone causes effects in target cells that inhibit further secretion of the hormone. Negative feedback is an important way of maintaining homeostasis—that is, keeping conditions within the body relatively constant over time.

Most hormones exert such powerful effects on the body that it would be harmful to have too much hormone working for too long. For example, suppose you have jogged several miles on a hot, sunny day and lost a pint of water through perspiration. In response to the loss of water from your bloodstream, your pituitary gland releases antidiuretic hormone (ADH), which causes your kidneys to reabsorb more water and produce a very concentrated urine (see Chapter 33). However, if you arrive home and drink a quart of Gatorade, you will more than replace the water you lost in sweat. Continued retention of this excess water could raise blood pressure and possibly damage your heart. Negative feedback ensures that when your blood water content returns to normal, ADH secretion is turned off and your kidneys begin eliminating the excess water (see Fig. 33-8). Negative feedback is also at work in the control of thyroxine secretion (see Fig. 35-9).

In a few cases, positive feedback controls hormone release. As mentioned in Chapter 29, contractions of the uterus early in childbirth cause the release of oxytocin by the posterior pituitary. The oxytocin stimulates stronger

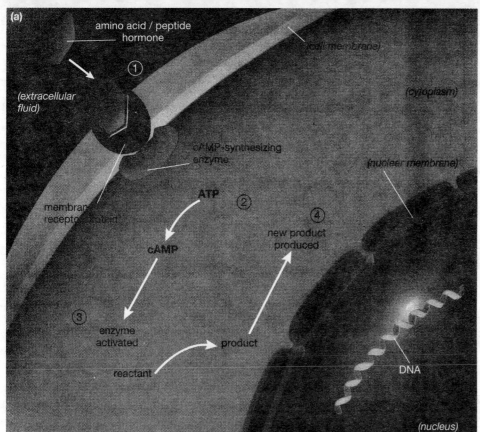

(a) amino acid / peptide hormone

(cell membrane)

(cytoplasm)

①

(extracellular fluid)

cAMP-synthesizing enzyme

(nuclear membrane)

membrane receptor protein

ATP ②

cAMP

④

new product produced

③

enzyme activated

product

reactant

DNA

(nucleus)

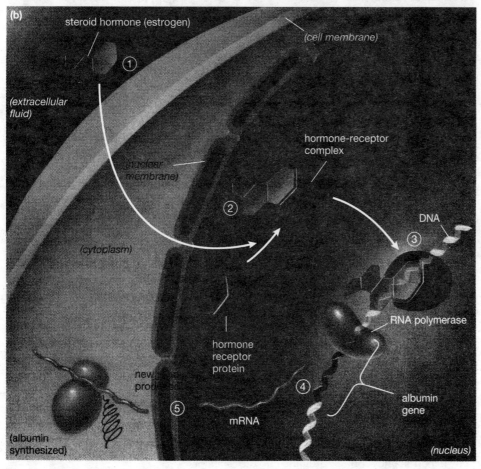

(b) steroid hormone (estrogen)

(cell membrane)

①

(extracellular fluid)

hormone-receptor complex

(nuclear membrane)

②

(cytoplasm)

DNA

③

RNA polymerase

hormone receptor protein

new products

⑤

④

mRNA

albumin gene

(albumin synthesized)

(nucleus)

Figure 35-2 Modes of action of hormones

(a) Non-lipid-soluble peptide and amino acid hormones bind to a receptor on the outside of the target cell membrane ①. Hormone-receptor binding triggers synthesis of cyclic AMP (cAMP) ②. Cyclic AMP in turn activates specific enzymes ③ that promote specific cellular reactions that produce new products ④. This cyclic AMP "cascade" may generate a variety of responses. Examples include an increase in glucose synthesis induced by epinephrine and an increase in estrogen synthesis induced by luteinizing hormone.

(b) Lipid-soluble steroid hormones diffuse readily through the cell membrane into the target cell ① and then into the nucleus where they combine with a protein receptor molecule ②. The hormone-receptor complex binds to DNA and facilitates the binding of RNA polymerase to promoter sites on specific genes ③, accelerating transcription of DNA into messenger RNA (mRNA) ④. The mRNA then directs protein synthesis ⑤. In hens, for example, estrogen promotes transcription of the albumin gene, causing synthesis of albumin (egg white), which is packaged in the egg as a food supply for the developing chick.

contractions of the uterus, which cause more oxytocin release, creating a positive feedback cycle. Simultaneously, oxytocin causes uterine cells to release prostaglandins that further enhance uterine contractions, another example of positive feedback. Both positive and negative feedback are involved in the interactions between mother and child during breastfeeding (see Fig. 35-5).

The Mammalian Endocrine System

Endocrinologists (biologists who study the endocrine system) are still far from fully understanding hormonal control in mammals. New hormones, or new roles for previously known hormones, are discovered nearly every year. What we might call the major endocrine glands and endocrine organs, however, have been known for many years. These are the hypothalamus-pituitary complex, the thyroid and parathyroid glands, the pancreas, the sex organs, and the adrenal glands (Fig. 35-1). Table 35-2 lists these and other glands, their major hormones, and their principal functions.

Mammals Have Both Exocrine and Endocrine Glands

Mammals have two types of glands: exocrine glands and endocrine glands (Fig. 35-3). **Exocrine glands** produce secretions that are released outside the body (*exo* means "out of" in Greek) or into the digestive tract (which is actually a hollow tube continuous with the outside world). Exocrine gland secretions are released through tubes or openings called **ducts**. The exocrine glands include the sweat and sebaceous (oil-producing) glands of the skin, the lacrimal (tear-producing) glands of the eye, the mammary (milk-producing) glands, as well as glands producing digestive secretions.

Endocrine glands, sometimes called ductless glands, release their hormones within the body (*endo* means "inside of"). An endocrine gland generally consists of clusters of hormone-producing cells embedded within a network of capillaries. The cells secrete their hormones into the extracellular fluid surrounding the capillaries. The hormones then enter the capillaries by diffusion and are distributed throughout the body by the bloodstream.

The Hypothalamus Controls the Secretions of the Pituitary Gland

The **hypothalamus** is a part of the brain that contains clusters of specialized nerve cells, called **neurosecretory cells**. Neurosecretory cells synthesize peptide hormones, store them, and release them when stimulated. The **pituitary** is a pea-sized gland that dangles from the hypothalamus by a stalk (Figs. 35-1 and 35-4, p. 686). Anatomically, the pituitary consists of two distinct lobes, or parts: the **posterior pituitary** and the **anterior pituitary**. The hypothalamus con-

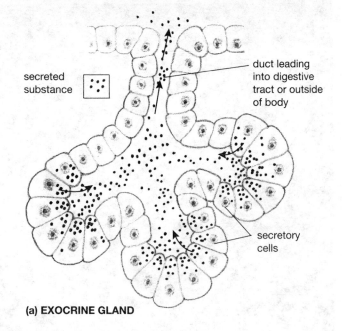

secreted substance

duct leading into digestive tract or outside of body

secretory cells

(a) EXOCRINE GLAND

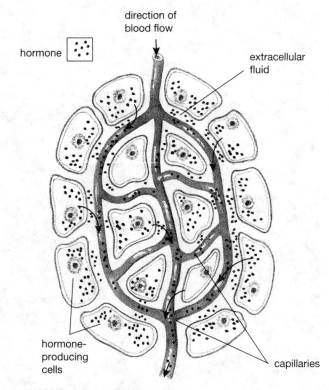

direction of blood flow

hormone

extracellular fluid

hormone-producing cells

capillaries

(b) ENDOCRINE GLAND

Figure 35-3 **The structure of exocrine and endocrine glands**

(a) The secretory cells of exocrine glands secrete substances into ducts that usually open outside the body (sweat glands, mammary glands) or into the digestive tract (pancreas, salivary glands). **(b)** Endocrine glands consist of hormone-producing cells embedded with a network of capillaries. The cells secrete hormones into the extracellular fluid from which they diffuse into the capillaries.

TABLE 35-2 ❊ *Mammalian Endocrine Glands and Hormones*

Endocrine Gland	Hormone	Type of Chemical	Principal Function
Hypothalamus (via posterior pituitary)	Antidiuretic hormone (ADH)	Peptide	Promotes reabsorption of water from kidneys; constricts arterioles
	Oxytocin	Peptide	In females, stimulates contraction of uterine muscles during childbirth, milk ejection, and maternal behaviors; in males, causes sperm ejection
Hypothalamus (to anterior pituitary)	Releasing and inhibiting hormones	Peptides	At least nine hormones; releasing hormones stimulate release of hormones from anterior pituitary; inhibiting hormones inhibit release of hormones from anterior pituitary
Anterior pituitary	Follicle-stimulating hormone (FSH)	Peptide	In females, stimulates growth of follicle, secretion of estrogen, and perhaps ovulation; in males, stimulates spermatogenesis
	Luteinizing hormone (LH)	Peptide	In females, stimulates ovulation, growth of corpus luteum, and secretion of estrogen and progesterone; in males, stimulates secretion of testosterone
	Thyroid-stimulating hormone (TSH)	Peptide	Stimulates thyroid to release thyroxine
	Growth hormone	Peptide	Stimulates growth, protein synthesis, and fat metabolism; inhibits sugar metabolism
	Adrenocorticotropic hormone (ACTH)	Peptide	Stimulates adrenal cortex to release hormones, especially glucocorticoids
	Prolactin	Peptide	Stimulates milk synthesis in and secretion from mammary glands
Thyroid	Thyroxine	Modified amino acid	Increases metabolic rate of most body cells; increases body temperature; regulates growth and development
	Calcitonin	Peptide	Inhibits release of calcium from bones
Parathyroid	Parathormone	Peptide	Stimulates release of calcium from bone; promotes absorption of calcium by intestines; promotes reabsorption of calcium by kidneys
Adrenal medulla	Epinephrine and norepinephrine (adrenaline and noradrenaline)	Modified amino acids	Increase levels of sugar and fatty acids in blood; increase metabolic rate; increase rate and force of contractions of the heart; constrict some blood vessels
Adrenal cortex	Glucocorticoids	Steroid	Increase blood sugar; regulate sugar, lipid, and fat metabolism; anti-inflammatory effects
	Aldosterone	Steroid	Increases reabsorption of salt in kidney
	Testosterone	Steroid	Causes masculinization of body features, growth

trols the release of hormones from both parts. The anterior pituitary is a true endocrine gland, composed of several types of hormone-secreting cells enmeshed in a network of capillaries. The posterior pituitary, on the other hand, is derived from an outgrowth of the hypothalamus.

The Posterior Pituitary Releases Hormones Produced by Cells in the Hypothalamus

The posterior pituitary contains the endings of two types of neurosecretory cells whose cell bodies are found in the hypothalamus. These neurosecretory cell endings are enmeshed in a capillary bed into which they release hormones to be carried into the bloodstream (Fig. 35-4). Two peptide hormones are synthesized in the hypothalamus and released from the posterior pituitary: **antidiuretic hormone (ADH)** and **oxytocin**.

Antidiuretic hormone, which literally means "hormone that prevents urination," helps prevent dehydration. As you learned in Chapter 33, ADH causes more water to be reabsorbed from the urine and retained in the body, by increasing the permeability to water of the collecting ducts of nephrons in the kidney. Interestingly, alcohol inhibits the release of ADH, greatly increasing urination, so a beer drinker may temporarily lose more fluid than he has taken in.

Other neurosecretory cells of the hypothalamus release oxytocin from their endings in the posterior pituitary. Oxytocin triggers the "milk ejection reflex" by causing contraction of muscle tissue within the breasts during lacta-

TABLE 35-2 ▪ *(Continued)*

Endocrine Gland	Hormone	Type of Chemical	Principal Function
Pancreas	Insulin	Peptide	Decreases blood glucose levels by increasing uptake of glucose into cells and converting glucose to glycogen, especially in liver; regulates fat metabolism
	Glucagon	Peptide	Converts glycogen to glucose, raising blood glucose levels
Ovaries[a]	Estrogen	Steroid	Causes development of female secondary sexual characteristics and maturation of eggs; promotes growth of uterine lining
	Progesterone	Steroid	Stimulates development of uterine lining and formation of placenta
Testes[a]	Testosterone	Steroid	Stimulates development of genitalia and male secondary sexual characteristics; stimulates spermatogenesis

Other Sources of Hormones

Digestive tract[b]	Secretin, gastrin, cholecystokinin, and others	Peptides	Control secretion of mucus, enzymes, and salts in digestive tract; regulate peristalsis
Thymus	Thymosin	Peptide	Stimulates maturation of cells of immune system
Pineal gland	Melatonin	Modified amino acid	Regulates seasonal reproductive cycles and sleep-wake cycles; may regulate onset of puberty
Kidney	Renin	Peptide	Acts on blood proteins to produce hormone (angiotensin) that regulates blood pressure
	Erythropoietin	Peptide	Stimulates red blood cell synthesis in bone marrow
Heart	Atrial natriuretic peptide (ANP)	Peptide	Increases salt and water excretion by kidneys; lowers blood pressure

[a]See Chapter 39, 40.
[b]See Chapter 32.

tion (breastfeeding). This reflex ejects milk from the saclike milk glands into the nipples (Fig. 35-5). Oxytocin also causes contractions of the muscles of the uterus during childbirth, helping to expel the infant from the womb.

Recent studies using laboratory animals indicate that oxytocin also has behavioral effects. In rats, for example, oxytocin injections cause virgin females to exhibit maternal behavior such as building a nest, licking pups, and retrieving pups that have strayed. Oxytocin may also have a role in male reproductive behavior. In several animals, oxytocin stimulates the contraction of muscles surrounding the tubes that conduct sperm from the testes to the penis, causing ejaculation.

The Anterior Pituitary Produces and Releases a Variety of Hormones

The anterior pituitary (see Fig. 35-4) produces six peptide hormones, four of which help regulate hormone production in other endocrine glands. Two of these, **follicle-stimulating hormone (FSH)** and **luteinizing hormone (LH)**, stimulate production of sperm and testosterone in males and eggs, estrogen, and progesterone in females. We will discuss the roles of FSH and LH in more detail in Chap-

ter 39. **Thyroid-stimulating hormone (TSH)** stimulates the thyroid gland to release its hormones, and **ACTH**, or **adrenocorticotropic hormone** ("hormone that stimulates the adrenal cortex"), causes the release of hormones from the adrenal cortex. We discuss the effects of thyroid and adrenal cortical hormones later in this chapter.

The remaining two hormones of the anterior pituitary, prolactin and growth hormone, do not act on other endocrine glands. **Prolactin**, in conjunction with other hormones, stimulates the development of the mammary glands (which are exocrine glands) during pregnancy. Suckling by the newborn infant then stimulates further release of prolactin, which in turn stimulates milk secretion. When the infant no longer suckles, prolactin secretion is turned off, and the ability to produce milk is lost within a few days.

Growth hormone regulates the growth of the body. Growth hormone acts on all the body's cells, increasing protein synthesis, fat utilization, and the storage of carbohydrates. During maturation, it has a stimulatory effect on bone growth, which influences the ultimate size of the adult organism. Much of the normal variation in human height is due to differences in secretion of growth hormone from the anterior pituitary. Too little growth hormone causes some cases of

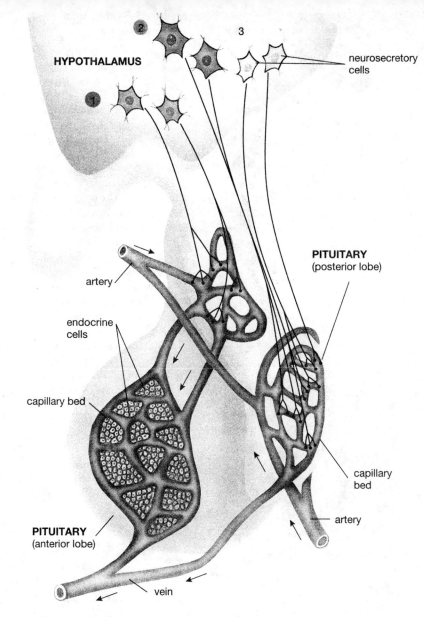

ANTERIOR LOBE	
Hormone	Target Organs
Follicle-stimulating hormone (FSH)	Gonads
Luteinizing hormone (LH)	
Thyroid-stimulating hormone (TSH)	Thyroid
Adrenocorticotropic hormone (ACTH)	Adrenal cortex
Prolactin	Mammary glands
Growth hormone	Most cells
POSTERIOR LOBE	
Hormone	Target Organs
Oxytocin	Uterus, mammary glands
Antidiuretic hormone (ADH)	Kidneys

Figure 35-4 **Anatomical relationships between the hypothalamus and pituitary**

The anterior lobe of the pituitary (left) consists of secretory cells enmeshed in a capillary bed. Release of hormones from these cells is controlled by releasing and inhibiting hormones produced by neurosecretory cells ① of the hypothalamus. These neurosecretory cells release their hormones into a capillary network directly "upstream" from the anterior pituitary (see Fig. 35-7). The posterior lobe of the pituitary (right) is an extension of the hypothalamus. Two types of neurosecretory cells, ② and ③, whose cell bodies are found in the hypothalamus, have cell endings on a capillary bed in the posterior lobe, where they release their hormones. The table shows the hormones of the anterior and posterior pituitary and their target organs.

dwarfism, whereas too much can cause gigantism (Fig. 35-6). Although in adulthood many bones lose their ability to grow, growth hormone continues to be secreted throughout life, helping to regulate protein, fat, and sugar metabolism.

A major advance in the treatment of dwarfism occurred when molecular biologists successfully inserted the gene for human growth hormone into bacteria, which churn out large quantities of the substance (see Chapter 14). Previously, tiny amounts were extracted from human cadavers at great cost. Now children with underactive pituitary glands who would previously have been dwarfs can achieve normal height.

Hypothalamic Hormones Exert Control over the Anterior Pituitary

Neurosecretory cells of the hypothalamus produce at least nine peptide hormones that regulate the release of hormones from the anterior pituitary. These peptides are called **releasing hormones** or **inhibiting hormones** depending on whether they stimulate or prevent the release of pituitary hormone (Fig. 35-7). Releasing and inhibiting hormones are synthesized in nerve cells in the hypothalamus, secreted into a capillary bed in the lower portion of the hypothalamus, and travel a short distance through blood vessels down the pituitary stalk to a second capillary bed surrounding the endocrine cells of the anterior pituitary (see Fig. 35-4). There, the releasers and inhibitors diffuse out of the capillaries and influence pituitary hormone secretion.

Because the releasing and inhibiting hormones are secreted very close to the anterior pituitary, they are produced only in minute amounts. Not surprisingly, they were extremely difficult to isolate and study. Andrew Schally and Roger Guillemin, American endocrinologists who shared the Nobel Prize in 1977 for characterizing several of these hormones, used the brains of millions of sheep

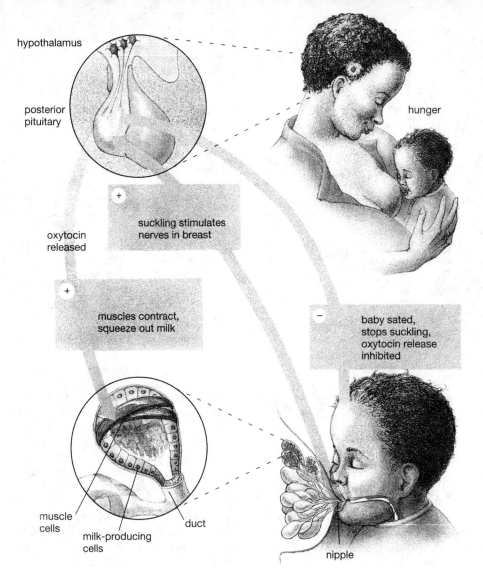

Figure 35-5 Hormones and breastfeeding

The control of milk letdown by oxytocin during breastfeeding is regulated by positive (+) and negative (–) feedback between the baby and its mother. The breast, or mammary gland, is an exocrine gland. Here, clusters of milk-producing cells surround hollow bulbs, where milk collects in lactating women. The bulbs are surrounded by muscle that can expel the milk through the nipple. Milk is expelled when suckling by the baby stimulates nerve endings that send a signal to the mother's hypothalamus, causing secretion of oxytocin into the bloodstream by the posterior pituitary. When oxytocin reaches the muscles surrounding the milk ducts, it causes them to contract and expel milk through the nipple. This cycle continues until the infant is full and stops suckling. With the nipple no longer being stimulated, oxytocin release stops, the muscles relax, and milk flow ceases.

and pigs (obtained from slaughterhouses) to extract enough releasing hormone to analyze.

The Thyroid and Parathyroid Glands Are Located in the Neck

In the front of the neck, nestled around the larynx, lies the **thyroid gland** (Fig. 35-8a). The four small discs of the **parathyroid glands** are embedded in the back of the thyroid.

The thyroid produces two major hormones, **thyroxine** and **calcitonin**. Thyroxine is an iodine-containing modified amino acid that raises the metabolic rate of most body cells. Calcitonin is a peptide important in calcium metabolism.

In juvenile animals, including humans, thyroxine helps regulate growth, stimulating both metabolic rate and the development of the nervous system. Cretinism, caused by undersecretion of thyroid hormone from birth, results in mentally retarded dwarfs. Fortunately, early diagnosis and thyroxine supplementation can prevent this tragedy. Pre-

cocious development in vertebrate animals is triggered by oversecretion of thyroxine. In 1912, in one of the first demonstrations of hormone action, a physiologist discovered that thyroxine can induce early metamorphosis in tadpoles (see "Evolutionary Connections: The Evolution of Hormones").

Thyroxine influences most of the cells in the body, elevating their metabolic rate. Its effects include increasing oxygen consumption and heart rate and stimulating the synthesis of enzymes that break down glucose and provide energy. In adults, an elevated metabolic rate seems to be involved in regulating body temperature and stress reactions. Exposure to cold, for example, greatly increases thyroid hormone production.

Levels of thyroxine in the bloodstream are finely tuned by negative feedback loops. Thyroxine release is stimulated by thyroid-stimulating hormone (TSH) from the anterior pituitary, which in turn is stimulated by a releasing hormone from the hypothalamus. The amount of TSH released from

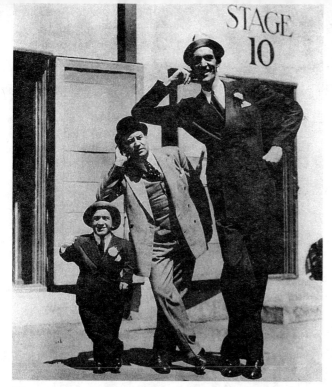

Figure 35-6   When the anterior pituitary malfunctions

An improperly functioning anterior pituitary can produce either too much or too little growth hormone. Too much can result in gigantism; too little causes dwarfism.

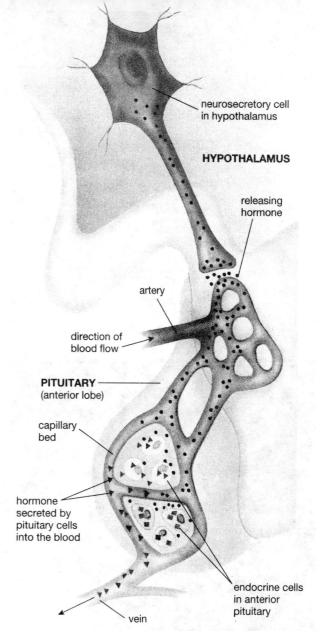

Figure 35-7   The hypothalamus controls the anterior pituitary

Hormone release from the anterior pituitary is under the control of releasing and inhibiting hormones from neurosecretory cells of the hypothalamus. Releasing hormones enter a capillary bed in the hypothalamus and travel downstream to capillaries in the anterior pituitary. There the releasing hormones contact the various endocrine cells of the pituitary. Only endocrine cells with matching cell membrane receptors respond to a given releasing hormone (see Fig. 35-2a), so each releasing hormone stimulates a particular type of endocrine cell to release its hormone while leaving other types unaffected.

the pituitary is regulated by thyroxine levels in the blood (Fig. 35-9): High concentrations of thyroxine inhibit the secretion of both the releasing hormone and TSH, thus inhibiting further release of thyroxine from the thyroid.

Iodine deficiency causes a reduction in thyroxine that stimulates dramatic growth of the thyroid (increasing the number of thyroxine-producing cells), an example of a feedback mechanism acting to restore normal hormone levels. The enlarged gland bulges from the neck, producing a condition called **goiter** (Fig. 35-8b). Goiter was once common in some regions of the United States, but widespread use of iodized salt has now all but eliminated this condition in developed countries.

Calcitonin, along with **parathormone**, the hormone secreted by the parathyroids, controls the concentration of calcium in the blood and other body fluids. Calcium is essential for many processes, including nerve and muscle function, so the calcium concentration in body fluids must be kept within narrow limits. Calcitonin and parathormone regulate calcium absorption and release by the bones, which serve both as a skeleton and as a bank into which calcium can be deposited or withdrawn as necessary. In response to low blood calcium, the parathyroids release parathormone, which causes release of calcium from bones. The parathyroids increase in size in pregnant and lactating women, thereby enhancing parathormone output and allowing the mother's

body to meet the extra demands for calcium imposed by the developing fetus and, later, milk production. If blood calcium levels become too high, the thyroid releases calcitonin, which inhibits the release of calcium from bones.

325

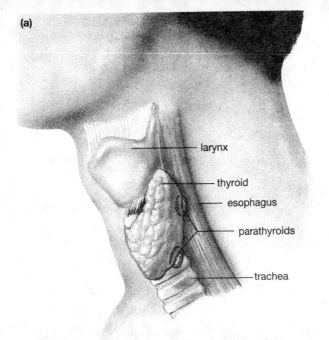

(a)

larynx

thyroid

esophagus

parathyroids

trachea

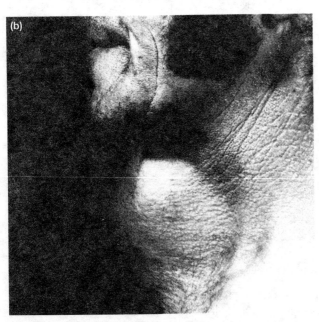

(b)

Figure 35-8   **The thyroid and parathyroid glands**

(a) The thyroid and parathyroid glands are located around the front of the larynx in the neck. (b) Individuals with iodine-deficient diets may suffer from goiter, a condition in which the thyroid becomes greatly enlarged.

The Pancreas Is Both an Exocrine and an Endocrine Gland

The **pancreas** is a double gland producing both exocrine and endocrine secretions (Fig. 35-10). The exocrine portion synthesizes digestive secretions that are released into the pancreatic duct and flow into the small intestine (see Chapter 32). The endocrine portion consists of clusters of cells, called **islet cells**, that produce peptide hormones.

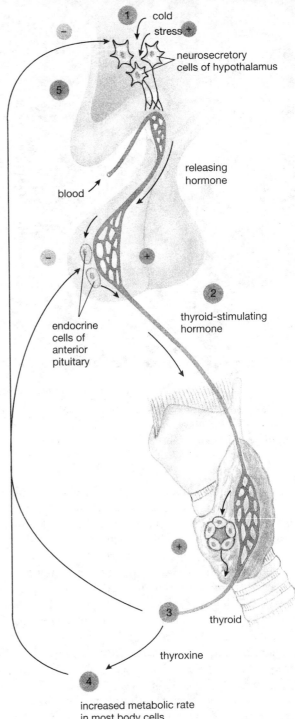

1 cold

stress

– +

neurosecretory
cells of hypothalamus

5

releasing
hormone

blood

– +

endocrine
cells of
anterior
pituitary

thyroid-stimulating
hormone

2

+

thyroid

3

thyroxine

+

4

increased metabolic rate
in most body cells

Figure 35-9   **Negative feedback in thyroid function**

Low body temperature or stress stimulates neurosecretory cells of the hypothalamus ①, whose releasing hormones trigger thyroid-stimulating hormone (TSH) release in the anterior pituitary ②. TSH then stimulates the thyroid to release thyroxine ③. Thyroxine causes increased metabolic activity in most cells of the body, generating ATP energy and heat ④. Both the raised body temperature and high thyroxine levels in the blood inhibit the releasing-hormone cells and the TSH-producing cells ⑤.

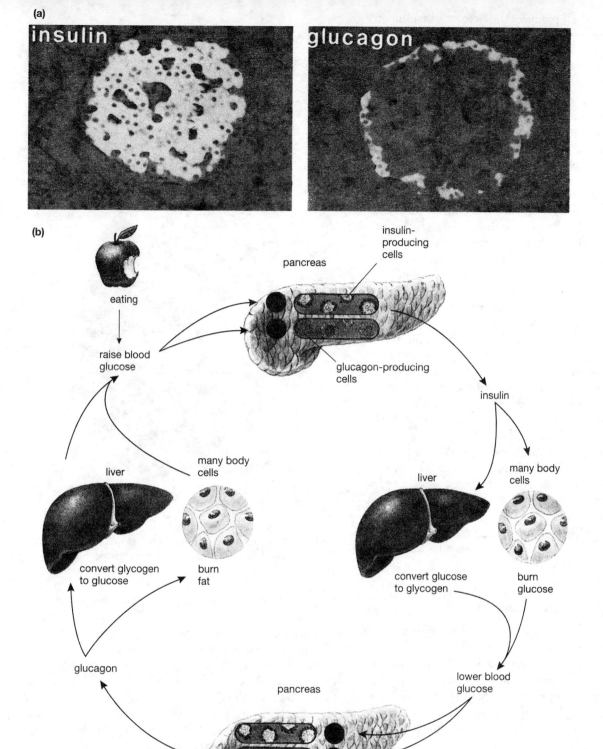

Figure 35-10 **The pancreas islets control blood glucose levels**

(a) The pancreatic islets contain two populations of hormone-producing cells, one producing insulin, the other glucagon. (b) These two hormones cooperate in a two-part negative feedback loop to control blood glucose concentrations. High blood glucose stimulates the insulin cells and inhibits the glucagon cells; low blood glucose stimulates the glucagon cells and inhibits the insulin cells. This dual control quickly corrects either high or low blood glucose levels.

One type of islet cell produces the hormone **insulin**; another type produces **glucagon**.

Insulin and glucagon work in opposite ways to regulate carbohydrate and fat metabolism. When blood glucose rises (for example, after a meal), insulin is released. Insulin causes most of the cells of the body to take up glucose and either metabolize it for energy or convert it to fat or glycogen (a starchlike molecule) for storage. By far the most important storage organ for glycogen is the liver. When blood glucose levels drop (for example, after a person skips breakfast or runs a 10-kilometer race), glucagon is released. Glucagon activates a liver enzyme that breaks down glycogen, releasing glucose into the blood. It also promotes lipid breakdown, releasing fatty acids that are metabolized for energy. Insulin, then, reduces blood glucose levels, whereas glucagon increases them; together they help keep blood glucose levels nearly constant.

Defects in insulin production, release, or reception by target cells result in **diabetes mellitus**, a condition in which blood glucose levels are high and fluctuate wildly with sugar intake. The lack of functional insulin in diabetics causes the body to rely much more heavily on fats as an energy source, leading to high circulating levels of lipids, including cholesterol. Severe diabetes causes fat deposits in the blood vessels, resulting in high blood pressure and heart disease; diabetes is an important cause of heart attacks in the United States. The fatty deposits in small vessels can also damage the retina of the eye, leading to blindness, and the kidneys, leading to kidney failure. Insulin supplements traditionally contained insulin extracted from the pancreases of cows and pigs, obtained from slaughterhouses. Recently, however, the gene for human insulin has been inserted into bacteria, allowing the production of large quantities of human insulin, which is now commercially available.

The Sex Organs Secrete Steroid Hormones

The male testes and female ovaries are important endocrine organs. The testes secrete several steroid hormones, collectively called **androgens**. The most important of these is **testosterone**. The ovary secretes two types of steroid hormones, **estrogen** and **progesterone**. The role of the sex hormones in development, the menstrual cycle, and pregnancy is discussed in Chapters 39 and 40.

The Adrenal Glands Have Two Parts That Secrete Different Hormones

Like the pituitary and pancreas, the adrenals (Latin for "on the kidney") are two glands in one: the adrenal medulla and the adrenal cortex (Fig. 35-11). The **adrenal medulla** is located in the center of each gland (*medulla* means "marrow" in Latin). It consists of secretory cells derived during development from nervous tissue, and its hormone secretion is controlled directly by the nervous

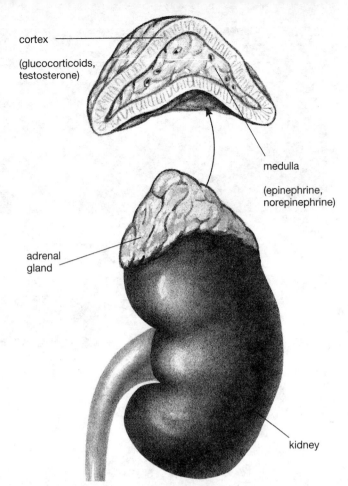

Figure 35-11   The adrenal glands

Atop each kidney sits an adrenal gland, which is a two-part gland composed of very dissimilar cells. The outer cortex consists of ordinary endocrine cells that secrete steroid hormones. The inner medulla is derived from nervous tissue during development and secretes epinephrine and norepinephrine.

system. The adrenal medulla produces two hormones, **epinephrine** and **norepinephrine** (also called **adrenaline** and **noradrenaline**), in response to stress. These hormones, which are modified amino acids, prepare the body for emergency action. They increase the heart and respiratory rates, cause blood glucose levels to rise, and direct blood flow away from the digestive tract and toward the brain and muscles. The adrenal medulla is activated by the sympathetic nervous system, which prepares the body to respond to emergencies, as described in Chapter 36.

The outer layer of the adrenal gland forms the **adrenal cortex** (*cortex* is Latin for "bark"). The cortex secretes three types of steroid hormones synthesized from cholesterol, called **glucocorticoids**. These hormones help control glucose metabolism. Glucocorticoid release is stimulated by ACTH from the anterior pituitary; ACTH release in turn is stimulated by releasing hormones produced by the hypothalamus in response to stressful stimuli, including trauma, infection, or exposure to extremes of temperature. In some respects, the glucocorticoids act similarly to glucagon, raising blood glucose levels by stimulating glucose production and promoting the use of fats instead of glucose for energy production.

You may have noticed that many different hormones are involved in glucose metabolism: thyroxine, insulin, glucagon, epinephrine, and the glucocorticoids. Why? The reason can probably be traced to a metabolic requirement of the brain. Although most body cells can produce energy from fats and proteins as well as carbohydrates, brain cells can burn only glucose. Thus, blood glucose levels cannot be allowed to fall too low, or brain cells rapidly starve, leading to unconsciousness and death.

The adrenal cortex also secretes **aldosterone**, which regulates the sodium content of the blood. Sodium ions, derived from salt in the diet, are the major positive ions in blood and fluid surrounding cells. The sodium ion gradient across cell membranes (high outside, low inside) is used in many cellular events, including the production of electrical signals by nerve cells (see Chapter 36). If blood sodium falls, the adrenal cortex releases aldosterone, which causes the kidneys and sweat glands to retain sodium. Then salt and other sources of dietary sodium, combined with aldosterone-induced sodium conservation, raise blood sodium levels again, shutting off further aldosterone secretion. Too much salt increases the osmolarity of blood and extracellular fluid, drawing water out of cells by osmosis and increasing extracellular fluid and blood volume. The result is a decrease in aldosterone release that allows the kidneys to excrete more sodium.

Finally, the adrenal cortex produces the male sex hormone testosterone, although normally in much smaller amounts than the testes produce. Tumors of the adrenal medulla sometimes lead to excessive testosterone release, causing masculinization of women. Many of the "bearded ladies" who once appeared in circus sideshows probably suffered from this condition.

Many Types of Cells Produce Prostaglandins

Unlike most other hormones, which are synthesized by a limited number of cells, prostaglandins are produced by many, perhaps all, cells of the body. They are modified fatty acids, synthesized by the cell from membrane phospholipids. Several prostaglandins are known, and probably a great many more await discovery. One prostaglandin causes arteries to constrict and stops bleeding from the umbilical cords of newborn infants. Another prostaglandin works in conjunction with oxytocin during labor, stimulating uterine contractions. Prostaglandin-soaked vaginal suppositories are currently used to induce labor. Menstrual cramps are caused by the overproduction of uterine prostaglandins, stimulating uterine contractions.

Some prostaglandins cause inflammation (such as occurs in arthritic joints) and stimulate pain receptors. Drugs such as aspirin and ibuprofen, which inhibit prostaglandin synthesis, can provide relief. Some prostaglandins expand

the air passages of the lungs, and one day asthma sufferers may benefit from research into this effect. Others stimulate production of the protective mucus that lines the stomach, a potential boon for ulcer patients. Research on this diverse and potent family of compounds is still in its infancy, but it promises many health benefits in the future.

Other Endocrine Organs Include the Pineal Gland, Thymus, Kidneys, Heart, and Digestive Tract

The **pineal gland** is located between the two hemispheres of the brain, just above and behind the brainstem (see Fig. 35-1). Named for its resemblance to a pine cone, the pineal is smaller than a pea. In 1646, the philosopher René Descartes described it as "the seat of the rational soul." Since then, scientists have learned more about this organ, although many of its functions are still poorly understood. The pineal produces the hormone **melatonin**, a modified amino acid. Melatonin is secreted in a daily rhythm, which in mammals is regulated by the eyes. In some vertebrates, such as the frog, the pineal itself contains photoreceptive cells, and the skull above it is thin, so the pineal can detect sunlight and thus daylength. By responding to daylengths characteristic of different seasons, the pineal appears to regulate the seasonal reproductive cycles of many mammals. Despite years of research, the function of the human pineal and of melatonin is still unclear. One hypothesis is that the pineal and melatonin secretion influence sleep-wake cycles. Improper pineal function may contribute to the depression that some people experience during the short days of winter.

The **thymus** is located in the chest cavity behind the breastbone, or sternum (see Fig. 35-1). In addition to producing white blood cells, the thymus produces the hormone **thymosin**, which stimulates the development of specialized white blood cells (T cells) that play an important role in the immune system (see Chapter 34). The thymus is extremely large in the infant, but begins decreasing in size after puberty.

The kidney, which plays a central role in maintaining body fluid homeostasis, has recently been recognized as an important endocrine organ as well. When the oxygen content of the blood drops, the kidney produces the hormone **erythropoietin**, which increases red blood cell production, as described in Chapter 30. The kidney also produces a second hormone, **renin**, in response to low blood pressure, such as may be caused by bleeding. Renin is an enzyme that catalyzes the production of another hormone, called **angiotensin**, from proteins in the blood. Angiotensin raises blood pressure by constricting arterioles. It also stimulates aldosterone release by the adrenal cortex, causing the kidneys to retain sodium, which in turn increases blood volume.

The heart seems an unlikely endocrine organ, but in 1981, a substance extracted from heart atrial tissue was found to cause an increase in the output of salt and water by the kidneys when injected into rats. Two years later, the active substance, **atrial natriuretic peptide (ANP)**, was described and its amino acid sequence determined. This peptide is released by cells in the atria of the heart when blood volume increases. Increased blood volume causes extra distension of the heart. Atrial natriuretic peptide causes reduction of blood volume by decreasing the release of both ADH and aldosterone. The pace of modern biomedical research is astonishing: Only 5 years after the factor was first detected in heart extract, clinical trials of synthetic ANP were started to test its value in treating high blood pressure and related problems.

The stomach and small intestine produce a variety of peptide hormones that help regulate digestion. These hormones include **gastrin**, **secretin**, and **cholecystokinin**, discussed in Chapter 32.

E V O L U T I O N A R Y C O N N E C T I O N S

The Evolution of Hormones

Not long ago, vertebrate endocrine systems were considered unique to our phylum, and the endocrine chemicals were thought to have evolved expressly for their role in vertebrate physiology. In recent years, however, physiologists have discovered that hormones are evolutionarily ancient. Insulin, for example, is found not only in vertebrates but also in protists, fungi, and bacteria, although research has not yet determined the function of insulin in most of those organisms. Protists also manufacture ACTH, although of course they have no adrenal glands to stimulate. Yeasts have receptors for estrogen but, of course, no ovaries.

Thyroid hormones have been found in certain invertebrates, such as worms, insects, and mollusks, as well as in vertebrates. Even among vertebrates, the effects of chemically identical hormones, secreted by the same glands, may vary dramatically from organism to organism. Let's look briefly at the diverse effects that the thyroid hormone thyroxine has on several different organisms.

Some fish undergo radical physiological changes during their lifetimes. A salmon, for example, begins life in fresh water, migrates to the ocean, and finally returns to fresh water to spawn. In the stream where it hatched, fresh water tends to enter the fish's tissues by osmosis; in salt water, the fish tends to lose water, becoming dehydrated. The fish's migrations, therefore, require complete revamping of salt and water control. In salmon, one of the functions of thyroxine is to produce the metabolic changes necessary to go from life in streams to life in the ocean.

In amphibians, thyroxine has the dramatic effect of triggering metamorphosis. In 1912, in one of the first demonstrations of the action of any hormone, tadpoles were fed minced horse thyroid. As a result, they meta-

morphosed prematurely into miniature adult frogs (Fig. 35-12). In high mountain lakes in Mexico, where the water is deficient in the iodine needed to synthesize thyroxine, natural selection has produced one species of salamander that has the ability to reproduce while still in its juvenile form.

Thyroxine regulates the seasonal molting of most vertebrates. From snakes to birds to the family dog, surges of thyroxine stimulate the shedding of skin, feathers, or hair. In people (who neither migrate, metamorphose, nor molt), thyroxine regulates growth and metabolism.

The use of chemicals to regulate cellular activity is extremely ancient. The diversity of life on Earth rests upon a conservative foundation: A relative handful of chemicals coordinate activities within single cells and among groups of cells. Life's diversity originated in part by changing the systems used to deliver the chemicals and by evolving new types of responses. Early in their evolution, animals developed a complement to hormonal communication that provides faster, more precise delivery of chemical messages: the nervous system. As we explain in the next chapter, the nervous system permits rapid responses to environmental stimuli, flexibility in response options, and ultimately consciousness itself.

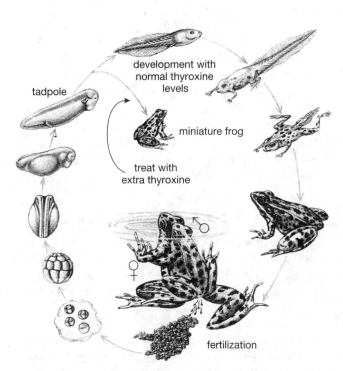

Figure 35-12 **Thyroxine controls metamorphosis in amphibians**

The life cycle of the frog begins with fertilization of the eggs (bottom); then development into an aquatic, fishlike tadpole; growth of the tadpole; and ultimately metamorphosis into an adult frog. Metamorphosis is triggered by a surge of thyroxine from the tadpole's thyroid gland. If a young tadpole is injected with extra thyroxine, it will metamorphose ahead of schedule into a miniature adult frog.

Animal Hormone Structure and Function

A hormone is a chemical secreted by cells in one part of the body that is transported in the bloodstream to other parts of the body, where it affects the activity of specific target cells.

Four types of molecules are known to act as hormones: peptides, modified amino acids, steroids, and prostaglandins.

Most hormones act on their target cells in one of two ways. Peptide hormones and modified amino acids bind to receptors on the surfaces of target cells and activate intracellular second messengers such as cyclic AMP and calmodulin. The second messengers then alter the metabolism of the cell. Steroid hormones diffuse through the cell membranes of the target cells and bind with receptor proteins in the cytoplasm. The hormone-receptor complex travels to the nucleus and promotes transcription of specific genes. Thyroid hormones also penetrate the cell membrane but diffuse into the nucleus, where they bind to receptors associated with the chromosomes and influence gene transcription.

Hormone action is often regulated through negative feedback, a process in which the hormone causes changes that inhibit further secretion of that hormone.

The Mammalian Endocrine System

Hormones are produced by endocrine glands, which are clusters of cells embedded within a network of capillaries. Hormones are secreted into the extracellular fluid and diffuse into the capillaries. The major endocrine glands of the human body are the hypothalamus-pituitary complex, the thyroid and parathyroid glands, the pancreas, the sex organs, and the adrenal glands. The hormones released by these glands and their actions are summarized in Table 35-2. Prostaglandins, unlike other hormones, are not secreted by discrete glands but are synthesized and released by many cells of the body. Other endocrine organs include the pineal gland, kidneys, heart, and the stomach and small intestine.

✖ K E Y   T E R M S

adrenal cortex	exocrine gland	pineal gland
adrenal medulla	goiter	pituitary
androgen	hormone	posterior pituitary
anterior pituitary	hypothalamus	prostaglandin
calmodulin	inhibiting hormone	releasing hormone
cyclic AMP	islet cell	second messenger
diabetes mellitus	neurosecretory cell	steroid
duct	pancreas	target cell
endocrine gland	parathyroid gland	thymus
endocrine system	peptide hormone	thyroid gland

✖ T H I N K I N G   T H R O U G H   T H E   C O N C E P T S

Multiple Choice

1. Steroid hormones
   a. alter the activity of genes
   b. trigger rapid, short-term responses in cells
   c. work via second messengers
   d. initiate open channels in cell membranes
   e. bind to cell surface receptors
2. Examples of posterior pituitary hormones are
   a. FSH and LH
   b. prolactin and parathormone
   c. secretin and cholecystokynin
   d. melatonin and prostaglandin
   e. ADH and oxytocin
3. Negative feedback to the hypothalamus controls the level of _____ in the blood.
   a. thyroxine   b. estrogen
   c. glucocorticoids   d. estrogen
   e. all of the above
4. The primary targets for FSH are cells in the
   a. hypothalamus   b. ovary
   c. thyroid   d. adrenal medulla
   e. pituitary
5. The kidney is a source of
   a. thyroxine and parathormone
   b. calcitonin and oxytocin
   c. renin and erythropoietin
   d. ANP and epinephrine
   e. glucagon and glucocorticoids

6. Hormones that are produced by many different body cells and cause a variety of localized effects are known as
   a. peptide hormones
   b. parathormones
   c. releasing hormones
   d. prostaglandins
   e. exocrine hormones

Review Questions

1. What are the four types of molecules used as hormones in vertebrates? Give an example of each.
2. What is the difference between an endocrine and an exocrine gland? Which type releases hormones?
3. When peptide hormones attach to receptors in target cells, what cellular events follow? How do steroid hormones behave by comparison?
4. Diagram the process of negative feedback, and give an example of negative feedback in the control of hormone action.
5. What are the major endocrine glands in the human body, and where are they located?
6. Describe the structure of the hypothalamus-pituitary complex. Which pituitary hormones are neurosecretory? What are their functions?
7. Describe how releasing hormones regulate the secretion of hormones by cells of the anterior pituitary. Name the hormones of the anterior pituitary and give one function of each.
8. Describe how the hormones of the pancreas act together to regulate the concentration of glucose in the blood.
9. Compare the adrenal cortex and medulla by answering the following questions. Where are they located within the adrenal gland? What are their embryological origins? What hormones do they produce? What organs do their hormones target? What homeostatic processes regulate blood levels of the respective hormones?

✖ APPLYING THE CONCEPTS

1. An enterprising student decides to do a science project on the effect of the thyroid gland on frog metamorphosis. She sets up three aquaria with tadpoles. She adds thyroxine to the water of one, thiouracil to a second, and nothing to the third. Thiouracil reacts with thyroxine inside tadpoles to produce an ineffective compound. Assuming the student uses appropriate physiological concentrations, predict what will happen.
2. Diabetes mellitus is common diabetes. Two other forms, adrenal and pituitary diabetes, are also characterized by high levels of blood glucose. What specific parts of regulatory cycles are disrupted in these latter forms to cause hyperglycemia?
3. Suggest a hypothesis about the endocrine system to explain why many birds lay their eggs in the spring and why poultry farmers keep lights on at night in their egg laying operations.
4. Anabolic steroids, used by risk-taking athletes and bodybuilders, are chemically related to testosterone. They increase bone and muscle mass and do seem to improve athletic performance. But anabolic steroids can cause liver problems, heart attacks, strokes, testicular atrophy, and personality changes in males. Females on anabolic steroids also have liver and circulatory problems. In addition, their voices deepen, their bodies develop more hair, and their menstrual cycles are disturbed. Explain how the same compound can produce testicular atrophy in males but virilism in females.
5. Some parents, interested in college sports scholarships for their children, are asking physicians to prescribe growth hormone treatments. Farmers also have an economic incentive to treat cows with growth hormone, which can now be produced in large quantities with genetic-engineering techniques. What biological and ethical problems do you foresee for parents, children, physicians, coaches, college scholarship boards, food consumers, farmers, the U.S. Food and Drug Administration, and bio-tech companies?

✖ FOR MORE INFORMATION

Atkinson, M., and MacLaren, N. "What Causes Diabetes?" *Scientific American*, July 1991.

Berridge, M. J. "The Molecular Basis of Communication within the Cell." *Scientific American*, October 1985. Both the "classical" cyclic AMP and more recently discovered second messengers convey information from cell surface receptors to DNA and cellular metabolism.

Guillemin, R., and Burgus, R. "The Hormones of the Hypothalamus." *Scientific American*, November 1972. The interaction between hypothalamus and pituitary is explored.

Sapolsky, R. "Stress in the Wild." *Scientific American*, January 1990. An interesting study of baboons showing the effects of hormones on stress responses.

Snyder, S. H. "The Molecular Basis of Communication between Cells." *Scientific American*, October 1985. Snyder describes the similarities and differences between neural and hormonal control systems in the body.

NET WATCH

On-line resources for this chapter are on the World Wide Web at:
http://www.prenhall.com/~audesirk (click on the table of contents link and then select Chapter 35).

11

INTELLIGENCE
AND TESTING

RENEE LIVED IN NORWICH WITH HER FAMILY. IT MIGHT HAVE BEEN CALLED AN EXTENDED, NO-PARENT FAMILY, FOR SHE LIVED WITH HER GRANDMOTHER AND two cousins.

The Grants, along with 30 other families, had been selected for study by a team of research psychologists from a nearby university, examining influences on the literacy of children in low-income communities. The team members were interviewing the families, observing the children, and administering various tests.

"Renee will do my homework if I sweep the kitchen floor for her," Tanya announced proudly to their visitor from the university, perhaps without fully appreciating the difference between housework and homework. They do *sound* alike. The visiting psychologist, on the lookout for the school dropout, was interested in all members of the household, including the grandmother.

Granny was virtually illiterate. In her late sixties, she was learning to read in a class held at the building where she cleaned offices every weekday evening. Granny looked forward to these classes. "The teacher is understanding," she explained.

"The best person I look up to is my grand-mother," Renee declared, "because when I want something, I get it. When I'm sick, she takes care of me. When I want to talk to her about something, she'll listen. She is like a mother to me."

Renee arrived at her grandmother's house almost ten years earlier, at age two. She was fol-lowed by her younger cousins, Tanya and Sharon. These three schoolgirls and Granny formed a close family unit, organizing their lives around the televi-sion set to a large extent. They shared their home with two long-term boarders and an intermittent stream of relatives who appeared and disappeared at a moment's notice. These transient kin seemed to have no more in common with one another, or with the Grant family, than people at a motel.

For more than 20 years, Granny had lived in the neighborhood, a low-income community, ethni-cally and linguistically mixed. She even lived in the same house, sent her children to the local school, and was sending her grandchildren there. She enjoyed watching them set out for school each day. That school was quite adequate as far as she was concerned.

Robin Henderson lived in the same neighborhood. As 12-year-old classmates in Mr. Barasch's sixth-grade class, she and Renee maintained a special friendship, although they came from quite different

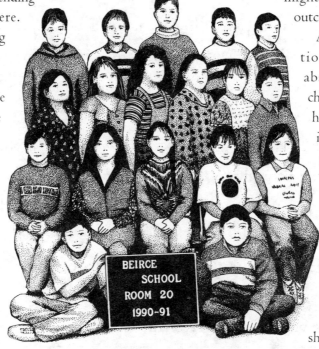

homes. Robin shared a meticulously neat and clean three-bedroom apartment with her nuclear family: both parents, two older brothers, and a younger sis-ter. For economic reasons, they had immigrated from Trinidad, and both parents held jobs outside the home.

In the Henderson household, furnished with books and magazines, schoolwork was considered most important. Ms. Henderson, in particular, held high educational aspirations for her children, an outlook that prompted her to criticize the Norwich schools from time to time. Robin was bright, and Ms. Henderson had committed herself to long-term career goals for all of her children (Snow, Barnes, Chandler, Goodman, & Hemphill, 1991).

The different intellectual abilities of Renee and Robin, the school dropout problem, and the learn-ing activities in Mr. Barasch's classroom offer a use-ful narrative about intelligence, testing, and related research questions. Renee, for example, caused some concern among her teachers. Her low scores on intelligence tests and her background in a largely nonliterate household placed her at risk for leaving school early. Would that happen? What might be done to prevent this outcome?

Amid these practical ques-tions, one long-standing abstract problem for psy-chologists and teachers alike has been the definition of intelligence. Today **intelli-gence** is most commonly defined as the capacity to learn from experience and to adapt to new sit-uations. This definition has the advantage of being applicable at vari-ous levels of the animal kingdom, but it does not show the complexity of the concept or the differences of opinion about it. Our discussion is therefore organized around four related controversies, presented in the context of the Grant family and their neighbors, the Hendersons.

First, we look at the testing movement. It began with the measurement of intelligence, still disputed today. Second, we consider extremes of intelligence, especially the question of appropriate schooling for children with retardation and giftedness. It has had a remarkably stormy history. Third, we examine diverse theories of intelligence, noting that psychologists themselves have been unable to agree on the basic nature of this concept. The fourth great controversy concerns the nature-nurture issue. Here we note the complex roles of heredity and environment in human development. In conclusion, we consider current views on a question that no longer appears controversial, at least for the moment: intelligence and aging. What happens to us intellectually as we grow older?

• THE TESTING MOVEMENT •

At the time of Granny's birth, in the first decade of this century, there were no significant psychological tests of any sort. Psychological characteristics were considered immeasurable. Intelligence, aptitude, and personality could not be measured in physical terms and therefore could not be measured at all—or so it was believed. No one would have seriously considered measuring Granny's intelligence, except a young Frenchman, Alfred Binet.

INTELLIGENCE TESTING

As director of the first psychological laboratory in France, Binet had been asked by the Ministry of Education to solve a practical problem. Which Parisian schoolchildren had insufficient ability to profit from normal classroom instruction? Decisions based solely on teachers' judgments were inap-

propriate because they could be influenced by extraneous factors: the child's conduct, appearance, family, and so forth. Binet therefore began to construct an **intelligence test,** broadly defined as an instrument for measuring a wide range of mental and some physical abilities, especially verbal, numerical, and social competence.

BINET'S EARLY SCALES. The fundamental idea in Binet's approach, which had not been attempted previously in any precise fashion, was to arrange a series of questions or problems in everyday life in order of increasing difficulty. He and his collaborator, Theophile Simon, therefore devised a number of different questions involving memory, attention, and visual discrimination. Then, by experimenting with children who were making normal progress at home and in school, they determined the difficulty of these tasks, discovering which of them could be performed by average children at each of the various age levels.

At the lowest level, for example, Binet moved around a dimly lit room with a lighted candle. No question was asked. Did the child follow the candle with its gaze, moving the eyes and head as necessary? In the intermediate range, a somewhat older child was asked to imitate gestures and obey brief requests: "Touch your nose." "Put this box on the table." At a still higher level, the child was asked to define words, remember numbers, and think abstractly. "Tell me what *pretend* means." "Say these numbers after me: 7, 4, 5, 2." Binet and Simon tested normal schoolchildren in these ways and then in 1905 published this collection of items (Binet & Simon, 1905).

Immediately, this test became a target of criticism. Detractors objected that it had an arbitrary zero point. A child who could not answer any questions nevertheless had *some* intelligence. Binet agreed, replying that his scale was not intended to be like physical measurement. His goal was merely to classify children according to ability, not to measure intelligence in absolute amounts. His test showed which children were most capable, least capable, of average ability, and so forth.

Others objected that the test did not assess inborn ability, apart from experience. Again Binet replied that his purpose had been misunderstood. His focus was on current intellectual performance, not its origins.

Psychiatrists and teachers also had grave doubts. How could a 40-minute test be more accurate than a longer interview or extended classroom experience? Binet's response was to ask them how they formed their conclusions, and it was clear that they also resorted to tests. But their tests were awkwardly applied, involved inconsistent scoring standards, and varied from one instance to another (Tuddenham, 1962).

To dispel further resistance, Binet devised an improved instrument, the 1908 scale, eliminating the weakest items and adding a variety of new ones. All of these items were identified according to age levels from 3 to 12 years. An item was included at the 5-year level, for example, because the average five-year-old child could pass it. It was too difficult for the average four-year-old and too easy for the average six-year-old. With this procedure the 1908 scale could be used to determine a child's mental age. The **mental age** (MA) is the level of mental ability of the average child at any given chronological age. All five-year-old children who are average in intelligence have a mental age of 5 years.

STANFORD-BINET SCALE. The Binet scales soon found advocates in the United States, especially at Stanford University in California. By discarding certain items, developing others, and changing the age levels, psychologists there in 1916 prepared a massive adaptation of this scale for the American population (Terman, 1916). This well-constructed test, the **Stanford-Binet Intelligence Scale,** became the leading intelligence test in the

AGE	SAMPLE ITEM
2	"Point to your toes."
6	"Tell me what's next: A minute is short; an hour is ___."
10	"Try to repeat these numbers: 8–9–4–2–6–1."
14	"How are 'begining' and 'end' alike?"
Adult	"What does this mean? 'The watched pot never boils?'"

TABLE 13-1 STANFORD-BINET INTELLIGENCE SCALE. As these illustrations show, test items for young children typically involve concrete activities, such as building with blocks or pointing to things. Those for older subjects are generally more abstract.

world. Now there are standard versions, adaptations, and short forms for different groups all over the globe (Prewett, 1992; Table 13–1).

A refinement to the concept of mental age was adapted from Germany. The child's cumulative age since birth, called the **chronological age** (CA), is also considered. Using the conventional formula, the mental age is divided by the chronological age to yield an **intelligence quotient** (IQ), which is simply a ratio of these two ages: IQ = MA/CA (100). A child with a chronological age of 10 and a mental age of 10 has an IQ of 100, for the result is always multiplied by 100 to remove the decimal point. Tests that yield intelligence quotients are constructed so that the average IQ is 100.

The advantage of the IQ is that it can be used to compare children of different ages, such as Renee, Tanya, and Sharon, all with different levels of ability. For example, a six-year-old child with a mental age of 8 would have an IQ of 133. Compared to age peers, this six-year-old child and a nine-year-old child with a mental age of 12 are equally bright (Table 13–2).

THE WECHSLER SCALES. Not long after the Stanford-Binet Intelligence Scale appeared, a group of psychologists at Bellevue Psychiatric Hospital in New York City experienced its shortcom-

$$IQ = MA/CA \times 100$$
$$= 8/6 \times 100 = 133$$
$$= 12/9 \times 100 = 133$$

TABLE 13–2 COMPUTATION OF IQ.
The conventional method of computing the IQ provides a rapid, close approximation to the modern deviation method, developed from statistical tables.

ings for work with their particular population, largely adults. These psychologists, in a hospital setting, under the direction of David Wechsler, began developing a test more suitable for clinical work. They focused on adults; they developed procedures for identifying different types of intellectual abilities; and in doing so, they recognized the disruptive role of adjustment problems, including psychiatric difficulties (Wechsler, 1939).

Appearing in 1939, this test became the forerunner of several revisions and extensions downward for younger subjects, now collectively called the **Wechsler Intelligence Scales.** The adult edition, used for people from the late teens to the mid-70s, is called the *Wechsler Adult Intelligence Scale (WAIS)* (1981). There is an edition for children, the *Wechsler Intelligence Scale for Children (WISC-III)* (1991). Another edition serves preschool children. In addition, there are Spanish versions, *Escala de Inteligencia Wechsler para Adultos (EIWA)* and another for children, *Escala de Inteligencia Wechsler para Niños (EIWN-Revisada)*, referred to later with respect to culturally sensitive testing.

In contrast to the Stanford-Binet, the Wechsler items are grouped into two large categories: verbal and nonverbal. The nonverbal category assesses intelligence without using words, an essential approach in cases of language handicaps. Then the items in these two major categories are divided into subtests. For example, the verbal subtests measure memory, vocabulary, verbal reasoning, and so forth. The nonverbal items measure capacity for spatial relations, perceptual speed, nonverbal reasoning, and the like (Figure 13–1).

Administration of a full Wechsler test provides an overall measure of intelligence, or IQ, including a *verbal IQ* and a *nonverbal IQ*, the latter also called *performance IQ*. In addition, scores on the separate subtests, when examined as a group, provide a profile of the individual's intellectual strengths and weaknesses. The capacity to generate these different profiles is an important characteristic of the Wechsler tests (Burgess, 1991).

EVALUATING TESTS

All children in Renee's sixth-grade class had been administered the vocabulary subtest of the Wechsler Intelligence Scale for Children. Renee never did well on these tests, a concern for her teachers, as well as members of the university research team. Some students, when tested once and then again

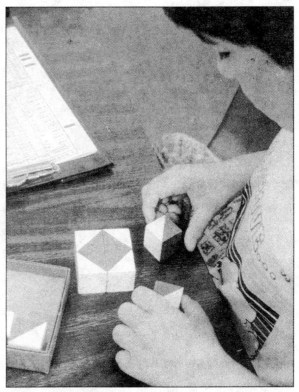

FIGURE 13–1 WECHSLER NONVERBAL ITEMS. The subject here is arranging colored blocks to form various patterns.

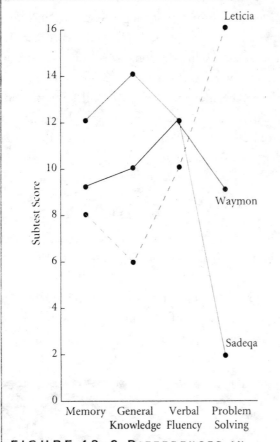

FIGURE 13–2 DIFFERENCES IN MENTAL ABILITIES. Each person achieved an average score of ten on four Wechsler subtests. However, their results form very different profiles, indicating that each overall IQ may represent diverse mental abilities.

four years later, actually obtained lower scores on the second occasion. These outcomes might have been influenced by the tendency of Mr. Barasch to use low-level textbooks. In any case, the scores were used for decisions about grade promotion and placement in reading groups (Snow et al., 1991).

Such tests can yield useful information about individuals (Figure 13-2). But they need adequate reliability, validity, and norms.

THE QUESTION OF RELIABILITY. Consider a man who is worried about his weight. Stepping on a scale, he notes that he weighs 160 pounds, an unexpected loss of 10 pounds. After stepping off the scale, he decides to weigh himself

a second time. The scale reads 158. Then, he tries his neighbor's scale, which is another version of his own model, and it gives a reading of 161. There is still some doubt in his mind, however. So he asks his neighbor to read the dial, and the neighbor reports a reading of 160.

This example illustrates the question of **reliability**, which concerns the consistency of test results—that is, the agreement among scores whenever the test is administered to the same people on several occasions.

One of Binet's early items asked the child which would be better to eat, a piece of wood or a piece of cake. If the child chose correctly on some trials and incorrectly on others, the item had low reliability. Assuming that the characteristic being measured remains constant, the answer should be the same on every occasion. Thus, **test-retest reliability** is determined by administering the test to a group of subjects, repeating the procedure later with the *same* subjects, and then comparing the two sets of scores. The test is reliable to the extent that each subject achieves the same score on both occasions.

Subjects taking a psychological test for the second time may recall their earlier answers, thereby generating an erroneously high measure of reliability. The approach here is to use **equivalent-form reliability**, which involves different versions of the same test, similar in content and structure but containing different questions. If the subjects achieve similar scores on the two versions, the test has high equivalent-form reliability.

To be useful, the answers must be scored. The issue here, called **interjudge reliability**, concerns consistency among examiners in scoring the same response. If two or more examiners award the same score to the same answer, the test item has high interjudge reliability. If not, it has low reliability and is of doubtful value.

These three types of reliability were illustrated by the man checking his weight. He stepped on his scale a second time, test-retest reliability. He tried his neighbor's version of the same scale, equivalent-form reliability. And he asked his neighbor to read the scale, a matter of interjudge reliability.

THE QUESTION OF VALIDITY. In evaluating any test, validity is the key issue. The concern in **validity** is whether a test measures what it purports to measure. A valid test accurately assesses the characteristic in question. For example, a valid test of sales ability measures sales ability, not something else.

There are many forms of validity but, among them, **face validity** is not true validity. It merely indicates that a test *seems* appropriate for its alleged purpose. The test looks like it works. In World War I, when aircraft pilots first engaged in warfare, it was decided that a good pilot would be calm and unperturbed in the face of the unexpected. Thus, it seemed that the gunshot-and-cold-cloth test would be useful. A pistol suddenly was fired near the unsuspecting candidate; later, a cold cloth was flung in his face. Hundreds of men were thereby rejected as pilots, for their reactions were judged to be too slow or too prolonged for good pilots. Later, during World War II, this test was studied further and found to be worthless. The startle pattern and hand tremors did not predict success or failure as a pilot. The cold-cloth-in-the-face test had nothing more than face validity (National Research Council, 1943).

Among the true types of validity, **predictive validity** makes a statement about the future; it attempts to forecast the performance of subjects at a later date, after they have received some form of training or other preparation. A test with significant predictive validity for aircraft pilots would identify candidates likely to profit most from pilot training.

In contrast, **concurrent validity** is concerned with the present; it indicates which subjects are best suited to perform a certain task right away, without further training. A test with high concurrent validity, for example, would identify the best person for immediate work as a translator of foreign languages or consultant in computer technology.

To determine the validity of a test, apart from face validity, it is necessary to have a *criterion*, which is a standard for judging the value of something. For a test of sales ability, sales records might be useful as a criterion. Many people would be administered the test of sales ability, and these results would be compared with their sales records. Did the people with high sales records earn high scores on the test? Did those who made few sales make low scores? If so, the test has some degree of validity for sales ability. It can identify or predict this characteristic.

However it is determined, validity generally is the most important characteristic of a test. If validity is reasonably high, ranging at least in the upper half of a scale from 0.00, meaning no validity, to 1.00, indicating perfect validity, then the test can be regarded as having some capacity for measuring what it claims to measure. Reliability coefficients are typically higher, but they do not provide any direct evidence of the validity of a test.

As a rule, a test that is valid, accurately measuring what it purports to measure, is also reliable—providing the same results on each occasion. In contrast, a test can be reliable, giving the same result each time, without measuring what it purports to measure. Requesting schoolchildren to race around the playground may produce much the same results each time, demonstrating reliability, but this test is not a valid measure of intelligence.

THE NEED FOR NORMS. The other concern is **norms,** which are standards or guidelines for interpreting a test score, developed from previous test scores. Norms are collections of prior scores that serve as reference points for determining what is normal, high, or low on a particular test or test item. Any score can be judged against this collection of scores.

When using a test, there may be a need for *national norms,* meaning scores that are representative of the population throughout the country. On other occasions, it may be more appropriate to use *local norms,* obtained from a specific group, such as the pilots for just one airline.

Using the national norms on a reading test, Renee was found to be more than a year below her expected grade level. Using the local norms for the Norwich public schools, she was closer to average. In decisions about schooling, hiring, and promotion, local norms may prove more helpful than scores from the general population (Darou, 1992).

TESTS AS TOOLS

Psychological tests are instruments for solving a problem. They provide a sample of behavior for making decisions about selection and placement. Is Ms. Henderson a promising candidate for a certain job at the bank? Is her oldest son in a school environment suited to his interests and abilities?

TYPES OF TESTS. Literally hundreds of new tests appear each year in our society, designed for all sorts of purposes. Their profusion is so great that catalogues of thousands of pages are needed to describe them, containing information on the publisher, price, and purpose, as well as on reliability, validity, and norms. The oldest of these catalogues, now in its eleventh edition, is the *Mental Measurements Yearbook* (Kramer & Conoley, 1992). It lists 18 categories of tests, summarized as five types, the first of which has been described already: intelligence, achievement, aptitude, interest, and personality.

The reader is perhaps all too familiar with the **achievement test,** which measures a person's current level of accomplishment in a particular field, ranging from Latin to landscaping. There are many national tests of this type, such as the *Wide Range Achievement Test,* used in Renee's school. When her

class was tested for word recognition, the students scored on the average 1.6 years below the national norms. In other words, their achievement was 1.6 years lower than that of the average student of their age throughout the country. Renee's level was still lower. She was a year and a half behind even her own classmates.

The capacity to learn is known as *aptitude.* An **aptitude test** measures probable accomplishment at some future date, after training. A test of flying aptitude should have high predictive validity. A test of flying achievement indicates a person's current ability as a pilot—right now, as the plane sits on the runway, ready for takeoff. It should have high concurrent validity. Electronic, mechanical, and clerical workers are the largest labor groups in the United States, and tests of these aptitudes are widespread (Figure 13–3).

There are no right or wrong answers on a vocational **interest inventory** because here people merely indicate their *preferences* for work-related activities.

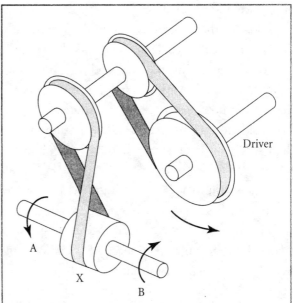

FIGURE 13–3 TEST OF MECHANICAL APTITUDE. With the driver moving in the indicated direction, determine the direction of rotation of axle *X.* In evaluating an answer, the examiner may consider the amount of time required and the probability of guessing correctly.

On the *Strong-Campbell Interest Inventory*, for example, a person reads a list of diverse occupations, school subjects, and hobbies and then for each item marks "Like," "Indifferent," or "Dislike." In vocational counseling, this information is used with a great deal of other background material, for it does not consider ability in any significant manner.

Finally, the **personality test** aims to provide a broad description of an individual, measuring characteristic habits, interests, attitudes, and other qualities, including forms of adjustment and maladjustment. Discussed at length in the next chapter, these tests tend to be broad and diverse, ranging from multiple-choice items to highly ambiguous stimuli, such as vague pictures and inkblots.

USING TESTS. All types of tests may be improperly used. The intention may be good but the practice poor. A test *must* be administered, scored, and interpreted appropriately. The misinterpretation of test scores is a most significant factor in the controversy over intelligence testing (Snyderman & Rothman, 1987; Figure 13–4).

Mr. Barasch used the Wide Range Achievement Test to establish reading groups of different levels, and Renee's performance on one test illustrates the potential danger. Her score was low, and in an interview with one of the psychologists studying the Norwich schools, she gave various explanations. She had been sick the day of the test. Moreover, she had forgotten her glasses. How could she answer the questions if she could not read them? She even recruited Granny to plead her case—so determined was she that the score should be ignored or the test administered again (Snow, 1991).

To summarize the testing movement in a positive way, at least three uses of psychological tests can be recommended without significant reserva-

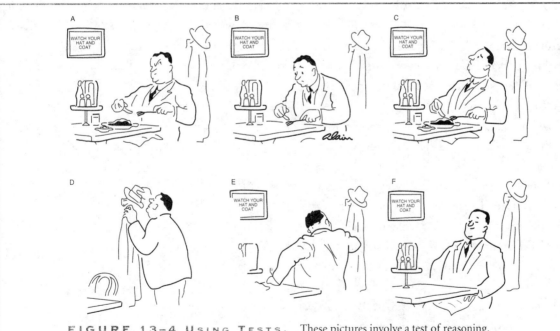

FIGURE 13-4 USING TESTS. These pictures involve a test of reasoning. Arrange them in a meaningful sequence. *Answer:* The arrangement considered correct is *D, F, C, A, E,* and *B*. However, *D* is sometimes placed last instead of first. The man is seen taking his coat and hat off the hook rather than hanging them up before eating. His dinner has been stolen, and he wants to leave before losing anything else. This reasoning lessens the joke, but the careful examiner is aware that the answer is not contradicted by evidence in the drawings.

tions. They appear to avoid most, if not all, of the limitations. First, individual tests can be useful for diagnosis. They can assist in any detailed study and understanding of one person. Second, group tests can be an efficient technique in research, useful for collecting large masses of data from many subjects. And third, group tests can be useful for identifying people with special talents. The reason is that high scores are typically more valid than low scores. People may perform below their level of ability for many reasons, but they can hardly perform above it. The superior scores can be noted and the others ignored (Jensen, 1980).

• EXTREMES OF INTELLIGENCE •

"You've got your assignment; it's time to start," Mr. Barasch said, beginning a classroom project on the computation of fractions.

"I don't like yellow paper," objected Renee, leaving her desk.

Borrowing some white sheets from classmates, she distributed them to her neighbors and kept one for herself. Then she raised her hand: "Hey, Mr. Barasch. I need help on number 16."

"Okay," he said, assisting her for a moment. As soon as he left, Renee and her neighbors began talking and giggling again.

Mr. Barasch became increasingly exasperated as the lesson continued, attempting to deal with too many students at one time, each with different needs and different abilities. Concerned that his students might be disruptive, he planned activities that were simple to supervise. One method was to ask students to read aloud. This approach of course failed to take into account their different abilities (Snow et al., 1991).

Mental abilities, and most other human characteristics, are distributed across a wide range, often according to the **normal distribution,** meaning a bell-shaped curve in which most scores cluster near

the center and the rest taper off uniformly to the extremes. On intelligence tests, the average IQ is 100, and the extremes of intelligence refer to people at the very ends of the intelligence continuum, comprising the upper and lower 2% of the general population (Figure 13–5).

Those in the lower 2%, with an IQ below 70, are people with **mental retardation** or *mental disability.* As a result, they learn more slowly than others and need more support in the learning environment. The intelligence of those in the upper 2%, with an IQ above 130, is called **mental giftedness.** Compared to others, they learn rapidly and easily, often by themselves. Whenever possible, special provisions are made for the education of both groups.

It should be noted that some people with normal or even high intelligence may have a **learning disability,** meaning a difficulty with some specific mental skill, such as reading, spelling, or mathematics. Some of these disabilities appear to be caused by perceptual deficits, others by defects in memory, many of which are not noticeable in daily life and therefore remain undetected for years, as claimed for Thomas Edison, among others. These disabili-

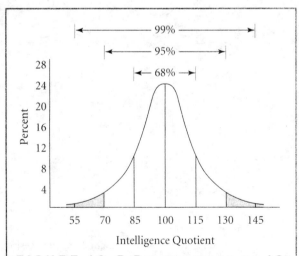

FIGURE 13–5 DISTRIBUTION OF IQ. The graph shows the approximate percentage of the general population at different points within the full range of IQs. The shaded areas represent the extremes of intelligence.

ties also may appear and disappear inexplicably, emphasizing the need for regular reevaluation of schoolchildren.

Mr. Barasch had made one provision for the differences in ability among his students. When the ten-o'clock bell rang, the six students at the highest reading level remained in his classroom—to use books with a restricted vocabulary, designed for sixth graders of *average* ability. Those in the middle and lowest groups filed into the hall, Renee included, and headed for the remedial classroom, although none of them had mental retardation. In the Norwich schools, there were special classes for those students (Snow et al., 1991).

MENTAL RETARDATION

An individual with mental retardation is described as having a handicap that ranges from mild to moderate to profound, depending on the IQ and other factors. In all cases, the focus is on treatment, not custodial care (Figure 13-6). However, before turning to that issue we should consider the causes of retardation, emphasizing that although the following factors are considered separately, they often act in combination (Scott & Carran, 1987).

GENETIC FACTORS. When retardation occurs extensively along family lines, it seems to be inherited. In such cases parents, children, and even grandchildren have received custodial care in the same institution. It should be noted, incidentally, that *incest,* sexual relations between people closely related in kinship, can be a cause of mental handicap. In these unions, the potential influence of detrimental recessive genes is sharply increased. It is no accident that the fear and stigma of incest have deep roots in human history (Jancar & Johnston, 1990).

Some instances of genetic retardation occur in **phenylketonuria** (PKU), transmitted by a recessive gene in both parents. This disorder can be diagnosed at an early age by testing the urine of new-

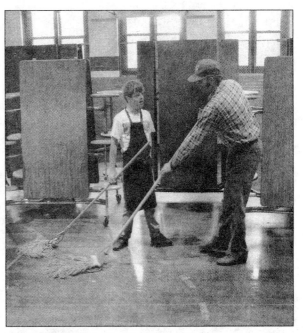

FIGURE 13-6 EDUCATION OF PERSONS WITH MENTAL RETARDATION. The instructor is using role playing to teach a student how to clean the floors. After demonstrating the correct procedure, the instructor asks the student to repeat this behavior using the same equipment.

born babies for the presence of phenylpyruvic acid, which interferes with brain functioning, producing mental sluggishness. If detected, the baby receives a controlled diet, removing the phenylpyruvic acid, and the disorder is alleviated. The symptoms also may be managed by ingestion of a phenylalanine-free dietary supplement (Hoskin, Sasitharan, & Howard, 1992).

The defect known as **Down's syndrome** is usually a condition of moderate retardation, due to a chromosomal disorder. A person with Down's syndrome has an extra twenty-first chromosome, and therefore the defect is sometimes called *trisomy 21.* The incidence of Down's syndrome increases sharply among the offspring of older mothers.

Still another form of genetic retardation, fragile X syndrome, is more common in males, accounting for 5–7% of all of their retardation, but it can also occur in females. So called because it is associated with a fragile site on the X chromosome, the **fragile X syndrome** involves difficulties in information processing, defective language, and deficits in social skills. Down's syndrome and fragile X syndrome are the most common forms of genetically based mental retardation (McEvoy, 1992; Zigler & Hodapp, 1991). Pharmacological treatment with folic acid often suppresses fragile X syndrome; it may even have a beneficial effect on cognitive and behavioral development (Curfs, Wiegers, & Fryns, 1990).

HEALTH FACTORS. In other cases, low intelligence is caused by some physical damage or disease in the pregnant woman or infant. These health problems include intoxication, brain injury, and malnutrition, and when a treatment is available, it is essentially medical. In one such disorder, **cretinism,** the individual is characteristically dwarfed, overweight, and lethargic, with an IQ that usually does not exceed 50. This problem may be related to underactivity of the thyroid gland in the mother or to nutritional deficiencies in her diet. If cretinism is diagnosed early and thyroxin is administered, sometimes this condition too can be alleviated.

A more widespread cause of mental retardation, perhaps a leading cause in the United States, is **fetal alcohol syndrome** (FAS), a cluster of traits including low birth weight, sleep disturbances, poor coordination, and low intelligence, found among infants born to mothers who consumed alcohol during the pregnancy. At one time, it was believed that this syndrome arose only through alcoholic mothers. It now appears that even very mild alcohol intake places the baby at risk (Phelps & Grabowski, 1992).

CULTURAL DEPRIVATION. Lack of normal learning experiences early in life, called **cultural deprivation,** can contribute to mental retardation. We saw this condition in the case of orphanage children left unattended and isolated for most of their childhood. They showed significantly less mental ability in adulthood than did a comparison group of children who, living in an institution with many older women, received considerable attention, stimulation, and learning opportunities (Skeels, 1966).

Over half of the children in Norwich, a small city in the northeastern United States, lived in deprived circumstances, as defined by eligibility for the free-lunch program. Only three towns in the state reported lower household incomes. Almost 25% of the students did not speak English as their native language, and many of the adults did not use literacy—reading and writing—to any significant degree. To learn to read, Renee and her cousins had to rely on a school system in which the dropout rate was increasing steadily (Snow et al., 1991).

The child deprived of early learning experiences not only fails to acquire certain necessary skills—and the conjectured brain development—but is also deprived of the intellectual tools for developing additional skills. Recognition of this "snowball effect" has prompted educational programs such as Head Start, designed to enable underprivileged children to develop to the best of their potential.

EMOTIONAL FACTORS. Intellectual functioning also can be disrupted by adjustment disorders, and many people with mental retardation experience emotional problems. The original handicap leads to frustration, which causes emotional upset, in turn engendering a further mental handicap.

One student in Mr. Barasch's class was handicapped for several reasons, including emotional factors. Very shy, he avoided his teachers and school assignments. Exposed to the frequent arguments of his parents, he was often ill or tardy at school. Assessing his chances of completing high school, his fifth-grade teacher called them "doubtful" (Snow et al., 1991).

EDUCATION OF PEOPLE WITH RETARDATION. Among several problems in educating people with retardation, one concerns children

344

who simply have some specific difficulty in a normal classroom. They are learning disabled, not mentally retarded, and usually have abilities too high for placement in special programs. In most schools, the aim is **mainstreaming,** which avoids complete separation of special-needs children and instead integrates them with other children through special provisions in the typical classroom. These provisions include greater structure, highly concrete materials, and a slower pace, including extra practice on specific tasks (Simpson & Myles, 1993; Springer & Coleman, 1992).

Children with mental retardation are often considered in three groups. The child who is *educable* is able to profit from instruction at some level of elementary school—learning academic, social, and occupational skills to the point of total or partial independence as an adult. The *trainable* child is not educable in the sense of achieving significant academic skills or social and occupational independence. This child can learn self-help skills, however, and can make limited contributions to work at home. For the *totally dependent* person, custodial care is required to fulfill personal needs and for survival.

MENTAL GIFTEDNESS

Popular belief in earlier days promoted the stereotype of a person with mental retardation as almost totally helpless, a myth that hopefully has been dispelled. Popular belief also gave a picture of the genius as physically weak and socially inferior, inept in almost everything except purely intellectual activity. Was this belief also a myth?

CHARACTERISTICS OF GIFTED PEOPLE. Lewis Terman, using Binet's instrument and others like it, decided to study this question. In fact, Terman, at Stanford University, was the chief force behind the development of the Stanford-Binet, and he identified over 1,000 schoolchildren with IQs ranging from 135 to 200. This group of

boys and girls, affectionately known as Termites, ranged from 3 to 19 years of age at the time. Terman hoped to determine the mental, physical, and personality characteristics of these intellectually gifted children.

Another purpose of this study was to observe human development throughout these people's lives, sometimes called *life span research*. The Termites were examined several times as children; they were examined again at 30 years of age; and altogether they have been studied intermittently for six decades. The oldest of all life span research, it has contributed significantly to developmental psychology and our understanding of gifted people.

Terman's findings completely contradicted the idea of the genius as a misfit. Compared with unselected children of the same age, the Termites were above average in popularity, cheerfulness, generosity, and fondness for being with large groups of people. In addition, they seemed healthier and had less mental illness. The deviation from the norm was upward in nearly all instances, a striking contrast to the popular stereotype of the socially inept child prodigy (Terman & Oden, 1947; Table 13–3).

At 30 years of age, the intellectual performance of the Termites was again in the upper 2% of the population, as much above the general adult level as it had been above the general child level earlier. Success in education and employment was much

TRAIT	PERCENT
Sense of humor	74
Cheerfulness	64
Self-confidence	81
Generosity	58
Leadership	70
Popularity	56
Fondness for groups	52

TABLE 13-3 TRAITS OF GIFTED PEOPLE. The table shows the percentage of gifted subjects who equaled or exceeded the mean for comparison subjects on each trait (Terman & Oden, 1947).

greater than one would expect in a random sample of adults of that same age (Terman, 1954).

PROBLEMS OF THE GIFTED. Experts also thought that gifted children were prone to certain problems in school, and Terman studied this question. He found that the traditional learning environment sometimes created a hardship for the gifted child, who must develop some tolerance for more typical learning rates and performance. But society must make adjustments, too. John Stuart Mill began to study Greek at age three. Charles Dickens wrote a tragedy before he was seven. Albert Einstein, at sixteen, discovered the paradox from which his theory of relativity was developed. With this precocity, tendencies to be independent and outspoken are likely.

Today we recognize that gifted people are a diverse group possessing special talents. Compared with other students, gifted individuals show a wider and less predictable range of abilities (Malone, Brownstein, von Brock, & Shaywitz, 1991; Sternberg, 1985). In particular, there is a need for programs to identify and assist gifted minority children. Given the unpredictability of special talents, these programs require precise multicultural assessment procedures (Ford & Harris, 1990).

EDUCATION OF THE GIFTED. Most students in Mr. Barasch's classroom regarded schoolwork as something to do when there were gaps in their conversations and entertainment. Robin Henderson was different.

"Oh, I know what 'puny' is," she said to Mr. Barasch, looking up from her work. "Very small."

"I want to start the story now," said Mr. Barasch. "Is everyone open to page 186?"

"Do we have to read aloud?" Kerry asked.

"Yes," announced Mr. Barasch firmly. "Robin, why don't you begin?"

Robin began the reading that day. Compared to the others, Robin read very well. She also finished assignments quickly and, on occasion, helped others with their work. Otherwise, there were no accommodations for her high level of ability (Snow et al., 1991).

Public education in the United States has concentrated largely on the typical student, aiming at mass education. There have been comparatively few large-scale programs for the gifted, who often go unattended. One argument against such programs lies in the diversity of American public school curricula, which allegedly provide the necessary enrichment opportunities already. Another states that gifted children will learn on their own, which is true to a substantial degree.

Those who promote special opportunities for the gifted raise a counterargument. They state that only by this procedure can we make the fullest use of human abilities, our most precious natural resource. It is also argued that special education for the gifted is in keeping with the basic American premise: Every student has the right to an education appropriate to his or her interests and abilities (Griggs, 1984).

As a rule, programs for the gifted involve enrichment, acceleration, or special classes, and each has its assets. In *enrichment* the child is encouraged to engage in additional schoolwork in related areas beyond the usual assignments. In *acceleration*, the child progresses to higher grades as rapidly as possible, according to mental age, not chronological age. And in *special classes*, the gifted child follows a curriculum that is faster in pace and less structured than that for the average child. Robin's school apparently did not have any extensive program of special classes for the gifted (Figure 13–7).

A rapid learner, Robin had a calmness and self-possession not evident among other students. Occasionally she showed real interest in schoolwork, asking questions, tutoring classmates, and so forth. Typically, however, she simply put her head down and slept at her seat. Mr. Barasch did not

346

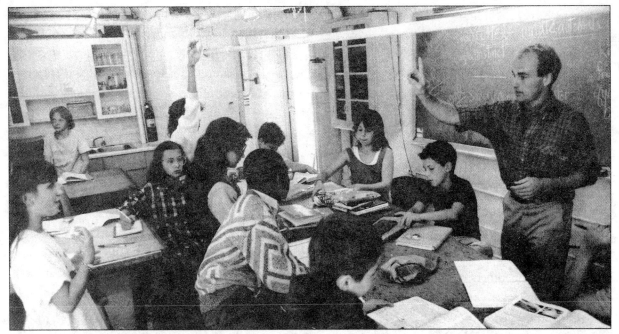

FIGURE 13-7 EDUCATION OF GIFTED PERSONS. In this special class, gifted students worked together, learning from one another. They conducted their own investigations of reflexes and instincts and shared their findings with their peers.

understand this lack of interest in school (Snow et al., 1991).

Two years earlier, in Ms. Pasquale's fourth-grade class, Robin had been distinctly more engaged in schoolwork. Ms. Pasquale was open, flexible, and challenging as a teacher. Her classroom included an extensive collection of books, maps, and teacher-constructed charts, guided by the needs of her students.

• THEORIES OF INTELLIGENCE •

Robin Henderson had lived in Norwich for six years, half of her life. Her father, a quiet man, held two jobs outside the home. He left decisions about the house and family to his wife, who worked in a savings bank. She was critical of the Norwich schools, complaining that they underestimated Robin's abilities (Snow et al., 1991).

We speak of Robin's mental abilities, for she had several talents—playing the clarinet, reading

poetry, writing stories for pleasure—and in the long-standing controversy over the nature of human intelligence, distinct types of intelligence have been increasingly recognized, especially in recent years. In the course of this controversy, psychologists have pursued two quite different paths, one older and more statistical, the other newer, broader, and more speculative.

PSYCHOMETRIC APPROACH

The first, known as the **psychometric approach,** aims to understand the mind, or *psyche*, through measurements of mental characteristics. It is based on the analysis of test results, dating back to Binet's early work.

Binet's effort produced a test far more widely acclaimed than he ever imagined, and it inaugurated the psychometric movement. Psychological tests became the means for discovering the nature of intelligence. This approach produced an efficient,

347

simple, and broad definition—which is also circular: Intelligence is what intelligence tests measure.

THE g AND s FACTORS.

After the Stanford-Binet and several other tests had been administered to many subjects, it was observed that the scores correlated with one another and that even the subtest scores were correlated. On this basis, an English psychologist, Charles Spearman, hypothesized that the different test items measured some common factor, called **general intelligence,** or g, and that many different skills involve this common factor. Mechanical ability, musical ability, mathematical ability, and others show a correlation with one another because certain amounts of g are required in all instances.

In addition to g, early theorists argued that each capacity calls for at least one **specific ability,** or s, which pertains to a particular field or skill. Facility in mathematics, for example, requires a certain amount of g and also specific mathematical abilities, such as ability to subtract, ability to multiply, and so forth, which would be the various s's in mathematical performance. Similarly, mechanical ability would require several mechanical s's, as well as a certain amount of g (Spearman, 1927).

PRIMARY MENTAL ABILITIES.

This view raised the possibility of some intermediate factors in intelligence, not as broad as g or as narrow as s. In mathematics, for example, perhaps a factor like number ability stood between general intelligence and the ability to subtract, to multiply, and so forth. If so, several such factors might account for most human intellectual capacity.

Analyses of many test scores can indicate which abilities are associated with one another and which are relatively independent. This statistical technique, called *factor analysis*, identifies the basic, irreducible factors in sets of test scores and it also reflects the psychometric approach. According to the *factorial approach*, intelligence is composed of a discrete number of factors, distinguishable because they do not correlate highly with one another.

Following this reasoning, two American psychologists, Louis and Thelma Thurstone, attempted to identify these intermediate factors. Through factor analysis, they defined seven *primary mental abilities,* readily measured by their tests. These were word fluency, number ability, verbal comprehension, memory, reasoning, spatial relations, and perceptual speed (Thurstone & Thurstone, 1941).

THEORY OF MULTIPLE INTELLIGENCES.

A more recent and controversial approach has been developed by Howard Gardner. He has postulated seven different kinds of intelligence, but his seven are *not* that seven—the seven primary mental abilities just mentioned. This approach is based on extensive research with people of special abilities, and it is controversial because it goes beyond mental functions. Stating that our traditional conception is too narrow, the theory of **multiple intelligences** addresses the broad spectrum of human abilities, including the arts, social relations, self-expression, and physical skills, as well as the traditional language and numerical abilities (Gardner, 1983).

These seven kinds of intelligence are: *linguistic,* evident in prose and poetry; *logical-mathematical,* demonstrated in mathematics, science, and philosophy; *spatial,* required in art, architecture, engineering, navigation, and related fields; *musical,* as in musical performance and composition; *bodily-kinesthetic,* essential in athletics, dance, and dramatic productions; *interpersonal,* shown in relations with other people; and *intrapersonal,* displayed in self-understanding, awareness of self, and so forth (Gardner, 1983). Clearly, these factors represent a much wider array of skills than do the older, more traditional tests of intelligence, even those in the factorial mode (Table 13–4).

One interesting difference among these factorial approaches concerns social intelligence. This

TYPE	OCCUPATION	EDUCATIONAL ACTIVITIES
Linguistic	Script writer	Storytelling, learning foreign languages
Logical-mathematical	Scientist	Playing chess, programming computers
Spatial	Sculptor	Designing tools, using a camera
Musical	Saxaphonist	Singing, listening to discs
Kinesthetic	Skater	Using athletic equipment, dancing
Interpersonal	Salesperson	Leading discussions, social activities
Intrapersonal	Self-knowledge	Keeping a journal, introspection

TABLE 13–4 MULTIPLE INTELLIGENCES. According to the theory of multiple intelligences, there are seven kinds of intelligence, each associated with certain occupations and educational activities, as illustrated by these samples. Traditional education focuses on linguistic and mathematical intelligence; the others are frequently overlooked in formal schooling (Armstrong, 1990).

ability holds a prominent place in the theory of multiple intelligences, especially in the interpersonal and intrapersonal domains, and yet it is ignored in other views. To ignore the social skills of someone like Renee Grant is to ignore her chief strength. As she reported to a member of the university research team, she began the study of Spanish by herself, not as a school subject but as a means of achieving better communication with friends (Snow, 1991). In the classroom, she was highly effective with peers, certainly a group leader, and maintained an almost collegial relationship with teachers. According to the theory of multiple intelligences, this ability should be considered a special factor in intelligence, along with linguistic ability, spatial ability, and so forth. Such views have become an important new line of inquiry among research psychologists (Riggio, Messamer, & Throckmorton, 1991).

One obvious problem with the psychometric or factorial approaches is the lack of agreement. Which are the basic factors? How many are there? Even after factor analysis, there is always some unexplained residue, perhaps because there is still some g factor present. Debate over the presence and significance of g in school and on the job continues even today (Ree & Earles, 1993; Sternberg & Wagner, 1993). Still another problem is that factors identified on a statistical basis must be labeled or

otherwise designated, a procedure that is sometimes arbitrary. In short, the factorial approach has failed to yield the specific factors of intelligence, even when the most sophisticated tests are used (Zachary, 1990).

COGNITIVE APPROACH

Modern investigations also have produced a new approach to theories of intelligence, one that arose through developments in cognitive psychology. Called the **cognitive approach,** or sometimes the *information processing approach,* it stresses how information is obtained, stored, and used—the mental operations in intelligent behavior. The focus is more on thought processes, less on test scores. The basic question is this: What cognitive processes, or strategies, do we employ when we behave in an intelligent fashion?

STRUCTURE-OF-INTELLECT MODEL.

Our discussion begins with an approach that falls between the factorial and information processing views. Developed and regularly modified by J. Paul Guilford over the course of his career, this comprehensive theory considers intellectual ability in three dimensions: how information is processed, called *operations;* what information is processed, called *contents;* and the results of this processing, called *prod-*

ucts. These dimensions are subdivided into six, five, and six parts, respectively, making a cubic model with 180 potential intellectual abilities, which define the **structure-of-intellect model** of intelligence (Guilford, 1988).

Characteristics of the operations dimension have been considered already in the chapters on perception, memory, and also thought and language. More than the others, this dimension focuses on information processing and presents the model as a cognitive theory. For example, one operation, *convergent thinking,* involves a search for a particular answer to a specific question. Which are the two largest rivers in Europe? The aim is to discover the solution generally recognized as the correct or best answer. This type of thinking is often assessed on standard tests of general information. Another operation, *divergent thinking,* procedes in different directions, seeking alternatives. What are several ways to travel around Europe without much money? The goal here is to create a number of alternatives. This form of thinking is commonly required on tests of creativity.

The contents dimension, closer to the psychometric approach, involves the various kinds of information that might be dealt with intellectually. It might include symbolic information, such as the letters and numbers in language and mathematics. It might involve behavioral information, colloquially called "body language," expressing unverbalized feelings. A very bright mathematician, for example, is not necessarily astute in understanding people.

Finally, the products dimension is concerned with results. What happens when someone performs certain mental operations on certain contents? One outcome is classes, in which two or more things are grouped together, as in concept formation. Another is systems, in which two or more things are organized in a special way, such as phrases in a sentence or postulates in a scientific theory. The products dimension is the form in which information is cast by the responding individual. Theoretically, all of the outcomes in any sort of problem solving should be found somewhere in this three-dimensional model (Guilford, 1975, 1988; Figure 13–8).

These studies have prompted the hypothesis that mental ability, like personality, shows increasing differentiation from birth through the most formative years. There may be a proportionately greater *g* factor in infants and more specific abilities in adulthood. This differentiation occurs partly on the basis of maturation, but it seems to be particularly sensitive to experience, as well.

CRYSTALLIZED AND FLUID INTELLIGENCE. By comparison, a very different theory illustrates the divergence among these views. Rather than 180, it identifies only two potential abilities, which at this point must come as a relief to the reader.

The first, **crystallized intelligence,** is based on an accumulation of knowledge about the world and an ability to apply it in solving *daily* problems. It includes facts, vocabulary, and expressive capacity. The individual with high crystallized intelligence generally is recognized as an expert in at least one field. Crystallized intelligence develops in everyday life, through learning in school, at work, around the house, and elsewhere.

The second type, **fluid intelligence,** is the capacity to solve *novel* problems not encountered previously, using rapid and accurate reasoning. These problems cannot be readily solved through prior experience; thus crystallized intelligence is not essential. Rather, fluid intelligence provides a rapid analysis of the novel problem and accurate processing of new information. In a word, fluid intelligence provides flexibility when dealing with novelty.

When you use a map successfully, solve an arithmetic problem, or spell *crystallized* correctly, crystallized intelligence is involved. Experience is a most significant factor. Fluid intelligence is required when you form an hypothesis about some

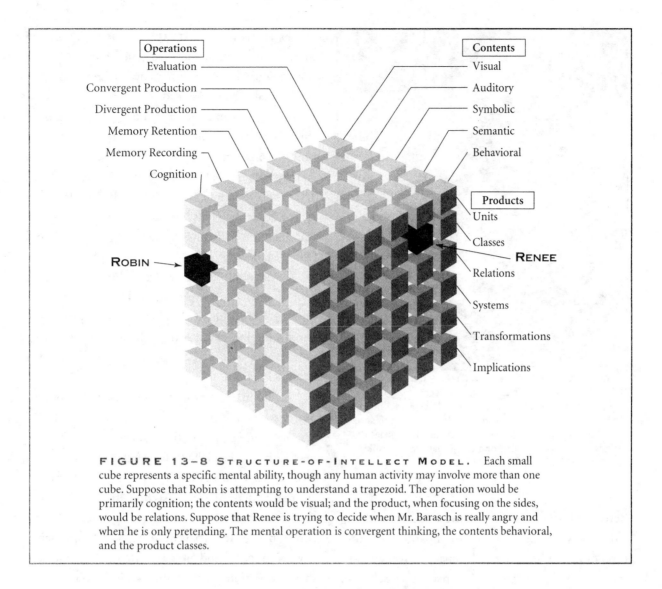

Operations
- Evaluation
- Convergent Production
- Divergent Production
- Memory Retention
- Memory Recording
- Cognition

Contents
- Visual
- Auditory
- Symbolic
- Semantic
- Behavioral

Products
- Units
- Classes
- Relations
- Systems
- Transformations
- Implications

ROBIN

RENEE

FIGURE 13–8 STRUCTURE-OF-INTELLECT MODEL. Each small cube represents a specific mental ability, though any human activity may involve more than one cube. Suppose that Robin is attempting to understand a trapezoid. The operation would be primarily cognition; the contents would be visual; and the product, when focusing on the sides, would be relations. Suppose that Renee is trying to decide when Mr. Barasch is really angry and when he is only pretending. The mental operation is convergent thinking, the contents behavioral, and the product classes.

novel problem or invent a new product. Flexibility is essential (Cattell, 1971).

TRIARCHIC THEORY. A final cognitive approach has gained attention because it is extremely broad and, at the same time, highly applicable to daily life. Developed by Robert Sternberg, the **triarchic theory** describes intelligence in three domains: componential, experiential, and contextual (Sternberg, 1985). The *componential* domain emphasizes the cognitive processes involved in typical intellectual pursuits, including school. This domain appears whenever someone answers the questions on standard tests of intelligence. Its name refers to such traditional components as perception, memory, and thinking.

The *experiential* domain turns in a different direction, focusing on the capacity to combine unique experiences in creative ways. Intelligence in this domain enables an individual to deal successfully with new situations and new tasks. To do so, the person must manage routine problems readily and easily, recognizing them as such and solving them almost without thought. This capacity leaves the individual with the interest, energy, and creativity necessary for success with novel problems.

Finally, there is the *contextual* domain, which, more than the others, is culturally or situationally

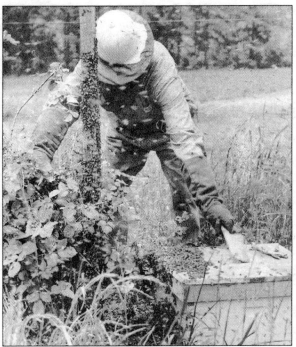

FIGURE 13-9 INTELLIGENCE AND KNOWLEDGE. The sailor is intelligent at sea, the cook in the kitchen, and the bee keeper around the hives. Knowing the habits of bees is a component of intelligence in this situation. But contextual intelligence is more than knowledge. It includes the capacity to find or create situations favorable to one's special abilities.

defined. It focuses on specific settings, ranging from the great outdoors to the boardroom, from the home to the street. Individuals with high contextual intelligence are able to place themselves in situations that require their particular talents, or they can modify settings to create a better match with their talents. Resourcefulness is vital (Figure 13–9).

The triarchic theory of intelligence aims to describe the intellectual abilities of all sorts of people in terms of these three domains, possessed in varying amounts. The students in Mr. Barasch's classroom, for example, could be approached in these ways. Robin's strength clearly lay in componential intelligence, despite her lack of interest in school. Renee was most capable in the contextual realm. With relatively little academic ability, she functioned very well in all sorts of situations outside school, especially social settings.

NONINTELLECTUAL FACTORS. As implied in the triarchic theory, intelligence should not be equated solely with mental operations. Nonintellectual factors are also involved, such as motivation, adjustment, and emotion. Intelligence, from this perspective, involves a value judgment; it is not only rational and purposeful but also directed to goals which are worthwhile (Scarr, 1981; Wechsler, 1975). For example, in the Norwich schools Robin lacked academic goals and values. In that sense, she did not have high functional intelligence in school (Snow et al., 1991).

These nonintellectual factors broaden the concept of intelligence a great deal. They also show the imposing problem of developing an adequate theory of intelligence. Fortunately, a concept can be quite useful even without a theory or a universally accepted definition.

In summary, we can conclude that the concept of *general* intelligence, prevalent at the turn of this century, perhaps has outlived its theoretical usefulness (Thorndike, 1990). Research today is guided along two complementary paths: the factorial approach, derived from psychometric studies, and the information processing approach, arising through cognitive psychology. Both approaches have been useful and are currently employed in further explorations of the nature of intelligence.

• NATURE-NURTURE ISSUE •

Parents provide our heredity *and* our early environment, quite a responsibility. There are exceptions, of course, as in the Grant family. Almost nothing is known about Renee's father, who was never mentioned around the house. After Renee's mother left the extended family years earlier, Renee rarely saw her (Snow, 1991).

Robin's mother, much involved in her children's schooling, had little formal education herself. Nevertheless, Ms. Henderson made rapid career advancement in a very short time. Her oldest son, after just a year in the United States, was a good student, reading well beyond his grade level. Ms. Henderson was concerned about her children's schooling because she knew that the roots of intelligence lie in the environment, as well as in heredity. Closed doors and a silent television during homework hours testified to this outlook (Snow et al., 1991).

Ideas on the origins of intelligence have prompted a long line of controversy dating back to Sir Francis Galton, a very bright Englishman, free from financial worries, who pondered the origins of his own high intelligence as he strolled the streets of London in 1882. He founded the first laboratory for studying mental abilities (Figure 13–10). Then he coined a phrase for the ensuing controversy. The **nature–nurture issue** refers to the debate over the contributions of heredity and environment, respectively, in the development of human abilities, especially intelligence, a controversy that continues even among experts today (Rushton, 1991; Vanderwolf & Cain, 1991).

Adding to the controversy have been mistakes, overzealous claims, and fraud on both sides. Sir Cyril Burt, an Englishman knighted for his research with identical twins, concocted data on behalf of the hereditarian view. Dr. Rick Heber, awarded several million dollars to augment intelligence among underprivileged children in Milwaukee, claimed massive changes in IQ, never issued a final report, and then was convicted of misusing federal funds (Page, 1986). These irregularities stand in marked contrast to the extensive and honest efforts that normally characterize scientific research throughout the world.

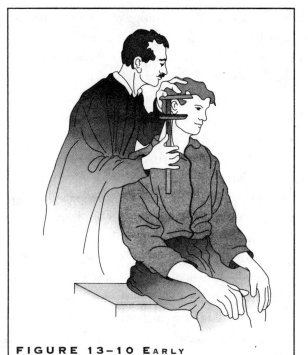

FIGURE 13–10 EARLY MEASUREMENT OF HUMAN CHARACTERISTICS. Sir Francis Galton established his first laboratory beside a fairgrounds but behind a trellis that merely allowed curious visitors to the fair to peek at the laboratory activities. He charged threepence for admission and did a thriving business. His assistants measured thousands of people for all sorts of physical and psychological traits.

STUDIES OF GROUP DIFFERENCES

Attempts to study the nature–nurture issue in large groups of human beings began most obviously in the United States during World War I, when more than 1,750,000 men were tested as they entered military service. The aim was twofold: to exclude those who were intellectually unfit and to place the others in positions most appropriate to their abilities. For these purposes, two group tests were developed: one verbal, known as the *Army Alpha*, and one nonverbal, the *Army Beta*. The outcome was a heated debate with political overtones, chiefly in the context of immigration laws.

THE POLITICAL ISSUES. One analysis of the Alpha scores echoed not only across the land but throughout the halls of Congress. Men from 16 countries were involved, and their scores showed sharp differences in intellectual ability. Those from countries in Northern and Western Europe were at the top of the scale, and those from nations in

Southern and Eastern Europe were toward the bottom. It was concluded, quite erroneously, that these national differences were due to hereditary factors (Kamin, 1974).

Subsequent inquiry disclosed that test performance was related to length of residence in the United States. Recent immigrants made low scores; those who had been here for 20 years made scores comparable to those of native-born American citizens, regardless of national background. The environmentalists, stressing the role of learning and experience in behavior, hailed this finding. It suggested that nurture, not nature, was the crucial factor.

But the hereditarians had another explanation. The Army Beta, a nonverbal test, constructed for people who did not speak English, also showed low scores for immigrants, and they were arriving in the United States in increasing numbers, much to the consternation of some observers. Again the environmentalists resisted this interpretation, claiming that exposure to the American culture was the crucial factor, even with a nonverbal test.

These data and interpretations from World War I began a long line of debate on group differences in intelligence, focusing on nationalities, racial groups, social classes, and the like. The history of this research is too long and political for inclusion here. The issue has been revived in contemporary form, however, with publication of *The Bell Curve*, a statistically based review of intelligence, genetics, and enthnicity in the context of social policy. It raised political as well as psychological questions about welfare procedures, affirmative action, and Head Start programs, provoking considerable controversy within and outside psychology (Hernstein & Murray, 1994).

Politics aside, most psychologists agree that intelligence has a genetic component and that, on conventional tests of IQ, certain subgroups score higher or lower than others. The interpretation of these differences is another matter. It seems clear that heredity contributes to within-group differ-

ences, but it is not yet apparent in what way, if at all, heredity contributes to among-group differences.

In either case, research findings alone cannot dictate social policy because political action requires judgments about goals and values. However, research findings may provide useful guidelines about the potential outcomes of various social policies (Arvey et al., 1994).

In Norwich and the surrounding area, for example, class differences were evident in the schools and homes. Towns less than 50 miles away, with the highest school budgets in the state, obtained the best, most inspirational teachers available. The low-level, uninspired approach characterizing Mr. Barasch's teaching occurred in other Norwich classrooms, resulting in a dropout rate of 25% among high school students. Whatever the sources of intelligence, in Norwich they generally were not nurtured at home or at school.

The Henderson home, however, seemed to provide some hope. Robin began the Norwich school system ahead of her grade level—although by the sixth grade she was showing a decline relative to national standards (Snow et al., 1991).

SEX DIFFERENCES. The question of sex differences in intelligence has not yet become controversial, partly because journalists have not focused on the small differences that do exist—magnifying them, debating them, or attributing them to various sources, biological or environmental. This question can be dispatched summarily because there is no significant difference between the sexes in *overall* intellectual capacity. This finding, suggested in small samples of women during World War II, has been corroborated in hundreds of studies of subjects ranging from grammar school children to psychiatric patients and college students (Kimura, 1992; Matarazzo, 1972).

There are, nevertheless, specific test items on which males and females perform differently. Binet and Terman, at the beginning of the testing movement, attempted to include in their tests an equal number of male-biased and female-biased items, or they tried to exclude such items entirely. This trend in test construction has continued, making it not surprising that large random samples of males and females score similarly on measures of general intelligence. Thus, there has been no controversy—yet.

These differences in specific abilities fit the popular notions. Women tend to perform slightly higher than men on tests of verbal fluency and perceptual speed; men tend to show somewhat greater success on tests of spatial relations and mathematical reasoning (Figure 13–11). It is not yet known whether these small but reliable findings for *specific* abilities reflect cultural or biological differences or both sets of factors in interaction (Hyde & Linn, 1988; Rosen, 1995). The influence of sex hormones on brain development begins very early in life, and during this sensitive period they may per-

manently alter brain function in ways yet to be understood (Kimura, 1990, 1992).

PROBLEMS IN MEASUREMENT. What can we say about these disparate efforts to identify hereditary and environmental factors in intelligence, whether they pertain to national, racial, social, or other characteristics? Beset with innumerable problems in measurement and testing, they leave us with respect for the complexities of this research.

In the first place, despite hopeful efforts with the Army Beta, it is virtually impossible to construct a **culture-free test** one in which the items do not favor any particular society. Some cultural factors inevitably become involved, even with the most carefully constructed nonverbal items. Robin, who spent her early years in Trinidad, came from a home that stressed reading and writing. Renee, born in the United States, lived in a home stressing work and social skills. Any test might favor one back-

---

TASKS FAVORING WOMEN

Perceptual Speed
Find the house that exactly matches the one on the left.

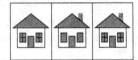

Verbal Fluency
Indicate another word that begins with the same letter, not included in the list.

Limp, Livery, Love, Laser, Liquid, Low, Like, Lag, Live, Lug, Light, Lift, Liver, Lime, Leg, Load, Lap, Lucid

Answers:
The house at the far right; Life or any other word beginning with L.

TASKS FAVORING MEN

Spatial Relations
A hole has been punched in the folded sheet. How will the sheet appear when unfolded?

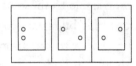

Mathematical Reasoning
In the space at the left, write the answer to the following problem.

If only 60% of seedlings will survive, how many must be planted to obtain 660 trees?

Answers:
The middle sheet; 1,100 seedlings.

FIGURE 13–11 GENDER DIFFERENCES IN MENTAL ABILITIES.
On most tests of intelligence, men and women perform similarly. These tasks illustrate some of the differences.

ground more than another. It might also favor one gender more than another, suggesting the need for a *gender-free* test as well.

Creating a test that is devoid of culture, gender, and other potential sources of bias appears to be an impossibility. For this reason, there have been attempts to eliminate all items influenced more by one culture than by another, thereby constructing a **culture-fair test** (Figure 13–12). As any test approaches the culture-fair ideal, however, it loses its capacity to predict performance in a specific situation, which is often the purpose of testing. A test equally appropriate for Trinidadians and New Englanders probably is not highly predictive of behavior in either culture.

The difficulties in developing culture-fair tests are also illustrated with the Escala de Inteligencia Wechsler para Adultos (EIWA). The Spanish Wechsler, mentioned earlier, is not merely a translation of the English version; it is an adaptation, involving many new items. However, Hispanic cultures are diverse, ranging from the Iberian peninsula to the South Pacific. This particular edition, developed in Central America, is not completely suitable for Spaniards or South Americans. Further, the test results are hardly comparable to those of the English version, even for highly bilingual people. When the two versions are used with the same bilingual subjects, the English version leads to an underestimation and the Spanish version to an overestimation of intelligence (Lopez & Taussig, 1991). Collectively, these findings point once again to the importance of **culturally sensitive testing,** meaning assessment procedures designed specifically to measure abilities and interests in a particular population or subgroup.

Still further, there is the inevitable problem of the confounded or mixed result. Highly intelligent parents provide their children with enriched environments, not only with reading materials and games but also in conversation. These children have a double advantage, a favorable heredity *and* a stim-

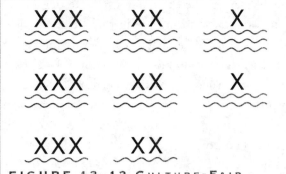

FIGURE 13–12 CULTURE-FAIR TEST. Fill in the blank space in the lower right corner. People from some cultures would be at a disadvantage in attempting this task. For this reason, such tests are often called *culture-reduced tests. Answer:* The solution is one cross above one wavy line.

ulating environment. Duller parents typically rear children in an impoverished environment. These children have a double disadvantage. Thus, the investigator cannot be certain of the influence of either factor.

Amid these difficulties, it appears virtually impossible to demonstrate conclusively the genetic basis of group differences in intelligence. Contemporary studies with sophisticated research designs have not shown any significant differences between groups that might be attributed solely to underlying genetic factors (Mackenzie, 1984; Weinberg, Scarr, & Waldman, 1992). Performance differences exist, but at this time there is no way of establishing sufficiently controlled conditions to determine the role of genetic factors in producing them.

METHODS OF ASSESSMENT

Today the basic question is no longer heredity *or* environment. Sometimes it is a question of emphasis, weighing the two sets of influences, and sometimes it is a question of interaction. How do heredity and environment unite to produce a certain outcome?

STUDIES OF IDENTICAL TWINS. Sir Francis Galton also inaugurated the study of identical twins, who have the same genetic makeup; therefore, these studies provide a control for hereditary factors. In many parts of the world, investigators have shown a relationship between the scores for members of twin pairs (Figure 13–13).

These results are commonly reported as a correlation coefficient, which provides a numerical indication of the degree of association between two variables. This coefficient, or numerical index, can vary from 0, meaning no relationship, to ±1.00, the maximum relationship. Overall, the correlations for numerous sets of identical twins are in the vicinity of .80, indicating a close relationship, or high agreement, between the scores, even when the two people have been reared apart. Correlations among fraternal twins, other brothers and sisters, and cousins are successively lower (Bouchard & McGue, 1981; Segal, 1985; Table 13–5).

This finding seems to support the hereditarian viewpoint, but there are two general objections. First, the correlation of .80 is less than perfect, demonstrating the influence of environmental factors as well. In fact, the impact of heredity in these

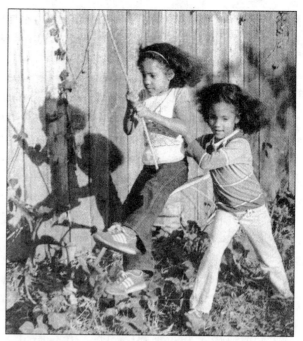

FIGURE 13–13 STUDIES OF IDENTICAL TWINS. When pairs of identical twins are studied for any characteristic, the research can accommodate both perspectives: heredity, looking for similarities, and the environment, looking for differences.

instances is estimated as the square of the correlation. Hence, the hereditary influence is assumed to account for about 64% of overall intelligence: .8 × .8 = .64. Second, this correlation of .80 is about equally distant between the approximately .60 correlation for fraternal twins, with no more common inheritance than ordinary siblings, and a perfect 1.00 correlation, which would occur if heredity were the only influence (Bouchard & McGue, 1981; Gottesman, 1963). Thus, even with identical twins, the environmental factor is clearly present.

When identical twins have been reared apart, generally one has not lived as a prince and the other as a pauper. Adoption agencies try to place foster children with adoptive parents who have comparable IQs. Hence, the environments of separated identical twins have not been very different. Under these circumstances, identical twins reared apart have shown greater similarity in intelligence than other siblings reared together (Bouchard, Lykken, McGue, Segal, & Tellegen, 1990).

RELATIONSHIP	GENETIC SHARING	CORRELATION
Identical twins, together	100%	.86
Identical twins, apart	100%	.72
Fraternal twins, together	50%	.60
Siblings, together	50%	.47
Siblings, apart	50%	.24
Cousins, apart	12½%	.15

TABLE 13–5 FAMILY CORRELATIONS IN INTELLIGENCE. The role of genetic factors is apparent in the higher correlations for identical twins than for any other relationship. The role of the environment is evident in the lower correlations for identical twins reared apart rather than together and for ordinary siblings reared apart rather than together. The table shows weighted average correlations (Bouchard & McGue, 1981).

HERITABILITY ESTIMATES. Studies in quantitative genetics have added some further understanding of the contribution of heredity, developing a concept known as the heritability estimate. The **heritability estimate** is a proportion or ratio representing the extent to which any given characteristic can be attributed to genetic factors, as opposed to *all* factors that might contribute to that characteristic. People exposed to *exactly* the same environment all of their lives would have a heritability estimate of 100% for all traits, meaning that all differences among them would be due to heredity. This condition of course is impossible.

In practice, heritability of intelligence is very difficult to estimate, and the figures vary widely. It is not surprising to find them ranging upward from 30% or so to as high as 80%. They are derived by studying similarities in intelligence, or any other characteristic, among subjects known to have the same or similar genetic backgrounds. Identical twins are a prime source of data. Other investigations have included brothers and sisters, parents and offspring, and even grandchildren, cousins, and other relatives.

STUDIES OF SIBLINGS. Investigations of family size and birth order have shed light on environmental influences. As a very *general* rule, the larger the family, the lower the *average* IQ among the siblings. The usual explanation focuses on the quality of the intellectual environment in the family, assuming that hereditary differences are randomized across birth order for the hundreds of thousands of subjects in these studies. When there is only one child or two siblings, each child can receive considerable stimulation from the parents. As the number increases, especially when there are more than four siblings, it becomes more and more difficult for the parents to provide special opportunities for mental development in each child (Pfouts, 1980).

The older children in a large family tend to have somewhat higher IQs than the younger children, a condition that has been substantiated in studies around the world (Wilson, Mundy-Castle, & Panditji, 1990; Zajonc & Markus, 1975). In their earliest years, the oldest siblings have early intellectual stimulation from parents more to themselves. Later-born children must share it from the beginning, sometimes with several siblings. On reading these words, do not swagger or thump your chest as a first-born, and do not slump in despair as a later-born child. You are no different than you were moments ago. Remember, too, that the average differences are *very* small and that, with the vicissitudes of life, there are countless exceptions.

Another advantage of being an older child lies with the opportunity to teach younger ones. We learn partly by instructing others, as Renee sometimes did with Tanya and Sharon. Renee also profited from the exclusive attention of her grandmother before Tanya and Sharon arrived in the household.

There are, of course, advantages for later-born children. One seems to lie in the social realm. Compared to older siblings, younger ones may be more skillful in managing interpersonal situations. Another advantage lies in the opportunity for learning physical skills, provided that the older siblings are willing to share their expertise. Younger children are also more likely to be independent, even rebellious (Sulloway, 1995). In addition, there is evidence that birth-order effects of all sorts diminish in adulthood, not a surprising outcome when we think of the profound influences of marriage, career, and other responsibilities in adult life (Schooler, 1972).

STUDIES OF COMPENSATORY EDUCATION. Another effort to study the nature–nurture issue has occurred in **compensatory education,** which attempts to provide early learning opportunities and an enriched environment for disadvantaged children. Some well-known programs of this sort include Head Start and A Better Chance

(ABC). They were founded with the expectation that an early enriched or remedial education would prove useful for disadvantaged children, compensating for even earlier environmental deficits.

Long-term follow-up studies of Head Start, one of the earliest and largest equal-opportunity programs in the United States, show several areas of favorable development among the graduates. The evidence for mental growth remains mixed, but these advantages are sometimes delayed (Figure 13-14). If the interventions continue, they may have a lasting effect (Besharov & Hartle, 1987; Kotelchuck & Richmond, 1987).

∾

NATURE–NURTURE INTERACTION

Today we realize that children can appear retarded and become retarded from being reared in deprived circumstances. The role of the environment, under-

estimated in many early studies of intellectual deficit, was apparent in the Grant family. Granny left school in the third grade. "I had to raise myself," she declared, an orphan early in life. Renee, already in danger of leaving school, was exposed to Granny's largely nonliterate household (Snow et al., 1991).

Considering all of the findings on identical twins, family constellations, and special education, what can we say about the contributions of heredity and environment to the intelligence of a given *individual?* Most psychologists would answer somewhat in this fashion: Heredity sets certain broad limits of potential intelligence, and environment determines the extent to which we achieve this potential. These limits are sometimes called the **reaction range,** referring to the genetically based limits or range of any inherited capacity, including intelligence. In a favorable environment, children should develop close to the peak

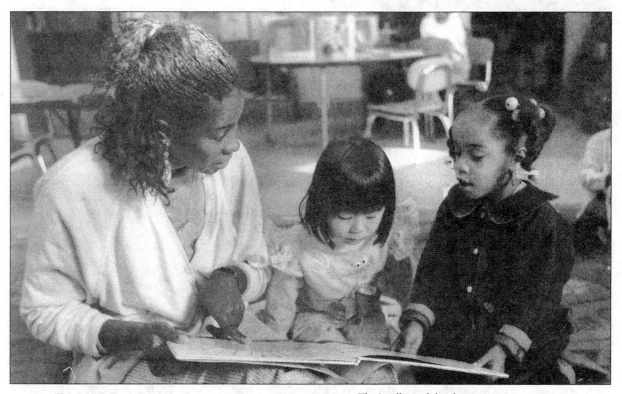

FIGURE 13–14 EARLY INTERVENTION. The intellectual developments produced by Head Start and similar programs are still debated. Personal and social gains have been well established, however, and these capacities are critical to successful functioning in adulthood.

of their intellectual reaction range. Those in less favored circumstances should reach a lower point in this range, which is assumed to be approximately 20 IQ points for the average individual (Figure 13–15). But even the limits of intelligence, according to some, may be influenced by the early environment.

Both factors, heredity *and* environment, are always present and operative for everyone. The impact of any particular heredity or any particular environment occurs within the context of the other. In this view, known as the **interaction principle,** heredity and environment inevitably influence one another. A favorable heredity may mean very little in a highly disadvantaged environment and vice versa. The outcomes from each source are interdependent. In a fundamental sense, everything interacts with everything else (Magnusson & Törestad, 1993).

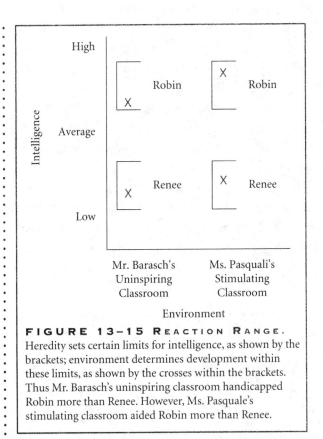

FIGURE 13–15 REACTION RANGE. Heredity sets certain limits for intelligence, as shown by the brackets; environment determines development within these limits, as shown by the crosses within the brackets. Thus Mr. Barasch's uninspiring classroom handicapped Robin more than Renee. However, Ms. Pasquale's stimulating classroom aided Robin more than Renee.

• INTELLIGENCE AND AGING •

Sitting on her front steps four years after her schooling with Mr. Barasch, 16-year-old Robin one day greeted an unexpected visitor, a woman from the research team at the local university, studying the Grants, Hendersons, and other Norwich families. She had returned for a follow-up interview.

Robin sat holding a baby. Her visitor inquired: "Oh, a new Henderson?" Robin replied, very assuredly, "Yes, this is *my* Henderson" (Snow, 1991).

Robin had dropped out of high school. Her new circumstances as a mother, and her prospects in life ahead, raise the question of intelligence and aging. What will happen to Robin intellectually? What will happen to Renee? Do people, as a rule, grow more intelligent as they grow older? When does a decline begin?

Psychology's earliest efforts to answer such questions inaugurated still another impassioned debate, arising largely through the research procedure employed at the time. Today two quite different methods are recognized: cross-sectional studies and longitudinal studies. Both are useful for examining changes in human characteristics during the life span; both have assets and limitations.

CROSS-SECTIONAL STUDIES

The first attempts to examine intellectual development during adulthood used **cross-sectional studies,** in which groups of subjects of different ages are tested simultaneously and then compared. Some subjects are 20 years of age, others 30, others 40, and so forth. A different group represents the population at each age level, and comparisons are made among them. In this method, Tanya and Sharon might be included with the children, Renee and Robin with the early adolescents, the Henderson parents in the late-forties group, Granny with the elderly, and so forth. Then the results for these different groups are compared.

Cross-sectional research began with military testing in World War I; it produced a dismal picture of American society and of immigrants as well. The average draftee, in his twenties, apparently had a mental age of 14. Many young men in the army at that time had not pursued a thorough education, and it was well known that physical ability begins to decline in the twenties. But this figure for mental age seemed unduly low (Yoakum & Yerkes, 1920).

Nevertheless, another investigation showed that maximum intellectual capacity usually occurred in the twenties and rarely after 30 years of age, although vocabulary showed the slowest decline (Wechsler, 1958). Still another cross-sectional investigation, this one in the 1950s, seemed to verify the earlier studies (Schaie, 1958).

Gradually, investigators began to adopt a skeptical view. Something was wrong—not the statistics but the procedure. In our rapidly changing society, younger subjects have a distinct advantage over older ones. Those in their thirties, for example, have received a better education than those in their fifties and seventies. The differences in performance between young and old subjects perhaps were due to gains by the younger people more than to a decline among the older people.

This phenomenon, now widely recognized in developmental research, is called the cohort effect. A *cohort* is a group of people who share an experience, typically because they are the same age or entered into some activity at the same time. People who were adolescents in the Roaring Twenties were a cohort, sharing that cultural experience, which was a different adolescence from that of people who were teenagers during the Great Depression or the Vietnam War. Whenever there is a difference in behavior or experience among generations that is not attributable to aging per se, but rather to some event such as education, disease, or economic hard-

ship, it is called a **cohort effect.** AIDS, drugs, and computers may produce a marked cohort effect when comparisons are made with other generations that did not experience these conditions. The advantage of the cross-sectional study is that it is relatively quick and efficient; people of different ages can be studied simultaneously. Its disadvantage lies in the potential for a cohort effect, meaning a difference that is not due to aging but rather to some other factor.

LONGITUDINAL STUDIES

The problem of the cohort effect was surmounted when another research approach was employed. Distinctly time-consuming, these investigations are called **longitudinal studies** because the same subjects are tested over and over again, at different ages, as they grow older. If Granny had participated in a longitudinal study, she would have been tested soon after birth, if possible, and then tested and retested during childhood, adolescence, adulthood, and into old age. Needless to say, such investigations are difficult to accomplish, for several years must pass and several testing sessions must be completed before significant effects can be observed.

Longitudinal investigations begun years ago have indicated a pattern quite different from that found using the cross-sectional approach. Studies of 768 Termites in adulthood showed that they, and their bright but generally less gifted spouses, experienced continuous growth in abstract thinking even up to age 50, their maximum age at the time (Bayley & Oden, 1955). Longitudinal studies of college graduates in England yielded similar results for vocabulary, spatial relations, numerical problems, analogies, and other forms of reasoning (Nisbet, 1957). Later studies showed no evidence of decline in overall test performance at least until the late sixties (Schaie & Willis, 1986).

But longitudinal studies are not without defect either. Ideally, the only difference between a longi-

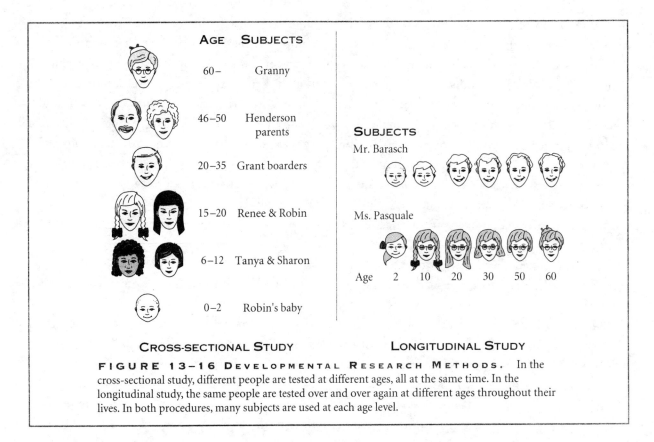

AGE	SUBJECTS
60–	Granny
46–50	Henderson parents
20–35	Grant boarders
15–20	Renee & Robin
6–12	Tanya & Sharon
0–2	Robin's baby

SUBJECTS

Mr. Barasch

Ms. Pasquale

Age   2   10   20   30   50   60

CROSS-SECTIONAL STUDY

LONGITUDINAL STUDY

FIGURE 13–16 DEVELOPMENTAL RESEARCH METHODS. In the cross-sectional study, different people are tested at different ages, all at the same time. In the longitudinal study, the same people are tested over and over again at different ages throughout their lives. In both procedures, many subjects are used at each age level.

tudinal subject at a younger and an older age is due to the general impact of aging per se, but subjects at the older ages are also benefiting from our expanding fund of knowledge and vastly improved methods of disseminating it (Emanuelsson & Svensson, 1990). Furthermore, there is a steady loss of the less healthy and less adjusted subjects, who no longer participate further in the research. In short, the advantage of the longitudinal study— avoiding a cohort effect by studying the same subjects throughout the developmental process—is offset by significant expenditures of time and money, as well as the potential for a biased sample of higher scores through improved education.

Thus, estimates are too low with the first approach, too high with the second. Each method has its assets and limitations (Figure 13-16).

One correctional procedure involves the use of comparison subjects with the longitudinal approach. These comparison subjects are tested at the same age as the longitudinal subjects were when they began the research or when they reached any later age under investigation. The difference in performance, if any, between the comparison subjects and the longitudinal subjects *at that same age*, years earlier, represents the amount of cultural change during that period. When this amount is subtracted from the performance of the longitudinal subjects, it corrects the data for cultural improvements. More sophisticated methods are also available, for one of the goals of developmental research is to take advantage of the longitudinal method while minimizing its drawbacks (Farrington, 1991; Verhulst & Koot, 1991).

This procedure was used in a longitudinal study of 96 male students who were tested as freshmen in 1919, again as alumni in 1950, and then once more in 1961. On the occasion of the final testing, 101 male freshmen at the same university were also tested, and the difference between their

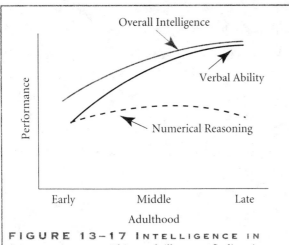

FIGURE 13-17 INTELLIGENCE IN ADULTHOOD. This graph illustrates findings in various studies. With adjustments for cultural change, the smooth lines indicate general trends, not specific patterns.

scores in 1961 and those of the earlier freshmen in 1919 represented the amount of cultural change. Thus, the gain of the alumni after 42 years was adjusted by this score, and overall, there was still an improvement in total ability. Verbal ability, in particular, increased markedly, remaining high at least through the fifties (Owens, 1966; Figure 13-17).

Other investigations have added confirmation, suggesting that intelligence may not reach its peak until the sixties or even later (Hertzog & Schaie, 1986). Then the different abilities show different rates of decline, with the major loss lying in the speed of response, followed by numerical ability (Honzik & MacFarlane, 1973; McCrae & Costa, 1987). However, the age of onset of this decline is significantly influenced by the person's intellectual interests and activities (Owens, 1966; Schaie, 1993).

IMPORTANCE OF EXPERIENCE

The subjects in the previous studies were college graduates, generally in vocations or avocations demanding a high level of mental activity. Among these individuals, a steady increase in intelligence can be expected for six or seven decades, especially in intelligence as a repository of information, skills, and problem-solving techniques acquired in daily life. As in all areas of human development, people exposed to a less favorable environment will experience an earlier peak ability and a slow but steady decline thereafter. One's occupation and mental activity are vital factors for continued mental growth in later adulthood (Owens, 1966; Schaie, 1993).

We leave the Grants and Hendersons with this finding in mind. Challenging mental activity is the critical factor in continued mental growth in the adult years.

The low expectation of her teachers was not the only reason Robin Henderson left school. The multiple bases of behavior suggest that other factors probably were involved as well. Clearly, her sexual activity played a role. Apparently another factor was her relationship with her mother, whom she described as "picky . . . not very nice, and impossible to please." Robin became resentful of her mother's attempts to encourage greater scholastic effort. With these factors in mind, there is considerable doubt that Robin, as a teenage mother, will ever complete a traditional high school program. Her definite intellectual potential may lie fallow or, in fact, begin to decline early in life. These doubts were expressed by the investigators who studied the children in 31 Norwich families. The influence of the home, they concluded, is the most powerful predictor of student achievement in school. The findings in many households are implicit in the title of their book on this research, *Unfulfilled Expectations: Home and School Influences on Literacy* (Snow et al., 1991).

There may be futher opportunities for Robin, however. Some programs for teenage parents have been highly successful, reducing the failure-to-finish rate from 80% to 38% (Clinchy, 1991). Robin certainly possesses the necessary componential intelligence, described earlier as an academic domain in the triarchic theory. For Robin, school assignments and tests were always easy—perhaps too easy. In a teenage parenting program she would pursue two courses of study: a traditional high school curriculum and instruction in parenting.

Participating in the same Norwich classrooms, Renee too had been assigned academic tasks below the average level but, with less capacity, she was less hindered by this lack of encouragement. While she drew meager academic assistance from her nonliterate grandmother, she obtained help from other students, joined an after-school program, and phoned a cousin across town when no other support was available. In these ways, Renee advanced through the Norwich system, and one day she graduated from high school, much to the delight of her very proud Granny. Afterward, she began looking for work for which she knew she was suited: "A people type of job" (Snow et al., 1991).

At some level, Renee understood her contextual intelligence, although she perhaps never encountered triarchic theory. Despite limited scholastic ability, Renee made the classroom into a favorable setting for herself, one that recognized her social competence. Almost brash with teachers on occasion, she nevertheless was selected as a teacher's aide and recognized as a class leader. In life after graduation, she should make the most of this practical intelligence, finding work situations in which it can be exercised or modifying a work setting to permit it to flourish.

And finally, we leave Granny, in her late sixties. She never graduated from elementary school, but she too had a practical intelligence, not unlike Renee. With common sense and a buoyant style, she had become an excellent model for her grandchildren, especially by going to class at night. This activity had two important benefits. First, she was demonstrating an attitude for all of her family: Learning never ends. Second, by providing herself with a challenging intellectual climate, she was forestalling a more rapid decline in her own mental abilities. In Granny's effort, all of us can find some inspiration.

• SUMMARY •

THE TESTING MOVEMENT

1. Intelligence is difficult to define, but most definitions generally refer to some aspect of flexibility or versatility of adjustment. Its measurement is often accomplished by individual intelligence tests: the Stanford-Binet and the Wechsler scales.
2. Well-constructed tests show high reliability, which refers to the consistency of subjects' scores. Successful tests must have high validity, which means that the test measures what it purports to measure. Norms are compilations of test scores that serve as guidelines for interpreting any particular score.
3. Tests are best understood as human tools, possessing assets and limitations. They can be useful for diagnosis, research, and screenings. Most important, the test user must exercise caution in the interpretation of test scores.

EXTREMES OF INTELLIGENCE

4. People with mental retardation, comprising the lower 2% of the population in measured intelligence, are classified as totally dependent, trainable, or educable. Causal factors in mental retardation include genetic factors, health factors, cultural deprivation, and emotional factors, which can accompany any sort of mental retardation.
5. Mentally gifted people comprise the upper 2% of the population in mental ability; generally they are more physically fit, socially adept, and traditionally

moral than the general population. Educational programs are less structured and proceed more rapidly than those for other children.

THEORIES OF INTELLIGENCE

6. In the psychometric approach to a theory of intelligence, the results of traditional intelligence tests are used to speculate on the nature of intelligence. The theory of multiple intelligences has identified seven kinds of intelligence: linguistic, logical-mathematical, spatial, musical, bodily-kinesthetic, interpersonal, and intrapersonal.

7. The cognitive approach stresses how information is obtained, stored, and used—the mental operations in intelligent behavior. The structure-of-intellect model postulates many distinct intellectual abilities. Crystallized and fluid intelligence stress the accumulation of knowledge and the capacity to solve novel problems, respectively. And the triarchic theory identifies three domains: componential, experiential, and contextual.

NATURE- NURTURE ISSUE

8. The nature–nurture controversy has a long history, extending through many studies of group differences. The question of the genetic basis of group differences is impossible to answer for several reasons, chiefly the absence of satisfactory tests.

9. Research on the nature-nurture issue involves comparison of identical twins reared apart; these studies have shown the influences of both heredity and environment, including a heritability estimate.

10. The influences of heredity and environment are always present, and they depend upon one another. Heredity sets broad limits, and environment determines the extent to which this intelligence is achieved. The key issue is their interaction.

INTELLIGENCE AND AGING

11. In studies of human development at different ages, two research methods are available. Cross-sectional investigations use different subjects at different ages. They are relatively quick and efficient, but they include the risk of a cohort effect.

12. Longitudinal investigations study the same subjects as they grow older. They avoid a cohort effect, but they are costly in terms of time and money.

13. When control procedures are used to correct for cultural changes, it is found that mental growth may continue into the sixth decade or later, providing that the individual is engaged in stimulating mental activities.

• WORKING WITH PSYCHOLOGY •

REVIEW OF KEY CONCEPTS

intelligence

The Testing Movement
  intelligence test
  mental age (MA)
  Stanford-Binet Intelligence Scale
  chronological age (CA)
  intelligence quotient (IQ)
  Wechsler Intelligence Scales
  reliability

test-retest reliability
equivalent-form reliability
interjudge reliability
validity
face validity
predictive validity
concurrent validity
norms
achievement test
aptitude test

interest inventory
personality test

Extremes of Intelligence
  normal distribution
  mental retardation
  mental giftedness
  learning disability
  phenylketonuria (PKU)
  Down's syndrome

fragile X syndrome
cretinism
fetal alcohol syndrome (FAS)
cultural deprivation
mainstreaming

cognitive approach
structure-of-intellect model
crystallized intelligence
fluid intelligence
triarchic theory

culturally sensitive testing
heritability estimate
compensatory education
reaction range
interaction principle

Theories of Intelligence
psychometric approach
general intelligence (*g*)
specific ability (*s*)
multiple intelligences

Nature–Nurture Issue
nature–nurture issue
culture-free test
culture-fair test

Intelligence and Aging
cross-sectional studies
cohort effect
longitudinal studies

❧ CLASS DISCUSSION/CRITICAL THINKING ❧

A NARRATIVE TWIST

Suppose that Renee, with her particular inheritance, had lived in the Henderson household. Suppose Robin, with her genetic makeup, had been a member of the Grant family. Speculate on the intellectual, social, and educational development of each girl at two stages, first as a student in Mr. Barasch's sixth-grade class and then four years later, when they would have been approximately 16 years old. Discuss the probable developmental changes experienced by each girl. Discuss the likely differences between the girls at each age. ❧

TOPICAL QUESTIONS

• *The Testing Movement.* You have been chosen to devise a nonverbal test identifying mentally gifted. Describe three sample items from your test.
• *Extremes of Intelligence.* Suppose typical students were educated as mentally gifted students. Would their intelligence be enhanced? Would it be diminished? Explain your reasons.
• *Theories of Intelligence.* Consider the factorial approach to intelligence. Develop a set of basic mental abilities that you feel encompasses the whole range of

intelligence. Defend your selection.
• *Nature-Nurture Issue.* To what extent is a culture-fair test possible? Write questions that might be considered for a culture-fair test.
• *Intelligence and Aging.* You are about to read an article on intelligence and aging among people with exceptional intelligence. Among which group, those with retardation or those who are gifted, would you expect to find the most variable changes in middle adulthood and old age? Why?

❧ TOPICS OF RELATED INTEREST ❧

The technique of correlation, which underlies the concepts of validity and reliability, is discussed in the chapter on statistical methods (18). The operations dimension of the structure-of-intellect model concerns memory (8) and thinking (9). The Skeels research in human development provides evidence for environmental influences on intelligence (12).

THE DEVELOPMENT OF AFFECTIONAL RESPONSES IN INFANT MONKEYS[1]

Harry F. Harlow and
Robert R. Zimmermann

Human beings have long observed the development of affection or love in the neonate and infant. It is an obvious fact that this early affection of the infant is first intimately bound to the mother and then gradually expands, through mechanisms by no means well known, to other human beings.

Observational evidence, often controlled, orderly, and systematic, has led scientists to speculate both on the nature of the early affectional responses and the development and generalization of these responses. Although experimental psychologists have given little attention to the fundamental nature or development of affection, their common theoretical position is that affection is a derived drive developed through the repeated association of the mother with reduction of the primary biological drives, particularly hunger and thirst.

A wide diversity of theoretical positions has been held by various psychoanalysts. Some, such as Klein (3), have emphasized the breast as an object for which the infant innately strives and connects, whereas others, including Winnecoot (7) and Ribble (5), have described broader innate needs relating to contact, movement, and temperature. Bowlby[2] has given approximately equal emphasis to primary clinging (contact) and sucking as innate affectional components, and at a later maturational level, visual and auditory following.

The role of visual and auditory following (imprinting) has been stressed by Lorenz (4) and other ethologists as primary innate mechanisms binding the infant bird and fish to the mother. Even if similar mechanisms exists in the primate, they appear at a later developmental stage and play less important roles than they do in lower animals.

There are many reasons for the absence of experimental analysis of the nature and development of affectional responses in the human infant. His motor capabilities are so limited at birth that there are few, if any, precise responses that can be measured and recorded, and by the time his precise responses can be measured, the antecedent determining variables have been obscured in a complex maze of confounded variables previously unmeasurable.

Fortunately, these difficulties are resolved in large part if we use the neonatal and infant macaque monkey as the subject for experimental analysis of basic affectional variables. It is possible to make precise measurements in this primate beginning at two to ten days of age, depending upon the maturational status of the individual subject at birth. The macaque infant differs for the human infant in that the monkey is more mature at birth and grows more rapidly, but the basic responses relating to affection, including nursing, contact, clinging, and even visual and auditory exploration, exhibit no fundamental differences in the two species. Even the development of perception, emotion, and learning capability follow very similar sequences.

In an effort to gain control over the lives of the monkeys used as subjects for affectional analysis, we separated these animals from their mothers six to twelve hours after birth and suckled them on tiny nursing bottles. Three years' previous experience with some sixty neonates, also separated from their mothers at birth, had demonstrated the complete feasibility of such procedures, for these earlier laboratory-raised monkeys were larger and healthier and had a higher incidence of survival than infants left to the care of their monkey mothers.

We had noted that the previous laboratory-raised babies showed strong attachment to the cloth pads (folded gauze diapers) which were used to cover the hardware-cloth floors of their cages. The infants clung to these pads and engaged in violent temper tantrums when the pads were removed and replaced for sanitary reasons. Such contact-need or responsiveness had been reported previously by Van Wagenen (6) and is reminiscent of the devotion often exhibited by human infants to their pillows, blankets, and soft, cuddly stuffed toys.

We took these observational data as the cue for the construction of two mother surrogates, one designed to be soft, the other to be rigid and unyielding. A cloth mother is made from a block of wood covered by sponge rubber and sheathed with terry cloth; the wire mother is made of hardware cloth, a substance entirely adequate to provide support and nursing capability. We presumed that the cloth and wire mothers would differ to the neonatal monkeys in no way other than the difference in contact comfort provided by the mother's body. Although we deliberately designed different faces for the two classes of mothers, responsiveness to the face matures at a later age than affectional responding.

In our initial experiment, the dual mother-surrogate condition, a cloth mother and a wire mother were placed in different cubicles attached to the infant's living cage. For four infant monkeys the cloth mother lactated and the wire mother did not, and for the other four this condition was reversed. In either condition the infant received all its milk through the mother surrogate as soon as it was able to maintain itself in this way. In the first few days, supplementary feedings were needed, but these could be eliminated after two or three days, except in the case of very immature animals. Thus, the experiment was designed as a test of the relative importance of the variables of contact comfort and nursing comfort. During the first fourteen days of life the monkey's cage floor was covered with a heating pad wrapped in a folded gauze diaper, and thereafter the cage floor was bare. The infant subjects were always free to leave the heating pad or cage floor to contact either mother, and the time spent on the surrogate mothers was automatically recorded. Figure 1 shows the total time spent on the cloth and wire mothers under the two conditions of feeding. These data make it obvious that contact comfort is a variable of overwhelming importance in the development of affectional responses, whereas lactation is a

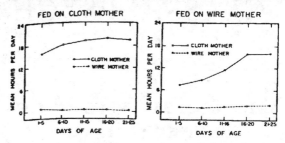

FIGURE 1 Time spent on cloth and wire mother surrogates.

variable of negligible importance. With age and opportunity to learn, responsiveness to the lactating wire mother decreases and responsiveness to the nonlactating cloth mother increases, a finding completely contrary to any interpretation of derived drive in which the mother-form becomes conditioned to hunger-thirst reduction. The persistence of these differential responses throughout 165 consecutive days of testing is evidence in Figure 2.

We were not surprised to discover that contact comfort was an important basic affectional or love variable, but we did not expect it to overshadow so completely the variable of nursing; indeed, the disparity is so great as to suggest that the primary function of nursing as an affectional variable is that of insuring frequent and intimate body contact of the infant with the mother.

One function of the real mother, human or subhuman, and presumably of a mother surrogate, is to provide a haven of safety for the infant in times of fear and anger. The frightened or ailing child clings to its mother, not its father, and this selective responsiveness in times of distress, disturbance, or danger may be used

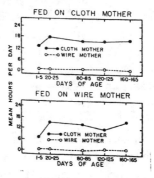

FIGURE 2 Long-term contract time on cloth and wire mother surrogates.

as a measure of the strength of affectional bonds. We have tested this kind of differential responsiveness by presenting to the infants in their cages, in the presence of the two mothers, various fear-producing stimuli such as the moving toy bear. The data on differential responsiveness are presented in Figure 3, and it is apparent that the cloth mother is highly preferred over the wire one, and this differential selectivity is enhanced by age and experience. In this situation, the variable of nursing appears to be of absolutely no importance; the infant consistently seeks the soft mother surrogate regardless of nursing condition.

Similarly, the mother or mother surrogate provides its young with a source of security, and this role or function is seen with special clarity when mother and child are in a strange situation. At the present time we have completed tests for this relationship on four of our eight baby monkeys assigned to the dual mother-surrogate condition by introducing them for three minutes into the strange environment of a room measuring six feet by six feet (also called the "open field test") and containing multiple stimuli known to elicit curiosity-manipulatory responses in baby monkeys. The subjects were placed in this situation twice a week for eight weeks with no mother surrogate present during alternate sessions and the cloth mother present during the others. A cloth diaper was always available as one of the stimuli throughout all sessions. After one or two adaptation sessions, the infants always rushed to the mother surrogate when she was present and clutched her, a response so strong that it can be adequately depicted only by motion pictures. After a few additional sessions, the infants began to use the mother surrogate as a source of security, a base of operations. They would explore and manipulate a stimulus and then return to the mother before adventuring again into the strange new world. The behavior of these infants was quite different when the mother was absent from the room. Frequently they would freeze in a crouched position. Emotionality indices such as vocalization, crouching, rocking, and sucking increased sharply, as shown in Figure 4. Total emotionality score was cut in half when the mother was present. In the absence of the mother some of the experimental monkeys would rush to the center of the room where the mother was customarily placed, and then run rapidly from object to object screaming and crying all the while. Continuous, frantic clutching of their bodies was very common, even when not in the crouching position. These monkeys frequently contacted and clutched the cloth diaper, but this action never pacified them. No difference between the cloth-mother-fed and wire-mother-fed infants was demonstrated under either condition. Four control infants never raised with a mother surrogate showed the same emotionality scores when the mother was absent as the experimental infants showed in the absence of the mother, but the controls' scores were slightly larger in the presence of the mother surrogate than in her absence.

Some years ago Butler (1) showed that mature monkeys enclosed in a dimly lighted box would open and reopen a door for hours on end for no other motivation than that of looking outside the box. We now have data demonstrating that neonatal monkeys show this same compulsive visual curiosity on their first test day in an adaptation of the Butler apparatus. Usually these tests are begun at ten days of age, but this same persistent visual exploration has been obtained in a three-day-old monkey during the first half-hour of testing. Butler (2) also demonstrated that rhesus monkeys show selectivity in rate and frequency of door-opening to stimuli of differential attractiveness in the visual field outside the box. We have utilized this principle of response selectivity by the monkey to measure strength of affectional responsiveness in our infants in the baby version of the Butler

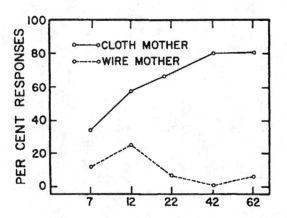

FIGURE 3 Differential resonses to the two mothers in fear tests.

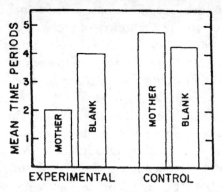

FIGURE 4 Emotionality index with and without the presence of the cloth mother.

box. The test sequence involves four repetitions of a test battery in which the four stimuli of cloth mother, wire mother, infant monkey, and empty box are presented for a thirty-minute period on successive days. The first four subjects in the dual mother-surrogate group were given a single test sequence at forty to fifty days of age, depending upon the availability of the apparatus, and only their data are presented. The second group of four subjects is being given repetitive tests to obtain information relating to the development of visual exploration. The data obtained from the first four infants raised with the two mother surrogates are presented in the middle graph of Figure 5 and show approximately equal responding to the cloth mother and another infant monkey, and no greater responsiveness to the wire mother than to an empty box. Again, the results are independent of the kind of mother that lactated, cloth or wire. The same results are found for a control group raised, but not fed, on a single cloth mother, and these data appear in the graph on the right. Contrariwise, the graph on the left shows no differential responsiveness to cloth and wire mothers by a second control group, which was not raised on any mother surrogate.

The first four infant monkeys in the dual mother-surrogate group were separated from their mothers between 165 and 170 days of age and tested for retention during the following nine days and then at thirty-day intervals for five successive months. Affectional retention as measured by the modified Butler box is given in Figure 6. In keeping with the data obtained on adult monkeys by Butler, we find a high rate of responding to any stimulus, even the empty box. But throughout the entire 160-day retention period there is a consistent and significant difference in response frequency to the cloth mother contrasted with either the wire mother or the empty box, and no consistent difference between wire mother and empty box.

Affectional retention was also tested in the open field during the first nine days after separation and then at thirty-day intervals, and each test condition was run twice at each retention interval. The infant's behavior differed from that observed during the period preceding separation. When the cloth mother was present in the post-separation period, the babies rushed rapidly to her, climbed up her body, clung tightly to her, and rubbed their head and face about her body. After this initial embrace and reunion, they played on the mother, including biting and tearing at her cloth cover; they rarely made any attempt to leave her during the test period, nor did they manipulate or play with the objects in the room, in contrast with their behavior before maternal separation. The only

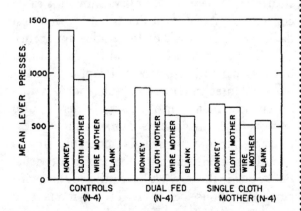

FIGURE 5 Differential responses to visual exploration.

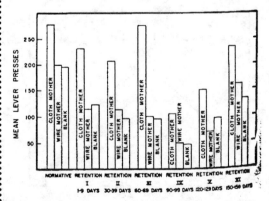

FIGURE 6 Retention of differential visual-exploration responses.

exception was the occasional monkey that left the mother surrogate momentarily, grasped the folded piece of paper (one of the standard stimuli in the field), and brought it quickly back to the mother. It appears that deprivation had enhanced the tie to the mother, and the contact-comfort need had become so prepotent that it overwhelmed the exploratory motives during the brief, three-minute test sessions. No change in these behaviors was observed throughout the 160-day period. When the mother was absent from the open field, the behavior of the infants was similar in the initial retention test to that during the pre-separation tests, but they tended to show gradual adaptation to the open-field situation with repeated testing and, consequently, a reduction in their emotionality scores.

In the last five retention test periods an additional test was introduced in which the surrogate mother was placed in the center of the room and covered with a clear Plexiglas box. The monkeys were initially disturbed and frustrated when their explorations and manipulations of the box failed to provide contact with the mother. However, all animals adapted to the situation rather rapidly, and soon they used the box as a place of orientation for exploratory and play behavior, made frequent contacts with the objects in the field, and very often brought these objects to the Plexiglas box. The emotional index was slightly lower than in the condition of the available cloth mothers, but it in no way approached the emotionality level displayed when the cloth mother was absent. Obviously, the infant monkeys gained emotional security by the presence of the mother even though contact was denied.

Affectional retention has also been measured by tests in which the monkey must unfasten a three-device mechanical puzzle to obtain entrance into a compartment containing the mother surrogate. All the trials are initiated by allowing the infant to go through a locked door, and in half the trials it finds the mother present and in half, an empty compartment. The door is then locked and a ten-minute test conducted. In tests given prior to separation from the surrogate mothers some of the infants had solved this puzzle and others had failed. The data of Figure 7 show that on the last test before sepa-

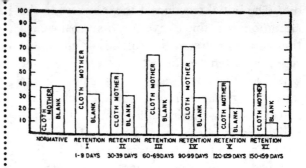

FIGURE 7 Retention of puzzle manipulation responsiveness.

ration there were no differences in total manipulation under mother-present and mother-absent conditions, but striking differences exist between the two conditions throughout the post-separation test periods. Even though there is an apparent trend for total amount of manipulation to decrease, the ratio of responsiveness to the mother-present and mother-absent conditions shows no sign of decreasing. Again, there is no interaction with conditions of feeding.

The over-all picture obtained from surveying the retention data is unequivocal. There is little, if any, waning of responsiveness to the mother throughout this five-month period as indicated by any measure. It becomes perfectly obvious that this affectional bond is highly resistant to forgetting and that it can be retained for very long periods of time by relatively little reinforcement of the contact variable. During the next year retention tests will be conducted at ninety-day intervals, and further plans are dependent upon the results obtained. It would appear that affectional responses may show as much resistance to extinction as has been previously demonstrated for learned fears and learned pain, and such data would be in keeping with those of common human observation.

We have already described the group of four control infants that had never lived in the presence of any mother surrogate and had demonstrated no sign of affection or security in the presence of the cloth mothers introduced in test sessions. When these infants reached the age of 250 days, cubicles containing both a cloth mother and a wire mother were attached to their cages. There was no lactation in these mothers, for the monkeys were on a solid-food diet. The initial reaction of the monkeys to the alterations was one of extreme disturbance. All the infants screamed violently and made repeated attempts to escape from the cage whenever the door was opened. They kept a maximum distance from the mother surrogates and exhibited a considerable amount of rocking and crouching behavior, indicative of emotionality. Our first thought was that the critical period for the development of maternally directed affection had passed and that these macaque children were doomed to live as affectional orphans. Fortunately, these behaviors continued for only twelve to forty-eight hours and then gradually ebbed, changing from indifference to active contact on, and exploration of, the surrogates. The home-cage behavior of these control monkeys slowly became similar to that of the animals raised with the mother surrogates from birth. Their manipulation and play on the cloth mother became progressively more vigorous to the point of actual mutilation, particularly during the morning, after the cloth mother had been given her daily change of terry covering. The control subjects were now actively running to the cloth mother when frightened and had to be coaxed from her to be taken from the cage for formal testing.

Objective evidence of these changing behaviors is given in Figure 8, which plots the amount of time these infants spent on the mother surrogates. Within ten days mean contact time is approximately nine hours, and this

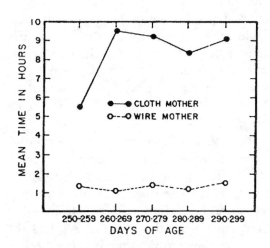

FIGURE 8 Differential time spent on cloth and wire mother surrogates by monkeys started at 250 days of age.

measure remains relatively constant throughout the next thirty days. Consistent with the results on the subjects reared from birth with dual mothers, these late-adopted infants spent less than one and one-half hours per day in contact with the wire mothers, and this activity level was relatively constant throughout the test sessions. Although the maximum time that the control monkeys spent on the cloth mother was only about half that spent by the original dual mother-surrogate group, we cannot be sure that this discrepancy is a function of differential early experience. The control monkeys were about three months older when the mothers were attached to their cages than the experimental animals were when their mothers were removed and the retention tests begun. Thus, we do not know what the amount of contact would be for a 250-day-old animal raised from the start with surrogate mothers. Nevertheless, the magnitude of the differences and the fact that the contact-time curves for the mothered-from-birth infants had remained constant for almost 150 days suggest that early experience with the mother is a variable of measurable importance.

The control group has also been tested for differential visual exploration after the introduction of the cloth and wire mothers, and these behaviors are plotted in Figure 9. By the second test session a high level of exploratory behavior has developed, and the responsiveness to the wire mother and the empty box is significantly greater than that to the cloth mother. This is probably not an artifact since there is every reason to believe that the face of the cloth mother is a fear stimulus to most monkeys that have not had extensive experience with this object during the first forty to sixty days of life. Within the third test session a sharp change in trend occurs, and the cloth mother is then more frequently viewed than the wire mother or the blank box, and this trend continues during the fourth session, producing a significant preference for the cloth mother.

Before the introduction of the mother surrogate into the home-cage situation only one of the four control monkeys had ever contacted the cloth mother in the open-field tests, and, in general, the surrogate mother not only gave the infants no security, but instead

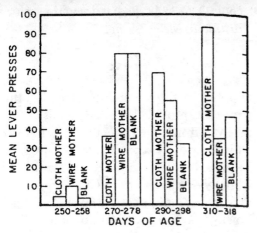

FIGURE 9 Differential visual exploration of monkeys started at 250 days of age.

appeared to serve as a fear stimulus. The emotionality scores of these control subjects were slightly higher during the mother-present test sessions than during the mother-absent test sessions. In Figure 10 the mean emotionality score for all the open-field tests given prior to the introduction of the surrogates to the home cage is compared with the mean of the fourth post-introduction test. In the absence of the cloth mothers the emotionality index in this fourth test remains near the earlier level, but the score is reduced by half when the mother is present, a result strikingly similar to that found for infants raised with the dual mother surrogates from birth. The control infants now show increasing object exploration and play behavior, and they begin to use the mother as a base

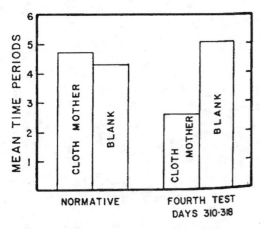

FIGURE 10 Differential emotionality scores in open-field test for monkeys started at 250 days of age.

of operations as did the infants raised from birth with the mother surrogates. However, there are still definite differences in the behavior of the two groups. The control infants do not rush directly to the mother and clutch her violently, but instead they go toward, and orient around, her, usually after an initial period during which they frequently show disturbed behavior, exploratory behavior, or both.

That the control monkeys develop affection or love for the cloth mother when she is introduced into the cage at 250 days of age cannot be questioned. There is every reason to believe, however, that this interval of delay depresses the intensity of the affectional response level below that of the infant monkeys that were surrogate-mothered from birth onward. In interpreting these data it is well to remember that the control monkeys had continuous opportunity to observe and hear other monkeys housed in adjacent cages and that they had had limited opportunity to view and contact surrogate mothers in the test situations, even though they did not exploit the opportunities. Finally, it should be remembered that neither surrogate was a nursing mother.

The researches which we have presented here on the analysis of affectional variables and the nature of their development in monkeys are of necessity incomplete inasmuch as the program was initiated only a year ago and the investigations cited were planned as pilot studies outlining a broad research field. In spite of the limitations certain facts stand out in sharp relief: Multiple objective techniques, reliable and with apparent face validity, can be devised to measure the infant's affectional ties. Even an appropriate inanimate mother surrogate can readily become an object loved with intensity and for a long period of time. Satisfactory body contact is an extremely strong affectional variable and may well prove to be the most important affectional variable for primates.

∾
REFERENCES

Butler, R.A. 1953. Discrimination learning by rhesus monkeys to visual exploration motivation. *Jour. Comp. Physiol. Psychol.* 46: 95–98.

_____. 1954. Incentive conditions which influence visual exploration. *Jour. Exp. Psychol.* 48: 19–23.

Klein, M. 1957. Envy and gratitude. London, Tavistock Publications.

Lorenz, K. 1937. The companion in the bird's world. *Auk* 54: 245–273.

Ribble, M. A. 1943. The rights of infants. New York, Columbia Univ. Press.

Van Wagenen, G. 1950. The monkey. In E. J. Farris (ed.), *The care and breeding of laboratory animals*. New York, Wiley.

Winnecoot, D.W. 1948. Pediatrics and psychiatry. *Brit. Jour. Med. Psychol.* 21: 229–240.

∾
NOTES

1. Support for the research presented in this paper was provided through funds received from the Graduate School of the University of Wisconsin, and from Grant M-722, National Institutes of Health, and from a Ford Foundation Grant.
2. Personal communication from Dr. John Bowlby, Tavistock Clinic, London, England.

❦ Journal Article Review Form ❦

Name _____ Date _____

Article Name: _____

Article Authors: _____

1. Why did the authors perform this study? (What question(s) did the authors want to answer?)

2. Identify the IV(s) and the DV(s) used in this study (Note: there may be more than one of each).

3. How was the welfare of human subjects or animal subjects safeguarded?

4. What were the major findings of this study?

5. Why were these results significant?

6. What would be a good follow-up to this study? (What study should be done next?)

1. According to Harlow, the trusting relationship that the child feels for the mother is called
   _____ and is generated by _____.
   a. bonding; the food rewards provided the child
   b. attachment; contact comfort
   c. dependence; the mother meeting the child's physical needs
   d. friendship; the mother playing with the child

2. A person who has some of the behavioral characteristics of both males and females is
   considered to be:
   a. hermaphroditic
   b. androgynous
   c. heterosexual
   d. homosexual
   e. bisexual

3. Which of the following are sex steroids:
   a. androgen   c. progesterone
   b. estrogen   d. all 3 are steroids

4. If a "genetic" human fetus with XX chromosomes is exposed to testosterone during the last
   trimester of pregnancy, "her" primary and secondary sex organs at 20 years of age will be:
   a. all male-like
   b. all female-like
   c. female-like except for the absence of ovaries
   d. a complex combination of male and female organs

5. The evidence for brain differences between men and women is that men have:
   a. higher levels of serotonin.
   b. enlarged size of all hypothalamic nuclei examined to date.
   c. different sizes of specific brain regions.
   d. little estrogen in their bloodstream.
   e. All of the above.

6. At six weeks after conception, the developing conceptus has formed a single gonad with two
   rudimentary reproductive systems. If sufficient testosterone is present, the _____
   system develops, and the _____ system shrinks.
   a. Mullerian; Wolffian   c. androgenic; estrogenic
   b. Wolffian; Mullerian   d. estrogenic; androgenic

7. One's sex or gender is determined by _____.
   a. one's internal and external reproductive organs
   b. whether the system that develops from the original single gonad is male or female
   c. one's brain structures and the behaviors that result from their activity
   d. a complex process of masculinization/feminization of all the above by the presence or
      absence of testosterone during the prenatal period

8. Which of the following would NOT support a hormonal or biological explanation of sexual
   orientation?
   a. In homosexual males, the anterior hypothalamus is the same size as in heterosexual
      females rather than the same size as heterosexual males.
   b. XY fetuses subjected to testosterone-blocking drugs during the latter half of their
      pregnancies are not all gay, but still many are homosexual.
   c. Homosexual males generally report that they have known they were "somehow different"
      from other males from the very beginning of their lives.
   d. Lesbian women often report that their sexual orientation was a "life choice" that
      occurred in their later years.

9. Having many behavioral characteristics of both gender is known as
   a. androgyny
   c. transsexualism
   b. gender confusion
   d. bisexuality

10. Which part of the autonomic nervous system allows you to calm down and resume normal functioning after an emergency is past?
    a. sympathetic
    c. interstitial
    b. parasympathetic
    d. endocrine

11. The master gland of the endocrine system is the _____; it secretes _____ directly into the bloodstream.
    a. posterior pituitary; excitatory neurotransmitters
    b. anterior pituitary; trophic hormones
    c. hypothalamus; endorphins
    d. adrenal glands; ions

12. What makes a test valid?
    a. It tests for intelligence.
    b. It tests what it is supposed to test.
    c. If someone gets a similar score the second time they take the same test.
    d. All of the above.

13. When we can demonstrate that a test actually measures what it is supposed to measure, we can say the test has _____.
    a. reliability
    c. validity
    b. norms
    d. common sense

14. Which of the following is true of the determinants of intelligence?
    a. it is almost totally determined by hereditary factors.
    b. it is environmentally determined and will change with the environment.
    c. it varies with environment until puberty, and then remains the same for the rest of your life.
    d. heredity sets a range for intelligence, and environment determines where within that range your intelligence falls.

15. Using numbers from 1 to 7, fill in the blanks the order in which gender develops.
    _____ chromosomal sex
    _____ brain sex
    _____ a single type of gonad appears
    _____ sex hormones secretions begin
    _____ male/female external reproductive organs
    _____ male/female internal reproductive organs
    _____ basis of sexual behavior is established

PART FOUR:
BEHAVIOR IN A MODERN WORLD

These days one often hears people saying the whole world seems to have gone crazy. Each of us may have harbored the same thoughts when reading the latest headlines about a terrorist bombing in a coffee shop or a respected member of the community charged with child sexual abuse. The suggestion is that the modern world in which we now live has generated deviant behaviors never known before. After calming ourselves a bit, most of us can agree that deviancy is not new. The historical record is full of innocent people being victimized by others. As discussed in the initial chapter of Part Four, psychologists and psychiatrists for many decades have been diagnosing and treating abnormal and deviant behaviors, also known as psychopathologies. Still, there do seem to be pressures in this modern world unknown previously—a crowded planet in which professional success is paramount in the minds of many, and drugs in the minds of a few. Better said, the pressures are not really new, crowds, drugs and stress surely have been with people since the beginnings. What may be new is the intensity of the pressures, that more of us have them and the means we have to deal with them. The latter is discussed in brief chapters here on drug categories and the modern medications developed as therapies to treat psychopathology. The Social Psychology chapter switches gears to speak to normal behaviors of quite sane people. There we will find principles uncovered by social psychologists on the ways people deal with other people. The final chapter reverts to the pathological, at least to the physiological toll taken by living in a high-stress environment. Hopefully, you will come away from Part Four with a better understanding of the age-old and the uniquely modern conditions leading to deviant behavior. Mostly, we hope you will end this part of the text with a bit of optimism because behavioral scientists have given us new knowledge to avoid the traps and new tools to treat the problems when they do emerge.

ᔫ ᔫ ᔫ ᔫ ᔫ ᔫ

12

ADJUSTMENT AND DISORDER

THE PAIR SAT BEHIND CLOSED DOORS. FINALLY, THE PSYCHIATRIST SPOKE AGAIN. "WHAT ELSE CAN YOU TELL ME?" SHE ASKED THE YOUNG MAN. "IS THERE anything else?"

"No, they just say 'Empty.' "

"Anything . . . anything more?"

"Well, sometimes they say—'Empty!' 'Hollow!' 'Thud!' "

Resigning herself to this impasse, the psychiatrist made some further notes, then tried to ask more productive questions. She asked the man about his home life. How was everything there? He described his wife and children affectionately and spoke of his parents in the same way.

When asked about his job, he explained that he was a pediatrician, expressing the pleasures of that work, as well as its burdens. Then he chatted about his hobbies.

Once more the psychiatrist inquired about the voices. Were they still there? The man nodded emphatically, "Yes!" Did they say the same things? He repeated: "Empty!" "Hollow!" "Thud!"

These remarks left the psychiatrist puzzled. The young man showed signs of a serious adjustment problem. He seemed to be suffering from hallucinations. At the same time, he appeared to be reasonably happy and living a productive life. He did not mention that he had been referred to the hospital by David Rosenhan. He was there seeking admission, which was all that mattered at that point.

After more questions and further doubt, the psychiatrist finished the interview and then led the young man down the hall to the nurse's station. He was admitted to the psychiatric ward, thereby initiating a surprising story about human adjustment useful in this chapter.

This chapter begins by examining the process of adjustment and then turns to the perplexing problem of determining abnormality. Afterward, the focus shifts to the major types of disorders. The chapter concludes with a discussion of adjustment and culture, for any view of adjustment must take into account cultural standards.

Throughout this chapter, beware of the *medical student syndrome*. Students in medicine and psychology often see themselves as displaying the symptoms they are studying. All of us have physical and psychological difficulties of some sort, and some of them may seem similar to topics discussed in this text. If you begin to think, as a result of this reading, that you have a particular adjustment problem not noticed previously, you are probably wrong. But if something has been bothering you and the following discussion increases your concerns, do not try self-diagnosis and do not ignore the problem any longer. Seek assistance.

• PROCESS OF ADJUSTMENT •

Adjustment is a continuous process, not a fixed or static state. Specifically, **adjustment** is the constant process of satisfying one's needs and desires as they emerge and reemerge throughout life. On this basis, no one achieves complete adjustment, at least not for long. Eventually, some need or desire arises, physical or psychological, and the individual seeks ways to deal with it. These concerns may be distinct and immediate, as in hunger or fear, or they may be difficult and lengthy, as in developing a vocational path in today's continuously changing society (Slee, 1993). As noted by Marcus Aurelius, an early Roman philosopher: The art of living is sometimes more like wrestling than dancing (*Meditations*, 7:61).

Many of us, dealing with our own adjustment problems, may overestimate the adjustment of others throughout the world. As we look around, there are people who seem to maintain a *normal adjustment*, healthy and free of conflict, acting within the acceptable standards of some group, without significant difficulty (Wolman, 1989). However, they are often people we do not know well. If we knew them better, we might decide that they too are wrestling, rather than waltzing through life (Figure 15–1).

DAVID ROSENHAN

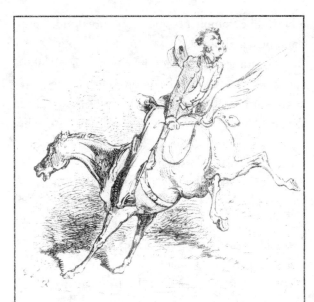

FIGURE 15-1 THE ART OF LIVING.
The psychology of adjustment attempts to assist people with problems of living and to understand why life for so many often becomes so difficult. The greatest of all arts, according to sages throughout the centuries, is the art of living appropriately.

THE ADJUSTMENT CONTINUUM

Adjustment is a continuous process and, in a general sense, it exists on a continuum. At one end there is the so-called adjusted person, who in many respects is ever-changing and ever-adapting, coping with problems and disappointments in life without excess stress and in a way that promotes progress. At the other end is the poorly adjusted person. In the extreme, this person may show signs of anxiety, aggression, or disordered thinking, perhaps like the young pediatrician just mentioned. He reported hearing unspoken voices, which were hallucinations, having no basis in reality, and he was admitted to the hospital. A person in this condition is less adaptive, responding in much the same way regardless of the circumstances, with the result that his behavior is often inappropriate.

However, the line between adjustment and maladjustment—normal and abnormal or functional and dysfunctional—is vague and variable. It depends on a number of factors, including the setting, culture, and era in which the individual lives, as well as the person's age, sex, and outlook on life. This idea appears intermittently throughout our discussion, as we examine various points on this continuum and consider the underlying factors.

Where on this continuum, for example, do we place Mahatma Gandhi? What about Joan of Arc, Florence Nightingale, Albert Einstein, Edgar Allan Poe, Wolfgang Amadeus Mozart, and countless others? What sort of medicine, government, law, education, literature, and music would be available if all of these and similar individuals were clearly at the adjusted end of the continuum?

VIEWS OF MENTAL HEALTH. Successful adjustment is sometimes referred to as mental health, another concept that is difficult to define. Insofar as adjustment is a continuous process, maintaining mental health is also a more or less constant process. Expressed the other way around, mental health is not a permanent state. All of us become a *bit* depressed from time to time. In a broad sense, criteria for **mental health** include feelings of well-being and accomplishments appropriate to one's abilities (Wolman, 1989).

Theorists of all sorts have offered more specific definitions. In the midst of his work with maladjustment, Sigmund Freud was asked to describe mental health. He quickly replied: "The capacity to love and to work." This response has been expanded by others into books and articles. Freud simply meant that the well-adjusted person finds fulfillment in both respects (Jones, 1957).

Abraham Maslow described the mentally healthy person in terms of self-actualization. Human beings constantly seek expression of their potential. Those developing and utilizing their capacities to the fullest are said to be self-actualizing (Maslow, 1970). Another humanistic psychologist, Carl Rogers, cited two dimensions of mental health: openness to experience and trust in oneself. These characteristics are not fixed and permanent; they are transient and fluid processes. With openness and trust, an individual may become a fully functioning person (Rogers, 1980). Clearly, Maslow and Rogers recognize the importance of feelings and also the realization of one's potential.

More recent conceptions of mental health focus on cognitive elements, including optimism and self-esteem. A person's outlook on life is not only an important characteristic but also a determinant of mental health (Scheier & Carver, 1992).

Recent research also has overturned earlier findings about the traditional male gender role in relation to mental health. There are positive features in the traditional masculine role, such as taking an active, achievement-oriented approach to life's challenges. There are also positive features in the traditional feminine role, such as experiencing satisfaction through intimate personal relationships. It now appears that androgynous people, possessing positive elements of traditional male and female response styles, are most likely to be regarded as mentally healthy (O'Heron & Orlofsky, 1990).

CRITERIA FOR MALADJUSTMENT. Consider the question of adjustment from a different context. Suppose a person becomes extremely depressed on being diagnosed with cancer. Is this response a normal reaction to a life-threatening illness? Or is it a psychological disorder? Could it be both?

In thinking about psychological disorders, there are many perplexing decisions, but in most societies two criteria define this end of the continuum. The first concerns personal discomfort, and sometimes this discomfort is obvious. The individual is clearly unhappy, unable to work, and unsuccessful with others. The complaints and demeanor loudly proclaim personal distress.

Sometimes this discomfort is not at all obvious, as when someone hears unspoken voices, suffers disturbing thoughts, or simply feels wretched. We are shocked to discover that a person who seems happy and successful has committed suicide, needed psychiatric assistance, become divorced, or simply confessed to a deep dissatisfaction with life, not evident to the casual observer. In the poet's words, Richard Cory was a gentleman, clean favored, schooled in every grace, and richer than a king: "And Richard Cory, one calm summer night, / Went home and put a bullet through his head" (Robinson, 1921).

The second criterion involves socially disruptive behavior. The maladjusted person disturbs other people, causing suffering of some sort. This outcome is obvious in a sudden rampage of destruction, but it also occurs in lesser forms. A person at the bus station regularly accosts anyone available, asking demanding, insulting, or incoherent questions. An adolescent sets fire to buildings with the intention of destroying property. Such people are not necessarily discontent with themselves; they may be judged as maladjusted or dysfunctional on the basis of the consequences for others.

All of us have experienced discomfort, and most of us have disrupted others in one way or another. Hence, it is the intensity and frequency of these conditions that define any point on the continuum. The psychiatrist in the mental hospital was faced with these questions during the interview with the pediatrician. Where did he stand on this continuum?

STATISTICAL AND CLINICAL APPROACHES. In making judgments about personal discomfort and disruptive behavior, psychologists tend to proceed along two lines. The first, a *statistical approach,* is concerned with the probabilities of various reactions. How rare is the feeling or behavior? How far does it deviate from the norm? Running naked in New York and fasting for weeks—statistically rare events—may reflect some psychological disturbance. However, they may not be signs of maladjustment at all. Madame Curie and Harry Houdini were statistically rare individuals, and they participated in statistically rare events in science and magic, but they would not be considered abnormal (Figure 15–2). The statistical approach does not take into account the usefulness or desirability of the behavior.

From the other perspective, the person is not judged merely on the basis of statistical probabilities or usual behavior. In the *clinical approach*, the decision rests on the qualitative judgment of a professional psychologist, psychiatrist, or group of such people. The premise here is that careful, well-trained clinicians can arrive at a more sensible, accurate conclusion than that obtained on the basis of sheer numbers. Fasting is statistically deviant, but it may serve a useful purpose, as part of a protest movement for social change, bringing attention to some form of injustice. Similarly, people who run naked in the street must be viewed in a given context. A rapid, public display of nudity, called streaking, has been a popular diversion on occasion in the last decades of this century. Some interpretation of each event is needed, and it can be accomplished by an experienced, conscientious professional.

These two approaches, statistical and clinical, are often used together, each with its special assets and limitations. In fact, the pediatrician was admitted to the mental hospital because hearing unspoken voices is a statistically rare event, and it is considered a serious clinical matter. Still another approach raises the issue of the lawfulness of the individual's behavior. Not of concern here, it offers a legal definition of abnormality.

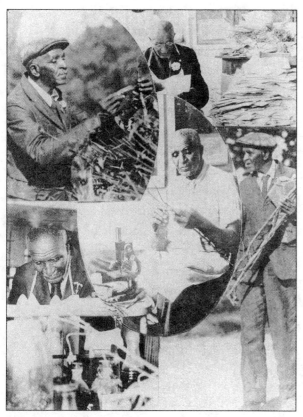

FIGURE 15–2 A STATISTICALLY RARE INDIVIDUAL. Born a slave and raised amid abject poverty, George Washington Carver became a renowned agricultural chemist, widely respected for literally hundreds of discoveries concerning uses and products of the peanut and potato. By these means, he greatly assisted poor farming communities in the South.

COPING EFFECTIVELY

We solve many adjustment problems in completely routine fashion, so much so that we may not realize we have surmounted a problem. Several basic ways of coping with personal problems were enumerated in the chapter on emotion and stress. They are relevant here. In this review, it should be remembered that these are normal and generally satisfactory adjustment reactions, although some are more useful than others.

The most effective approach is *to deal directly with the problem*, taking some direct action to change or eliminate it. In fact, direct action is the only method of really solving the problem. The pediatrician apparently went to the hospital to take direct action on the problem of unspoken voices. Once in the hospital, he was faced with a different problem—adjusting to that institutional setting.

Deprived of many conveniences, the hospitalized patients found ways to deal with their barren environment, making it more comfortable and interesting. One patient used a heating unit on the ward as a personal clothes dryer. Another requested a second serving at lunch—to be consumed later as "afternoon tea." Still another urinated into the laundry bin to save a trip to the toilet: "Those clothes were dirty anyway" (Rosenhan, 1973). The latter habit, a dubious practice from the viewpoint of health standards, illustrates socially disruptive behavior.

If the problem is insoluble, then indirect methods must be used, and there are several indirect, positive methods of coping. One such method is *to think about the problem differently.* In reframing the problem, also called *cognitive restructuring,* the individual looks at the problem from a new perspective. It is defined as more tolerable, less disruptive, or simply unimportant. A hospitalized person might decide that the institution is really not so bad after all—offering free food, shelter, and a chance to do some extensive thinking without disruptive telephone calls. Besides, the state pays some of the bills.

Another problem for the patients involved relations with the hospital staff. In doing their work, the staff often behaved in ways that rejected the patients, ignoring their attempts to make contact (Table 15–1). For the patients, one means of dealing with this rejection was to think about it differently. They might have decided that they should only expect routine assistance from the overworked staff. They might have looked forward instead to personal relations with family, friends, and other patients.

In addition, the individual can attempt *to relieve the stress reaction.* These techniques include two rather opposite approaches—complete relaxation and vig-

TYPE OF RESPONSE	PSYCHIATRISTS	NURSES
Moves on, averts head	71%	88%
Makes eye contact	23%	10%
Pauses and chats	2%	2%
Stops and talks	4%	1%

TABLE 15–1 RESPONSE TO PATIENTS BY HOSPITAL STAFF. These results, obtained from several hospitals, show the reaction of 13 psychiatrists and 47 nurses when a patient tried to initiate contact with them. Altogether, there were 185 attempts to contact the psychiatrists and 1,283 attempts to contact the nurses (Rosenhan, 1973).

orous exercise. The former includes muscle relaxation, breathing control, and visualization techniques in which one imagines relaxing scenes. The latter involves weight training, aerobics, and athletic competition, all of distinct value for reducing stress. They not only relax the body and relieve tension but also, by restoring normal balance, they offer the individual greater opportunity for using cognitive methods (Figure 15–3). The rested and controlled individual may think of a new plan.

One of the most common and useful indirect methods of handling problems is employed by almost everyone at one time or another. A *sense of humor* keeps one's problems in perspective—or at least puts them into the context of circus music, which seems to play in the background of all of our lives. Humor permits a person to acknowledge and to deal with events that are otherwise too difficult to be borne directly (Vaillant, 1992). People who can laugh at their troubles have in part mastered those troubles.

☙

INEFFICIENT COPING

We respond to everyday problems of adjustment in diverse ways. Most of these reactions are not statistically rare or clinically prominent, and they typically do not involve significant personal discomfort or disruption of others. They are routinely employed by all of us from time to time.

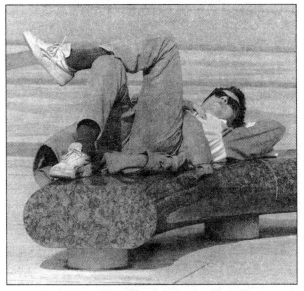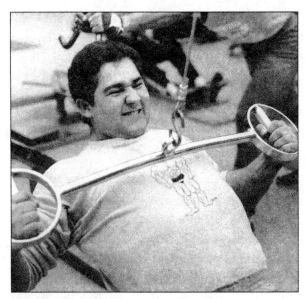

FIGURE 15-3 REDUCING STRESS. Complete relaxation and vigorous exercise can regulate disrupted biological processes and provide a refreshed mental state; they are often recommended for use in coordinated fashion.

But they may be inefficient. They may drain our energy, cause needless expenditure of time, prevent us from finding better solutions, and even make us more troubled. To what extent are they inefficient and damaging? The answer of course depends on their degree and duration.

DEFENSE MECHANISMS. Redefining the situation and using exercise, relaxation, and humor are conscious efforts to deal with an insoluble problem. According to many psychologists, we also use a method of which we are less aware. A **defense mechanism** is an unconscious means of dealing with anxiety, based on self-deception. As noted in the previous chapter, the basic defense mechanism is **repression,** a process of forgetting by which unpleasant thoughts are excluded from awareness, without the intention to do so. An individual who has seriously embarrassed, offended, or harmed someone else may be completely unable to remember that event, no matter how hard he or she tries. And certainly an individual who has been molested may be unable to remember it (Briere & Conte, 1993; Clark, 1993). This reaction differs from

suppression, which is a *conscious* attempt to avoid certain thoughts or actions and therefore not a defense mechanism in the traditional sense. The individual, aware of the offensive act, simply tries to think about something else, thereby blocking out the memory.

Since Sigmund Freud developed the concept, lists of defense mechanisms have become many and varied, depending on the strictness of the definition, especially the role of repression. However, certain defense mechanisms appear on all lists: rationalization, reaction formation, and projection, discussed in the previous chapter, as well as displacement, denial, and sublimation.

In **displacement,** an emotional reaction intended for a certain person or object is shifted to some other target. An adult frustrated in love with another adult may lavish extraordinary affection on a niece or nephew. A child, angered by parental restrictions, may break a toy. When the feelings and behavior are hostile, this reaction is often called *displaced aggression,* meaning that the attack is directed to a less threatening object rather than the source of its origin, which may be too threatening to confront. For such behavior to be considered a defense mechanism, rather than simply misdirected retaliation, the motives for aggression must be unconscious.

When some event is too difficult to confront, the mechanism may be **denial,** which is a refusal to recognize certain aspects of reality. An alcoholic person may deny his addiction or refuse to believe that extensive drinking can produce certain physical ailments.

Anxiety is often most successfully managed by **sublimation,** for here unacceptable impulses are directed toward socially approved targets. An aggressive person might become a crime fighter or trial lawyer. A sexually frustrated person might develop a program of sex education for teenagers or create sensuous art forms (Table 15–2).

Using any defense mechanism, especially repression, requires a constant expenditure of energy because the unconscious thoughts are always seeking expression. According to psychoanalysis, so much energy goes into the effort of excluding unwanted thoughts from awareness that repressed people are often stiff, inflexible, tired, and readily upset. They have relatively little energy left over for the tasks of daily life, to say nothing of unusual tasks, such as creativity. In other words, the process of repression occurs at the cost of considerable energy and flexibility.

Nevertheless, the use of defense mechanisms may be advantageous in two respects. Through repression, we may forget some of our most difficult problems and traumatic experiences. Through other defense mechanisms, especially sublimation, we may find partially effective ways of dealing with them.

DECREASED RESPONSIVENESS. After coping ineffectively with problems, human beings sometimes abandon their efforts, displaying lethargy and helplessness instead. They give up

MECHANISM	DEFINITION	ILLUSTRATION
Repression	Unconsciously excluding anxiety-provoking thoughts from awareness	A man who was sexually abused as a child cannot recall the traumatic incidents.
Rationalization	Finding false reasons to justify one's own behavior	A rejected author declares that he would not cooperate with that publisher anyway.
Reaction formation	Counteracting an unconscious impulse with the opposite reaction	Resenting her responsibility for elderly parents, a woman nurtures them intensely.
Projection	Attributing to others one's own unacceptable traits	A reckless auto racer declares that he drives well; other drivers are dangerous.
Displacement	Transferring an emotional reaction onto a less threatening target	Forsaken by his father, a boy directs his admiration and respect to a teacher.
Denial	Refusing to accept reality; rejecting evidence	A teenager decides that pregnancy is impossible, even without contraception.
Sublimation	Channeling basic impulses into more useful, creative expressions	An aggressive, defiant man devotes himself to the war on poverty.

TABLE 15–2 TRADITIONAL DEFENSE MECHANISMS. All defense mechanisms involve unconscious processes. Sublimation is generally considered more effective than the others because the repressed impulses are directed into socially useful activities.

hope, too defeated even to express resentment. In a hospital or jail, at work or in school, a person may feel overwhelmed and cease responding.

We do not know if the pediatrician reacted this way during his hospitalization. We do know that immediately after admission, he no longer claimed to hear voices and began taking notes on what he observed. He found that most patients sat or dozed in the lounge area, partly because of the medication they were given, partly because they had become dispirited (Rosenhan, 1973). If sufficiently frustrated by any uncontrollable circumstance, a person may display this adjustment reaction—some form of decreased responsiveness, becoming listless or apathetic.

In an experimental study, dogs were placed in a suspension harness that allowed some freedom of movement, and they all received a brief, mild shock. Some could not terminate it, but others could do so by pressing a nearby panel. Then each dog was placed individually in an open compartment without a harness, where another electric shock occurred. It was found that the dogs that had previously learned to escape the shock by pressing the panel readily jumped a barrier and thereby escaped the new shock. The others, although they could move about freely, usually whined and settled into a position to endure the shock, making no escape movements. Their earlier **learned helplessness,** in which they could do nothing to alleviate a stressful situation, apparently induced them to become lethargic later (Seligman, 1975; Seligman & Maier, 1967).

Certain ghetto situations may be analogous to the conditions of learned helplessness among animals. Poverty-stricken people may seem too lazy to do anything about their situation, but perhaps, like the dogs in harness, they have learned—rightly or wrongly—that there is nothing they can do to change it. After years of learned helplessness, they have stopped trying. The concept of laziness is inappropriate, just as it is in so many cases of homelessness (Goodman, Saxe, & Harvey, 1991; Olson & Schober, 1993).

RESORTING TO FANTASY. The inactive individual has not necessarily ignored the problem. Sometimes the problem is solved inwardly, by wishful thinking and dreams called **fantasy.** In imagination, a person may accomplish all sorts of feats, finding true love, vanquishing a rival, and overcoming an insurmountable obstacle (Figure 15–4). In *The Secret Life of Walter Mitty* a meek, ineffective man becomes a ship's captain in a raging storm, a brilliant surgeon directing an unprecedented operation, a courageous wartime hero, and so forth, all merely in his own thoughts while standing in the rain, caught in heavy traffic, or otherwise running errands for his mother (Thurber, 1983).

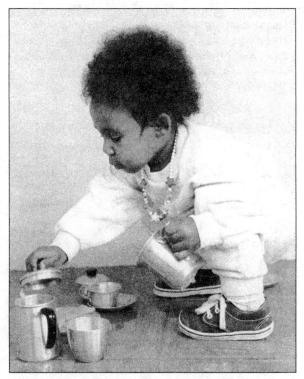

FIGURE 15–4 ENGAGING IN FANTASY. In fantasy play, a child may be trying out adult roles not readily available. Fantasy in this context represents a constructive force in personality development.

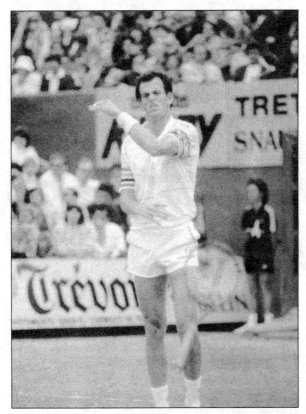

**FIGURE 15–5 DISPLACED
AGGRESSION.** This tennis player throwing his racquet clearly illustrates displaced aggression. The tennis racquet did not cause the problem. He has just missed a crucial point.

Everyone engages in fantasy. Such activities are not necessarily deviant. In fact, fantasy is often a major step in creative problem solving. It is a sign of maladjustment only when it becomes a persistent substitute for reality.

AGGRESSION AND REGRESSION.
Unsuccessful coping may result in aggressive behavior. People sometimes become abusive, break rules, argue, or criticize others. Or they assault someone physically. Aggression may be directed toward the source of frustration, toward an object or innocent person—as in displaced aggression—or even toward oneself (Figure 15–5).

As emphasized in the chapter on emotion and stress, aggression may be provoked by a variety of causes, and it is associated with many forms of maladaptive behavior, including substance use, impulse-control disorders, and the antisocial personality. Serious forms of aggression are discussed later in this chapter.

When other responses prove inadequate, people sometimes engage in **regression,** meaning that they move backward, repeating behavior that was satisfying or more appropriate at an earlier stage of development. Regression is childish behavior. Following the birth of a new brother or sister, an older child may revert to crying, baby talk, or bedwetting, and may even strike the newcomer, attempting to regain parental attention. Such behavior is not limited to children. Husbands sometimes attempt to dominate their wives, and wives their husbands, by sulking, weeping, and threats of harm to themselves if they do not get their way. If not directly aggressive, the regressed individual may be passively so, refusing to do something until his or her wish is granted.

As we turn to the question of abnormality, we should note again that adjustment lies on a continuum and is a continuous process. Aggression, regression, and the other previously discussed reactions, if chronic and extreme, would be considered abnormal. Similarly, some of the reactions to be considered next, although generally more deviant, are not completely debilitating.

• DETERMINING ABNORMALITY •

In the more disruptive adjustment disorders, we encounter less direct, less efficient problem solving. The individual is approaching abnormality, or mental disorder, a most important and complex issue in psychology. Its complexity is readily evident when even experts acknowledge that they have no adequate definition for the various boundaries of *mental disorder* (American Psychiatric Association, 1994).

Regardless of what definition we use, the pediatrician was a fraud. He *was* a pediatrician, one of eight people entering mental hospitals on the East Coast or West Coast, but he did not hear unspoken voices and experienced no psychiatric symptoms. He and the others sought admission under false pretenses, as part of a secret plan to investigate psychiatric hospitals. These five men and three women included a student, painter, housewife, psychiatrist, and three psychologists, as well as the pediatrician. David Rosenhan, a psychologist at Stanford University, was among them. Prior to their attempts to gain admission, all had been judged normal in an independent clinical evaluation. During the admissions interview, they gave only a false name, a false occupation when necessary, and the false complaint of hearing voices. Otherwise, there were no further alterations of any facts.

They entered 12 hospitals altogether, for some were admitted to more than one institution. All of them sought admission for the purpose of discovering whether expert clinicians could distinguish normal from abnormal behavior. In addition, they wanted to investigate conditions in mental hospitals. These pseudopatients were members of a research program called the *Rosenhan study*, after the chief investigator (Rosenhan, 1973).

This well-known research immediately demonstrated its major point: Experts can be fooled; they may make mistakes. It also suggested that psychiatric diagnosis is a complex process.

∾

THE DIAGNOSTIC CHALLENGE

When the Rosenhan deception was announced, it caused a titanic uproar. The press, always in search of a story, applauded this mischief, for it ridiculed psychiatry, clinical psychology, and the whole process of diagnosis. Psychiatry was quackery. Imagine! Hospitalizing perfectly normal people.

The professionals were outraged, naturally. This research, if it could be called that, revealed absolutely nothing new. It merely confirmed what everyone knows: Careful, hardworking experts in any field can be tricked by unscrupulous people.

And sober-minded folk saw in this duplicity certain defects and something of merit. Honest professionals had been treated fraudulently and perhaps unfairly, but this ruse clearly pointed to shortcomings in the diagnostic process. Rosenhan emphasized this point in his report, entitled *On Being Sane in Insane Places* (1973). If people are sane but in a place for the insane, even the experts may regard them as insane.

SELF-REPORT IN DIAGNOSIS. The hospitalization of the Rosenhan pseudopatients showed an important characteristic of the diagnostic process. It can be significantly influenced by what the patient says about his or her life. If the individual is not socially disruptive, the decision about abnormality rests with the patient's self-report of personal discomfort: "I am unhappy." "I hear voices." Clinical psychologists and psychiatrists have long known how dependent they are on the patient's self-report, and the Rosenhan research confirmed this view.

The same condition applies whenever someone seeks assistance in physical health, law, education, or any other field. A person wishing to obtain poor advice or a wrong diagnosis simply supplies false information. The Rosenhan study showed nothing new about fraud, although it did highlight the difficulty of diagnosis and did demonstrate the need for care in taking a patient's self-report at face value.

The fact that allegedly normal individuals were diagnosed as abnormal does *not* deny the validity of the diagnostic process or the relevant concepts, just as our difficulty in defining these terms does not repudiate our use of the ideas. Hot differs from cold, beautiful from ugly, and day from night, though there is no critical event of separation in any case. We argue about the distinction between life and death, and yet the value of these concepts is not refuted. In short, useful distinctions can be made between normal and abnormal, sanity and insanity, though clinicians can be fooled and certainly there are difficult cases.

LIMITATIONS OF THE DIAGNOSTIC PROCESS. Our lack of knowledge of the causes of mental disorder is an obvious limitation in the diagnostic process. As recently as the early twentieth century, people showing deviant behavior were thought to be possessed by the devil and described as *mad*. Later they were called *insane* and *abnormal*, but these terms were detrimental to the individual. When the concept of **mental illness** was introduced, it indicated a mental disorder of physical or psychological origin sufficiently severe to require professional assistance (Wolman, 1989). It also implied that the disturbed person has some disease analogous to physical illness.

By the middle of the twentieth century, this interpretation of the problem was criticized by an outspoken, dissident psychiatrist, Thomas Szasz. Calling disturbed people ill merely justified medical practice, he claimed. He popularized a new expression: "the myth of mental illness." It resisted the idea that psychological disorders are no different from physical disorders and that professional intervention is necessary to provide a cure. Szasz's replacement term, *problems in living*, has not been adopted, partly because it is more cumbersome (Szasz, 1974). Nevertheless, his assault on psychiatric practices became the early roots of movements for patients' rights and changes in the field (Smith, 1986).

In addition, the diagnostic labels focus on symptoms rather than causes. It is for this reason that the Rosenhan study provided such uniform results: The pseudopatients simply matched their behavior to the diagnostic symptoms. Claiming to hear nonexistent voices, they were admitted to a psychiatric ward. After they stopped reporting the voices, they were discharged. This focus on symptoms persists because it is useful in organizing clinical knowledge and in treating certain patients, but it does not further our understanding of the underlying psychological processes (Fernald & Gettys, 1980; Persons, 1986).

Sooner or later, the diagnostic label becomes a stigma, branding the individual as a social misfit or malcontent, but here the problem is in society. It is the culture, not the diagnosis or the label per se, that stigmatizes the person, as evident in the violent portrayal of psychological disorders on television. Most people with severe disorders are not dangerous but rather socially isolated and inept. The enormously detrimental effects of this portrayal are seen in the fear it arouses in the family, friends, neighbors, and coworkers of the individual.

One demonstration of the power of psychiatric labeling employed videotaped interviews of people said to be attending a mental health center. On the tapes, they were introduced as normal, undiagnosed, or schizophrenic—meaning a serious abnormal behavior. Each label was applied to each person in one context or another, and the tapes were rated by three groups of college students. It was found that a person labeled as schizophrenic was inevitably rated as deviant in social skills. Individuals not so labeled were not described as deviant. Some consolation was found among 30 trained social workers. They did not succumb to the labels, making their ratings without this potential bias influencing their judgments (O'Connor & Smith, 1987).

There are no simple solutions to these problems. Forms of maladjustment have been conceptualized in many ways, none of which has been highly successful. Earlier in this century a psychoanalytic concept, **neurosis,** was widely used to indicate a broad array of disorders characterized primarily by anxiety, experienced directly or indirectly. Except in psychoanalysis, the concept of neurosis has been largely abandoned, chiefly because it is too broad, lacking a clear definition. Moreover, psychoanalysis is only one of several major perspectives on psychological disorders.

DIAGNOSTIC MANUAL FOR MENTAL DISORDERS. Today the most definitive diagnostic source is the fourth edition of the *Diagnostic and Statistical Manual of Mental Disorders (DSM-IV)*, published in 1994 by the American Psychiatric Association. This edition, like its predecessors, includes a wide range of diagnostic categories (Table 15–3).

Any conception of mental disorders has social and professional significance. The *Diagnostic and Statistical Manual* is a social document with implications for health status, legal competence, disability payments, and so forth. Furthermore, the diagnostic labels may influence people's perception of a person's worth. Thus, the debate continues over just which patterns of behavior belong in the manual and how they should be presented (Nathan, 1991; Wilson & Walsh, 1991).

Disorders in Infancy, Childhood, or Adolescence
Delirium, Dementia, and Amnesic Cognitive Disorders
Mental Disorders Due to a General Medical Condition
Substance-Related Disorders
Schizophrenia and Other Psychotic Disorders
Mood Disorders
Anxiety Disorders
Somatoform Disorders
Factitious Disorders
Dissociative Disorders
Sexual and Gender Identity Disorders
Eating Disorders
Sleep Disorders
Impulse-Control Disorders
Adjustment Disorders
Personality Disorders

TABLE 15–3 MAJOR DIAGNOSTIC CATEGORIES. This table shows the major categories in the *Diagnostic and Statistical Manual, IV.* All categories include numerous subcategories.

In its almost 900 pages, the *DSM-IV* ignores **insanity,** a legal term indicating that someone is not of sufficiently sound mind to be responsible for his or her conduct. Insanity is a critical legal concept because it means someone does not know right from wrong and therefore is not responsible for wrongdoing. For corrective action, this person is referred to the mental health system rather than the prison system.

DIAGNOSTIC PERSPECTIVES

The focus in *DSM-IV* is on symptoms, but clinicians inevitably become concerned about origins of mental disorders. As they formulate treatment plans, they recognize several theoretical perspectives on causal factors, reflecting systems of psychology considered earlier: the biological, psychoanalytic, behavioral, and cognitive. Many clinicians adopt an eclectic perspective, using diverse elements from each of these and other viewpoints.

For example, one section of the *DSM-IV* describes impulse-control disorders, such as *kleptomania* and *pyromania*, an inability to resist stealing for pleasure and setting fire for pleasure, respectively. Still another impulse-control disorder involves **pathological gambling,** a persistent tendency to take risks with money, leaving the outcome largely to chance. This habit can cause more than loss of money and disruption of family and vocational life. It can result in forgery, fraud, embezzlement, and related illegal acts. This problem is especially disastrous for people with marginal incomes. Unfortunately, those who can least afford to lose the money—with the least education and least secure employment—are most likely to gamble it away (Volberg & Steadman, 1988, 1989). As the racehorse gambler said, "I'm going to the track today and hope I come out even—because I really need the money."

Pathological gambling may or may not begin

with some inherited predisposition, but according to the *biological view,* changes may take place within the nervous system as gambling continues. Initially, the gambler seeks action, an aroused state. Casino gamblers often report euphoria as the dice are rolled for a bet. Racetrack bettors describe a heart-stopping excitement when the announcer calls: "They're off!" The pathological element apparently arises in the need to maintain or increase this excitement, which is produced by increasingly greater risks, presumably associated with changes in brain chemistry. There is biological evidence that in some people the central nervous system is under-aroused and therefore highly responsive to further stimulation (Eysenck, 1990). In sensation-seeking behavior, discussed in the previous chapter, people search for thrilling, even dangerous stimulation (Zuckerman, 1990).

A very different perspective is adopted in the *psychoanalytic view,* which regards pathological gambling as symbolic of some underlying, unconscious problem, a symptom of earlier, unresolved personal issues. For many psychoanalysts, pathological gambling is a regression to the powerlessness of childhood. The hoped-for fortune is the parental figure to which the childlike gambler appeals for love, protection, and other forms of assistance (Cordery, 1987). In fact, loss of a parent in the early years and inconsistent discipline are characteristics associated with pathological gambling.

In the *behavioral view,* any response intermittently reinforced is difficult to extinguish. The gambler keeps betting because every so often there is a pay-off. This occasional reinforcement is sufficient to maintain the behavior. Or the act itself may be reinforcing, apart from the payoff. The individual gambles because this behavior relieves feelings of helplessness, anxiety, or depression (American Psychiatric Association, 1994).

Modern social science is characterized by a widespread concern with information processing.

On this basis, the *cognitive view* of pathological gambling focuses on the gambler's fallacy, which is an overestimation of the odds of winning. The individual erroneously decides that after ten consecutive losses, for example, the odds of winning on the very next chance are increased. Regardless of the fallacy, if gambling continues an increasingly risky pattern is likely to develop, with larger and larger bets, attempting to undo the series of losses. The mental processes responsible for this behavior involve various thought distortions, including denial, superstitions, and even over-confidence (American Psychiatric Association, 1994).

Pathological gambling is distinguished from social gambling, which occurs with colleagues, lasts for a specific period, and is based on predetermined, acceptable losses. It also differs from professional gambling, in which calculated risks are taken under a strict code of discipline. Cultural variations in the type and extent of gambling are observed throughout the world.

• TYPES OF DISORDERS •

After entering the hospitals, the Rosenhan pseudopatients immediately stopped claiming to hear unspoken voices. Instead, they behaved normally, engaging the real patients and staff in conversation and, according to plan, taking notes on what took place in the hospital. This note-taking was a primary research goal, and it showed, among other results, that the real patients recognized normality better than did the professional staff. At least they were more suspicious of the Rosenhan pseudopatients (Table 15–4).

The hospital environment included patients with all sorts of backgrounds and diagnoses, but relatively few of them would be classified according to the first two or three categories in the following sequence of psychological disorders. As a rule, anxiety and somatoform disorders do not require hospitalization, or at least extensive hospitalization.

ANXIETY DISORDERS

The predominant feature in an anxiety disorder is, of course, anxiety. Among all of the disorders in the *DSM-IV,* these occur most frequently, and they most closely represent what used to be called *neurosis.* The most common forms include generalized anxiety, phobia, posttraumatic stress, and the obsessive-compulsive disorder.

GENERALIZED ANXIETY DISORDER.

When a person experiences excessive worry for no apparent reason, and this condition has existed for at least six months, it may be referred to as a **generalized anxiety disorder.** This intense concern about circumstances that do not appear to warrant such anxiety is also accompanied by irritability, disturbed sleep, or some other related symptom. The person may say, "I'm really worried, but I don't know why. I have no reason to be, but I am."

Muscle tension is one of the prominent symptoms, evident in trembling, twitching, fatigue, and restlessness. In addition, there may be sweating and hot flashes or chills. At work or in moments of relaxation, the individual may feel irritable or keyed up or may have difficulty concentrating (American Psychiatric Association, 1994). However, this diagnosis does not apply if the anxiety seems to be due to some other mental disorder or to some organic factor, such as a thyroid condition or caffeine intoxication.

SPECIFIC PHOBIA. Unreasonable fear of some clearly discernible object or event, sufficient to interfere with an individual's work or social endeavors, is known as a **specific phobia.** Unlike the individual experiencing generalized anxiety, the phobic person knows what he or she fears and avoids that object or event. These reactions often involve animals: dogs, cats, insects, snakes, and rodents (Figure 15–6). Other specific phobic reactions involve strangers, blood, closed spaces, and air travel. They do not include fear of humiliation in social situations, referred to as *social phobia,* which involves difficulty speaking to strangers, using public places, and engaging in group behavior.

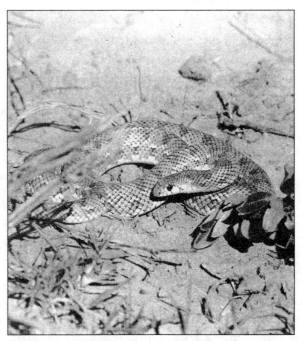

FIGURE 15–6 ORIGINS OF PHOBIAS. Phobias involving wild animals, insects, darkness, and heights are interpreted from various theoretical perspectives. In the behavioral approach, the phobia arises through association with some anxiety-provoking situation. In the psychoanalytic tradition, the phobic reaction is a symbolic expression of unconscious conflict. In the biological or evolutionary perspective, the phobia reflects a genetic predisposition from earlier times in which such events represented real dangers.

Sigmund Freud's case of Little Hans is a classic description of a specific phobia. A healthy five-year-old boy one day began to cry and refused to go for his usual walk. The next day he cried and refused again. Finally, he explained to his mother that he was afraid of horses, a fear that was inexplicable because the boy had never been kicked, bitten, or otherwise harmed by a horse. Eventually he could not go outside at all and complained that a horse might come into his room (Freud, 1909).

For any phobia, the degree of impairment depends partly on the environment. Little Hans was highly incapacitated because horses appeared throughout Vienna in his day. Snake phobias generally are not a problem for city dwellers; elevator phobias are of little significance in the country. Phobias in the general population range from agoraphobia, fear of open spaces, to zoophobia, fear of animals. However, people seldom seek treatment—perhaps because their avoidance reaction has become an accepted habit, part of everyday life, while therapy is an unknown condition and therefore even more threatening.

POSTTRAUMATIC STRESS DISORDER.

Another form of anxiety is not confined to a specific context. It can appear almost any place. Whenever someone re-experiences a severely disturbing event, thereby becoming intensely anxious again, the condition is called **posttraumatic stress disorder.** It is initiated by a memory, nightmare, flashback, or some other reminder of the original, terrifying incident. Rape victims, disaster survivors, and military personnel with wartime experiences have all reported this syndrome. Often it includes an insensitivity or numbness to people and events reminiscent of the painful experience, thereby disrupting the individual's capacity for intimacy, sexual desire, and close relationships.

The puzzling part of this disorder is that the memories do not fade. The brain's capacity for forgetting seems somehow disrupted. Speculation concerns the role of the amygdala in anxiety, apparently the most fundamental human emotion (Davis, 1992). There is also speculation that traumatic memories may be more readily stored in the right hemisphere, presumably involved in processing affect (Schiffer, Teicher, & Papanicolaou, 1995).

OBSESSIVE-COMPULSIVE DISORDER.

Most people experience some thoughts and actions of a recurring nature. We may think about an embarrassing experience over and over, unable to forget it, or we may expend too much effort writing and rewriting an inconsequential letter. When such ritualistic behavior requires considerable expenditure of time or its omission causes marked distress, it may be considered an **obsessive-compulsive disorder.** The essential feature is some persistent yet useless thought or action, consuming more than an hour daily (American Psychiatric Association, 1994).

The recurrent thought is called an *obsession*, and it causes pronounced anxiety. A repetitive thought of contamination, perhaps through eating improperly washed food, is an example. A recurrent act, such as constantly arranging and rearranging a linen closet, is known as a *compulsion*, and it serves to reduce anxiety. Excessive drinking and gambling are sometimes referred to as compulsive, but this usage is not in accordance with diagnostic standards. There is an obvious purpose in these repetitive behaviors; they are not completely useless activities.

Compulsive people often emerge as checkers or cleaners. Checkers ensure that the doors are locked, the clothes hung properly, the faucets turned off, or the plants watered, and then they check on their checking, again and again. Cleaners endlessly wash their hands, polish their shoes, sweep the floor, and rinse the sink, scrubbing and cleansing everything to the point where daily life is significantly disrupted. All of us check and clean in limited ways.

In obsessive-compulsive cases, these behaviors become overpowering habits, experienced in adult life by slightly over 2% of the population (American Psychiatric Association, 1994).

SOMATOFORM DISORDERS

The essential feature in a **somatoform disorder** is a physical symptom, a malfunction of the body, or *soma*, which cannot be fully explained by any medical condition. The symptom appears instead to be related to psychological stress, particularly inappropriate social learning and family problems (Ader & Cohen, 1993; Mullins & Olson, 1990). There is no faking or false claim, as with the Rosenhan pseudopatients.

In one form, called *somatization disorder*, the individual has multiple somatic complaints extending over several years, usually beginning in the teens, rarely later than the twenties. Without any identifiable physiological defect to account for the symptoms, the afflicted individual may seek medical care from several sources, sometimes simultaneously, with complaints about gastrointestinal, reproductive, cardiopulmonary, and other problems, as well as assorted aches and pains. The individual always has a series of *vague physical ailments*, if not of one sort, then of another.

In contrast, the *conversion disorder* is more specific, involving a persistent loss or alteration of a certain physical function. There is an inexplicable loss of muscle control or sensitivity in a *specific organ* of the body (Figure 15–7).

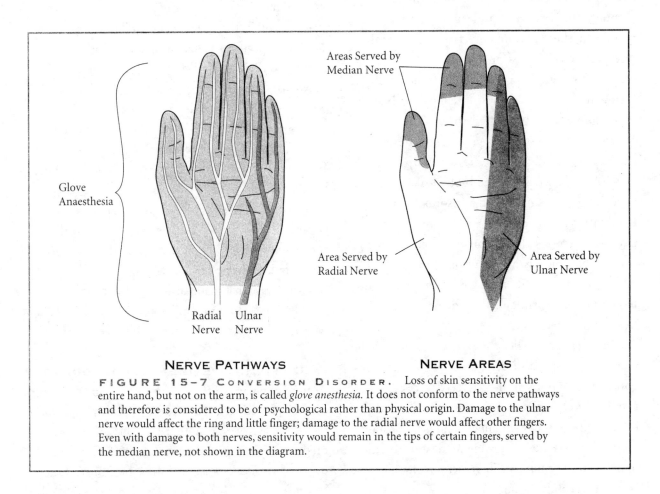

Glove Anaesthesia

Radial Nerve   Ulnar Nerve

Areas Served by Median Nerve

Area Served by Radial Nerve

Area Served by Ulnar Nerve

NERVE PATHWAYS   **NERVE AREAS**

FIGURE 15–7 CONVERSION DISORDER. Loss of skin sensitivity on the entire hand, but not on the arm, is called *glove anesthesia*. It does not conform to the nerve pathways and therefore is considered to be of psychological rather than physical origin. Damage to the ulnar nerve would affect the ring and little finger; damage to the radial nerve would affect other fingers. Even with damage to both nerves, sensitivity would remain in the tips of certain fingers, served by the median nerve, not shown in the diagram.

By definition, there is no known neurophysiological basis for these physical ailments, but two psychological mechanisms are suggested to account for them. There is the *primary gain,* which is the alleviation of anxiety from some other source. The underlying psychological disturbance, which is the real problem according to psychoanalysis, is kept out of awareness. The *secondary gain* involves some additional advantage, apart from disguising the fundamental problem. This gain may be achieved in the form of sympathy or gifts from others, or it may enable the afflicted individual to avoid some distasteful task.

The concept of secondary gain is central to the behavioral interpretation of somatoform disorders. According to the reinforcement principle, the individual's symptoms are maintained through the attention and support offered by people in the environment. The psychoanalytic interpretation focuses on repression and conversion of the earlier problem into some symbolic form, in this case a physical symptom. Nausea, for example, may be related to unconscious oral concerns. The biological perspective points out that the somatization disorder appears in 10–20% of all first-degree biological female relatives of a woman with this disorder (American Psychiatric Association, 1994). And the cognitive view stresses diverse mental events possibly responsible for this maladaption (Dodge, 1993). As expected, the different viewpoints stress different factors, although they demonstrate overlapping concerns.

In a related problem, *hypochondriasis,* there is no marked physical disorder but rather an excessive concern over one's health. Everyday coughs and cramps are considered symptoms of a dreaded disease. The person has an "illness phobia," constantly worried about health problems despite medical opinion to the contrary. This reaction appears to be partly by secondary gain.

DISSOCIATIVE DISORDERS

Some reactions to stress are characterized by forgetting or blocking out pervasive portions of one's life. In the dissociative disorder, there is a disruption of memory, consciousness, perception, or identity. Two or more aspects of the personality no longer appear connected. They seem to function independently, and yet they coexist, as in amnesia, fugues, and the dissociative identity disorder.

AMNESIA AND FUGUE. Loss of memory too pervasive to be considered ordinary forgetting is called *amnesia.* A case of **dissociative amnesia** involves extensive memory loss, presumably on a psychological basis, with no observable physical cause. This memory failure may pertain to any traumatic event in the individual's lifetime, and it may involve a specific setting, such as the workplace, or it may be more general. In either case, the individual remains in familiar surroundings and is otherwise reasonably adjusted.

Sometimes an individual cannot remember his or her name, family, or friends, and no one within hundreds of miles seems to know this person. This condition is known as a *fugue,* meaning a "flight." In a typical **dissociative fugue,** which also has no known organic basis, the person has experienced extreme memory loss and has moved some distance from home. In a sense, he or she has done in a serious and dramatic way what many of us may want to do occasionally—just go away and forget everything for a while.

DISSOCIATIVE IDENTITY DISORDER. A more popularized form of forgetting involves the **dissociative identity disorder,** in which a person seems to have two or more personality states. Previously called *multiple personality,* it is fictionally depicted in *Dr. Jekyll and Mr. Hyde* by Robert Louis Stevenson. A real-life account appeared in the book

The Three Faces of Eve, describing a woman with three personalities: Eve White, an unhappy housewife; Eve Black, a high-spirited, sexy young woman; and Jane, a dignified, cultured person (Thigpen & Cleckley, 1954). In her autobiography about these personalities, Chris Sizemore described several traumatic incidents with dead people in early childhood, from which she retreated in horror. It seemed to her at the time that someone else was viewing these scenes, not her. After an extensive course of therapy, during which one of the personalities sometimes displaced another in the middle of the treatment session, she eventually developed into an integrated adult with a single personality (Sizemore & Pittillo, 1977).

Many cases have been cited recently, including people accused of crimes who report that the deed was committed by their "other personality." Such claims raise perplexing legal questions about competence to stand trial, the insanity plea, and even malingering (Lewis & Bard, 1991). In forensic settings, it may be almost impossible to distinguish this disorder from clever deceit (Dinwiddie, North, & Yutzy, 1993).

Hypotheses about the origins of the dissociative identity disorder have ranged from childhood trauma to family disorders, but some form of self-hypnosis may be involved. To deal with severe conflict, such as sexual abuse or parental suicide, the child perhaps develops separate selves or personalities, each with its own awareness and memories (Confer & Ables, 1983; Figure 15–8).

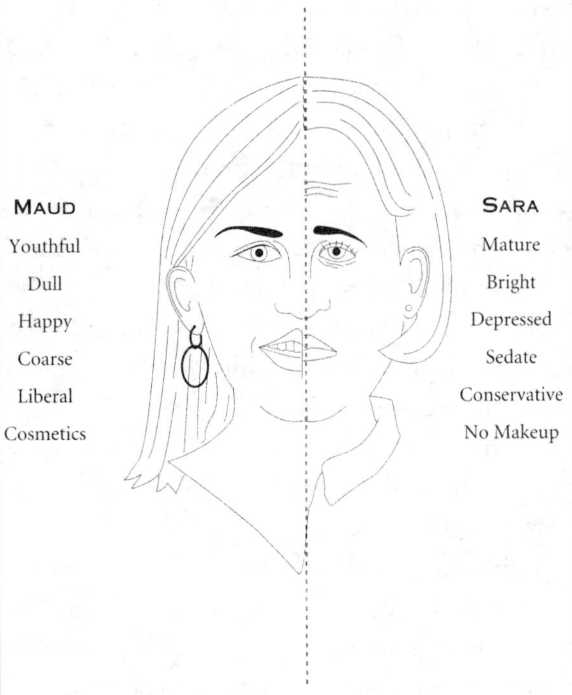

FIGURE 15–8 DISSOCIATIVE IDENTITY DISORDER. Maud and Sara were two different personalities in one woman's life. They alternated control of the same body (From Lipton, 1943).

MAUD
Youthful
Dull
Happy
Coarse
Liberal
Cosmetics

SARA
Mature
Bright
Depressed
Sedate
Conservative
No Makeup

MOOD DISORDERS

On the hospital wards, the Rosenhan pseudopatients soon discovered that no one cared what they did, provided that they caused no problem. Hence, most of them made their observations and completed their records openly, writing on standard tablets in dayrooms and elsewhere, describing how patients and staff dealt with crowding, medical procedures, and work routines. In some cases, the conditions were good and the staff laudable. In others, the situation was deplorable (Rosenhan, 1973).

Many of the patients on the ward suffered from one of two different disorders, both of which deserve careful consideration. The essential characteristic of the first, a mood disorder, is a prolonged, very deep feeling that influences one's entire outlook on life. The second, schizophrenia, involves primarily disordered thought. Alterations in thinking and mood are present in virtually all serious maladjustment, but exaggerated or inappropriate emotions are most obvious in mood disorders.

MAJOR DEPRESSIVE DISORDER. When feelings of intense disappointment and helplessness about life continue for at least two weeks, or there is a loss of pleasure in virtually all activities for an equal period, the condition may be a **major**

depressive disorder. However, these feelings must be accompanied by other symptoms, such as weight loss, fatigue, insomnia, agitation, a feeling of guilt, inability to concentrate, and so forth.

Extreme depression may result in complete loss of hope and, in dire cases, suicide. Women are more than twice as likely as men to attempt suicide, not a surprising condition inasmuch as they are more prone to depression (Strickland, 1992). Men are three or four times more likely to commit the act, however, partly because they use more potent weapons, such as guns and ropes, rather than poison or pills.

Suicide rates are highest among older people with little money, no friends, and poor health, but they are also high, and on the rise, among adolescents, especially those maintaining high aspirations or using illegal drugs. Recognition of these characteristics, particularly quiet depression, is essential in suicide prevention (Shneidman, 1981). Prescriptions on how to commit suicide, intended for terminally ill people, have raised further controversy in this area.

BIPOLAR DISORDER. Other mood disorders are characterized by sharp mood swings or up-and-down feelings. When an extremely excited or manic episode is preceded or followed by depression, the condition is called a **bipolar disorder.** The emotions may fluctuate rapidly from one pole to the other, or they may stay for some time at one extreme.

In the *manic episode* the individual may be extremely happy, singing at the top of his voice, or irritable, moving quickly in unrestrained fashion. Sometimes there is a flight of ideas; the individual goes off rapidly on one tangent, then another, and then another, as each idea occurs. In the *depressive episode* the person loses interest in life, including eating and other pleasurable activities, shows a loss of energy, and complains of worthlessness. Self-destructive acts and suicidal thoughts also may be present.

The manic and depressive conditions may alternate in a variety of ways, but the manic episode is usually sudden in onset, commonly the first phase of a bipolar disorder. The depressive episode is characteristically more prolonged, and recovery is more gradual. Today extreme mania and depression are seldom seen in mental hospitals because medications are used to stabilize the patient's emotional condition. But not all who suffer this condition are responsive to medication, and symptoms sometimes appear in spite of this treatment.

VIEWS OF DEPRESSIVE DISORDERS. Heredity is a major consideration in the biological view of depressive disorders. Studies of identical twins and adopted children support this outlook. Identical twins show similarity in depression. Neither or both members tend to be susceptible. Adopted children who display mood disorders tend to have biological parents with these disorders (Wender, Kety, Rosenthal, Schulsinger, Ortmann, & Lunde, 1986). Evidence for a neuropsychological factor is found in the rhythms of the bipolar disorder. When people suddenly become depressed or euphoric for no apparent reason, internal factors are believed to be at work, linked to brain chemistry. Norepinephrine and serotonin are neurotransmitters involved in arousal, awareness, and cognitive functions, and therefore it is hypothesized that depression may involve a depletion of these substances. In fact, medications that enhance the supply of norepinephrine and serotonin have been found to diminish depression (Schildkraut, Green, & Mooney, 1985).

From the psychoanalytic perspective, a major contributor to the depressive disorder is unconscious anger. This resentment, which cannot be openly expressed, has been turned toward the self, complicating the problem because then the individual experiences anger in both directions, outward and inward. The outward targets of this anger may be responsible for real or imagined rejection in childhood, or they may be deceased people, prompting resentment and anger over the loss (Fenichel, 1982).

The behavioral view is more parsimonious, attributing the reaction to changes in the environment, which no longer offers support for habitual behaviors. Divorce, death, retirement, being fired, reaching menopause, and countless other events result in a loss of reinforcement. The individual ceases to respond, and the related behaviors gradually disappear (Lewinsohn, 1974). The outcome is that other people cease even their normal reactions or they express sympathy, both of which augment a vicious cycle, resulting in less and less responsiveness on the part of the individual. Depression, in the behavioral view, arises through a lack of reinforcement in the environment.

Cognitive theorists also have interpretations of these disorders, especially mood disorders. Focusing on attributional style, one view states that people become depressed because they engage in self-blame, searching for evidence to confirm their worthlessness (Beck, 1976; Beck & Freeman, 1990). In another view, cognitive theorists suggest that the key factor is the individual's perception that events are out of his or her control, a view consistent with the principle of learned helplessness. A depressed person decides that nothing can be done about the situation. These two views are hardly compatible. People should not engage in self-blame, which is the basis of the first theory, if events are uncontrollable, as stated in the second interpretation. As so often happens in psychology, there are research findings to support both views (Benassi, Sweeney, & Dufour, 1988; Sweeney, Anderson, & Bailey, 1986).

Such findings are not surprising for two reasons. There are different types of depression, and different thought processes may be associated with each. Expectation, self-esteem, and explanatory style—optimism or pessimism—are important determinants of mental health, and they may even contribute significantly to physical health (Adler & Matthews, 1994).

SCHIZOPHRENIA

All of the Rosenhan pseudopatients, amid their bold research and note-taking, eventually gained a discharge. Their hospitalizations ranged from 7 to 52 days, with an average of 19 days (Rosenhan, 1973).

Here we find a lesson in the Rosenhan study that is just the opposite of what was intended. It was not evidence against clinical practice. Rather, it was further proof that the diagnostic system works, at least for apparently serious cases (Spitzer, 1975). When the patients feigned abnormality, they were incarcerated. When they abandoned their symptoms, they were discharged. The average hospitalization was 19 days, and the decision to discharge was made some days earlier in each case. When one considers the unpredictability of symptoms in almost any psychiatric disorder, slightly more than two weeks seems to be a reasonable period for a change in diagnosis (Farber, 1975).

Nevertheless, one of the fraudulent patients was hospitalized for almost two months. For someone behaving in a normal fashion, hospitalization for this period could have seemed quite a while.

The pseudopatients faked a disorder known as **schizophrenia,** which includes any of these symptoms: hallucinations, delusions, disorganized speech, disorganized behavior, and lack of responsiveness to the surroundings. Fundamentally it is a distortion of reality. The *hallucinations* are false perceptions, such as seeing images or hearing voices that have no objective basis. The Rosenhan subjects succeeded in their strategy because they made such a firm claim about this characteristic of the schizophrenic condition. They pretended to be having hallucinations. The *delusions* are false beliefs. The delusional person may think that he is the head of the institution in which he is a patient or that he has detected poison in his food. Inappropriate emotional responses also may appear, and incoherent speech is a common characteristic.

However, most schizophrenic people are not wildly crazy, despite suggestions in the mass media. Their condition may not even be noticeable on superficial contact, and it often fluctuates. Sometimes only close observation shows the deficits in thinking (Taylor & Abrams, 1984).

For the pseudopatients in the Rosenhan study, the diagnosis in every case was the same, a psychotic disorder, specifically schizophrenia. This general term, **psychotic disorder,** or *psychosis,* has several different definitions, all indicating a very serious, highly incapacitating mental state, includ-

ing loss of contact with reality, as well as delusions, hallucinations, and other fundamental disturbances (American Psychiatric Association, 1994). In a legal context, this condition is insanity. From a lay perspective, the person is crazy. Schizophrenia is the most widely publicized psychotic reaction, but there are others, including pure delusional disorders, substance-induced psychotic disorders, and those due to a general medical condition, such as thyroid malfunction, infection, or brain injury (Figure 15–9).

SIGNIFICANCE OF THE SYMPTOMS.

Schizophrenic symptoms are likely to appear first in adolescence or early adulthood, and they may develop over a long period. This condition is called *chronic schizophrenia,* for the individual has been maladjusted for years, in minor or major ways, and eventually the condition is recognized as schizo-

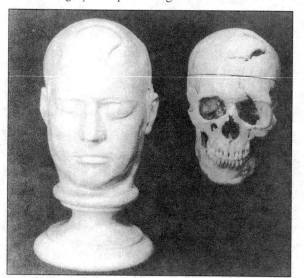

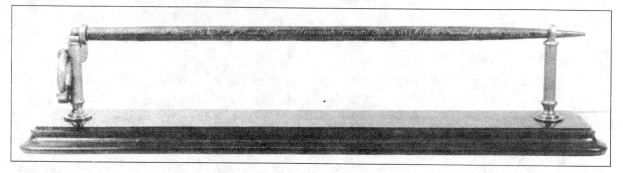

FIGURE 15–9 BRAIN DAMAGE AND PSYCHOTIC DISORDER. On the unlucky 13th of September 1848, an explosion sent a 13-pound, 4-foot crowbar completely through the head of Phineas Gage, a railroad foreman in Vermont. Miraculously, he recovered physically, but afterwards he was extremely obstinate, unrealistic, and emotional. Known earlier as a well-controlled, successful man, his friends simply said he was "no longer Gage" (Harlow, 1869). The crowbar, preserved in a museum, entered under the left cheekbone and exited from the left frontal lobe.

phrenic. In *acute schizophrenia*, the condition appears abruptly, apparently in response to some sudden stress, such as losing one's spouse, job, or life savings. While the origins of schizophrenia are uncertain, the prognosis is most favorable when the symptoms develop suddenly, over a short term.

Schizophrenic symptoms can be described in another twofold category that has significance for prognosis. These categories are positive and negative, which in this context do not indicate good and bad. Instead, **positive symptoms** are behavioral excesses: hallucinations, delusions, incoherent speech, and aggressive behavior. The **negative symptoms** are behavioral deficits: loss of interest in the world, absence of emotional expression, inattention, and lack of speech. Among schizophrenic people, those with positive signs are regarded as having more promise for treatment and recovery than those with negative signs (Andreasen, Flaum, Swayze, Tyrrell, & Arndt, 1990; Fenton & McGlashan, 1991; Figure 15–10).

SUBTYPES OF SCHIZOPHRENIA. In earlier days, classifications included certain subtypes of schizophrenia, now not widely emphasized. Some people show the *disorganized type,* displaying disorganized behavior, disorganized speech, and inappropriate feelings in certain situations. When not completely immobile for long periods of time,

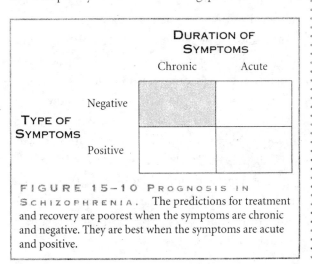

FIGURE 15–10 PROGNOSIS IN SCHIZOPHRENIA. The predictions for treatment and recovery are poorest when the symptoms are chronic and negative. They are best when the symptoms are acute and positive.

the *catatonic type* may endlessly repeat certain gestures, facial expressions, or words, often in a highly excitable, even violent manner. Today the catatonic condition is viewed as a motor dysfunction occurring in diverse psychiatric problems, sometimes associated with medications prescribed for other symptoms (Rogers, 1991). For many people with schizophrenia, the diagnosis is *undifferentiated type* because the symptoms cannot be readily classified or represent some mixture of other types.

The *paranoid type* of schizophrenia is usually the most difficult to diagnose because there is no disorganization or catatonia; instead, the individual speaks quite lucidly and convincingly, often about a central theme. On closer inspection, it may become clear that the theme is based on irrational premises. These premises may involve delusions of persecution, in which the person wrongly believes that people are trying to harm him. Or they may involve delusions of grandeur, in which he believes himself to be an extraordinarily important person.

Regardless of the specific symptoms and subtypes of schizophrenia, the Rosenhan research demonstrated a humanitarian dimension in our psychiatric services. *All* of the pseudopatients were hospitalized. When someone requests or seems to need hospitalization, that condition is taken very seriously. Hence, the admitting officers in the Rosenhan study cannot be judged too harshly. The appearance of the pseudopatients at the hospital door was certainly an implicit sign that they were seeking help. Things are as they should be—proof of a condition dangerous to oneself or others normally is not required for admission to a hospital (Blair, 1973).

DANGER OF LABELS. In all instances except one, the Rosenhan pseudopatients were discharged with the diagnosis *schizophrenia in remission,* indicating that the symptoms somehow had disappeared without treatment. This label, contrary to what one might hope, does not mean that the person is cured or has recovered. It simply indicates that no schizophrenic symptoms are currently present, and here we encounter another lesson from the Rosenhan study: the dangers of psychiatric labeling.

The most disconcerting finding in this research is that this label would have stayed with the patients, indicating that they were or had been schizophrenic, psychotic, or whatever label one prefers. It undoubtedly would have influenced others' reactions to them in their later lives had they not used pseudonyms. Sometimes it was significant on the ward, where normal behavior was wrongly interpreted to coincide with the diagnostic label. One would hope instead that the early diagnosis would have been modified in accordance with later evidence or that it might have been a deferred diagnosis, recognizing that the early symptoms were unclear (Farber, 1975).

In fairness to the professionals in the Rosenhan study, schizophrenia in remission is relatively rare as a discharge diagnosis. Most patients are still disturbed when released from the hospital, allowed to go home under outpatient care, with the use of medication, accompanied by family or friends. Being disturbed does not necessarily require further hospitalization, just as physical illness does not imply that hospitalization is necessary. In this sense, the discharge diagnosis of schizophrenia in remission is more understandable.

SEARCH FOR CAUSES. What makes people suddenly leave the world of accepted reality and enter one of their own making? The frank answer is that we do not yet know. This question is one of the most puzzling of all in clinical psychology. Significant progress may occur only when it is recognized that schizophrenia, as the term is currently employed, may represent not one but a wide variety of brain disorders. On this basis, different investigators, all studying different aspects of schizophrenia, may in fact be studying quite different illnesses (Heinrichs, 1993).

To describe how various factors interact in psychotic disorders, psychologists often refer to a *diathesis-stress model.* This rather imposing label can be readily understood, for *diathesis* simply means an inherited predisposition to a certain disease. The meaning of *stress* is obvious. Thus, the **diathesis-stress model** states that the origins of schizophrenia, or other *serious* mental disorders, lie in a combination of factors including, on the one hand, a genetic predisposition and, on the other hand, stressful environmental conditions that cause this predisposition to become manifest. An individual with a marked hereditary predisposition may show a schizophrenic reaction under relatively mild environmental pressures; a person without this genetic potential may not show schizophrenia even in highly adverse circumstances. In a favorable setting, neither person will manifest the disorder (Monroe & Simons, 1991).

In this model, the genetic factors are specific to the disorder; the environmental factors are not specific. The environmental stress is common to many types of adjustment problems (Fowles, 1992).

There is substantial evidence that heredity plays a role, especially in schizophrenia, as supported by studies of identical and fraternal twins. Since identical twins have the same inheritance, schizophrenic reactions, if based on heredity, should show a higher correspondence than in fraternal twins. A number of studies support this conclusion. When one twin experiences a schizophrenic condition, the chances of the other twin becoming schizophrenic are approximately five times greater for identical than for fraternal twins (Gottesman & Shields, 1966; Table 15–5). In schizophrenic and nonschizophrenic twins, there are also marked differences in the development of subcortical brain areas (Torrey, Bowler, Taylor, & Gottesman, 1994).

	IDENTICAL TWINS		FRATERNAL TWINS	
COUNTRY	NUMBER OF PAIRS	PERCENT BOTH SCHIZOPHRENIC	NUMBER OF PAIRS	PERCENT BOTH SCHIZOPHRENIC
United States	174	69	296	11
United Kingdom	37	65	60	13
Sweden	11	64	27	15
United States	41	61	53	13
Japan	55	60	11	18
Germany	19	58	13	0
United Kingdom	24	42	33	9
Denmark	7	29	31	6
Norway	8	25	12	17
Weighted average		62		12

TABLE 15–5 TWINS AND SCHIZOPHRENIA. This investigation summarized the results of many twin studies throughout the world. For all countries, the percentage of instances in which both twins were schizophrenic was much larger for identical than for fraternal pairs, showing the influence of genetic factors (Gottsman & Shields, 1966, 1982).

Further hereditary evidence comes from foster children adopted shortly after birth, some having a biological parent diagnosed as schizophrenic and others with apparently normal parents. In these cases, the rate of schizophrenia or borderline schizophrenia is significantly higher for the children having a biological parent diagnosed as schizophrenic. Since both groups have foster parents with apparently comparable childrearing methods, the difference in schizophrenic reactions seems to suggest an inherited condition (de Marchi, 1991). However, the mode of inheritance of schizophrenia is still not understood (Baron, 1986; Knight, Knight, & Unguari, 1992).

From a neurophysiological perspective, it is postulated that dopamine, a neurotransmitter involved in brain arousal and motor activity, may play a key role in schizophrenia. According to the **dopamine hypothesis,** a schizophrenic condition is caused by unusually high levels of dopamine or is the result of a brain unusually responsive to normal amounts of this neurotransmitter. Evidence for this hypothesis is found in cases of overdoses with amphetamines, which stimulate dopamine activity. Even in normal individuals, sufficient quantities of amphetamines can provoke a psychoticlike reaction. Similarly, minimal injections of a stimulant that produces dopamine have prompted temporary but increased schizophrenic symptoms in people who are mildly schizophrenic already (Davis, 1974). Drugs known to block dopamine have been effective in reducing schizophrenic symptoms (McGeer & McGeer, 1980). In addition, postmortem studies and brain scans support the dopamine hypothesis (Davis, Kahn, Ko, & Davidson, 1991). Collectively, these investigations have resulted in steady progress in understanding the neurobiology of dopamine systems, but it still has not been demonstrated that dopamine itself is a fundamental cause of schizophrenia (Healy, 1991).

Brain scans and imaging techniques capable of revealing brain structure and function have added biochemical evidence (Andreasen, 1988). With regard to structure, they show a degeneration of neural tissue in the cerebral cortex of people diagnosed with schizophrenia, most prominent in those with long-standing schizophrenic symptoms (Jernigan et al., 1991). In function, they show diminished activity in the brains of people with schizophrenia, compared with normal brains, especially in the frontal lobes (Weinberger & Kleinman, 1986). Whether a cause or a consequence, such defects coincide with what might be expected in this disorder.

Investigators concerned with environmental influences regard many of these studies quite differently. In the identical-twin studies, for example, they point out that when one twin is schizophrenic, the other is not inevitably schizophrenic, although their inherited structures are exactly the same. Similarly, some foster children born to normal parents develop borderline schizophrenic reactions. Schizophrenia may occur through recessive genes, but child-rearing practices and the context of the schizophrenic behavior also may be highly influential factors.

Within the family, difficulties arise when the child and parents are unsuccessful in communicating with one another. This problem is viewed broadly as **communicative deviance,** in which the parents criticize or ignore the child, contradict themselves, or otherwise communicate in an unintelligible fashion. A review of almost three decades of research on the family environment and psychopathology has provided some support for this viewpoint, showing that disturbances among family members are associated with schizophrenic and affective disorders in the offspring (Goldstein, 1988).

Research has shown, furthermore, that relapse into a schizophrenic condition is distinctly related to emotion in a family. The degree to which the family expresses hostility to and overinvolvement with a former patient is called **expressed emotion** (Hooley, 1985). Patients who return to a home with high expressed emotion are several times more likely to relapse than those who return to a home without critical or overly involved family members (Leff & Vaughn, 1981).

Poverty is a related condition. Many studies have demonstrated that the greater the poverty and population density, the greater is the incidence of schizophrenia. Two causal interpretations seem involved. According to one view, lower-class communities engender schizophrenia through frustration and social disorganization. According to another, schizophrenic individuals migrate to impoverished urban areas as part of a process of social selection. In either case, poverty involves stress, and exposure to stress is regarded by many investigators as an important contributor to this disorder (Coyne & Downey, 1991).

In summary, hereditary, biochemical, and environmental factors all appear influential, again illustrating the theme of the multiple bases of behavior. Diverse factors *combine* in various ways to produce a psychotic condition (Gallagher, Jones, & Barakat, 1987). The current view is that genetic factors may play a significant predisposing role while environmental or biological factors serve as precipitating events.

PERSONALITY DISORDERS

The pseudopatients in the Rosenhan study attempted to portray a schizophrenic condition. They succeeded in this deceit because their chief symptom was a concern about another reality, a claim that could not be contradicted by objective evidence. They heard voices that no one else could hear. For most people in our society, such voices would be a source of serious personal discomfort.

At the beginning of this chapter, two criteria were cited as defining maladjustment: personal discomfort and socially disruptive behavior. We now turn to socially disruptive behavior, which also exists on a continuum.

The **personality disorder** is a persistent and inflexible pattern of behavior that deviates from cultural expectations and, stable over the years, results in distress for colleagues and associates, as well as for the afflicted individual. People with this disorder wear out their relationships with others by their relentless and excessive demands. They are recognized for the havoc and exasperation they cause others, more than for their own sense of distress.

They are considered in several subcategories, three of which illustrate the inflexibility of the established pattern.

ANTISOCIAL PERSONALITY DISORDER.

The essential feature of the **antisocial personality disorder** is a chronic disregard for social order and legal restraints. The individual tends to violate the rights of others in some significant way. In earlier days, this individual was called a *psychopath* or *sociopath*. For this diagnosis, the individual must be at least 18 years of age. Otherwise the problem is considered a chronic disorder of childhood, or it is not yet of sufficient duration to be regarded as a personality disorder.

Among men, in whom the antisocial personality disorder is more common, the typical early signs include persistent lying, thefts, vandalism, fighting, truancy, and low school achievement. In adult life, an important symptom is the inability to sustain a consistent work record, evident in unemployment, absenteeism, and departure from the job without notice, much like the truancy and poor school performance of earlier years. Antisocial personalities may be likable on superficial contact and may hold important positions at work. In such cases, the problem usually has not been sufficiently severe to interfere with the necessary schooling.

BORDERLINE PERSONALITY DISORDER.

An individual with the diagnosis of **borderline personality disorder** usually demontrates instability in self-image, mood, and personal relationships, sometimes showing characteristics close to schizophrenic and mood disorders, prompting the term *borderline*. For brief periods the person may seem out of contact with reality, but the hallmark is instability—sudden, dramatic shifts in regard for others. A new acquaintance is viewed as a supportive, caregiving person and then abruptly considered cruelly punitive. An old lover or friend is idealized and romanticized one moment, criticized and slandered the next. Often the intense emotional displays have no obvious external cause.

People with this disorder are potentially self-damaging. They may impulsively engage in pathological gambling, unsafe sex, careless driving, or binge eating. Recurrent suicidal gestures or self-mutilation may occur, initiated as an effort to avoid separation or abandonment, real or imagined, from someone perceived as important to them.

NARCISSISTIC PERSONALITY DISORDER.

According to a Greek myth, Narcissus fell in love with himself (Figure 15–11). Unable to fall in

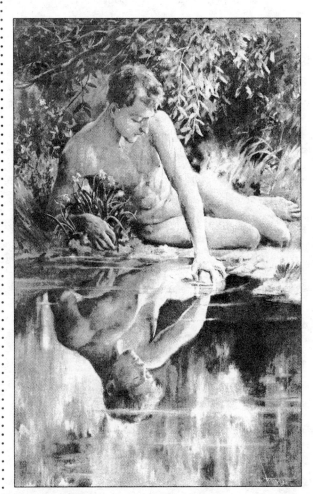

FIGURE 15–11 NARCISSISTIC PERSONALITY DISORDER. Gazing too fondly at his own reflection, Narcissus thereby gave his name to a personality disorder. It is characterized by a sense of self-importance and a strong need for admiration from others.

love with the beautiful nymph Echo, he fell in love instead with his own image reflected in a pool of water. Individuals with a **narcissistic personality disorder** have experienced a similar fate; they are intensely focused on themselves. Unable to take the perspective of another person, they have instead a sense of entitlement, demanding privileges yet denying them to others. As a result, they fail to form mature and satisfying relationships with coworkers and other colleagues.

A key element in the narcissistic personality disorder is an exaggerated concern over how one appears to others. Guided by their wish to impress others, such persons are more concerned with their image and importance than with how they and others feel. Even with a distinguished record of achievements and successes, they persistently seek attention and approval from others (Lowen, 1983).

Among all psychiatric classifications, personality disorders of all types are commonly misdiagnosed, partly because they are not well understood, partly because the subtypes may overlap. Furthermore, the characteristics central to personality disorders clearly exist on a continuum, from mild expressions to pathological extremes. The gentler expressions are present in normal or slightly eccentric individuals. The clinician's judgment of the duration, frequency, and intensity of impairment is a critical factor in the diagnosis.

VIEWS OF CAUSAL FACTORS. As in schizophrenia, one set of causal factors may lie in the individual's genetic background. Adopted children whose mothers have been diagnosed as antisocial personalities, in comparison with adopted control children, show a significantly higher rate of antisocial behavior, despite leaving the mother in infancy (Crowe, 1974). Underactivity of the nervous system may be involved. Antisocial personalities, in terms of brain function, apparently are not as readily aroused as more normal individuals. They are uniformly slower in all sorts of reaction time, which is a measure of arousability (Pfeiffer & Maltzman, 1974). Consequently, such people may engage in actions that yield more than normal excitation.

Family structure may be an influential factor, especially when no other adequate social attachments are available to the developing personality. If the parents and others are rejecting or neglecting, sometimes the young person uses antisocial behavior to gain attention (Loeber & Dishion, 1983).

Delinquent and criminal behaviors are not confined to antisocial personalities. People in any condition may transgress against society.

The causes of the borderline and narcissistic disorders are also far from understood. Learning appears to be significantly involved in the former condition because fears of abandonment or rejection by others are so prominent. For the latter, the environment also may play a significant role, for this disorder seems to be increasing in recent years. Some writers have suggested that Western culture, with its emphasis on success, individualism, and power, encourages the narcissistic personality disorder (Lasch, 1978; Lowen, 1983).

• ADJUSTMENT AND CULTURE •

After the pseudopatients were released from the hospital, all was not quiet for long in psychiatric admissions offices. David Rosenhan announced another investigation. Within three months, fraudulent people would try again to gain admission to one of the twelve hospitals in the original research. This time Rosenhan was giving the staffs a clear warning. Could they detect the frauds? Rosenhan called this part of his research the "challenge study."

Like their predecessors, these pseudopatients would feign certain symptoms. Clearly, they needed to display behaviors deemed abnormal or deviant in our culture, and here we return to the issue considered at the beginning of this chapter: What is abnormal? There we considered statistical and clinical judgments and the dual criteria of personal discomfort and socially disruptive behavior. Here, at the close of this chapter, we recognize a broader determining factor—the influence of culture.

Suppose the pediatrician in the admissions office claimed intense anxiety about his penis receding into his body, thereby causing his death. Would he have been accepted for psychiatric treatment? The answer probably would depend on the amount of anxiety expressed—unless the examiner were someone with experience in Asian cultures. This condition, not considered a mental disorder in this country, is included in the *Chinese Classification of Mental Disorders*. Called *koro*, it is known by various local terms throughout southern and eastern Asia (American Psychiatric Association, 1994).

Suppose the pseudopatient who was a college student claimed that her brain was fatigued. This malady, *brain fag*, arising from too much thinking, might well elicit psychiatric attention in West Africa but perhaps not so readily in the United States. Similarly, *taijin kyofusho* is a distinctive Japanese phobia that one's body parts are offensive in form, odor, or movement. Included in the Japanese diagnostic system, it resembles our social phobia in certain ways; at the same time, this comparison shows that concepts of normal and abnormal are inevitably culture bound.

∾

ASSESSING ADJUSTMENT

Suppose you are in a restaurant and someone nearby protests against the food. He complains loudly and then hurls his fork across the room. Still upset with the menu, he throws himself on the floor, pounding his fists. Tears come to his eyes, and he begins to shout. What do you think of *his* behavior? You regard it as abnormal—until you find out that this patron is two years old.

When a clinician ponders any psychological disorder, two questions came immediately to mind: What is the person's age? And gender? No

statement about diagnosis or prognosis can ignore these factors.

Today, with greater awareness of cultural diversity, a third characteristic becomes relevant immediately: cultural background. To understand the significance of all of these factors—culture, age, and gender—the following discussion considers two additional psychological disorders. The aim is to show that what is deviant in one culture, at one age, or for one gender is not necessarily deviant for another.

SUBSTANCE-RELATED DISORDERS. Cultures around the world vary widely in the degree to which the consumption of psychoactive substances is regarded as abnormal or illegal. A **psychoactive substance** alters the mental processes in some marked way, chiefly by depressing or stimulating activity in the central nervous system or by producing alterations in perception.

The chief feature in *substance dependence* is the chronic inability to regulate consumption of a drug, medication, or toxin—resulting in disturbances in thought, behavior, and biological functioning. Caffeine dependency is not included, chiefly because few heavy coffee drinkers have difficulty switching to substitutes (Figure 15–12).

SOURCE	CAFFEINE
Coffee, brewed, 6 oz	100 mg
Coffee, instant, 6 oz	65 mg
Soda, caffeinated, 12 oz	45 mg
Tea, 6 oz	40 mg
Analgesic, 1 tablet	35 mg
Chocolate, 1 bar	5 mg

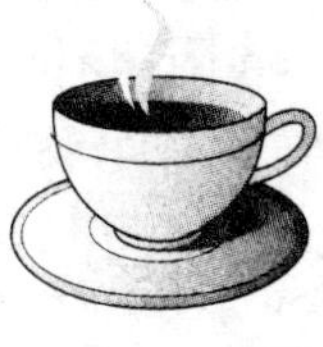

FIGURE 15–12 CULTURE AND CAFFEINE. Throughout the world, caffeine is the most widely consumed psychoactive drug. The average intake in developing countries is less than 50 milligrams per day, but in Sweden and England the average exceeds 400 milligrams per day.

All other substance-related disorders fall into the category of *substance abuse*, a residual category that does not involve dependency. Someone binges wildly on a particular substance every few weekends; someone else continues drinking alcohol despite a warning about damage to the liver. Both are symptoms of substance abuse but there is no clear dependency (American Psychiatric Association, 1994).

Some social groups, such as Muslims, show a low incidence of alcoholism because this substance is forbidden in their society; others, including large populations in Western nations, show high rates. In Asian cultures, alcohol-related disorders are relatively infrequent, due partly to physiological factors. In Chinese, Japanese, and Korean populations, a biochemical predisposition sometimes operates against alcohol consumption by producing adverse physiological reactions, such as heart palpitations and a flushed skin condition (American Psychiatric Association, 1994).

Age plays a role in alcoholism throughout the world. Consumption is highest among people between 18 and 30 to 40 years old, a condition that holds for all mood-altering substances. After middle age, and especially among elderly people, biological changes result in decreased consumption. Greater susceptibility to alcohol's depressant effects causes more severe intoxication, thereby creating related physiological problems (American Psychiatric Association, 1994).

Gender differences in alcoholism are readily evident among young people. In the United States, they show a ratio of males to females reaching 5 to 1. However, the ratio changes substantially at older ages, for women begin drinking more heavily later in life. Incidentally, due to their lower percentage of body water and lower metabolic rate for alcohol, they tend to acquire a higher blood alcohol concentration than do men and therefore are at greater risk for health-related consequences (American Psychiatric Association, 1994).

SEXUAL DISORDERS. Sexual activities also vary widely depending on culture, age, and gender. Certain modes of satisfaction, infrequent in one population, may become highly significant in another or for subgroups or individuals.

Disturbances in the normal sexual response cycle, including sexual desire and psychophysiological changes, are the defining characteristics of **sexual dysfunction.** Typically, there is a disturbance in both respects, the sense of pleasure and the physiological activities. This disruption is most evident in men in the form of erectile disorder and premature ejaculation. The chief problem for women is an orgasmic disorder or general lack of responsiveness (Bhugra, 1987).

Judgments about these disorders must consider the person's background. In some societies, sexual responsiveness in the female is considered relatively insignificant; the main concern is fertility. In other cultures, males experience problems which are less frequently encountered in the United States. In India, *dhat* refers to severe anxiety and somatic concerns associated with ejaculation, accompanied by a fear of complete loss of semen (American Psychological Association, 1994). In all cultures, diminished sexual interests are associated with aging, although there are wide individual differences.

The essential feature of a **paraphilia** is sexual attraction to some object or event not normally associated with sexual arousal. The term is derived from *para*, meaning "beyond," and *philia*, indicating a tendency or attraction toward something. There are intense sexual urges or fantasies concerning nonhuman objects, nonconsenting partners, and the suffering or humiliation of some human being. The individual may engage in a variety of these behaviors with a variety of people (Abel & Osborn, 1992). This problem is extremely serious when a nonconsenting partner is involved, adult or child.

When the attachment is to an object, arousing sexual urges or fantasies, the condition is called *fetishism*. Leather items and underwear are common fetishes, although sometimes the attraction is to a smell, sound, or other stimulus. In two paraphilic practices, *sadism* and *masochism*, sexual excitement is attained from delivering and receiving punishment, respectively. Sexual arousal apparently is derived from the total control, or lack of control, over another person, thereby facilitating the expression of various sexual fantasies. The critical legal issue here is the consent or willingness of another adult.

Paraphilic practices that figure prominently in the press involve the display or observation of sex organs, usually by men. In *exhibitionism*, a person obtains sexual gratification by showing his or her organs to others, including strangers. This behavior, is considered an offense in the street. Its counterpart, *voyeurism*, involves sexual pleasure from observing others' sex organs or sexual behavior. Again, peeking without consent invites arrest as a Peeping Tom.

Here again, adjustment is on a continuum, for these reactions clearly relate to normal behaviors. Seeing and being seen are natural aspects of sharing between sexual partners; exhibitionism and voyeurism expand these responses. The dominance and submission of sadists and masochists are outgrowths of the give-and-take basic to sexual intercourse. Even a fetish is an extension of normal behavior, for the focus of the sexual response is broadened to include something in addition to or other than the individual's partner.

For these reasons, the diagnosis of paraphilias across cultures is decidedly complicated. A behavior considered abnormal in one setting may be acceptable elsewhere (Figure 15–13). Gender differences are quite stable, however. Paraphilias everywhere are far more common in men than in women (American Psychiatric Association, 1994).

For the sake of completeness, it should be noted that the *DSM-IV* also includes the extremely rare **gender identity disorder,** a strong desire to be, or insistence that one is, of the opposite sex, apart from any perceived cultural advantage, and a persistent distress about one's own sex or gender role.

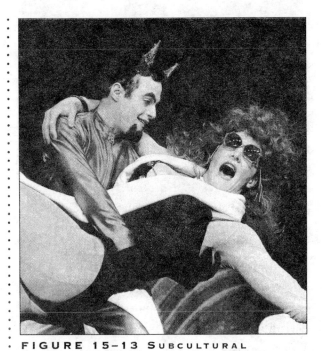

FIGURE 15–13 SUBCULTURAL NORMS. Decisions about abnormality and maladjustment are complicated by subcultural norms. Each year 16 men in this college club, producing a highly regarded musical show, dress in and act the parts of women. This cross-dressing is not considered a paraphilia, called *transvestism*, unless the men obtain sexual excitement from wearing women's clothes. Former club members include John F. Kennedy and Franklin Delano Roosevelt.

Adults with this disorder are preoccupied with the wish to be a member of the other sex. Men with this disorder are three times more common than women and seem to suffer more from peer rejection (Shane & Shane, 1995).

CULTURAL RELATIVISM

During the period of the challenge study offered by David Rosenhan, 193 patients were admitted to the psychiatric ward of the selected teaching and research hospital. Of these, approximately 20% were judged with high confidence by at least one staff member to have been feigning schizophrenic symptoms. How successful was this staff in meeting Rosenhan's challenge? Not very—no Rosenhan pseudopatient sought admission during this interval (Rosenhan, 1973).

This further deception showed once again that assessing psychological disorder is a complex, challenging task. When factors of culture are included, it becomes even more so.

All societies must deal with psychological disorders, and certain behaviors are unacceptable throughout most of the civilized world. These include homicide, rape, theft, arson, treason, and assault and battery, all destructive to the social order. Other behaviors, less aggressive, are regarded quite differently in different societies. Polygamy has been the custom in certain Middle Eastern societies; nakedness is accepted in diverse cultures; and prostitution is practiced openly in many parts of the globe. All these behaviors are considered deviant, if not illegal, in much of contemporary Western society.

The term **cultural relativism** indicates that there are no universal standards for judging many social phenomena. The standards for virtue, beauty, justice, and adjustment are culture-bound; they have a particular meaning in a particular environment.

Behavior considered normal in one society may be regarded as abnormal in another (Figure 15–14).

DIFFERENCES AMONG SUBCULTURES. The marked differences among subcultures, even in the same society, are illustrated by a man from the Ozark Mountains. He received a call from God to preach in his community, and his efforts were received with considerable enthusiasm. Soon he was called by God to a neighboring community, and then to another, and he was warmly received on each occasion. His growing reputation eventually prompted him to accept a call to St. Louis. There he was received with less enthusiasm—and a call by the police, who arrested him for disturbing rush-hour traffic (Slotkin, 1955). Lauded and encouraged in one environment, he was considered deviant and socially disruptive in another.

Hearing voices that no one else can hear, like the Rosenhan pseudopatients, is not a sign of disturbed behavior in all cultures. In some, it may even

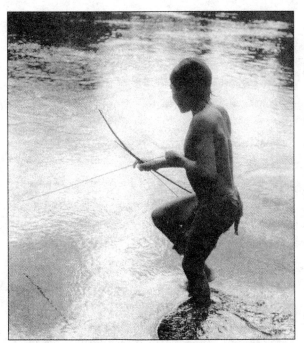 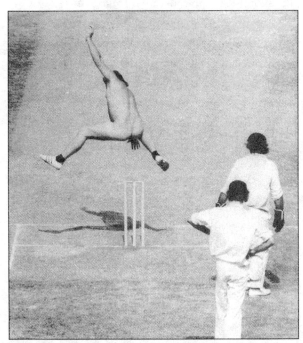

FIGURE 15–14 CULTURAL RELATIVISM. The culture plays a critical role in decisions about deviance. Nakedness is not cricket during a match.

be regarded as an honor. A delusion in one society may be a belief in another, and the trance state is regarded very differently in different cultures (Westermeyer, 1987). Such differences emphasize once again that there can be no universal definition of good adjustment and poor adjustment. Anyone stating such a definition is simply expressing a preference for a particular social or ethical order (Smith, 1986; Szasz, 1970).

DIFFERENCES AMONG ERAS. Standards also change from one era to the next within a given culture, especially a highly developed one. Our ideas about nakedness, nonmarital cohabitation, and homosexuality have changed a great deal from those of two generations ago. When compared with the first part of this century, ours seems a very different world indeed. Similarly, our views about what constitutes rape, child abuse, and discrimination are constantly being revised, and there have been continuous efforts to change the grounds for divorce and the insanity plea in legal issues. All such classifications must be tentative, reflecting cultural standards and the tentative nature of knowledge (Sue & Sue, 1987).

The *DSM-IV* is simply a momentary point in an ongoing process, indicating the criteria for our particular era. There is relativity across cultures and also within the same culture over time.

At some future date, the Rosenhan study should be of interest to historians, for the observations of the pseudopatients provided considerable information on life in a twentieth-century mental hospital—the crowded conditions, inadequate medical procedures, and sometimes good, sometimes poor staff–patient relations (Rosenhan, 1973). They showed that many responses of the patients were normal or reasonable reactions to confinement, as they tried to avail themselves of any small opportunity to improve their circumstances: pilfering biscuits from the dining hall, making friendships with the staff, and feigning illness to receive special treatment. Frequent trips to the gymnasium did not necessarily indicate an interest in vigorous exercise. More commonly, they offered a chance for a surreptitious snooze on the soft mats.

The Rosenhan study also may seem a bit puzzling to historians, for it contends that the sane cannot be distinguished from the insane. To demonstrate this point, Rosenhan selected eight accomplices, all allegedly normal. He then selected symptoms that would realistically portray them as abnormal, the voices saying "Empty!" "Hollow!" and "Thud!" Finally, he asserted that all of these accomplices behaved in a normal fashion once they gained admission to the ward. These claims about normal and abnormal may seem a bit incongruous in a study attempting to demonstrate that the two conditions cannot be distinguished from one another.

• SUMMARY •

PROCESS
OF ADJUSTMENT

1. Adjustment is a continuous process; individuals constantly strive to satisfy physiological or psychological motives. Adjustment also exists on a continuum from well adjusted to poorly adjusted.

2. An individual can attempt to cope with an adjustment problem in many ways: direct action, cognitive restructuring, relaxation techniques, vigorous exercise, and a sense of humor.

3. Inefficient coping responses include defense mechanisms, which are unconscious means of dealing with anxiety: repression, displacement, denial, and sublimation. Other reactions include lethargy, fantasy, aggression, and regression.

DETERMINING ABNORMALITY

4. The labels for poorly adjusted people have changed considerably with the passage of time, reflecting greater acceptance of the problem, but eventually any label becomes derogatory. The latest diagnostic manual, *DSM-IV*, includes a wide range of classifications.

5. Four common views of maladjustment include: the biological, giving attention to the neurophysiological bases of behavior; the psychoanalytic, emphasizing unconscious processes; the behavioral, focusing on reinforcement in the environment; and the cognitive, pointing to the mental processes responsible for maladaptive behavior.

TYPES OF DISORDERS

6. The various anxiety disorders include: generalized anxiety disorder, in which there are no specific symptoms except anxiety; specific phobia, which involves an incapacitating fear of a harmless object; posttraumatic stress disorder, a reminder of some terrifying event; and obsessive-compulsive disorder, with recurrent thoughts and/or actions.

7. In the somatoform disorder, it is assumed that psychological stress has played a role in producing bodily symptoms. The somatization disorder involves multiple complaints often vaguely identified. In the conversion disorder, there is a more specific loss or alteration of a physical function.

8. The various dissociative disorders include: amnesia, which involves pervasive forgetting with no evidence of brain damage; fugue, in which the individual may be discovered far from home with no memory of his or her past; and dissociative identity disorder, a dramatic form of forgetting in which the individual demonstrates various personalities.

9. The mood disorder is associated with emotional turmoil, especially a deep feeling of elation or depression. One form, the major depressive disorder, involves intense feelings of helplessness and disappointment; another is the bipolar disorder, characterized by extreme elation or alternating periods of elation and depression.

10. The chief characteristics of schizophrenia, a psychotic reaction, include hallucinations, delusions, and incoherent speech. The person is out of contact with reality and usually requires hospitalization. Heredity, biochemical, and environmental factors all seem involved in these disorders.

11. In a personality disorder, some trait or set of traits prevents the individual from fulfilling expected social roles. These include the antisocial personality disorder, violating others' rights; the borderline personality disorder, characterized by instability; and the narcissistic personality disorder, preoccupied with the self.

ADJUSTMENT AND CULTURE

12. Substance-related disorders involve the consumption of psychoactive materials in a fashion that interferes with daily life. Sexual disorders are of three types. Sexual dysfunction involves an inhibition of interest or performance in the full sexual response. Paraphilias involve attraction to stimuli not normally part of sexual arousal. In gender identity disorder, a person strongly desires to be a member of the opposite sex.

13. The concept of cultural relativism indicates that certain abstract concepts have meaning only in relation to the standards of a given society. Behavior considered normal in one culture may be regarded as abnormal in another.

• WORKING WITH PSYCHOLOGY •

REVIEW OF KEY CONCEPTS

Process of Adjustment
adjustment

mental health
defense mechanism

repression
suppression

displacement
denial
sublimation
learned helplessness
fantasy
regression

Determining Abnormality
mental illness
neurosis
insanity
pathological gambling

Types of Disorders
generalized anxiety disorder

specific phobia
posttraumatic stress disorder
obsessive-compulsive disorder
somatoform disorder
dissociative amnesia
dissociative fugue
dissociative identity disorder
major depressive disorder
bipolar disorder
schizophrenia
psychotic disorder
positive symptoms
negative symptoms
diathesis-stress model

dopamine hypothesis
communicative deviance
expressed emotion
personality disorder
antisocial personality disorder
borderline personality disorder
narcissistic personality disorder

Adjustment and Culture
psychoactive substance
sexual dysfunction
paraphilia
gender identity disorder
cultural relativism

✍ CLASS DISCUSSION/CRITICAL THINKING ✍

A NARRATIVE TWIST

Imagine that the Rosenhan study were repeated today using the same symptoms. Would the rate of admission to the hospitals be the same or different? Why? In reaching a decision, consider the current practices in mental health centers, role of the insurance industry, and possible influence of Rosenhan's research on subsequent psychiatric admissions. Then imagine that today's pseudopatients might falsely claim instead to be victims of childhood sexual abuse. Would this approach influence the outcome of the study? Explain the reasons for your answer. ✍

TOPICAL QUESTIONS

• *Process of Adjustment.* Should

political and social activists, leading marches and sit-ins and organizing dissent, be considered maladjusted for their socially disruptive behavior? Explain your view. Think about Walter Mitty, who regularly resorted to fantasy simply to make daily life a bit more pleasant, imagining himself in all sorts of heroic situations while accomplishing mundane tasks. Does this response solve problems, obscure them, or in fact create problems? Explain how it may play a role in any of these outcomes.

• *Determining Abnormality.* Suppose a woman snores mildly at night, but it significantly disrupts the sleep of her bedtime companion. If she seeks treatment for this problem, which does not disturb her, should

she be eligible for insurance coverage? Is her snoring a significantly abnormal condition to warrant medical reimbursement?

• *Types of Disorders.* Speculate on some specific diagnostic problem underlying the development of the *DSM-IV*, such as the criteria for a certain phobia or somatoform disorder. Which criteria of maladjustment should be regarded as most significant? Why? In view of social biases and cultural norms, which interest groups, if any, should be given special consideration?

• *Adjustment and Culture.* How does cultural relativism play a role in the ratings of films as PG, R, and X? Are some criteria universal, pertaining to all cultures? Explain your view.

✍ TOPICS OF RELATED INTEREST ✍

Methods of dealing with stress are described in connection with emotion (11). Repression is discussed in several other contexts: memory

(8), motivation (10), personality (14), and therapy (16). Aggression is considered with regard to emotion (11). The systems of psychol-

ogy relevant to diagnostic perspectives have been presented on several occasions, beginning in the opening chapter (1).

13

DRUG CLASSIFICATION

&

GENERAL ISSUES ADDRESSED IN THIS CHAPTER

- Criteria for grouping the different classes of drugs
- Various categories of a behaviorally based drug classification scheme
- Categories of the legal classification of drugs

INTRODUCTION

A comprehensive list of all drugs is a formidable task, however, this task is successfully accomplished in certain books like Goodman and Gilman's *The Pharmacological Basis of Therapeutics.*[1] As we have discussed in chapter 1, it is difficult for a drug molecule to cross the blood-brain barrier and enter the brain. Most drugs will not be able to cross the barrier, thus most drugs do not exert a direct influence on brain functioning. Some drugs, however, may directly affect the peripheral nervous system, specifically the sympathetic and/or the parasympathetic arousal system and, by so doing, will indirectly influence the central nervous system. We will focus our attention on the drugs that have a significant impact on behavior, which then presents the problem of organizing those drugs into common groups.

CATEGORIZATION OF DRUGS THAT AFFECT THE CENTRAL NERVOUS SYSTEM

One can create a drug category system based on the specific actions of a class of drugs on specific brain functioning. This sounds logical except that the mechanism of action of many drugs has not been well-described nor understood (for example, in alcohol and marijuana). Thus, at this time in drug research, there is no sufficient data base to categorize all drugs by their direct effects on brain functioning.

One can create a scheme based on the behavior elicited by a class of drugs. One major problem with this criterion, as we shall see in our discussion of sedatives in chapter 6, is that one drug can elicit a variety of different behaviors, depending on the dose and on the tolerance of the user.

Another way of classifying drugs is by the medical use of a particular class of drug. There are medical situations for which certain drugs have been found to be most useful. The *Physicians' Desk Reference* (PDR)[2] is a compendium of drugs for which physicians and other professionals with prescription-writing privileges can use in medical treatment. A casual examination of the PDR reveals a unique classification of these medicinal agents, which focuses on the presentation of symptoms of particular disorders. This type of categorization is useful to the medical practitioner who is seeking information concerning a specific drug, but it is not useful to the student who wishes to determine how drugs influence the brain's mediation of behavior. Moreover, there are drugs that are not legitimately prescribed for medical treatment that need to be categorized because of their effects on behavior. Thus, this single criterion is also lacking.

The drug categorization we will use does not depend exclusively on any one of these criteria, but enforces the criteria as is appropriate for the specific drug in question.

Sedatives and Hypnotics—CNS Depressants

These drugs are grouped together because of their similar effects on depressing behavior. Even though these drugs share the common ability to cause intoxication, the way they alter brain functioning is not the same. Each drug has its own unique mechanism of action on the brain. The different subclasses of the sedatives/hypnotics include:

a. Barbiturates (phenobarbital, secobarbital, etc.)
b. Benzodiazepines (Valium®, Librium®, triazolam, alprazolam, etc.)
c. Other non-barbiturate sedatives (methaqualone, meprobamate, etc.)
d. Newer non-benzodiazepines (buspirone hydrochloride, alpidem, etc.)
e. Ethanol (alcohol)
f. Cannabis (marijuana, hashish)
g. Antihistamines

Chapter 4 will deal with the principles of the sedatives/hypnotics. However, since alcohol is such a pervasive drug in Western culture, there will be a separate treatment in chapter 5 of those issues surrounding it. Likewise, the seemingly permanent controversy that surrounds cannabis (marijuana) will be treated separately in chapter 6.

Opiates—Drugs That Alter the Brain's Pain Processing

The drugs in this category share the common property of acting on a specific class of brain receptors.

a. Natural opiates (morphine, codeine, etc.)
b. Synthetic opiates
   1. similar in structure to the opiates (heroin, Percodan®, etc.)
   2. not similar in structure to the opiates (methadone, Demerol®, etc.)
c. Opiate antagonists (naloxone, naltrexone, etc.)

The special issues concerning these drugs will be discussed in chapter 7.

Stimulants—Drugs That Produce Behavioral Arousal

The principal criterion for grouping these particular drugs is their common outcome of behavioral arousal. The specific mechanism of action varies for each of the different types of stimulants.

a. Amphetamine (including methamphetamine)
b. Cocaine (including synthetic cocaines)
c. Methylxanthines (caffeine, theophylline, and theobromine)
d. Drugs used to treat hyperactivity (Ritalin®, pemoline)

421

    e.   Over-the-counter appetite suppressants (phenylpropanolamine hydrochloride)

    f.   Khat—a naturally occurring stimulant, similar to amphetamine

These drugs will be discussed in chapter 8.

Drugs Used to Treat Mental Disorders

The drugs included in this category have proven useful in the treatment of specific mental disorders. There are two main classes of these particular drugs:

    a.   Drugs used to treat affective disorders, such as depression and/or mania. (There are several classes within this one subclass):

        1.   Tricyclic antidepressants (imipramine, amitriptyline, desipramine hydrochloride, etc.)

        2.   The newer "heterocyclic" antidepressants (fluoxetine—Prozac®, sectraline-zoloft)

        3.   Monoamine oxidase inhibitors (tranylcypromine sulfate—Parnate®)

    b.   Drugs used to treat psychosis (for example, schizophrenia):

        1.   Phenothiazines (chlorpromazine—Thorazine®, thioridazine—Mellaril®, etc.)

        2.   Butyrophenones (haloperidol—Haldol®)

Not only are there special issues involved in this type of drug administration, but also these drugs have provided a wealth of information about the nature of neural communication. They will be discussed in chapter 9.

Hallucinogens

The drugs in this category share the unusual behavioral outcome of inducing hallucinations. They can be further divided into the following classes:

    a.   Agents that have a molecular structure similar to serotonin (lysergic acid diethylamide (LSD), psilocin, etc.)

    b.   Agents that have a molecular structure similar to norepinephrine (mescaline, 3,4 methylenedioxymethamphetamine—"ecstasy")

    c.   Agents that do not fall into the first two subclasses (ibotenic acid, phencyclidine hydrochloride—"angel dust")

These drugs are surrounded by controversy and create a great deal of concern. The special issues of hallucinogens will be discussed in chapter 10.

Drugs Used for Anesthesia

There is a class of drugs that alter brain functioning and have proven to be quite effective in producing an anesthetic state for surgical procedures. Anesthesia is a reversible loss of sensation that is usually but not always accompanied by a loss of consciousness. Anesthetics fall into several subclasses:

    a.   Gaseous anesthetics (nitrous oxide)

    b.   Volatile anesthetics (agents that are liquids at room temperature, such as ether and halothane)

    c.   Parenterally administered anesthetics (barbiturates, ketamine hydrochloride)

TABLE 3.1 Drug Classification

SEDATIVE AND HYPNOTICS—CNS DEPRESSANTS	OPIATES	STIMULANTS	DRUGS USED TO TREAT MENTAL DISORDERS
Barbiturates (phenobarbital, secobarbital, etc.)	Natural opiates (morphine, codeine, etc.)	Amphetamines (including methamphetamine)	Tricyclic antidepressants (imipramine, amitriptyline hydrochloride, desipramine hydrochloride, etc.)
Benzodiazepines (Valium®, Librium®, triazolam, alprazolam, etc.)	Synthetic opiates (heroin, methadone, Demerol®)	Cocaine (including synthetic cocaines)	The newer "heterocyclic" antidepressants (fluoxetine—Prozac®, trazodone hydrochloride)
Other nonbarbiturate sedatives (methaqualone, meprobamate, etc.)		Methylxanthines (caffeine, theophylline, and theobromine)	Monoamine oxidase inhibitors (tranylcypromine sulfate—Parnate®)
Ethanol (alcohol)		Drugs used to treat hyperactivity (Ritalin®, pemoline)	Phenothiazines (chlorpromazine—Thorazine®, thioridazine—Mellaril®, etc.)
Cannabis (marijuana, hashish)		Over-the-counter appetite suppressants (phenylpropanolamine hydrochloride)	Butyrophenones (haloperidol—Haldol®)
Antihistamines			

HALLUCINOGENS	DRUGS USED FOR ANESTHESIA	DRUGS USED TO TREAT EPILEPSY
Structurally similar to serotonin (LSD, psilocin, etc.)	Gaseous anesthetics (nitrous oxide)	Hydantoins (diphenylhydantoin—Dilantin®)
Structurally similar to norepinephrine (mescaline, MDMA—"ecstasy")	Volatile anesthetics (ether, halothane)	Barbiturates (phenobarbital)
Other agents (ibotenic acid, phencyclidine hydrochloride—"angel dust")	Parenterally administered anesthetics (barbiturates, ketamine hydrochloride)	Carbamazepine
		Valproic acid

423

The development of anesthetic agents is a colorful and engaging story, and the reader is urged to pursue this history in further readings. Because these drugs are so specifically used, this class will not be discussed in the text.

Drugs Used to Treat Epilepsy

One of the most common neurological disorders successfully managed with medication is epilepsy. The drugs that have proven effective in altering brain functioning to offer relief from this disorder can be divided into the following classes:

a. Hydantoins (diphenylhydantoin—Dilantin®)
b. Barbiturates (phenobarbital)
c. Carbamazepine
d. Valproic acid

The use of these drugs is restricted to the therapeutic situation of seizure control, which will not be discussed in this text. Although easily available, these drugs are rarely abused, with the exception perhaps of the barbiturates, which will be discussed in chapter 6.

LEGAL SCHEME

There is another drug classification that merits attention. In an attempt to limit the availability of potentially dangerous drugs to the public, laws have evolved that impose a structure to the distribution of drugs, as well as penalties for not complying with this scheme.

The particular evolution of our current drug control legislation is fascinating. As a fledgling nation, drug control was nonexistent, and the importation of all drugs was uncontrolled and unrestricted. By the late 1800s, for example, the use of opiates in a host of "tonics" and other medicinal products lead the United States, as a nation, to develop an intense consumption of opiates. The unrestricted use of cocaine at this time also grew, both in legitimate medical treatment, with endorsements from high-profile professionals, and also recreationally, in levels that were drawing concern. Legislators both locally and nationally, motivated to protect the public from the perceived harm of chronic intoxication from these drugs, responded by drafting specific drug legislation. Thus began an evolution of laws to deal with the problems of drug importation, distribution, and availability in general. The dynamics involved in this particular part of American history are covered in depth by David Musto in *The American Disease—Origins of Narcotic Control*[3].

The present federal legislation that deals with the control of drugs is the Comprehensive Drug Abuse Prevention and Control Act, passed in 1970. This law divides drugs into five categories or "schedules," according to the perceived risk of developing a dependency on that drug. As with any legislation, there are a great many factors involved in the conception and actual wording of a law. One of the main motivating factors in any legislation is the pressure exerted by the constituency of an elected legislator. In other words, the impressions of the public are at times more influential in drafting legislation than the actual facts surrounding an issue. In the case of drug legislation, the public perception (including the perceptions of a legislator) of the dangers of a substance are often shaped not by scientific data but rather by newspaper and television accounts of drug issues. Thus, there are some peculiarities to the schedule system, which hopefully will be adjusted by subsequent legislation. However, it is important to remember that regardless of any scientific pharmacological data that may argue the specific merits of a particular drug, this is the law. While some may choose to work for modifications, the public is still subject to its regulations and penalties.

The following is the drug categorization, according to the Comprehensive Drug Abuse Prevention and Control Act of 1970:

Schedule I

The drugs in this category have the highest risk for the development of drug dependency and are drugs that have no accepted medical use in treatment. Drugs in this schedule include:

1. Heroin, LSD, mescaline, peyote, psilocybin
2. Certain morphine preparations—benzylmorphine, dihydromorphinone hydrochloride, morphine methylsulfonate
3. Marijuana

The drugs in this schedule are the "forbidden" drugs and cannot be obtained by prescription. These drugs can be obtained for scientific research following the submission and approval of a research grant.

Schedule II

The drugs in this category also have the highest risk for the development of drug dependency, however these drugs are accepted by the medical community for treatment. Drugs in this schedule include:

1. The opiates—opium, morphine, codeine, methadone, meperidine hydrochloride (Demerol®), oxycodone hydrochloride (Percodan®)
2. The stimulants—amphetamines, methamphetamines, methylphenidate hydrochloride (Ritalin®)
3. Certain barbiturates—pentobarbital (Nembutal®), secobarbital (Seconal®), and amobarbital (Amytal®)

These drugs can be obtained legally only by prescription.

Schedule III

The drugs in this category have a risk for the development of moderate physical drug dependency or a high psychological dependency. Drugs in this schedule include:

1. Preparations that contain limited quantities of opiates (i.e., morphine, codeine)
2. Phencyclidine (also known as "angel dust")
3. The barbiturates not classified in schedules II or IV

Schedule IV

The drugs in this category have only a slight risk for the development of mild physical or psychological drug dependency. Drugs in this schedule include:

1. The barbiturates—phenobarbital and methylphenobarbital
2. Meprobamate
3. The benzodiazepines—diazepam (Valium®) and chlordiazepoxide (Librium®)

Schedule V

The drugs in this category have even less risk for the development of mild physical or psychological drug dependency than do the drugs in Schedule IV. Drugs in this schedule include the barbiturates—phenobarbital and methylphenobarbital.

As you can see, this particular categorization of drugs is based on the potential of a drug to be "abused" and not based on behavior per se. Thus, this breakdown of drugs will not be useful in examining the issues of drugs and behavior.

The exclusion of alcohol or tobacco in our current schedule system, which is based on the "abuse" potential of drugs, merits a comment. Alcohol is such a part of Western culture and tobacco is such a part of American culture that many individuals do not consider either a "drug." In fact, the federal government deals with ethanol and tobacco in the same way our founding fathers did in the late 1700s. The legislation relating to alcohol and tobacco concerns the collection of taxes and falls under the jurisdiction of an agency called the Alcohol, Firearms, and Tobacco (AFT), a division of the U.S. Department of Treasury.

In the following chapters, we will examine the various drug classes and specific drugs as they relate to the alteration of brain functioning and subsequent changes in behavior. There are general issues that are illustrated clearly by some classes of drugs, and there are some unique topics concerning specific drugs.

REVIEW EXAM

1. How are drugs categorized in the Physicians' Desk Reference (PDR)?
2. Name the five types of sedatives/hypnotics.
3. Give at least one example of each of the five types of sedatives/hypnotics.
4. Give one example of a naturally occurring opiate.
5. What is the difference between the two types of synthetic opiates?
6. Give at least one example of the two types of synthetic opiates.
7. Name five types of stimulants.
8. List specific examples of three of these stimulant types.
9. List the two main classes of drugs used to treat mental disorders.

426

10. Name two subtypes of each of the main classes of drugs used to treat mental disorders.
11. Give one specific example for each subtype of each of the main classes of drugs used to treat mental disorders.
12. What are the differences between the types of hallucinogens?
13. List specific examples of each type of hallucinogen.
14. Name the types of drugs used for anesthesia.
15. Name the types of drugs used for treating epilepsy.
16. What are the criteria for a drug to be classified as Schedule I?
17. What are the criteria for a drug to be classified as Schedule II?
18. List specific examples of drugs in Schedules I and II.
19. What is the difference in the criteria between Schedule III and IV?

REFERENCES

1. GOODMAN, L., & GILMAN, A. (1990). *The Pharmacological Basis of Therapeutics* (8th ed.). New York: Macmillan Publishing Co.
2. BARNHART, E. (ED.). (1993). *Physicians' Desk Reference.* New Jersey: Medical Economics Co. Inc.
3. MUSTO, D. (1987). *The American Disease—Origins of Narcotic Control.* New York: Oxford University Press.

14
Drugs Used to Treat Mental Disorders

GENERAL ISSUES ADDRESSED IN THIS CHAPTER

- The serendipitous discovery of the antipsychotics
- The principal symptoms of schizophrenia
- Variability in the absorption and clearance of the antipsychotics
- How antipsychotics block dopamine receptors in the brain
- A review of brain dopamine systems and dopamine receptor types
- Behavioral and nonbehavioral consequences of the antipsychotic medication
- The four common adverse behavioral motor problems associated with antipsychotic medication
- The dopamine theory of schizophrenia
- The significance of the new antipsychotic—clozapine
- The principal symptoms of mood disorder
- How the traditional tricyclic antidepressants alter brain functioning
- How the monoamine oxidase inhibitors and heterocyclic antidepressants alter brain functioning
- Behavioral and nonbehavioral consequences of the antidepressant medications
- The cheese reaction to the monoamine oxidase inhibitors
- The various adverse behavioral effects associated with the tricyclic antidepressants
- The monoamine and beta-adrenergic theories of mood disorders
- Electroconvulsive shock therapy (ECT)
- The concerns surrounding Prozac®
- Behavioral and nonbehavioral consequences of lithium medication
- How lithium alters brain functioning
- Adverse effects associated with lithium medication

LIST OF DRUGS

I. Antipsychotic Medications
    1. Phenothiazines—Chlorpromazine (Thorazine®)
        a. Thioridazine (Mellaril®)
        b. Trifluoperazine hydrochloride (Stelazine®)
        c. Fluphenazine (Prolixin®)
    2. Butyrophenones—Haloperidol (Haldol®)

II. Antidepressant Medications
    1. Tricyclic Antidepressants
        A. Secondary Amines
            a. Desipramine (Norpramin®)
            b. Nortriptyline (Aventyl®)
            c. Protriptyline (Vivactil®)
        B. Tertiary Amines
            a. Imipramine (Tofranil®)
            b. Amitriptyline (Elavil®)
            c. Doxepin (Sinequan®)
    2. Monoamine Oxidase Inhibitors—Tranylcypromine sulfate (Parnate®)

3. Heterocyclic Antidepressants—Trazodone (Desyrel®)
   a. Fluoxetine (Prozac®)
   b. Sertraline (Zoloft®)

III. Lithium

INTRODUCTION

Up to now, we have been reviewing how drugs influence behavior in a variety of medicating and illicit situations. In this chapter, we find the unique situation in which drugs are used to improve the abnormal behavior of individuals with psychological pathologies. In chapter 4 we saw that the treatment of anxiety disorders typically uses the benzodiazepines and, more recently, newer drugs such as the azopirones (buspirone), the imidazo-pyridines (zolpidem), and the cyclopyrrolones (suriclone and zoplicone). This chapter will focus on severe mental illness, specifically psychoses and affective disorders (depression and mania). They will be discussed separately, since different drugs are used to treat each condition. In addition, lithium is discussed specifically. Let us begin with psychoses.

ANTIPSYCHOTIC MEDICATIONS

The antipsychotics have been referred to as the major tranquilizers, which is not an accurate term. It implies that they only help calm individuals who are uncontrollably agitated. While this is true in some cases, this class of drug accomplishes more. The antipsychotics also help withdrawn and behaviorally retarded individuals in that they help them become less withdrawn and exhibit *more* behavior. Thus, the term tranquilizer really does not convey the full behavioral scope of these drugs.

HISTORY

One major class of antipsychotic medication is the phenothiazines. The discovery of their antipsychotic properties was accidental. Phenothiazine, first synthesized in 1883 in a chemical study of dyes, was initially examined as a possible medication for treating clinical conditions like parasitic worms and also as an antihistamine in the 1940s.[1] Around this time, in France, a naval surgeon named Laborit was experimenting with different drug combinations, which included antihistamines, to extend and strengthen anesthesia.[2] In the 1950s, Laborit tried a new antihistamine, chlorpromazine (Thorazine®), and discovered a peculiar behavioral outcome. Chlorpromazine had the unique characteristic of producing tranquilization in patients without loss of consciousness.[2] Patients' apparent lack of concern about their immediate environment was called artificial hibernation or the hibernation syndrome, or a *lobotomie pharmacologique.*[3] These observations eventually led clinicians to experiment with using chlorpromazine to calm agitated mentally disordered patients. In the next few years, the ensuing clinical trials, done first on manic patients then on other types, including schizophrenics, led to the discovery that chlorpromazine was a potent antipsychotic with effects not seen previously with any drug.[4] It was in a 1952 report that Daly and his colleagues coined the term "neuroleptic" for drugs that reduced neurological activity.

Around this time, in 1953, a young physician returned to work in his family's small pharmaceutical company. Because of limited facilities and resources, he developed a strategy that is the basis for designer drugs today, namely to take a known drug, slightly modify its structure, then test it as a "new" drug. The opiate drug meperidine (Demerol®) was modified and two compounds were developed: one was diphenoxylate, or Lomotil®, a potent antidiarrheal drug and another was an analgesic.[1] This analgesic was further modified until ultimately a drug was developed which had a profile, based on tests with animals, that was similar to other antipsychotic drugs. This drug, a variant of meperidine, is called haloperidol (Haldol®). It was first tested clinically in 1958 and found to be even more potent an antipsychotic than chlorpromazine, thus, by the 1960s, haloperidol was a common medication in Europe.[1] It is interesting that the two major classes of antipsychotic medications were both discovered accidentally.

Since this time, many medications have been synthesized and, with only one noted exception, all of the newer medications are no more effective than the original drugs.[5]

CLASSIFICATION OF SCHIZOPHRENIC DISORDERS

Schizophrenia, the most common form of psychosis, is actually a group of disorders. The DSM-II-R categorizes the schizophrenias into five essential subtypes, based on the specific symptoms shown by each. They are:

1. Disorganized type
2. Catatonic type
3. Paranoid type
4. Undifferentiated type
5. Residual type

Symptoms include the following:

1. Hallucinations. These are disturbances in perception in which the person experiences a perception in the absence of actual stimuli. Although hallucinations may occur in any sensory modality, auditory hallucinations are most common.
2. Delusions. These are distortions of reality that lead to misevaluations and erroneous conclusions. A common example of delusions are ideas of reference, in which personal significance is attached to unrelated events, like the evening newscaster is thought to be talking directly to the patient, trying to get a message to him or her.

432

3. Disturbances of thought, language, and communication. The logic and reasoning exhibited by these patients is faulty and is reflected in their speech. Their language is severely impaired and difficult to follow because of the odd associations.

4. Disturbances of emotion. This can be seen as either tremendous swings, from happy to sad, triggered by situations that would not normally elicit such a strong response or seen as a person's having little emotion, or flat affect.

ABSORPTION, DISTRIBUTION, AND EXCRETION

The phenothiazines and haloperidol are both readily absorbed from the GI tract, making the enteral oral route the easiest and most convenient route of administration. Parenteral injection routes, typically intramuscular (IM) and intravenous (IV) also are used in some situations in which a more rapid onset of effects is required. For example, an oral dose of chlorpromazine will achieve peak blood levels in about two hours, whereas a parenteral IM dose will have peak blood levels in fifteen minutes.[6] However, regardless of the route, the antipsychotic drugs, compared to other drug classes, have the greatest variability in terms of dose, absorption, and other therapeutic indicators.[1] Table 9–1 shows the total twenty-four-hour drug dose for several typical antipsychotic medications. Note that the daily dose range for chlorpromazine (Thorazine®) is 50 mg to 400 mg, whereas the daily dose for haloperidol (Haldol®) is only 2 mg to 6 mg.

Absorption from a single oral dose also has a great deal of variability, not only from one person to another but also in the same individual from one single dose to another.[3] Even after chronic daily administration of 300 mg of chlorpromazine* for one month, the blood levels of chlorpromazine measured in thirty-two patients showed a twelvefold difference between the lowest and highest values.[3]

The half-life of the antipsychotics also is quite variable among subjects, with some estimates of half-life being in the four-to-six hour range[1] and other estimates in the ten-to-twenty hour range.[6] The antipsychotics are very lipid-soluble and as such will tend to accumulate in fat depots and have biphasic clearance profiles from the blood. For chlorpromazine, the biphasic clearance is first rapid, with a half-life of approximately two hours and then is slower, with an approximate half-life of thirty hours.[6]

The antipsychotics are metabolized primarily by the enzymes in the liver and excreted primarily by the kidneys in the urine, but small quantities are sequestered in the bile and excreted in the feces.[6] Chlorpromazine and trifluoperazine (Stelazine®) have many metabolites, several of which are active.[3] Haloperidol (Haldol®) and other selective antipsychotics are metabolized entirely to nonactive metabolites. If drug administration is discontinued for chlorpromazine, for example, the actual drug levels in the blood will of course drop, but the metabolites will linger and be detectable in the urine for several months.[3]

---

*Chlorpromazine is perhaps the most extensively studied of the antipsychotic medications. Much less can be said about the other specific drugs in this class.

TABLE 9–1 Relative doses of typical antipsychotic drugs (for people who are not hospitalized)

ANTIPSYCHOTIC DRUGS	DOSE RANGE (TOTAL MG/DAY)
Chlorpromazine (Thorazine®)	50–400
Trifluoperazine (Stelazine®)	4–10
Haloperidol (Haldol®)	2–6

MECHANISMS OF ACTION

The antipsychotic drugs affect not only the brain but also the peripheral nervous system. In the PNS, antipsychotic drugs have two principal actions: 1. They block acetylcholine (ACh) receptors; and 2. They block alpha-adrenergic receptors.[6] As we shall see, these effects on the PNS account for many of the effects listed in the section below.

Effects on the central nervous system. Even though the phenothiazines and the butyrophenones are structurally dissimilar, the antipsychotic drugs, as a class, share a common mechanism of action on the brain—they block dopamine receptors. The better an individual drug is at blocking dopamine receptors, the more efficient that drug will be in the clinical treatment of psychoses.[7] This correlation is so strong that the success of a drug in human clinical use can be predicted with a great deal of accuracy, based on dopamine receptor blocking done in animal tissue studies.[8] This robust effect has led to the so-called dopamine theory of schizophrenia. Simply stated, this hypothesis essentially proposes the following: Since the drugs that are effective in treating psychoses have as their principal action the blockage of brain dopamine receptors, then psychoses, like schizophrenia, may be the result of abnormally overactive brain dopamine systems. We will consider this hypothesis in more detail later. Figure 9–1 illustrates the structural similarity between the dopamine molecule and a typical antipsychotic chlorpromazine. By turning the chlorpromazine molecule ninety degrees, one can better see the physical commonality in these two molecules. Brain dopamine systems and the various brain dopamine receptors will be reviewed next.

Dopamine Systems

Recall from chapter 2 that there are several specific brain nuclei whose cells use dopamine as a neurotransmitter. The three most prominent are:

1. The nigrostriatal dopamine pathway. Its cell bodies are in the nucleus of the substantia nigra in the midbrain. Its axons are sent to two nuclei, the striatum, in the telencephalon. This system is critically involved in motor behavior and is the system that is damaged in Parkinson's disease.
2. The mesolimbic and mesocortical systems. Its cell bodies are in the ventral tegmentum in the midbrain. Its axons are sent to either the prefrontal cerebral cortex (mesocortical system) or to a variety of limbic nuclei (mesolimbic system). This system seems to be involved in emotional behavior and may be the brain system that is abnormal or functioning abnormally in psychoses. This is the target system for antipsychotic medication.

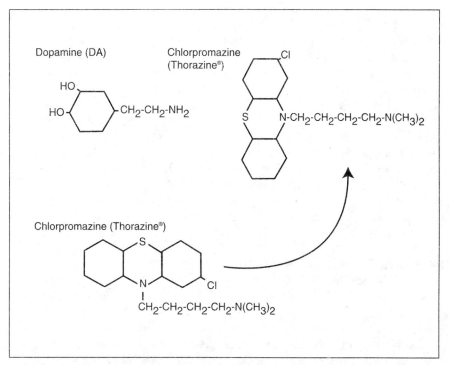

FIGURE 9–1 The Similarity of Chlorpromazine to Dopamine
By turning the molecular structure of chlorpromazine, one can better see how its center portion is similar in structure to dopamine.

3. The tubero-infundibular system. Its cell bodies are in the hypothalamus just above the pituitary. Its axons are sent a short distance to an area that has a special blood vessel link with the pituitary. Essentially, this system plays a role in the hypothalamus-pituitary interactions that maintain appropriate hormone levels in the blood.

All of these systems use dopamine as a neurotransmitter, thus all of their targets have dopamine receptors at those particular synapses. While the most likely systems that may be pathological in psychoses are the mesolimbic and mesocortical systems, the antipsychotic medications, with the possible exception of clozapine, will block dopamine receptors in all of these systems, resulting in a variety of motor problems (see the Adverse and Toxic Effects section later in this chapter). However, there are several types of receptors for dopamine, and the antipsychotics affect them differently.

Dopamine Receptor Types

There have been six dopamine receptor subtypes that have been characterized in the brain: D_1, D_{2a}, D_{2b}, D_3, D_4, and D_5.[9] These different subtypes can be functionally classified by how they are affected by the antipsychotics and anatomically by where they are found in the brain. The D_1 and D_5 receptors are not blocked very well by the phenothiazine and butyrophenone antipsychotics. Both of the D_2 receptors are the principal sites of action for the phenothiazines and butyrophenones. These receptors are found in the cerebral cortex, in critical limbic structures involved with emotion, and in the striatum, which is involved with motor behavior. In addition to being on the postsynaptic surface, the D_{2b} receptors appear to be on the presynaptic terminals of the dopamine cells and act as inhibitory autoreceptors for them. The D_3 and D_4 receptors also are found in limbic areas and in the cerebral cortex, but not in motor areas like the striatum. The phenothiazine and butyrophenone antipsychotic medications show very little binding to the D_3 and D_4 receptor types. However, clozapine, one of the newer antipsychotic medications, blocks the D_3 and D_4 receptors best and only weakly blocks the D_2's receptor types. It is this differential blockade of dopamine receptors that results in clozapine treatment having very few motor problems commonly associated with the more traditional antipsychotic medications.

NONBEHAVIORAL AND BEHAVIORAL CONSEQUENCES OF ANTIPSYCHOTIC DRUGS

There is a variety of effects of the antipsychotics that relates to their anticholinergic properties, including dry mouth or decreased salivation, constipation, and blurred vision.[3] The blocking of alpha-adrenergic receptors by the antipsychotics results in some distinctive cardiovascular effects, like an increased heart rate (tachycardia), a mild decrease in blood pressure, postural hypotension*,[6] and peripheral vasodilation, which causes mild hypothermia.[10] The severity of these effects varies among the particular antipsychotic medications.

Behaviorally, the antipsychotics typically induce a tranquilized state without loss of consciousness, a condition that was originally termed artificial hibernation—an indifference to the immediate environment. Some of the antipsychotics, chlorpromazine in particular, will induce sedation, whereas some, like trifluoperazine, are more likely to induce agitation.[3]

Of course, the most profound behavioral effect of these drugs is the relief of psychotic symptoms in mentally disordered patients. Even though discovered by accident, the success of this class of drugs in the treatment of psychoses is an accomplishment of enormous importance. Prior to this alternative, care of severely mentally disordered patients was essentially only custodial. These drugs have brought patients back into life and within reach of conventional therapy.

The symptoms that appear to respond well to the antipsychotic drugs include hallucinations, acute delusions, hostility, flat affect, and general withdrawal.[6] Moreover, these drugs also seem to alleviate the primary core symptoms, such as thought disorder and paranoia, although this has been challenged by some.[3] Clearly, the

*Also referred to as orthostatic hypotension, this term refers to the condition in which a person experiences lightheadedness or dizziness when standing up from a sitting or reclined position.

antipsychotic medications do not actually cure psychoses, but rather are an absolutely essential part of a treatment strategy that helps control the disorder.

In addition to treating various psychotic conditions, the antipsychotic medications also have been used to treat Tourette's syndrome, a disorder in which the patient has uncontrolled motor tics, sudden nonverbal vocalizations like barks and grunts, and unpredictable outbursts of foul language.[1] Antipsychotic drugs also have been used to treat nausea and vomiting due to a variety of causes.[6]

WITHDRAWAL AND TOLERANCE

Since antipsychotic drugs are used to reverse or correct a given set of behaviors that are already established in a patient, the issues of drug dependency and withdrawal are somewhat complex. Certainly, if antipsychotic medication is discontinued the psychotic behavior invariably returns. This does not constitute a withdrawal syndrome, since it was present prior to the administration of the drug. When directly examined in animals, there is virtually no withdrawal syndrome associated with the discontinuation of antipsychotic medication, and with the exception of some muscle discomfort, the same is true for humans.[6]

Tolerance develops for the sedation often seen with antipsychotic medications and cross-tolerance develops between the antipsychotics.[6] Tolerance does not develop to the antipsychotic relief these drugs render, which means that the dose does not have to be increased over the years of treatment.

ADVERSE AND TOXIC EFFECTS

In terms of lethality, the antipsychotics are remarkably safe. It is difficult for adults to die from overdoses of antipsychotics alone. For example, a single dose of 10,000 mg (that is, 10 grams) of chlorpromazine did not result in death.[6] However, there is a rare condition called the malignant syndrome, in which following antipsychotic medication a person experiences rigidity, fever, and hypertension, among other symptoms, which may progress to coma and even death.[11]

Another relatively rare reaction to antipsychotic medication is agranulocytosis, which is a severe decrease in white blood cells, usually in response to a fever. Although this can become a potentially fatal reaction, if detected in its early stages recovery is quick and complete. The incidence rate of agranulocytosis ranges from reports of one case in 10,000 for antipsychotic medications in general,[6] eleven cases in 1,000,[12] and eighteen cases in 3,000[13] for patients specifically receiving chlorpromazine. Typically, this reaction occurs in the first three months of treatment.[14]

A less severe adverse reaction to antipsychotic medications is skin photosensitivity,[6] abnormal accumulations of pigment in the skin[3] and, in some cases, the eye.[1]

By far the most significant type of adverse effect associated with the antipsychotics is a variety of abnormal motor behaviors, most of which occur soon after antipsychotic treatment has begun. The incidence of some motor disturbance induced by medication has been reported to be as high as 90 percent of all people who receive this medication[15] and one of the major reasons why patients do not comply with drug treatments.[16] Four of the most common reactions are reviewed next.

Acute Dystonia or Dystonic Reactions

Dystonia is a syndrome of sustained muscle contraction that usually results in bizarre appearances, depending on the muscle groups involved.[17] When dystonia affects the muscles of the face, the patient may grimace or the jaw may spasm open or closed. When the neck muscles are affected, the neck might be severely twisted or pulled either forward or backward. The muscles of the trunk also can be affected, resulting in odd postural stands. In addition, the tongue muscles can be the site for dystonia. One of the characteristics of dystonia is that the patient can often exert some control over the muscle spasm by touching the affected area, so that a dystonic reaction can be ended by the patient.

The risk of developing dystonia is highest within the first five days of beginning antipsychotic treatment.[18] Parenteral administration, either IV or IM, of anticholinergic agents like benztropine (Cogentin®) or antihistamines like diphenhydramine (Benadryl®) can provide immediate relief of these symptoms.[19] However, the most effective treatment of this antipsychotic-induced dystonia is to gradually discontinue the medication, which is not always an option given the severity of the psychoses being treated.[20]

Akathisia

Akathisia refers to a compulsion to move. There is no specific muscle group involved, nor is there a specific motor behavior, but rather akathisia is an intense feeling of restlessness experienced by the patient. Acute akathisia is the most common of the early-onset motor abnormalities induced by the antipsychotic medications.[21] The incidence rate is approximately 20 percent for patients placed on antipsychotics.[22] One study reported an incidence rate of 75 percent.[23] It usually occurs within five to forty days after the onset of antipsychotic medication.[18] Akathisia usually is seen as a constant movement by the patient, such as continuous pacing, shifting the weight from one foot to the other, continually crossing and uncrossing the legs when seated, changing one's stance, etc. These symptoms often are interpreted incorrectly as anxiety or as a worsening of the psychotic condition. The only clearly effective treatment for akathisia is a reduction in or discontinuation of the medication, which as mentioned earlier, may not be a realistic option in the overall treatment of a psychotic individual.

Parkinson Syndrome or Parkinsonism

Within five to thirty days after antipsychotic medication has been initiated, a patient may express a disorder that is indistinguishable from true Parkinson's disease in its clinical symptoms. The typical signs which characterize Parkinson's disease are akinesia or bradykinesia, rigidity, and tremor at rest.[24] Tremor at rest may often disappear or be reduced when purposeful activity is engaged in, but the condition becomes more intense during times of stress. Bradykinesia is a lack of spontaneous movement due to difficulty initiating voluntary movement. Rigidity is the result of an increase in muscle tone to the point that passive movement of limbs is resisted. The akinesia associated with Parkinson's Syndrome is especially debilitating, since it may often express itself as a lack of emotion, diminished gesturing, impaired social ability, and a general lack of concern.[19] The treatment for this drug-induced condition is the same as the treatment for true Parkinson's disease. There are several anticholinergic medications that have proven helpful. Two in particular include benztropine (Cogentin®) and procyclidine (Kemadrin®).[19]

The causal pathology in Parkinson's disease is a loss of cells in the substantia nigra, which use dopamine as a neurotransmitter (see chapter 2 and the section Dopamine Systems preceding). The antipsychotic medications mimic this disorder because their primary action is to block dopamine receptors, thus those motor areas in the brain which have dopamine receptors for the input of the substantia nigra also are blocked. The result, both in true Parkinson's disease and in the recipient of antipsychotic medication is that critical motor processing takes place without input from the substantia nigra.

Tardive Dyskinesia

As the name implies, this is a late-onset motor disorder that occurs after a relatively long time on antipsychotic medication. There is no doubt that the longer a person is given antipsychotic medication, the greater the risk for developing tardive dyskinesia. However, it has been extremely difficult to precisely describe the parameters of this relationship. Prospective studies have reported incidence rates for tardive dyskinesia that increase with drug exposure time.[25,26,27,28] Figure 9–2 summarizes the cumulative rates.

Tardive dyskinesia is a disorder that involes involuntary abnormal movements, typically of the mouth and tongue, for example, lip smacking and pursing, and the tongue darting out of the mouth. In some cases, other parts of the body are affected, such as the limbs. One peculiar aspect of this motor disorder is that the patient can voluntarily control the symptoms by attending to them.[18] The proposed mechanism for tardive dyskinesia is that following prolonged blockage of dopamine receptors, some aspect of the dopamine system may become hypersensitive or supersensitive.[29]

Unlike the other behavioral adverse reactions listed earlier, this syndrome may be irreversible in some patients.[18] This is an especially important issue since there is no effective treatment for tardive dyskinesia. The only accepted successful treatment strategy has been to discontinue the medication, which of course runs the risk of having the original psychosis emerge.[30]

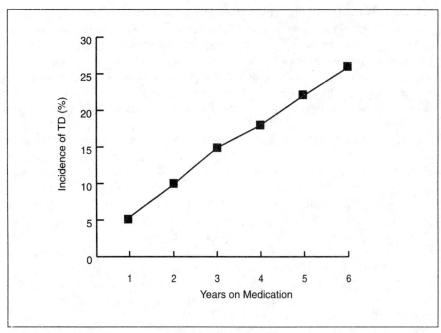

FIGURE 9–2 Incidence Rates of Tardive Dyskinesia
The longer a person is maintained on antipsychotic medication, the greater the risk for developing tardive dyskinesia. (The box marks the incidence rate after only three years of chronic antipsychotic medication.)

SPECIAL ISSUES

The Dopamine Theory of Schizophrenia

Essentially, this theory proposes that schizophrenia specifically and psychoses in general are the result of overactive dopamine systems in the brain. The initial support for this theory came from the two following facts: 1. Those drugs that offer the most effective relief from this disorder block dopamine receptors; and 2. Overstimulating the dopamine systems in the brain with stimulants leads to the amphetamine psychosis (see chapter 8). The more recent research efforts which support the dopamine theory of schizophrenia have resulted in ambiguous findings.

The New Generation Antipsychotics

Clozapine is a new antipsychotic that may mark the most significant advance since the initial development of antipsychotic medication. Compared to traditional antipsychotics, clozapine has been reported to be more effective in the treatment of psychoses,[31,32] and induces fewer[33] and less tardive dyskinesia.[34] Not only has clozapine been shown to be more effective than traditional antipsychotics like chlorpromazine,[35] but it also has been shown to be effective in patients who do not respond to the typical antipsychotic medications.[36]

The significance of this relatively new, so-called atypical antipsychotic lies in clozapine's unique property of blocking the D_3 and D_4 dopamine receptor types, while having only a minimal effect on the D_2 receptor type.[9] The motor effects following antipsychotic medication are due primarily to the D_2 receptors in motor systems like the nigrostriatal pathway.[37] The phenothiazines and haloperidol block the D_2 receptors in these motor areas as effectively as they block D_2 receptors in the limbic/emotional areas. Clozapine, on the other hand, does not bind to the D_2 receptors in these motor areas very well,[38] thus does not cause the motor problems seen with the more traditional antipsychotics.

Clozapine appears to have two other significant effects on brain functioning. It blocks the specific serotonin receptor types 5HT2 and 5HT1c.[39] It is not clear if this action of clozapine relates to either its antipsychotic properties or its lack of motor effects. Clozapine also blocks muscarinic acetylcholine receptors.[40] As we have seen, the use of anticholinergic drugs seems to alleviate the motor problems of antipsychotic medications. By having this built-in feature, clozapine may itself correct for any detrimental D_2 receptor blockade.

Even though clozapine may not have the motor problems associated with the other antipsychotic medications, it does have other adverse effects, the most serious being agranulocytosis. While the occurrence of agranulocytosis can happen with conventional antipsychotics, the rate is much higher with clozapine, approximately 1 to 2 percent.[41] The development of agranulocytosis induced by clozapine use follows a similar time course as that of the conventional antipsychotics, namely within the first few months of treatment.[36]

Other less severe adverse effects associated with clozapine treatment include seizure, increased heart rate, hypotension, weight gain, and increased salivation.[33]

ANTIDEPRESSANTS

The affective disorders are disorders of mood, like depression and mania. The incidence rate of these debilitating disorders can be as high as 10 percent of the general population of Western countries.[42] As with the antipsychotic medications, the discovery of the drugs used to treat affective disorders were discovered accidentally.

Basically, there are four classes of drugs used in the treatment of affective disorders:

1. Traditional tricyclic antidepressants (TCA)
2. Monoamine oxidase inhibitors (MAOIs)
3. Newer heterocyclic antidepressants
4. Lithium

Since lithium is used to treat mania, in particular, it will be discussed in a separate section.

HISTORY

The parent compound for the tricyclic antidepressants was synthesized in 1889. It was not until the 1940s that a derivative, imipramine, was examined as a possible antihistamine. When the findings were released that another suspected antihistamine, chlorpromazine, actually had antipsychotic effects, imipramine was tested again in 1958. Khun found that imipramine was not an effective antipsychotic but did seem to render relief to the depressed patients in the sample.[43] Since then there have been numerous studies indicating how effective tricyclic antidepressants are in the treatment of affective disorders.

Around this time, the serendipitous discovery of the antidepressant properties of another drug also were made. The drug, iproniazid, which was developed and being used to treat tuberculosis, had another effect—patients who received it experienced an elevation in mood, to the point of euphoria. It soon was discovered that iproniazid severely hampered the action of an enzyme—monoamine oxidase (MAO). By 1957, the successful use of monoamine oxidase inhibitors (MAOIs) to treat depression was reported.

There was another serendipitous discovery that also happened around this time. Hypertensive patients had been given a drug called reserpine, which seemed to cause these otherwise normal patients to experience profound depression. While this discovery did not directly impact the development of newer drugs, it provided another set of data which supported the monoamine theory of affective disorders.

CLASSIFICATION OF MOOD DISORDERS

The basic behavioral disturbance in this disorder is a profound alteration of mood. This alteration can be expressed as a pathologically depressed, elevated, or manic mood. In the depressed mood, the main symptoms include a profound loss of pleasure, an intense apathy, nonintentional change in weight (increase or decrease), change in sleep (either insomnia or hypersomnia), suicidal ideation or thoughts of death. In the manic mood, the main symptoms include feelings of grandiosity, periods of excessive talking, decreased need for sleep, distractibility, and engaging in risky behavior (financial, business, or sexual indiscretions). There are five basic subclassifications of these disorders, depending on the occurrence of a manic period: 1. bipolar disorder; 2. major depressive disorder (formerly referred to as unipolar); 3. cyclothymic disorder; 4. bipolar disorder NOS (not otherwise specified); and depressive disorder NOS.

ABSORPTION, DISTRIBUTION, AND BIOTRANSFORMATION

As a group, the antidepressant drugs used to treat mood disorders, formerly referred to as affective disorders, are readily absorbed from the GI tract. The TCAs are usually completely absorbed from an oral administration within ten hours and peak plasma concentrations are reached within two hours.[44] Distribution is fairly even throughout body compartments except in the case of imipramine, in which there is an unusually high concentration in the brain.[44]

Biotransformation for both TCAs and MAOIs is done in the liver. The metabolism of many of the TCAs produces active metabolites. For example, imipramine metabolism yields desimipramine; amitriptyline metabolism yields nortriptyline; doxepin metabolism yields nordoxepin. Although these metabolites are active, their role in the clinical effectiveness of the TCAs has yet to be determined.[6] Typically, the metabolism of the MAOIs does not yield active metabolites.

The following is a representative sample of the half-lifes of the TCAs:[45]

1. Imipramine—thirteen hours
2. Amitriptyline—fifteen hours (Nortriptyline—thirty-one hours)
3. Desipramine—eighteen hours
4. Doxepin—seventeen hours
5. Protriptyline—seventy-eight hours
6. Trazadone—five hours
7. Fluoxetine—forty-eight hours (and as long as six days after chronic treatment)[46]
8. Sertraline—twenty-four hours[46]

EFFECTS ON THE CENTRAL NERVOUS SYSTEM

Tricyclic Antidepressants

The TCAs can be subdivided into two categories according to their molecular structure and precise action on synaptic functioning in the brain. Structurally, the TCAs can be subdivided into two classes:

1. TCAs with one methyl group (CH_3), referred to as secondary amines—specifically, desipramine and protriptyline
2. TCAs with two methyl groups, referred to as tertiary amines—specifically, imipramine, amitriptyline, doxepin, and clomipramine[47]

After a neuron has fired, it releases neurotransmitter molecules into the synaptic cleft to interact with special postsynaptic receptors on the target surface. Neurons must then engage a mechanism to terminate this action and get ready for the next firing (i.e., the next action potential) (see chapter 2). Neurons in the brain that use the monoamines, namely norepinephrine (NE), dopamine (DA), or serotonin (5HT) as neurotransmitters terminate the action of their neurotransmitter molecules by a reuptake process. The released neurotransmitter molecules that are in the synapse are actively taken back into the presynaptic terminal by an active membrane transport mechanism. The TCAs block this reuptake system. The result of the TCAs' hampering of this reuptake process is that the neurotransmitter molecules remain on the postsynaptic receptors longer. Thus, the principal functional consequence of TCAs is the immediate enhancement of monoamine transmission. Recall from our discussion of the stimulants that one of the mechanisms of the action of amphetamines is also a hampering of the reuptake process in monoamine neurons.

It is important to note that the specific monoamines are affected differently by the TCAs. The TCAs belonging to the one methyl group, secondary amines, namely desipramine and protriptyline, block the reuptake of norepinephrine (NE) much more efficiently than serotonin (5HT). The TCAs belonging to the two methyl group, tertiary amines, that is, imipramine, amitriptyline, doxepin, and clomipramine, block the reuptake of serotonin (5HT) much more efficiently than norepinephrine (NE). Appreciate that both norepinephrine and serotonin reuptake systems are blocked by the TCAs. The main difference between the subclasses of TCAs is one of relative degree.

Monoamine Oxidase Inhibitors

As their name implies, these drugs block the enzyme monoamine oxidase (MAO). This enzyme exists in the presynaptic terminal of the neurons that use monoamines as neurotransmitters. This enzyme will break down monoamine neurotransmitter molecules in the cytoplasm, not yet in the synaptic vesicle. By breaking down so-called free-floating neurotransmitter molecules, MAO decreases the absolute amount of molecules available for packaging into synaptic vesicles. Ultimately then, MAO regulates the amount of neurotransmitter molecules that are released when the cell fires. By inhibiting this action of MAO, the MAO inhibitors (MAOIs) will cause the release of more monoamine neurotransmitter molecules with each action potential.

Heterocyclic Antidepressants

These newer medications, like fluoxetine (Prozac®) and maprotiline, are like the traditional tricyclic antidepressants in that they also block the reuptake process of certain monoamine neurons. These drugs are different because they have been developed to be even more specific to one monoamine system than are the traditional TCAs. For example, maprotiline is approximately 600 times more selective for blocking NE reuptake than 5HT reuptake, compared to desipramine,[48] and fluoxetine is approximately 30 times more effective in blocking the reuptake of serotonin than NE reuptake.[48] Sertraline (Zoloft®), like fluoxetine (Prozac®), is another specific serotonin reuptake blocker.

Note that for all three classes of antidepressants, the immediate effect on brain functioning is the enhancement of communication with those neurons that use monoamines as a neurotransmitter.

The long-term consequences of blocking monoamine reuptake, whether NE or 5HT, may be one of the causal factors in the clinical efficacy of these antidepressant medications. This will be discussed later in the Special Issues section.

BEHAVIORAL EFFECTS

There are few behavioral effects of antidepressant drugs in those individuals who are not suffering from clinical depression, and these can be characterized as generally unpleasant. There may be sedation, decrease in blood pressure, and dry mouth.[6] Doxepin may be more sedating than imipramine in these control populations.[47] This is especially striking considering that amphetamines and cocaine also block monoamine reuptake (see chapter 8), yet the antidepressants do not induce the euphoria of the stimulants. This suggests that it may be the other actions of the stimulants which account for their high reinforcing properties.

In patient populations that are depressed, the antidepressants will relieve the symptoms of their depression. A characteristic common to all of the antidepressant medications is that there is a ten-to-fourteen day delay from the onset of taking the medication and the onset of clinical relief. The elevation of mood as a result of the alleviation of depression is not euphoric, such as with the stimulants cocaine and amphetamines, but rather is an absence of severe depression. While the antidepressant medications have consistently been shown to be more effective than placebo treatments, approximately 30 percent of patients will not positively respond to these medications.[47] The considerably high spontaneous improvement rate, approximately 31 percent in populations receiving only the placebo,[49] or other nonpharmacological interventions, indicate that mood disorders are a heterogeneous collection of disorders with a variety of treatment strategies available to the attending practitioner.

WITHDRAWAL

The withdrawal symptoms from abruptly stopping tricyclic antidepressant medications are similar to a severe flu reaction: headache, chills, diarrhea and vomiting, abdominal cramps, dizziness, insomnia, and irritability.[50]

Abrupt withdrawal from MAOI medication has not been considered a serious problem.[51] The symptoms include nausea, headaches, palpitations, sweating, and muscle weakness.[52]

ADVERSE AND TOXIC EFFECTS

General Toxicity

Unlike the antipsychotics, overdoses of the TCAs can be fatal. This is especially problematic when one considers that one of the common characteristics of the population being treated with TCAs is suicidal tendencies. Suicides are common with TCA medication.[53] If given more than a week's supply, a depressed patient will have enough of the drug to achieve a fatal overdose,[6] so care must be exercised to prevent this situation. The MAOIs also are quite lethal at doses well within the availability of the patient.[54]

The TCAs induce a variety of effects on the autonomic nervous system. They include: dry mouth, increased heart rate (tachycardia), decreased blood pressure (hypotension), postural hypotension, constipation, dizziness, vomiting,[53] and urinary retention.[6]

The MAOIs have a similar profile of autonomic effects as do the TCAs. These signs include: dizziness, postural hypotension, dry mouth, constipation, difficulty in urination, inhibited orgasm, and impotence.[53] A massive overdose can result in convulsions and death.[6]

The most serious toxic reaction to the MAOIs is a hypertensive crisis sometimes referred to as the "Cheese Reaction." Our food sometimes contains certain agents called "pressor" agents which if left uncontrolled would elicit the sympathetic nervous system to rapidly raise blood pressure. Normally, there is MAO in the liver and in the gut to metabolize these compounds in our food and thus prevent this increase in blood pressure.[54] When MAOIs are given in the treatment of depression, all MAO is inhibited including this peripheral MAO. Thus the consumption of foods rich in these pressor agents would lead to a sharp increase in blood pressure. Tyramine, a product of the fermentation process, is the most common dietary pressor agent responsible for a MAOI induced hypertensive reaction. Foods rich in tyramine include: aged cheeses especially cheddar and Swiss, red wines, red wine vinegars, beer, homemade yogurt, and any food with Brewer's yeast.[54] Thus the term "Cheese" reaction is not accurate.

There are three progressively more severe stages to this reaction.[53]

1. Stage one: Sudden throbbing headaches are commonly reported, along with nausea, vomiting, and sweating. These signs may disappear within a few hours if no further tyramine-containing food is ingested.
2. Stage two: Severe hypertension, palpitations, and chest pains, along with headache and sweating, and potential collapse are seen here.
3. Stage three: All of the above symptoms are experienced, as well as intracranial bleeding, which is fatal.

Drugs that induce sympathetic reactions, like amphetamines and cocaine, also precipitate a hypertensive crisis if taken in combination with MAOIs.[53]

Tricyclic Antidepressants

There are several adverse behavioral consequences with the tricyclic drugs.

1. Aggression. There are certain people with personality disorders who are at risk for showing increased aggression in response to antidepressant medication. One study reported that almost half of the patients with previously diagnosed borderline personality disorder showed increased paranoia and became more suicidal, hostile, and impulsive

446

while on antidepressant drugs.[55] This medication-induced increased aggression appears to occur only in those individuals who may be predisposed to aggression prior to the medication.[51]

2. Weight gain. Weight gain is one of the more common effects of chronic antidepressant medication.[56] The incidence of either weight gain and/or carbohydrate craving may be as high as 50 percent in certain populations.[51]

3. Jitteriness syndrome. Just after the initiation of antidepressant medication, typically those drugs which have a more direct effect on the norepinephrine system, like imipramine, desipramine, and protriptyline,[56] the patient sometimes will suddenly experience an intense feeling of restlessness, increased energy, and irritability.[57] This usually will resolve within a day.[58]

4. Sleep effects. The TCAs will reliably suppress REM sleep.[59] This effect is immediate and seems to correlate with the eventual clinical effectiveness in treating the depression.[60] There also is an increase in nocturnal myoclonus, which is the strong leg contraction or kick that occurs during sleep.[61] This effect appears to occur with those antidepressants that more directly affect the serotonin system, such as clomipramine.[62] The patient is usually unaware of this nocturnal myoclonus and it is the patient's bed partner that brings this condition to the attention of the attending physician.[62]

The MAOIs have similar adverse behavioral effects as do the TCAs, including weight gain,[51] suppressing REM sleep,[59] inducing mania,[63] and even antisocial behavior, in some rare cases.[64]

SPECIAL ISSUES

The Monoamine Theory of Affective Disorders

Essentially, this theory suggests that affective disorders like depression are the result of a chemical, that is a neurotransmitter, imbalance or deficit in the brain. Specifically, the monoamine theory holds that affective disorders are the result of either an underactive monoamine system in the brain or that levels of monoamine neurotransmitter molecules in the brain are too low. The monoamine theory is based on a variety of sources, including the initial observations of patients treated with reserpine and the MAOI iproniazid (see above), as well as the later evidence that successful medications that reverse depressive symptoms all seem to enhance monoamine activity. The major shortcoming of this theory is that it fails to explain why there is a ten-to-fourteen day delay from the onset of taking medication to the onset of clinical improvement. The medications typically enhance monoamine systems immediately, yet the person does not experience relief for two weeks.

Recent advances in the technology of directly studying specific receptors in the brain have led to an alternate theory.

The Beta-Adrenergic Theory of Affective Disorders

There are two specific receptor types for norepinephrine—the alpha- and beta-adrenergic receptors. Each has a distinctive distribution in the peripheral nervous system and the central nervous system. It is important to consider a general charac-

447

teristic shared by most receptors, that is, not all of them are functional at any one point in time. In other words, a given population of receptors will have a portion that is not active, and the brain will regulate just how many receptors are active according to its needs.

One long-term consequence of chronic antidepressant medication is the decreased number, referred to as a down regulation, of beta-adrenergic receptors in the brain.[65] This down regulation, which takes approximately ten to fourteen days to accomplish, is found not only with drugs that block the reuptake of norepinephrine but also with a variety of antidepressants that do not directly alter norepinephrine. The specific serotonin reuptake blockers, like fluoxetine (Prozac®) and sertraline (Zoloft®), also cause the eventual down regulation of beta-adrenergic receptors in the brain, as do the MAOIs and even the nonpharmacological treatment ECT.[65] Thus, it appears that the norepinephrine and serotonin systems in the brain interact with each other in such a way that altering one will impact the other, and the common outcome for these medications centers around the beta-adrenergic receptors in the brain. For example, the administration of both fluoxetine and desipramine not only enhanced the antidepressant results of the medications, but also was one-third faster than either medication alone.[66]

Recent research has been describing the precise role of serotonin in the clinical effectiveness of antidepressants. Traditional tricyclic antidepressant medications and ECT, in addition to the down regulation of beta-adrenergic receptors, will also enhance serotonin receptor sensitivity on the cerebral cortex,[67] specifically the 5-HT1A serotonin receptor.[68] It appears that the serotonin-norepinepherine interaction that may mediate the clinical relief of antidepressant medications is a down regulation of the beta-adrenergic receptors and an increase in serotonin receptor activity.[69] Postmortem biochemical analyses of the brains of suicide victims indicate that the prefrontal cortex has lower levels of 5HT transport activity[70] and higher beta-adrenergic receptor binding.[71]

Electroconvulsive Shock Therapy (ECT)

Based on the observations of the Hungarian physician von Meduna in the early 1900s, it was believed that seizures protected patients from severe psychiatric pathology, thus the strategy of inducing seizures for therapeutic reasons began. At first, seizures were pharmacologically induced, but in 1938 the use of electroconvulsive techniques were introduced into clinical medicine.[72] Originally, ECT was done without anesthesia or other medications. The procedure now involves the use of muscle relaxants and some anesthesia to prevent bone fractures during the convulsions and to prevent anxiety surrounding the procedure.[72] The optimal ECT schedule is considered to be a series of two seizures a week for three to four weeks.[73] Bilateral ECT, that is, causing the entire brain to go into seizure, is slightly more effective than unilateral ECT, which causes only one hemisphere of the brain to go into seizure.[74] Modern ECT is considered safe and effective,[75] with positive response rates as high as 95 percent.[74] ECT is believed to induce more rapid relief than the standard two-week delay of the antidepressants, which becomes critical when dealing with some suicidal patients. However, this alleged rapid clinical response and success in suicidal patients has not been observed by all.[47] Although ECT has been suggested for patients who do not respond to antidepressant medications, the positive response rate to ECT by medication-resistant patients is quite low, around 50 percent.[76]

Despite the new ECT techniques, which obviate many of the major problems with ECT, there remain two significant concerns. First, ECT will invariably induce confusion and a loss of memory surrounding the ECT treatment, which becomes progressively more severe with increased sessions.[72] Second, without additional pharmacological support, the relapse rate of patients with successful ECT six months later is significantly higher than with those patients with additional antidepressant medication.[77]

The precise mechanism by which ECT provides clinical relief is not known. However, ECT, like traditional antidepressant medication, does cause a down regulation of beta-adrenergic receptors[65] and enhances 5HT sensitivity in the cerebral cortex.[67]

Concerns Surrounding Prozac®

Despite press accounts of aggressive and suicidal effects induced by fluoxetine (Prozac®), controlled examinations of these allegations do not support these observations. The adverse behavioral effects associated with the traditional antidepressants do not appear to be different than those attributed to Prozac®. One study examined over 1,000 cases of patients medicated with Prozac® and found no differences between Prozac® and other antidepressant medications in the incidence of new suicidal ideation.[78] As discussed earlier, the occurrence of aggressive behavior following the administration of antidepressant medication is restricted to certain patient populations that have borderline personality disorders. This effect is not specific to fluoxetine but rather to this class of medication.

It is important to remember that one of the core symptoms of severe affective disorders include suicidal ideation. The practitioner must always be vigilant to its appearance at any time during the course of treatment.

LITHIUM® AND MANIA

The antidepressant medications listed earlier are not useful in the treatment of mania. Lithium is the principal medication that will effectively treat mania, with a success rate as high as 95 percent.[74] In addition, lithium may even prevent the occurrence of bipolar swings into depression from a manic phase.[79]

HISTORY

The discovery of lithium was not as serendipitous as the other medications discussed in this chapter. In Australia, in the 1940s, John Cade developed a hypothesis stating that mania was the result of some endotoxin produced by manic patients. Using an animal model, Cade found that the urea from the urine of manic patients was one toxic substance. His subsequent experiments to increase the solubility of urates led to the discovery of lithium as a potential sedating candidate.[80] Although Cade's initial clinical trials of using lithium on manic patients were overwhelmingly successful, it took almost twenty years before the worldwide medical community accepted its use in the treatment of mania. There were several reasons for this unusually long delay.[47] The initial Cade clinical reports were published in local Australian medical journals, not the more widely read international journals. The use of lithium as a sodium substitute in the 1940s resulted in several fatalities, casting a negative shroud on this drug. Financially, lithium could not be patented, thus it was not commercially profitable for drug companies. Despite these difficulties, the use of lithium in treating mania has become the first-line medication worldwide.

ABSORPTION, DISTRIBUTION, AND EXCRETION

Lithium is almost exclusively given orally. It is completely absorbed from the GI tract, is almost entirely excreted by the kidney at a moderate rate, and has a half-life of approximately twenty-four hours. The excretion of lithium is influenced by the sodium balance in the patient. When sodium intake is low, lithium is retained longer. If sodium intake is increased, lithium is excreted more rapidly.[80] Lithium tends to accumulate in the kidneys.[79]

BEHAVIORAL AND NONBEHAVIORAL EFFECTS

In nonmanic individuals, lithium may elicit subjective feelings of fatigue, lethargy, and decreased ability to concentrate, as well as decreased memory functioning.[79] In the manic patient, lithium can help control manic episodes and even prevent the occurrence of future manic swings.[74] For the manic patient, this means that they are able to experience a level of control over their positive emotions that was not previously there. It is important to note that, like the antidepressants, lithium has a six-to-ten day delay from the onset of medication and relief of symptoms.[47]

Lithium has a poor therapeutic index, which means that the dose required to relieve manic symptoms is very close to adverse and even toxic levels. At clinical dose levels, manic patients will typically experience the effects mentioned above and more. The most frequently observed side effect to lithium therapy is tremor, which is typically seen early in treatment and will abate within the first two weeks of treatment.[81] Other signs include dry mouth, frequent urination,[74] and GI tract upset, seen as nausea, vomiting, or diarrhea, due to the fact that lithium irritates the GI tract.[80]

EFFECTS ON THE CENTRAL NERVOUS SYSTEM

Lithium has a variety of effects. Precisely which one(s) account for the clinical relief of mania has yet to be determined. Lithium, a positively charged ion, can substitute for other positively charged ions like sodium, potassium, calcium, and magnesium,[79] all of which play critical roles in brain functioning. Lithium can be transported by the sodium-potassium-ATPase pump in neurons,[79] which maintains the proper ionic environment of the neuron so it is able to communicate. Lithium enhances the reuptake of norepinephrine (NE) at the synapse and may even decrease the amount of NE released when the cell fires.[80] Lithium will also decrease the synthesis and release of acetylcholine (ACh) at those synapses that use ACh.[79] It increases the reuptake of serotonin as well.[80] The amount of calcium in the presynaptic terminal is a necessary factor in the release of any neurotransmitter, and lithium will decrease the amount of calcium available presynaptically.[79] Which of these effects, if any, is responsible for the clinical actions of lithium is not known.

WITHDRAWAL

There are no reports of any withdrawal syndrome associated with the abrupt discontinuation of lithium treatment.

TOXIC EFFECTS

We have listed some of the adverse effects usually observed with lithium treatment. As we have also mentioned, clinical doses of lithium are close to toxic levels. The first symptoms that precede a toxic reaction to lithium are a worsening of the hand tremor or having the tremor spread to other parts of the body, incoordination, inability to articulate, due to spasticity in the muscles used for speaking, disorientation, muscle twitching, dizziness, and involuntary contractions of the face muscles.[79]

If the condition is allowed to continue, severe lithium toxicity would elicit confusion, convulsions, delirium, and eventually coma and death.[79] This is why monitoring the patient and blood levels of lithium is so important during treatment.

REVIEW EXAM

1. What is the hibernation syndrome?
2. Describe the difference between hallucinations and delusions.
3. Name the typical routes of administration for the antipsychotic medications.
4. What are the common half-lifes for the antipsychotics?
5. What are the specific effects of the antipsychotics on the PNS and CNS?
6. What are the dopamine systems that may be involved in psychotic behavior?
7. Characterize the dopamine receptors that are affected by the antipsychotic medications.
8. Name three nonbehavioral effects following antipsychotic medication.
9. Which psychotic symptoms seem to respond to the antipsychotic medications?
10. Characterize each of the four motor problems associated with the antipsychotic medications.

11. Describe the dopamine theory of schizophrenia.

12. How does clozapine differ from the other antipsychotic medications?

13. Describe the principal symptoms of depressed and manic mood disorders.

14. Compare the half-life of traditional tricyclic antidepressants to that of Prozac® and Zoloft®.

15. Describe how the two types of tricyclic antidepressants alter brain functioning at the synapse.

16. How do the newer heterocyclic antidepressants alter brain functioning at the synapse?

17. Describe the withdrawal symptoms associated with the antidepressants.

18. Describe the nonbehavioral adverse effects of the tricyclic antidepressants and of the MAOIs.

19. Describe the three stages of the cheese reaction.

20. Describe two of the four adverse behavioral effects associated with the antidepressants.

21. Compare the monoamine theory of mood disorder with the beta-adrenergic theory of mood disorder.

22. What are the main advantages and disadvantages of electroconvulsive shock therapy (ECT)?

23. How does sodium intake influence lithium excretion?

24. Name the subjective feelings that lithium elicits from normal nonmanic individuals.

25. How does lithium alter brain functioning?

26. What are the signs that precede a toxic reaction to Lithium®?

REFERENCES

1. HOLLISTER, L. (1977). Antipsychotic medications and treatment of schizophrenia. In J. Barchas, P. Berger, R. Ciaranello, & G. Elliot (Eds.), *Psychopharmacology: From Theory to Practice* (pp. 121–150). New York: Oxford Press.

2. RIFKIN, A. (1987). Extrapyramidal side effects: a historical perspective. *Journal of Clinical Psychiatry,* 48 (Suppl. 9), 3–6.

3. LADER, M. (1983). Antipsychotic drugs. In *Introduction to Psychopharmacology* (pp. 51–67). Kalamazoo, MI: The Upjohn Co.

4. DELAY, J., DENIKER, P., & HARL, J. (1952). Utilisation en therapeutique psychiatrique d'une phenothiazine d'action centrale elective. *Annals of Medical Psychology,* 110, 112–117.

5. HOLLISTER, R. (1987). Strategies for research in clinical psychopharmacology. In H. Meltzer (Ed.), *Psychopharmacology: The Third Generation* (pp. 31–38). New York: Raven Press.

6. BALDESSARINI, R. (1980). Drugs and the treatment of psychiatric disorders. In A. Gilman & L. Goodman (Eds.), *The Pharmacological Basis of Therapeutics* (6th ed., pp. 391–447). New York: Macmillan Publishing Co., Inc.

7. CREESE, I., BURT, D., & SNYDER, S. (1976). Dopamine receptor binding predicts clinical and pharmacological potencies of antischizophrenic drugs. *Science,* 192, 481–482.

8. CREESE, I. (1985). Receptor binding as a primary drug screen. In H. Yamamura, S. Enna, & M. Kuhar (Eds.), *Neurotransmitter Receptor Binding* (pp. 189–233). New York: Raven Press.

9. KANDEL, E. (1991). Disorders of thought: schizophrenia. In E. Kandel, J. Schwartz, & T. Jessell (Eds.), *Principles of Neural Science* (3rd ed., pp. 853–868). Norwalk, CT: Appleton and Lange.

10. BYCK, R. (1975). Drugs and the treatment of psychiatric disorders. In A. Gilman & L. Goodman (Eds.), *The Pharmacological Basis of Therapeutics* (5th ed., pp. 152–200). New York: Macmillan Publishing Co., Inc.

11. MELTZER, H. (1973). Rigidity, hyperpyrexia, and coma following fluphenazine enanthate. *Psychopharmacologia,* 29, 337–346.

12. CARFAGNO, S., & MCGEE, J. (1961). Granulocytopenia due to chlorpromazine: a report of 11 cases. *American Journal of Medical Science,* 241, 44–54.

13. PISCIOTTA, A., EBBE, S., LENNON, E., METZGER, G., & MADISON, F. (1958). Agranulocytosis after administration of phenothiazine derivatives. *American Journal of Medicine, 25,* 210–223.
14. HOLLISTER, L. (1958). Allergic reactions to tranquilizing drugs. *Annals of Internal Medicine, 49,* 17–29.
15. CASEY, D. (1991). Neuroleptic drug-induced extrapyramidal syndromes and tardive dyskinesia. *Schizophrenia Research, 4,* 109–120.
16. VAN PUTTEN, T. (1974). Why do schizophrenic patients refuse to take their drugs? *Archives of General Psychology, 31,* 67–72.
17. FAHN, S. (1988). Concept and classification of dystonia. In S. Fahn, C. Marsden, & D. Caline (Eds.), *Advances in Neurology* (pp. 2–8).
18. KLEIN, D., GITTELMAN, R., QUITKIN, F., & RIFKIN, A. (Eds.). (1980). *Diagnosis and Drug Treatment of Psychiatric Disorders: Adults and Children* (2nd ed., pp. 174–214). Baltimore, MD: Williams & Wilkins.
19. LAVIN, M., & RIFKIN, A. (1992). Neuroleptic-induced Parkinsonism. In J. Kane & J. Lieberman (Eds.), *Adverse Effects of Psychotropic Drugs,* (pp. 175–188).
20. BURKE, R. (1992). Neuromuscular effects of neuroleptics: dystonia. In J. Kane & J. Lieberman (Eds.), *Adverse Effects of Psychotropic Drugs* (pp. 189–200). New York: Gilford Press
21. BARNES, T. (1992). Neuromuscular effects of neuroleptics: akathisia. In J. Kane & J. Lieberman (Eds.), *Adverse Effects of Psychotropic Drugs* (pp. 201–217). New York: Gilford Press
22. AYD, F. (1961). A survey of drug-induced extrapyramidal reaction. *Journal of the American Medical Association, 175,* 1054–1060.
23. VAN PUTTEN, T., MAY, P., & MARDER, S. (1984). Akathisia with haloperidol and thiothixene. *Archives of General Psychiatry, 41,* 1036–1039.
24. BIANCHINE, J. (1980). Drugs for Parkinson's disease: centrally acting muscle relaxants. In A. Gilman & L. Goodman (Eds.), *The Pharmacological Basis of Therapeutics,* (6th ed. pp. 475–493). New York: Macmillan Publishing Co., Inc.
25. YASSA, R., NAIR, V., & SCHWARTZ, G. (1984). Tardive dyskinesia: a two-year follow-up study. *Psychosomatics, 25,* 852–855.
26. SALTZ, B., WOERNER, M., KANE J., LIEBERMAN, J., ALVIN, J., BERGMANN, K., BLANK, K., KOBLENZER, J., & KAHANER, K. (1991). Prospective study in tardive dyskinesia in the elderly. *Journal of the American Medical Association, 266,* 2402–2406.
27. KANE, J., WOERNER, M., WEINHOLD, P., WEGNER, J., & KINON, B. (1984). Incidence of tardive dyskinesia: five-year data from a prospective study. *Psychopharmacology Bulletin, 20*(3), 387–389.
28. KANE, J., WOERNER, M., & BORENSTEIN, M. (1986). Integrating incidence and prevalence of tardive dyskinesia. *Psychopharmacology Bulletin, 22*(1), 254–258.
29. GERLICH, J., REISBY, N., & RANDRUP, A. (1974). Dopaminergic hypersensitivity and cholinergic hypofunction in the pathophysiology of tardive dyskinesia. *Psychopharmacologia, 34,* 21–35.
30. KANE, J., & LIEBERMAN, J. (1992). Tardive dyskinesia. In J. Kane & J. Lieberman (Eds.), *Adverse Effects of Psychotropic Drugs* (pp. 235–245). New York: Gilford Press
31. CONLEY, R., SCHULZ, S., BAKER, R., COLLINS, J., & BELL J. (1988). Clozapine efficacy in schizophrenic nonresponders. *Psychopharmacology Bulletin, 24*(2), 269–274.
32. KANE, J., HONIGFELD, G., SINGER, J., & MELTZER, H. (1989). Clozapine for the treatment-resistant schizophrenic: results of a U.S. multicenter trial. *Psychopharmacology, 99,* S60–S63.
33. SAFFERMAN, A., LIEBERMAN, J., KANE, J., SZYMANSKI, S., & KINON, B. (1991). Update on clinical efficacy and side effects of clozapine. *Schizophrenia Bulletin, 17,* 247–262.
34. LIEBERMAN, J., SALTZ, C., JOHNS, C., POLLACK, S., BORENSTEIN, M., & KANE, J. (1991). The effect of clozapine on tardive dyskinesia. *British Journal of Psychiatry, 158,* 503–510.
35. CLAGHORN, J., HONIGFELD, G, & ABUZZAHAB, F. (1987). The risks and benefits of clozapine versus chlorpromazine. *Journal of Clinical Psychopharmacology, 7,* 377–384.
36. MELTZER, H. (1992). Pattern of efficacy in treatment-resistant schizophrenia. In H. Meltzer (Ed.), *Novel Antipsychotic Drugs* (pp. 33–46). New York: Raven Press.
37. SEEMAN, P., LEE, T., CHAN-WONG, M., & WONG, K. (1976). Antipsychotic drug doses and neuroleptic/dopamine receptors. *Nature, 261,* 717–718.
38. FARDE, L., WIESEL, F., NORDSTROM, A., & SEDVALL, G. (1989). D-1 and D-2 dopamine receptor occupancy during treatment with conventional and atypical neuroleptics. *Psychopharmacology, 99,* S28–S31.

453

39. MELTZER, H. (1992). The mechanism of action of clozapine in relation to its clinical advantages. In H. Meltzer (Ed.), *Novel Antipsychotic Drugs* (pp. 2–13). New York: Raven Press.

40. MILLER, R., & HILEY, C. (1976). Antimuscarinic properties of neuroleptics and drug-induced Parkinsonism. *Nature, 248,* 596–597.

41. KRUPP, P., & BARNES, P. (1989). Leponex-associated agranulocytopenia: a review of the situation. *Psychopharmacology, 99,* S118–S121.

42. HENINGER, G. (1993). The biologic basis of major affective disorders: an overview. In *Neurobiology of Affective Disorders* (pp. 2–6). New York: Raven Health Care Communications, a division of Raven Press.

43. KHUN, R. (1958). The treatment of depressed states with G22355 (imipramine hydrochloride). *American Journal of Psychiatry, 115,* 459–464.

44. LADER, M. (1983). *Introduction to Psychopharmacology* (pp. 68–89). Kalamazoo, MI: The Upjohn Co.

45. BENET, L., & SHEINER, L. (1980). Design and optimization of dosage regimens: pharmacokinetic data. In A. Gilman & L. Goodman (Eds.), *The Pharmacological Basis of Therapeutics* (6th ed., pp. 1675–1737). New York: Macmillan Publishing Co., Inc.

46. VAN HERTEN, J. (1993). Clinical pharmacokinetics of selective serotonin reuptake inhibitors. *Clinical Pharmacokinetics, 24(3),* 203–220.

47. KLEIN, D., GITTELMAN, R., QUITKIN, F., & RIFKIN, A. (Eds.). (1980). Review of the literature on mood-stabilizing drugs. In *Diagnosis and Drug Treatment of Psychiatric Disorders: Adults and Children* (2nd ed., pp. 268–408). Baltimore, MD: Williams & Wilkins.

48. FRAZER, A. (1993). Regionally selective effects in brain of typical and atypical antidepressants. In *Neurobiology of Affective Disorders* (pp. 17–21). New York: Raven Health Care Communications, a division of Raven Press.

49. KLERMAN, G., & COLE, J. (1965). Clinical pharmacology of imipramine and related antidepressant compounds. *Pharmacology Reviews, 17,* 101–141.

50. SHATAN, C. (1966). Withdrawal symptoms after abrupt termination of imipramine. *Canadian Psychiatric Association Journal, 11* (suppl.), S150–S158.

51. FRENKEL, A., QUITKIN, F., & RABKIN, J. (1992). Behavioral side effects associated with antidepressants and lithium. In J. Kane & J. Lieberman (Eds.), *Adverse Effects of Psychotropic Drugs* (pp. 111–127). New York: Gilford Press

52. PALLADINO, A. (1983). Adverse reactions to abrupt discontinuation with phenelzine. *Journal of Clinical Psychopharmacology, 3,* 206–207.

53. KLEIN, D., GITTELMAN, R., QUITKIN, F., & RIFKIN, A. (Eds.) (1980). Side effects of mood-stabilizing drugs and their treatment. In *Diagnosis and Drug Treatment of Psychiatric Disorders: Adults and Children* (2nd ed., pp. 449–492). Baltimore, MD: William & Wilkins.

54. MCGRATH, P., & HARRISON, W. (1992). Cardiovascular effects of monoamine oxidase inhibitor antidepressants and Lithium. In J. Kane & J. Lieberman (Eds.), *Adverse Effects of Psychotropic Drugs* (pp. 298–317). New York: Gilford Press

55. SOLOFF, P., GEORGE, A., NATHAN, R., SCHULZ, P., & PEREL, J. (1986). Paradoxical effects of amitriptyline on borderline patients. *American Journal of Psychiatry, 143,* 1603–1605.

56. COLE, J., & BODKIN, J. (1990). Antidepressant drug side effects. *Journal of Clinical Psychiatry, 51,* 21–26.

57. ZITRIN, C., KLEIN, D., & WOERNER, M. (1980). Treatment of agoraphobia with group exposure in vivo and imipramine. *Archives of General Psychiatry, 37,* 63–72.

58. ZUBENKO, G., COHEN, B., & LIPINSKI, J. (1987). Antidepressant-related akathisia. *Journal of Clinical Psychopharmacology 7,* 254–257.

59. KUPFER, D., SPIKER, D., COBEL, P., & MCPARTLARD, R. (1978). Amitriptyline and EEG sleep in depressed patients. *Sleep, 1(2),* 149–159.

60. KUPFER, D., SPIKER, D., COBEL, P., NEIL, J., ULRICH, R., & SHAW, D. (1981). Sleep treatment prediction in endogenous depression. *American Journal of Psychiatry, 138,* 429–434.

61. LIPPMAN, S., MOSKOVITZ, R., & O'TUAMA, L. (1977). Tricyclic-induced myoclonus. *American Journal of Psychiatry, 134, 90–91.*

62. *CASAS, M., GARCIA-RIBERTA, C., ALVAREZ, E., UDINA, C., QUERALTO, J., & GRAU, J. (1987). Myoclonic movements as a side effect of treatment with therapeutic doses of clomipramine. International Clinical Psychopharmacology, 2, 333–336.*

63. PICKAR, D., MURPHY, D., COHEN, R., CAMPBELL, I., & LIPPER, S. (1982). Selective and non-selective monoamine oxidase inhibitors: behavioral disturbances during their administration to depressed patients. *Archives of General Psychiatry, 39,* 535–540.

64. SHEEHAN, D., CLAYCOMB, J., & KOURETAS, N. (1980–81). Monoamine oxidase inhibitors: prescription and patient management. *International Journal of Psychiatry in Medicine, 10,* 99–121.
65. SULSER, F. (1993). The aminergic "link hypothesis" of affective disorders: a molecular view of therapy-resistant depression. In *Neurobiology of Affective Disorders* (pp. 7–12). New York: Raven Health Care Communications, a division of Raven Press.
66. NELSON, J., MAZURE, C., BOWERS, M., & JATLOW, P. (1991). A preliminary open study of the combination of fluoxetine and desipramine for rapid treatment of major depression. *Archives of General Psychiatry, 48,* 303–307.
67. DE MONTIGNY, C. (1984). Electroconvulsive shock treatments enhance responsiveness of forebrain neurons to serotonin. *Journal of Pharmacology and Experimental Therapeutics, 228,* 230–234.
68. CHAPUT, Y., DE MONTIGNY, C., & BLIER, P. (1991). Presynaptic and postsynaptic modifications of the serotonin system by long-term administration of antidepressant treatments: an in vivo electrophysiological study in the rat. *Neuropsychopharmacology, 5,* 219–229.
69. DE MONTIGNY, C. (1993). Is the serotonin system still a promising target for the future of pharmacotherapy of affective disorders? In *Neurobiology of Affective Disorders* (pp. 22–26). New York: Raven Health Care Communications, a division of Raven Press.
70. MANN, J., & ARANGO, V. (1992). Integration of neurobiology and psychopathology in a unified model of suicidal behavior. *Journal of Clinical Psychopharmacology, 12* (suppl.), 2S–7S.
71. MANN, J. (1993). The organization of noradrenergic and serotonergic receptor systems in the cerebral cortex of suicide victims: implications for the pathogenesis of suicidal behavior and depression. In *Neurobiology of Affective Disorders* (pp. 26–30). New York: Raven Health Care Communications, a division of Raven Press.
72. GULEVICH, G. (1977). Convulsive and coma therapies and psychosurgery. In J. Barchas, P. Berger, R. Ciaranello, & G. Elliott (Eds.), *Psychopharmacology: From Theory to Practice* (pp. 514–526). New York: Oxford Press.
73. SHAPIRA, B., CALEV, A., & LERER, B. (1991). Optimal use of electroconvulsive therapy: choosing a treatment schedule. *Psychiatric Clinics of North America, 14*(4), 935–946.
74. DAVIS, G., & GOLDMAN, B. (1992). Somatic therapies. In H. Goldman (Ed.), *Review of General Psychiatry* (3rd ed., pp. 370–390). Norwalk, CT: Appleton and Lange.
75. KHAN, A., MIROLO, M., HUGHES, D., & BIERUT, L. (1993). Electroconvulsive therapy. *Psychiatric Clinics of North America, 16*(3), 497–513.
76. DEVANAND, D., SACKEIM, H., & PRUDIC, J. (1991). Electroconvulsive therapy in the treatment-resistant patient. *Psychiatric Clinics of North America, 14*(4), 905–923.
77. SEAGER, C., & BIRD, R. (1962). Imipramine with electrical treatment in depression—a controlled trial. *Journal of Mental Science 108,* 704–707.
78. FAVA, M., & ROSENBAUM, J. (1991). Suicidality and fluoxetine: is there a relationship? *Journal of Clinical Psychiatry, 52,* 108–111.
79. LADER, M. (1983). Lithium. In *Introduction to Psychopharmacology* (pp. 90–94). Kalamazoo, MI: The Upjohn Co.
80. SACK, R., & DE FRAITES, E. (1977). Lithium and the treatment of mania. In J. Barchas, P. Berger, R. Ciaranello, & G. Elliott (Eds.), *Psychopharmacology: From Theory to Practice* (pp. 208–225). New York: Oxford Press.
81. LEMUS, C., & LIEBERMAN, J. (1992). Neuromuscular effects of antidepressants and lithium. In J. Kane & J. Lieberman (Eds.), *Adverse Effects of Psychotropic Drugs* (pp. 165–174). New York: Gilford Press

15
SOCIAL BEHAVIOR

STACY CRAWLED OUT OF HER SLEEPING BAG BEFORE
DAWN AND JOINED HER COMPANIONS AT THE SIX-FOOT
STONE ALTAR. THE SHERPAS WERE ALREADY THERE
sprinkling rice, chanting softly, and burning branches of juniper. They
certainly were not going to miss the ceremony. After all, they had built
the altar to assist them in challenging Chomolungma, the mightiest
mountain in the world.

The dozen or so Americans laid on the shelf of that altar their
most precious possessions at the moment—chocolate candies, raisins,
flags and pennants, and bottles of whiskey. The Sherpas offered up
sampas, which are balls of barley flour, standard fare at the Pujah, a
Buddhist blessing ritual.

Although the Americans did not understand the Pujah, they were taking
no chances. It *might* help—when they faced the towering masses of ice and
snow, the shrill whistle of blizzard winds, and the sudden roar of an
avalanche. Appealing to Buddha and the mountain gods for a safe passage

up Mount Everest, the Western name for Chomol-ungma, seemed like quite a good idea. Moreover, this ceremony reminded everyone that they were a team. Especially when they entered the Khumbu Ice Fall, 2,000 feet of sheer, vertical ice, the success of any one climber would depend on the cooperation of all. Of those who attempt this passage, many do not return.

Meanwhile, an American research group of psychologists and physiologists from the University of Washington went about its own business, preparing to assess the climbers on this expedition. People at high altitudes quickly lose control of mental and physical capacities, due to lack of oxygen, and the research team wanted to investigate these conditions. Knowing they would not ascend Everest beyond the second base camp, they were generally less concerned about satisfying the mountain gods.

While the climbers in the American expedition reflected on the challenge ahead, the Sherpas chanted and chanted, at times in wild crescendos, at times in low murmurs, like quiet prayers. Occasion-ally, they called to the Americans, asking them to throw handfuls of rice into the sky, as further offerings to Buddha.

When the ceremony was over, the American climbers frivolously tossed barley flour at one another, producing billowy white clouds suggestive of the blizzards ahead. Then they smeared flour on their hair and faces. The white streaks symbolized a long, happy life, and they were eager to do whatever might contribute to that outcome. Afterward, they posed for a photograph. Seemingly happy and confident, their smiles and besmirched faces belied the dangers that lay ahead (Allison, 1993).

The Sherpas were more reserved. They knew the mountains well, living in Nepal, among the Himalayas, between the borders of China and India. Often hired as porters and guides for climbing, they also knew the importance of teamwork on these expeditions.

What would happen on this expedition as friendships formed and personal difficulties arose? Who would climb with whom on the summit teams? Would Stacy Allison reach the top of the

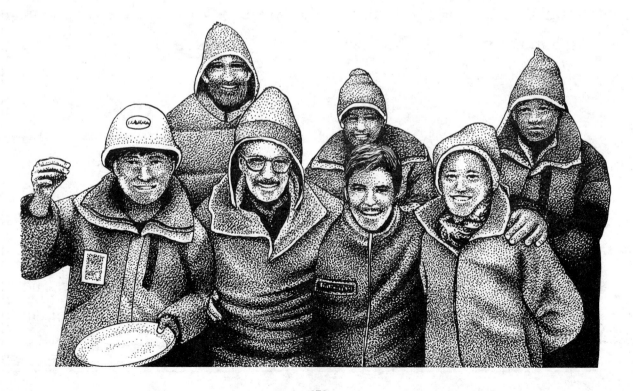

world? Would she be the first American woman to do so? Would cultural differences emerge?

Behaviors of this sort, and the related interactions, are the substance of social psychology. Simply defined, **social psychology** is the study of individuals in groups, specifically the ways in which human beings interact with one another. The Everest expedition provides a helpful background for this discussion because it includes interactions among men and women from two cultures and three groups: the American climbers, the Sherpa guides and porters, and the Washington research team.

We begin this chapter by examining attitudes, considered by some psychologists as a first principle in social behavior. Then we study a more exclusively social issue, social cognition. How do we interpret information about other people? At the next stage, we consider interpersonal attraction, our preferences for relationships with specific people.

The discussion then turns from the individual to the group, focusing on the conditions and outcomes of social influence: conformity, compliance, obedience, and altruism. Finally, we consider fundamental group processes, as individuals interact within the group setting.

• ATTITUDES •

One of the most widely used concepts in social psychology, an *attitude* is difficult to define. For this reason, and because attitudes cannot be observed directly, some psychologists ignore them. They study only overt behavior rather than make assumptions about inner states that allegedly influence behavior. The position adopted in this text, and by many social psychologists today, is that attitudes are important and can be usefully defined (Dillard, 1993). An integral part of an individual's interactions with others, an **attitude** is a tendency to make an evaluation, reflected in three basic components: thinking, feeling, and acting (Olson & Zanna, 1993).

Thinking, the first component, obviously involves a thought or belief about something. Stacy Allison believed that mountaineering is a healthy, inspiring activity, especially if pursued with proper knowledge and caution. What about her feelings?

Stacy immediately became excited by any opportunity to climb challenging mountains. This general excitement also became differentiated into more specific feelings, such as enthusiasm, confidence, and anticipation. And third, what about her actions? She reacted in a predictable, consistent manner. At the first opportunity, she signed on for an Everest expedition. In fact, she signed up twice, for her first effort proved to be a bitter, wrenching failure.

A year earlier, with three other American climbers, she had almost reached the peak of Mount Everest. After spending seven nights in an atmosphere too thin to support sustained life, they remained pinned down by an autumn blizzard, the worst on Mount Everest in 40 years. At that altitude, the human digestive system cannot readily utilize nourishment, and the climber's muscles begin to atrophy. At dawn the next day, the team members asked themselves: "One more day?" One member, barely able to eat breakfast, shook his head. "If I don't go down today," he said, "I'm not going to get down." As the climbers began their descent, they hid their anguish, and for Stacy that disappointment was acute. The others were men. If the team had advanced those last 3,000 feet, she would have been the first American woman to reach the peak of Mount Everest (Allison, 1993).

Clearly, Stacy Allison had a positive attitude toward mountaineering, even in the face of this disappointment. It showed in her thinking, feeling, and acting. These three components are also described as cognitive, affective, and behavioral components.

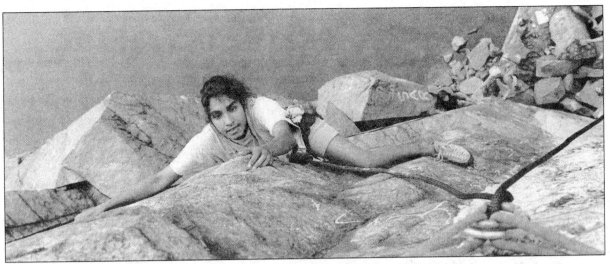

FIGURE 17-1 COMPONENTS OF ATTITUDE. The behavioral component of an attitude often is not readily displayed, especially in comparison with the cognitive and affective components. Among people with favorable attitudes toward mountaineering, only a few regularly climb mountain peaks.

FORMING ATTITUDES

How do attitudes develop? The obvious answer is that they arise initially through contacts with our parents, early teachers, and other adults. Later, peers and friends influence the various components (Figure 17-1). But the basic question still stands: By what processes do attitudes develop?

DIRECT INSTRUCTION AND MODELING. In the most obvious instances, attitudes are formed by direct instruction. A small girl was informed that she would have tapioca for lunch. She replied: "I don't like that." Then she asked, "What is it?" She had been told by her older sister that tapioca has a disagreeable taste, a form of direct instruction. Attitudes toward mountaineering, religious ceremonies, and social psychology develop in the same way. Direct instruction can play a significant role, as it did for Stacy in her adolescent years, but it is far from the whole story.

Sometimes the instruction is indirect. People teach one another merely by what they do. Siblings, parents, friends, public figures, and total strangers can influence our attitudes in this way—by acting as models. A *model* is someone who demonstrates the proper performance, intentionally or otherwise. During college, Stacy observed a park ranger nimbly scaling the summit of a rocky ledge. Watching her, Stacy decided that being a mountaineer was "everything I wanted to be" (Allison, 1993).

Children who observe their elders happily eating grasshoppers want to eat grasshoppers too. Those who notice adults befriending strangers tend to develop positive attitudes toward strangers. In this process, called *modeling*, discussed in the chapter on learning, one person learns by following the example of another.

CLASSICAL AND OPERANT CONDITIONING. Suppose a parent who wears a certain cologne is also kind and helpful to his child. Through the pairing of this odor with kindness, food, play, and so forth, the child eventually develops a positive attitude toward the cologne. Associated with good outcomes, this event becomes favorable too. You may recognize this process as classical conditioning.

An early study of this process used the names

for various nationalities—German, Swedish, French, and Dutch. They were paired with positive, negative, or neutral words. Later, after many pairings, an attitude questionnaire was administered regarding these nationalities. It was found that each nationality was perceived as positive, negative, or neutral, depending on its previous associations (Staats & Staats, 1958). Today there is abundant evidence of this sort (Kuykendall & Keating, 1990).

Suppose the child wore the cologne one day, and his family complimented him on it. If so, this behavior of wearing perfume was reinforced, and it was likely to reappear. The process here is operant conditioning, for behaviors that produce positive consequences tend to be repeated. While Stacy was mountaineering in Yosemite National Park one summer during college, her behavior certainly produced positive consequences. She felt the rhythm of the climb, the whispering of mountain breezes, and the sun on her back. She felt as free as a hawk that happened to be riding an updraft of air above her. As she expressed it, "The world was in harmony" (Allison, 1993).

ROLE OF COGNITION. Attitudes also can be developed or changed through the way we think about things—without direct instruction, modeling, or any significant conditioning. Thought is involved in all of those processes, and sometimes thought alone is the basis for attitude formation.

Suppose a young man receives a grade of 40 on a mathematics exam. Thinking that 44 is the maximum score, he regards his work favorably. Then he discovers that 60 is the maximum score, and his attitude toward his score promptly becomes unfavorable. Both attitudes are developed simply on the basis of reasoning, as he compares himself with an absolute standard and perhaps with other students, as well. Cognitive processes can be fundamentally involved in the development of attitudes (Chaiken & Stangor, 1987).

MEASUREMENT OF ATTITUDES. Regardless of their origins, how can we measure attitudes toward mountaineering or mathematics? A common method involves a *Likert rating scale,* in which printed statements concerning the issue are each accompanied by a scale of three to seven intervals, ranging from extremely negative to extremely positive. The subjects indicate their attitude toward each statement by marking a position on the scale. Likert scales are relatively easy to construct and score, but they can be readily faked (Table 17-1).

A very different approach employs modern electronic equipment for assessing heart rate, skin conductance, and even pupillary changes. Less subject to fabrication, physiological reactions are becoming more important as measures of attitudes (Tesser & Shaffer, 1990).

But there are problems here, too. First, a pounding heart and increased rate of breathing indicate that the reaction is a strong one, but we do not know whether it is positive or negative. Second, there are large individual differences in emotional expression. Some people, when aroused, experience a pounding heart; others develop sweaty palms; and still others show neither response, but their voices rise instead. Third, many measures, such as pupillary changes, require highly controlled conditions or elaborate apparatus. And finally, to the

---

1. Mountaineering is a worthwhile activity.
   SA   A   (MA)   MD   D   SD
2. Climbing mountains builds character.
   SA   (A)   MA   MD   D   SD
3. For an experienced person, climbing Mount Everest can be a safe form of recreation.
   SA   A   MA   MD   (D)   SD

SA = Strongly agree   MD = Mildy disagree
A = Agree   D = Disagree
MA = Mildly agree   SD = Strongly disagree

TABLE 17–1 AN ATTITUDE SCALE. A full attitude scale would include many items of this sort. The subject's reponse to each item is assigned a value ranging from +3 to −3, excluding 0. The scores for the circled responses here would be +1, +2, and −2. Hence, the total score is +1.

extent that the person being tested can concentrate on something else, the results may be misleading. Altogether, several physiological, psychological, and behavioral measures must be combined for the most effective measurement of attitudes.

CONSISTENCY IN ATTITUDES

Ralph Waldo Emerson remarked: "A foolish consistency is the hobgoblin of little minds." Most of us develop and maintain attitudes that are in agreement with one another, however. Several theories of attitude formation and change are based on this principle of consistency.

EARLY VIEWPOINTS. Among these theories, the oldest is called **balance theory** because it stresses that people seek a balanced or harmonious state among their attitudes. In college, Stacy met a young woman named Evelyn, and they became friendly. Both of them were learning mountaineering and enjoying it immensely. There were positive relationships all around; a balanced state existed. As this friendship developed, they discovered that neither of them liked their college studies. A balanced state still existed, for they liked each other and both disliked college.

Suppose a husband favors gun control and his wife does not, and yet they have a very satisfying marital relationship. Here there is imbalance. Neither person's attitude is supported by the other,

whom he or she likes (Alessio, 1990; Heider, 1946; Figure 17–2).

Another approach goes a step beyond balance or harmony. It regards attitudes as changeable and considers the probable outcome of these changes. Specifically, **congruity theory** states that attitude shifts occur in the direction of increased consistency (Osgood, Suci, & Tannenbaum, 1957). A woman mildly against day care finds that a lawyer she much admires is in favor of day care. It is hypothesized that her attitude toward him will become less positive and her attitude toward day care less negative. The degree of change should not be equal, however, unless the different attitudes are of the same strength. A greater shift is expected in the milder attitude. If she is not particularly concerned about day care and feels strongly about the lawyer, then her attitude toward day care should undergo the greater change in strength and direction.

In one study, 604 people from the general population were interviewed by telephone and asked their views on the quality of clothes available for purchase at various places of business. These places ranged from major department stores to off-price discount warehouses. As predicted by congruity theory, perception of the wearing apparel was decidedly influenced by the type of business with which it was associated. When offered for sale by department stores, brands of clothing were rated significantly higher than when available at discount and chain stores (Morganosky, 1990).

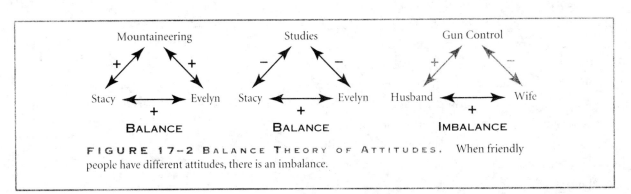

FIGURE 17–2 BALANCE THEORY OF ATTITUDES. When friendly people have different attitudes, there is an imbalance.

DISSONANCE THEORY. The third approach, dissonance theory, goes beyond the degree or direction of attitude change within an individual. It emphasizes instead the psychological processes by which inconsistency is resolved. This theory is called **cognitive-dissonance theory** because the individual's cognitions are dissonant or inconsistent, and the person is motivated to dispel this state of tension in various ways.

Consider what happened when people opposed to the use of electric shock agreed to administer shocks to others as part of a research project. Before the experiment, they experienced directly the amount of shock that the subjects would receive and rated its painfulness. After the experiment, in which they shocked other people, they again rated the painfulness of the shock. Can you make a prediction based on dissonance theory? In the second rating, did they increase or decrease their estimate of the painfulness of the shock? It had been anticipated that the subjects, after administering the shock to other people, would then rate it as less painful, and this prediction was supported (Brock & Buss, 1962).

More recently, householders in one group were informed about the inconsistency between their attitudes toward conservation and their high consumption of electricity. Those in a second group were simply informed that they were high consumers of electricity. Still others were sent information on how to conserve electricity. After two weeks, energy consumption was measured once again in all groups. It was found that among the 272 subjects, those in the first group, with high dissonance, conserved more electricity than those in any of the other groups (Kantola, Syme, & Campbell, 1984).

According to this research, dissonance can be reduced through rationalizing, perceiving selectively, changing one's behavior, or seeking new information. The subjects in the first experiment apparently were rationalizing or engaging in selective perception when rating the second shock as less painful. Those in the study on energy consumption changed their behavior. There is, of course, no dissonance if the individual does not perceive any inconsistency (Table 17-2).

TECHNIQUES OF PERSUASION

Apart from theory, everyday life in this country includes many practical techniques for developing and changing attitudes, especially through the mass media. They are vital not only to salespersons and swindlers but also to educators, counselors, health officials, and people concerned with public welfare. They urge us to drive safely, avoid drugs, dispose of litter and, of course, mail holiday gifts early.

THEORY	EMPHASIS	EXAMPLE
Balance	Harmony among an individual's attitudes	Wendy loves her sister Stacy, who enjoys mountaineering. Wendy mildly disapproves of mountaineering. There is imbalance.
Congruity	Attitude shift within an individual	Wendy feels strongly about her sister. She is only mildly against mountaineering. Thus, her attitude toward mountaineering will shift in a positive direction.
Cognitive dissonance	Resolving inconsistency among attitudes	Wendy feels some tension because her attitudes are inconsistent. She decides that she needs more information on the dangers of mountaineering.

TABLE 17-2 THEORIES OF ATTITUDE CONSISTENCY. Wendy maintained a loving relationship with her sister Stacy, and yet she had a mild dislike of mountaineering. Each of the three major theories of attitude consistency approaches Wendy's situation somewhat differently.

Mountaineers cannot finance major expeditions themselves, as Stacy soon discovered. They must persuade individuals and manufacturers to donate supplies, equipment, and funds. For this purpose, both Everest teams, based in Seattle, used an assortment of techniques addressing the three basic elements in communication: the source, audience, and message.

SOURCE CHARACTERISTICS. It has been almost 20 centuries since Aristotle wrote in his *Rhetoric* that the *ethos*, or credibility, of the communicator is the most important single factor in the persuasiveness of a communication, and most subsequent research supports this view (McGuire, 1985; Zimbardo & Lieppe, 1991). The crucial elements in credibility are trust and expertise. Don Goodman, organizer of the second expedition, had both of these qualities. Using his good-natured integrity and experience in climbing Everest, he gained considerable financial support from private corporations and public appeals (Allison, 1993).

Credibility also came from the University of Washington, which assembled the research group accompanying the expedition. High-altitude mountaineering is of special interest to investigators in psychology and physiology because the environment is extreme, yet natural. Learning and other thought processes are impaired at high altitudes due to the lack of oxygen in vital brain areas (Nelson, Dunlosky, White, Steinberg, Townes, & Anderson, 1990). One aim of the Washington research team was to study human thought under hypoxia, a condition of oxygen deficiency sometimes resembling alcohol intoxication.

The importance of source credibility is clearly recognized by television advertisers. They hire professional athletes to endorse sneakers, movie stars to endorse skin creams, and sedentary types to promote hemorrhoid treatments. An integral factor in the acceptance of the message, however, is the perceived intent of the communicator. Therefore, unsolicited common folk actually outstrip sports heroes and other celebrities in popularity for endorsement of products. These neighborly individuals presumably have no ulterior motives! And they ask for a lower endorsement fee.

AUDIENCE CHARACTERISTICS. A second concern, after the credibility of the communicator, is the participation of the audience. Here again, early studies established a principle that is still accepted today: Audiences tend to have the most positive attitudes toward events in which they have become most involved—through discussions, clapping, singing, and so forth. Sports teams, musical shows, and political speakers all utilize this principle, as did the Everest expeditions. The members involved the press in question-and-answer sessions, held rallies, and encouraged interested individuals to participate in fund-raising (Allison, 1993).

The importance of participation was demonstrated in a classic study during World War II. Choice cuts of meat were scarce, and attempts were made to persuade people to use less-preferred meat products. In one research program, some shoppers listened to a lecture on using these products. Other shoppers were involved in a group discussion about the problems they might experience in using such foods and how they might overcome them. At a later date, the investigators checked to discover the effectiveness of the two presentations. They found the discussion method far superior for promoting a change in attitude and behavior (Lewin, 1947).

Modern investigators have taken this question one step further, assessing the importance of the audience's predisposition to become active or passive. Hence, a dozen commercials were presented to 252 undergraduates serving as subjects. Each commercial was either open-ended, in which some issues were left to be considered by the interviewer, or closed-ended, raising no unanswered points. As predicted, when the audience was predisposed to be active and involved, the open-ended commercials stimulated more favorable reactions than the closed-ended ones. With uninterested audiences, there was little difference between the two appeals (Sawyer & Howard, 1991).

MESSAGE CHARACTERISTICS. The importance of message characteristics depends on the source and audience, and vice versa, as implied already. Nevertheless, a fundamental question arises in nearly all efforts at persuasion: To change an audience's attitude, should the message give the full story, telling both sides, or not? To persuade someone to accept viewpoint *A*, should viewpoint *B* be included or ignored?

Except in the case of very simple messages, such as those merely promoting a common product, the most lasting effect is achieved by presenting the desired view, the opposite view, and then counterarguments against the opposite view. In this way, the audience is inclined toward *A* and prepared against future propaganda on behalf of *B*, the opposing viewpoint. A *two-sided presentation*, in which the speaker discusses both the pros and cons of each side, can provide immunization against later exposure to opposing viewpoints. This balanced approach appears to be particularly important for audiences of high intelligence and for hostile or neutral audiences, who need to hear both sides of the issue (McGuire, 1985).

From another perspective, most messages can be divided roughly into two types. Those that appeal to thought and reason use a central route; they go directly to the point and substance of the issue. Those that employ extraneous appeals, such as songs and celebrities and slogans, follow a peripheral route; the approach is roundabout and more emotional. Which route is favored? Research has shown that an enduring attitude change is most likely fostered by the central route. To develop or change a *complex* attitude, we need to think about the proposition, elaborate on it, and consider the details. This finding supports the *elaboration-likelihood model* of persuasion, which states that when the audience is intelligent and motivated, a direct appeal to thought, reason, and mulling things over will be the better route to persuasion. When the audience is less able and willing, rules of thumb and short cuts will be more effective (Petty & Cacioppo, 1986).

Many messages include both approaches. In her fund-raising efforts, Stacy stressed the specific facts of the expedition and used an emotional appeal, trying to make the prospective giver "feel the poetry of the climb" (Allison, 1993).

FEAR-AROUSING MESSAGES. Among all the questions about message characteristics, the use of fear has received the most research attention (Olson & Zanna, 1993). One form of common sense states that warnings about dangers should aim to instill a high level of fear. An announcement might show alcohol, a crashed car, and a graveyard. Another might show a cocaine addict describing her broken life. A competing form of common sense states that unpleasant messages are rejected or ignored; only positive appeals are heeded. A message low in fear arousal might show an animated embryo thanking its mother for not using alcohol or cigarettes (Reeves, Newhagen, Maibach, Basil, & Kurz, 1991).

This debate has a long history with mixed results, for several factors are influential, one of which is the subjects' initial level of fear. If it is high, a further increase may produce an immobilized state or an avoidance reaction, thus impeding change. If it is low, arousing fear may stimulate action in the desired direction. Hence, campaigns against AIDS and drug abuse, for example, must take into account the original level of anxiety in the target population (Sherr, 1990).

A related vital factor is the extent to which the message contains instructions on the correct or desired behavior. Messages low in fear arousal generally contain more detailed instructions and advice than those high in fear arousal. Therefore, other things being equal, they may be more likely to lead to constructive behavior (Reeves et al., 1991).

In summary, these techniques of persuasion reflect the basic theme of this book: the multiple bases of behavior. An audience may be persuaded by the credibility of the source, participation in the presentation, balance of the presentation, and arousal of fear, which in turn depends on the initial level of fear and the amount of instruction in the message. Behavior is influenced by many factors within and outside the individual.

• SOCIAL COGNITION •

After the Pujah blessing ceremony, the camp alarms went off at 2:00 A.M., and the ascent began that day, August 29. The climbers wanted to complete most of the day's work before the sun heated and loosened the ice. Donning boots and head lamps, they began setting a zigzag route through the ice fall. Jim Frush, leader on the mountain, encouraged group efforts and team spirit. Working together under the constant threat of avalanches, the members became more and more aware of one another.

This awareness brings us to a prominent topic in social psychology, **social cognition,** concerned with how people interpret information about other people, their relationships, social events, and social institutions. Social cognition is the inner, individual dimension of social behavior and experience.

FORMING IMPRESSIONS

The expedition included two hard-working physicians, Steve Ruoss and Geoff Tabin, both in their early thirties, quick-witted, and experienced at high altitudes. Steve was a bit taller; Geoff was bearded; and they both wore the usual climber's garb (Allison, 1993).

What do we think about these members of the expedition? What are they like? We have only their clothes, physical appearance, and occupations on which to make a judgment. This problem, called *person perception,* refers to the ways in which we perceive and understand another individual. Part of social cognition, it appears to be an extremely complex activity, raising questions about unconscious as well as conscious processes (Figure 17–3).

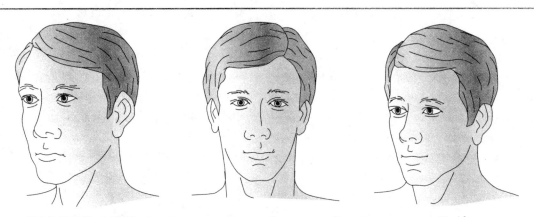

FIGURE 17–3 AWARENESS AND PERSON PERCEPTION. Decide which face is most attractive and indicate the reasons for your choice. Subjects performing this task typically prefer the center face, with normal proportions, rather than the one on the left or right, with the eyes too high or too low, respectively. In repeating this task with many different faces and explaining the reasons for their choices, subjects commonly select the normal face but do not refer to the proportions. In other words, they seem to utilize information about the faces that is not immediately accessible to their awareness (Hill & Lewicki, 1991).

INFLUENCE OF CENTRAL TRAITS. Especially when dealing with strangers, we dislike ambiguity. We try to resolve the uncertainty as soon as possible, and therefore we sometimes form an impression based on little evidence. If we arbitrarily decide, for example, that one of these mountaineers is cold and aloof and that the other is warm and personable, then we may soon find ourselves jumping to other conclusions about them.

This characteristic, degree of social warmth, also called the *warm–cold dimension*, is highly influential in our estimates of other personal traits; therefore, in social psychology it is called a **central trait.** Central traits are instrumental in the way we perceive other people; they are *not* necessarily the *basic traits* of the individual, discussed in the chapter on personality. Research on central traits has shown that a person described as intelligent, skillful, industrious, cold, determined, practical, and polite is considered significantly different from one described in exactly the same way, except with the substitution of *warm* for *cold.* The warm–cold dimension greatly influences our judgment about whether the person is generous, happy, good-natured, and even important. Other traits have not shown this effect. The substitution of *blunt* for *polite,* for example, does not change the overall rating significantly (Asch, 1946).

Another characteristic that is certainly central and therefore influences other people's reactions is *insane, schizophrenic,* or *crazy.* Once a person has been so labeled, even normal behaviors tend to be perceived as deviant (Rosenhan, 1973).

A perceptual error of this sort is known as the **halo effect,** meaning that a favorable or unfavorable judgment about one characteristic prompts similar judgments about other characteristics of this same person, regardless of the objective situation. Suppose Geoff proves to be highly intelligent, an admirable quality. The halo effect prompts us to assume that he possesses other esteemed traits. The halo effect even operates with beauty. Beautiful people tend to be judged as more intelligent than people of the same intelligence who are less attractive (Hatfield & Sprecher, 1986).

OUT-OF-ROLE BEHAVIOR. Another way of forming impressions relies on unusual or unexpected behavior. For example, some members of the Everest expedition, those with the most experience, signed on as summit climbers. They expected or hoped to make the last stage of the ascent, reaching the very top of the mountain. Others joined as support climbers; with less experience, they agreed to stay at the lower levels, assisting the summit teams. Besides Stacy, clearly a summit aspirant, there were two other women on the expedition. One of them, Peggy Luce, was inexperienced. "I don't mind being a support climber," she said, acknowledging her background. "I just want to go" (Allison, 1993).

Scaling Mount Everest is not a straightforward task. It begins when support climbers and summit climbers establish a large base camp at the bottom of the mountain, followed by four or so intermediate camps partway up the mountain. After the fourth camp has been set, two or three summit climbers attempt to reach the top of the mountain.

Suppose, instead, that one of the support climbers decides to make a sprint for the summit. What would be your impression of this person? You might decide that this person is bold and unruly. Why? The reason is that this response would involve out-of-role behavior. A role is a pattern of behavior associated with a particular position, and *out-of-role behavior* is a response not expected from someone in that position. A support climber should not suddenly ignore agreements and behave instead like a summit climber. If this behavior occurred, it would seem to be a characteristic of that individual.

In one experiment, the subjects listened to a tape in which people sometimes showed the behavior expected of a job applicant and sometimes showed out-of-role behavior, making irrelevant comments and asking inappropriate questions. When these people acted contrary to the expected role, the judges perceived them as showing their true colors (Jones, David, & Jergen, 1961). Not called forth by any obvious aspect of the external situation, out-of-role behavior is assumed to be a function of underlying personal characteristics.

USING STEREOTYPES

A major reason for the interest in attitudes among early social psychologists was their relevance for stereotypes and prejudice. Recently, with greater sensitivity to cultural differences, there has been a resurgence of research interest in these topics (Olson & Zanna, 1993).

The attempt to climb Mount Everest involved two major cultural groups, North Americans and Sherpas. Among the Americans, there were subgroups of summit climbers and support climbers, and they differed in age, experience, and the goal of climbing to the top of the world. Also, there was the research team, distinguished by its academic interests.

The Sherpas, people of Tibetan stock, live on the southern side of the Himalaya Mountains. They are dark-skinned, possess powerful lungs, and demonstrate considerable mountaineering ability. Knowing that Karma was a Sherpa, in fact manager of the Sherpas on this expedition, we might decide that he too was an agile climber.

A view of this sort, based on an oversimplified perception or rigid generalization, is known as a stereotype. In a **stereotype,** certain traits are assigned to an individual simply because that person is a member of a particular social group—an occupational group, race, nationality, or other category of people. According to stereotypes, Italians are passionate; the upper class is snobbish; librarians are prim and proper; and psychologists . . . well . . . er . . . they like to write about stereotypes. In

fact, as the head Sherpa on this expedition, Karma was regarded as overweight, sloppy, and too dedicated to Nepalese beer to be a notable climber (Allison, 1993). He did *not* fit the stereotype.

What characteristics are used in forming stereotypes? Just as you would expect, they are immediately accessible: gender, age, and race. On this basis, one would expect physical appearance to be an important basis for stereotypes, and such is the case (Fiske, 1993).

STEREOTYPES AND PREJUDICE. In addition to stereotypes, our ideas about people are sometimes based on considerable emotion without much thought. This reaction is known as a **prejudice,** which is an attitude, usually negative, toward something or some members of a group, developed without objective evaluation. The topic in question has been prejudged. Like other attitudes, a prejudice has three components—cognitive, affective, and behavioral—but the latter two dominate, especially the affective component. Also, like other attitudes, a prejudice may be formed through modeling, conditioning, and direct instruction. We can be prejudiced for or against people who drink beer, become physicians, or pursue any other lifestyle.

Stereotypes and prejudices differ in at least two related ways. The former are more cognitive, concerned with thinking; the latter are more affective, concerned with feelings. Consequently, and this is the second difference, stereotypes can be relatively neutral; prejudices are essentially positive or negative, usually negative (Hilton & von Hippel, 1996).

STEREOTYPES AS FACILITATING. A great deal has been written about stereotypes, and there has been considerable reluctance among educated people to think in terms of these categories. Nevertheless, we all use them in dealing with people. We make generalizations about adolescents, used-car dealers, scientists, and kings—all from the perspectives of our different subcultures. Without some generalizations, life would be difficult indeed; we would have to start from the zero point in each new situation (Figure 17-4).

The psychologists on the Washington research team, for example, behaved according to occupational stereotypes. They administered questionnaires to climbers at different altitudes, aiming to discover the ways in which oxygen deprivation influenced climbers' memories and judgments about their memories.

If you are to be a host for the weekend, you want to know whether your guest is a child, a guide from the Maine woods, or a city lawyer. Then you plan to bob for apples, serve apple strudel, or visit the Big Apple. These decisions are also based on stereotypes.

Thirty people serving as judges were asked to predict the occupational interests of six strangers. In one instance, the predictions were based on the information that each person was a typical male or female undergraduate at a certain university. In

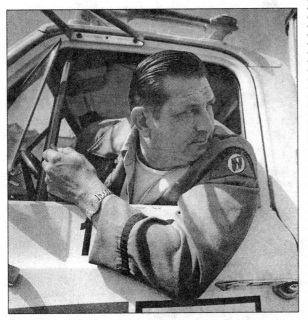

FIGURE 17-4 USING STEREOTYPES.
Make some guesses about this man's favorite activities. Select two: reading fairy tales, watching football games, going to sewing class, playing with his dog. Generalizations about truck drivers *may* aid in first impressions, but the observer must be prepared to revise them on the basis of contrary evidence.

another instance, predictions were made after each stranger appeared separately before the judges and completed simple tasks, such as drawing on the blackboard, building a house of cards, and describing the room. When the two predictions were compared, it was found that those based on the stereotypes were significantly more accurate than those based on observations of each individual's expressive behavior. The clues provided by the behavior were either ignored or misunderstood by the judges (Gage, 1952).

These results suggest that in forming first impressions, knowledge of a stereotype may be superior to brief observation. The crucial factor, of course, is the accuracy of the stereotype. If you are seeking porters and climbers to assist in an Everest expedition, you would be wise to search among the Sherpas.

STEREOTYPES AS DEBILITATING.
Despite the possible advantage of stereotypes in forming first impressions, their limitations must be kept firmly in mind. First, their accuracy may be overrated or unknown. Second, although a stereotype may have some validity for a group of people, the chances are considerably less that it applies to a given individual. Contrary to a popular stereotype, not every psychologist is a bearded fellow with rumpled clothes and a foreign accent. And many are only mildly eccentric. Not all Sherpas are able mountaineers, as Karma demonstrated.

Third, and most important, some stereotypes involve **ethnocentrism,** the belief that other cultures are necessarily odd, immoral, or inferior because they do not share the standards of one's own culture. For many years, people living in the United States described countries with fewer technological developments as backward. The damaging consequences of such a viewpoint need not be elaborated. As a native of one of these countries wryly explained to a missionary, in a popular cartoon: "It's not that my country is underdeveloped but perhaps that yours is overdeveloped."

Furthermore, as stereotypes become increasingly affective, they become prejudices. In *sexism*, for example, one gender is considered inferior to the other, rather than different from it. In *ageism*, it is considered better to be young than old. The elderly are not valued for their experience but rejected for their lack of strength and quickness, both mental and physical. Cultures differ widely in ageism, as is evident in comparisons among China, Nepal, and the United States.

CULTURAL PLURALISM. The term **culture** refers to the totality of beliefs and behavior patterns characteristic of a particular group. These may include language, customs, and religion, as well as age, racial background, and other factors.

The difficulty of cross-cultural understanding is evident in a comparison between common aphorisms in the United States and Japan. One well-known piece of advice in this country states: "The squeaky wheel gets the oil." The Japanese have a different saying: "The nail that stands out gets pounded down." In the collectivist cultures of Eastern societies, individual differences are minimized. In many Western societies, people take pride in being distinguished (Triandis, McCusker, & Hui, 1990). In the United States, people tend to develop an *individual self*, in which personal traits are more important than group memberships. Japanese commonly develop a *relational self*, identifying themselves as group members first and then as individuals.

Cultural differences in the United States are heightened by differences among our ancestors, including Native Americans, African-Americans, and European colonists, as well as the enormous diversity among later immigrants. According to the melting pot theory, it was assumed that features of these subcultures would melt away, becoming assimilated into a new, unique, and homogeneous culture, that of the United States. This outcome has not occurred, partly because people are proud of their heritage and partly because some subcultures were denied ready assimilation into the dominant society. Instead, the new metaphor is a mosaic. The social ideal is *cultural pluralism*, in which differences among subcultures are recognized, accepted, and valued (Figure 17-5).

Faced with this challenge, our society is encouraging **multicultural awareness,** meaning sensitivity to and acceptance of differences among subgroups or subcultures, regarding them as equally viable approaches to human civilization. Multicultural awareness is essentially the opposite of ethnocentrism. As we move toward a global economy, culturally sensitive research becomes essential to the integrity of psychology (Graham, 1992).

As it turned out, awareness of other cultures was inevitable on the south side of Mount Everest

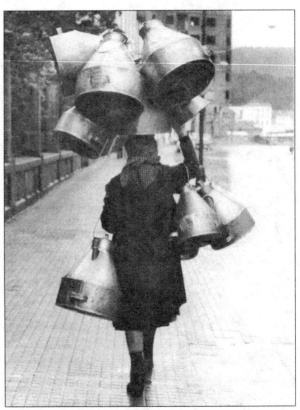

FIGURE 17-5 CULTURAL DIFFERENCES. Necessity is the mother of invention, prompting certain skills in one culture not found in another.

470

during Stacy's second expedition. Groups from several nations sought or built routes to the summit. A team of Koreans cooperated with the Americans. The French became three parties, traveling together but climbing separately. The Czechs and New Zealanders formed a joint team, and the Spaniards struggled to find their place among these diverse groups.

∽

ATTRIBUTION THEORY

The third woman climber on the American expedition was Diana Dailey, a very athletic person in her mid-forties and ever mindful of her fitness. Popular opinion pointed to her as most likely to become the first American woman to reach the peak of Mount Everest. Overflowing with energy, Diana rarely stopped training and spoke in a friendly manner to everyone (Allison, 1993).

How did the other members of the expedition *decide* about her personality? What thought processes did they use? Here we are concerned not with impressions of other people but rather with how they are formed.

The aim of **attribution theory** is to understand how people explain others' and their own behavior. Behavior can be attributed to dispositions within the individual, to factors in the environment, or to both conditions (Kelley, 1967; Zuckerman & Feldman, 1984).

ASSIGNING CAUSES. Let us look at the fact that Diana trained incessantly. The expedition members might have decided that this behavior occurred because she had high standards and was conscientious. In a **dispositional attribution**, the causes of behavior are assigned to traits or dispositions within the individual. Diana behaved that way because she was that way; she was simply and naturally energetic.

Alternatively, her teammates might have decided that she exercised constantly because she

was new to the expedition and uncertain of her place in it. After becoming established, she would be more relaxed. Then, too, perhaps she wanted to be the first American woman to scale Everest, an opportunity that might come her way. In a **situational attribution,** the causes of behavior are assigned to the circumstances, not to the individual.

In making this decision, three factors are influential. The first, consistency, concerns the regularity with which the behavior occurs. If Diana exercised intensely every day, which she did, then we would be inclined to maintain the dispositional attribution. A second factor, consensus, raises the question of whether other people behave the same way. If no other member of the expedition engaged in such extensive exercise, including newcomers, then there is further evidence for the dispositional attribution. And finally, the concern in distinctiveness is whether or not this behavior occurred in other contexts (Kelley, 1967). If Diana trained constantly back in Seattle and elsewhere, even before the expedition became possible for her, then the dispositional attribution would have still further confirmation.

OVERATTRIBUTION EFFECT. It would be nice to say that when the evidence is mixed, people carefully weigh all factors and arrive at a wise decision, but such is not the case. In judging *other people's behavior*, we tend to overestimate the importance of personality characteristics. This tendency to overlook the influence of the situation in judging other people's behavior, and to overemphasize personal traits instead, is sufficiently pervasive in our culture that it has been called the **overattribution effect**—also known as the *fundamental attribution error*. Observing Diana's strenuous efforts at physical conditioning on the mountain, her teammates might have assumed that she had received financial inducements to become the first American woman to climb Mount Everest, that she was trying to impress other climbers, or that she had been threatened with dismissal if she did not do well. As a rule, we do not make these sorts of assumptions because we have not observed the relevant background factors. Rather, we note the individual's behavior and assume that she is invariably that way. We decide that Diana is always highly energetic and conscientious (Table 17–3).

Evidence for the overattribution effect has been obtained in many ways. In one instance, college men were asked to cite the reasons for selecting their major fields of study and for being attracted to their girlfriends. They tended to use slightly more situational explanations, referring to factors outside themselves. They explained: "Investment banking pays well" or "She's affectionate." Quite different attributions were made, however, when they were asked to explain why a *friend* chose a particular major and girlfriend. The reasons here were much in favor of the dispositional attributions, meaning factors within the individual. They cited their friend's need for this or that job or girlfriend (Nisbett, Caputo, Legant, & Mareck, 1973).

In an industrial setting, 36 managers of various businesses evaluated themselves and their employees on the job, and these ratings also gave evidence of the overattribution effect. The managers used more dispositional attributions in explaining their employees' behavior than in evaluating their own performances (Martin & Klimoski, 1990). According to the managers, the employees behaved that way because they *were that way* rather than because of the circumstances.

As always, a caution is necessary, and in this case it concerns the matter of culture. Research has indicated that people from cultures stressing *independence*, such as the United States and England, are more likely to engage in overattribution than are people from cultures stressing *interdependence* and group relations, such as Hong Kong, Japan, and India (Markus & Kitayama, 1991; Smith & Whitehead, 1984). In other words, dispositional attributions are more typical in Western cultures; situation attributions are somewhat more typical in Eastern cultures (Lee, Hallahan, & Herzog, 1996; Miller, 1984b; Schuster, Fosterling, & Weiner, 1989).

SELF-SERVING PERCEPTIONS. Knowing a great deal about their own personal circumstances, people in independent cultures tend to explain *their own* behavior from the opposite perspective. They often attribute their reactions to the circumstances, displaying a situational bias, especially in unfavorable circumstances. In situations of spouse abuse, for example, the aggressors tend to attribute their behavior to external causes. The spouse was irresponsible, unfaithful, or hostile, and the beating was administered for that reason (Overholser & Moll, 1990).

Suppose a new employee criticized his boss and

Concept	Process	Example
Dispositional attribution	Assigning the causes of behavior to the individual	Diana trains constantly because she is that way, always energetic.
Situational attribution	Assigning the causes of behavior to the situation	Diana trains constantly because she is new to the expedition.
Overattribution effect	Underestimating the influence of the situation in judging others' behavior	Diana trains constantly because she is very energetic; there are no significant situational factors.

TABLE 17–3 BASIC CONCEPTS IN ATTRIBUTION THEORY. The overattribution effect occurs when we attend only to the most dominant cues available—in this case, Diana's energetic training efforts.

then was fired. Falling prey to the overattribution effect, he might report that his boss was ignorant, unfair, and dishonest. Similarly, falling prey to the self-serving bias concerning his own behavior, he would likely explain that his criticism of his boss was called forth by the circumstances. He probably would not conclude that he was an argumentative, fault-finding individual, as might his coworkers.

When husbands and wives estimated how much each of them contributed to several household chores, the combined totals for each pair usually exceeded 100% because the partners overestimated their own contributions. They were not around when the spouse took out the trash, cleaned out the closet, and worked out the budget. They knew very well when they did these tasks themselves (Ross & Sicoly, 1979). This response is not an attribution bias, for the concern is not with the causes of someone's behavior. Rather, it has been called an *egocentric bias,* showing once again that we have our own self-centered perceptions about the trash, the closets, the budgets, and other details of this world.

• INTERPERSONAL ATTRACTION •

With this background in attitudes and social cognition, we now consider our preferences for living and working with certain people, a condition called **interpersonal attraction.** Among the diverse members of the Everest expedition, who might be attracted to whom? What factors might be involved in these preferences? How do they operate?

FACTORS IN ATTRACTION

On a cold, dark, windswept mountain, most of us would be at least mildly attracted to a strong, experienced mountaineer, but in more routine circum-stances other factors are prominent. We generally seek health, beauty, wisdom, and wit; they are obvious determinants of attraction. We cannot always have what we want, however, and with this reservation in mind, there are two basic determinants of attraction: similarity and familiarity.

DEGREE OF SIMILARITY. When a large, outspoken woman marries a small, quiet man, people say, "Opposites attract!" Here we encounter a commonsense view that does not make sense. It usually ignores many basic similarities between the partners. Indeed, the members of this couple probably speak the same language, have a similar level of intelligence, and share ideas about ethics, religion, and politics. If they are going to continue to be compatible, they should have similar ideas about handling money and avocational interests, as well. They may even have a common concern about physical size, each finding some consolation in the other's dimensions. When one considers all the marriages and friendships one knows, and all possible dimensions of individual differences, it is clear that opposites do *not* attract.

A fun-loving but slightly anxious man may enjoy the company of a confident but reserved woman. The expression about opposites attracting perhaps notes some exceptions, or it refers to less important characteristics. If not, there would be many more marriages and friendships between elderly, sophisticated intellectuals and youthful, uneducated peasants from other cultures.

According to the **matching hypothesis,** the members of a couple are usually about equal in physical attractiveness, whatever their individual standards of beauty. This hypothesis has been supported in research with both dating and married couples (Wong, McCreary, Bowden, & Jenner, 1991). In one study, the photographs of members of 99 married couples were rated individually for physical attractiveness by a panel of judges. Then the two scores for each couple were compared. Afterward, the photographs for each sex were mixed and then paired on a random basis, creating 99 randomly matched couples from the same photographs. When the ratings for these randomly paired couples were compared, they showed much less similarity than the ratings for the married couples. The marital partners were also more similar in other ways, apart from appearance (Murstein, 1972).

If the members are not approximately equal in attractiveness, then the less attractive person usually offers some compensating quality. This trade-off, discussed previously in the context of equity theory, states that in the marketplace of interpersonal relations we develop and maintain a relationship only if the outcome is at least what we feel we deserve, weighing all of our attributes against the norms of society.

Members of a couple also tend to be similar in intelligence. Highly intelligent and marginally intelligent people generally do not seek one another's company. Common interests also play a vital role. All told, it is likely that in any marriage, friendship, or even social gathering, there are many more important similarities than differences in attitudes, interests, and abilities (Figure 17–6).

On the lower slopes of Everest, the expedition scientists—psychologists and physiologists—tended to associate with one another, just as the mutual interests of the climbers, struggling to extend a route up the mountain, caused them to be attracted to one another. Although rivals in one sense, Stacy and Diana maintained a closer relationship with each other than they did with the scientists.

DEGREE OF FAMILIARITY. Our preference for certain people is indisputably related to another major factor: familiarity. Among occupants of an apartment complex, for example, a pronounced relationship was found between friendship patterns and distances between apartments, even when the distances were no more than ten yards (Festinger, Schachter, & Back, 1950). In other words, presence makes the heart grow fonder, despite Shakespeare's famous line about absence.

In modern society, familiarity is not necessarily a function of proximity. With the telephone, magazines, videos, and television, familiarity can be gained even at a distance. To improve their chances for election, political candidates seek almost any sort of exposure. There is so much evidence that attraction increases with familiarity that this finding has been called a general law of human behavior. If you want someone to like you, hang around as much as possible. It should help.

In one instance, a mixed list of the names of 200 public people and 40 nonexistent people were rated on a like–dislike scale, and a marked direct relationship was discovered between the familiarity of the figure and the favorability of the ratings (Harrison, 1969). In another instance, the mere anticipation of familiarity increased liking for another person. College students in this study met in groups,

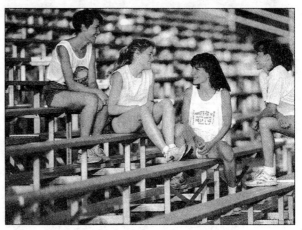

FIGURE 17–6 SIMILARITY AND ATTRACTION. Your friends generally share your interests, as well as your intelligence, age, and background. Similarity is an extremely powerful factor in interpersonal attraction.

expecting to work afterward with some students and not with others. Although exposure was equal, the ratings for likability of anticipated partners were significantly higher than those for anticipated nonpartners (Darley & Berscheid, 1967).

This general law extends even to events and ideas. People exposed frequently to certain passages of music liked those passages more than others to which they had been exposed less frequently (Zissman & Neimark, 1990). College students exposed to situations requiring negotiations rated the most familiar situations as most likely to be settled by agreement (Druckman & Broome, 1991).

It has been said that women fall in love by way of their ears and men by way of their eyes. By whatever means, we usually fall in love with our neighbors, or at least with people we know well.

LONG-TERM RELATIONSHIPS

Similarity and familiarity are vital factors in attraction. In long-term relationships, other factors become prominent, especially psychological characteristics. Styles of loving were discussed in the chapter on emotion; the focus here is on the continuation and dissolution of relationships.

SELF-DISCLOSURE IN THE RELATIONSHIP. In a two-person, loving relationship, the passionate dimension declines relatively early, as noted already, often replaced by other forms of love, most notably companionate love. What fosters this development? One critical issue is successful communication. It is often the foundation of a long-term relationship (Brehm, 1992).

Within this communication, self-disclosure is perhaps the foremost issue. When people communicate intimate thoughts, desires, and memories about themselves, the process is called **self-disclosure.** Efforts to study self-dis-

closure constitute a prominent research theme in current studies of interpersonal relationships (Kelley, 1991).

One of the major findings is the *reciprocity* in self-disclosure. The amount of information disclosed *to* a friend, colleague, parent, or partner is closely related to the amount of information disclosed *by* that person. As one person makes disclosures, the other is prompted to react similarly. This process strengthens their familiarity with one another, a fundamental dimension of attraction (Miller, 1990; Figure 17-7).

Timing is important. Self-disclosure will not invariably strengthen a relationship. Especially at the outset, a person engaging in much self-disclosure may appear lacking in discretion and thereby disrupt the developing friendship (Levin & Gergen, 1969). The longer the relationship exists, and the more it is based on significant mutual events rather than trivial ones, the more likely it is that self-disclosure will strengthen the personal bond.

"I wasn't the easiest woman to get to know," Stacy said of herself. Eventually she met a man named David Shute; he made it easier. "He moved slowly," she said of their conversations, "and waited for me to catch up." Then she added, referring to self-disclosure: "Sometimes it took a while for me to get up the courage to round the corner, but

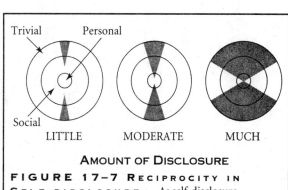

AMOUNT OF DISCLOSURE

FIGURE 17-7 RECIPROCITY IN SELF-DISCLOSURE. As self-disclosure continues, it increases in depth and breadth. In reciprocal fashion, each partner stimulates the other to react in this way (Adapted from Brehm, 1992).

successful, the person must become emotionally responsive and engage in self-disclosure (Betz & Fitzgerald, 1993).

This masculine resistance to therapy is especially significant because masculinity is hazardous to health. Under conditions of stress, the socialization of men tends to restrict their responses to consuming drugs, driving rapidly, acting aggressively, and other self-destructive behaviors. Greater readiness to engage in a therapeutic relationship presumably would reduce these physical and psychological risks (Eisler & Blalock, 1991).

Men and women traditionally develop self-esteem in different ways. Men commonly do so through competition, outdoing their peers. Women more often obtain self-esteem through personal relations (Joseph, Markus, & Tafarodi, 1992). But conditions are changing. Stacy prided herself on building her own home, and she clearly gained self-esteem from her success in mountaineering. Gender differences in gaining esteem are rapidly diminishing in many parts of the United States (Fried-Buchalter, 1992; Sancho & Hewitt, 1990).

Gender differences should not be expected to disappear, however. Gender is the most basic of all human categories (Banaji & Prentice, 1994).

• SOCIAL INFLUENCE •

At this point, we should be explicit about the transition taking place in this chapter. We have been moving steadily away from the individual toward people in interaction. Our earlier emphases were on attitudes, social cognition, and interpersonal attraction—how people think about and perceive others. The forthcoming emphases are on social influence and group processes—how people interact with one another in a group setting.

Interactions among members of the Everest team changed markedly after the four inter-mediate camps had been set, for then it was time for the big push to the summit, a dangerous trek in that rarefied air. Only two or three members could climb together, and Jim, as leader, selected these smaller summit teams. He chose Steve and Stacy to accompany him on the first team, much to their irrepressible joy. Diana did not hide her displeasure over her assignment to the second team. Geoff was one of a pair of climbers on the third. Except for the first team and Peggy, who knew she belonged on the fourth team, these results were a widespread source of dissatisfaction. As Stacy acknowledged, "Any leader who puts himself on the first summit team, no matter the circumstances, is bound to face criticisms" (Allison, 1993).

The term **social influence** refers to the ways in which people modify one another's behavior or experience, intentionally or otherwise. These actions range from the unspoken expectations of group membership to an explicit request from an individual. Jim's assignment of climbers to summit teams resulted in reluctant compliance by those involved, an instance of very direct social influence.

TENDENCY TO CONFORM

In established groups, there is agreement on many behaviors, such as patterns of dress, speech, religious outlook, sexual behavior, and so forth. Even in spontaneously formed groups, this agreement is evident and the pressure toward conformity can be significant. In **conformity,** an individual adopts the thoughts or behaviors of a social group *without* any direct pressure to do so.

On the Everest expedition, a plastic pink flamingo was used to mark the entry of the meeting area at base camp, perhaps because it provided such a clear contrast to its surroundings. Moreover, all members of the American party carried a tiny toy flamingo in their packs. This trinket served no

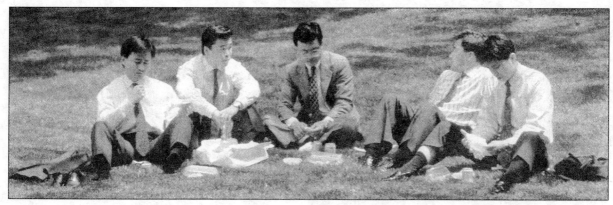

FIGURE 17–8 CONFORMITY IN DAILY LIFE. Acceptance by others is a fundamental goal at all ages. It is achieved partly by adherence to group customs and interests.

obvious purpose. No one was explicitly asked to carry it; the members did so spontaneously. In these ways, they displayed conformity. They voluntarily adopted an implicit social code (Figure 17-8).

Conformity is influenced by **social norms,** which are unstated expectations indicating what social behavior is usual or typical. People generally do not wish to violate a norm or standard, even when there is no direct pressure to behave like others.

In a series of experiments some years ago, conducted by a social psychologist, Solomon Asch, American college students were asked to make judgments about the length of vertical lines. Seven men made these simple judgments aloud, one by one, in a group setting, but the sixth person in the sequence was the only true subject. The other people were Asch's accomplices and, without the true subject's knowledge, on many trials they all intentionally made the same incorrect guess. Perhaps for the first time in his life, the true subject suddenly found the evidence from his senses contradicted by the unanimous opinion of the majority (Figure 17–9).

The results were impressive. Even in this simple task, only about one-fourth of the subjects completely resisted the others' answers, making no errors, and they remained doubt-ridden throughout the investigation. Among those who yielded, some were influenced occasionally. Others followed the unanimous but incorrect opinion on every trial, showing complete acquiescence to group pressure. Later, it was found that they grossly underestimated their degree of conformity (Asch, 1956).

Experiments with French and Norwegian subjects supported these findings, although the two groups performed somewhat differently. Subsequent studies showed these same results among Arabian and British students. On these bases, the powerful influence of a unanimous group on the behavior of an individual, resulting in conformity, is now known as the *Asch effect.* Some mixed results have appeared in recent years, perhaps owing to social change, making the Asch effect a topic of continued interest in contemporary psychology (Amir, 1984; Friend, Rafferty, & Bramel, 1990; Larsen, 1990).

These results should not suggest that conformity is undesirable. Think of the impossibility of maintaining any social group if people did not conform to certain standards. Nonconformity, furthermore, does not necessarily indicate independence. Some people adopt the contrary view regardless of the issue. They are called *counterdependent* because their views are determined by the norm, although in the opposite direction.

Uncertainty may play a role in a special type of conformity. In a crowd or mob scene, people sometimes lose their sense of individual responsibility,

478

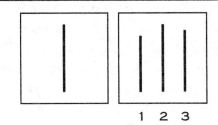

FIGURE 17–9 CONFORMITY IN THE LABORATORY. The task was to match the single line on the left with the line of the same length from the card at the right, some distance away.

engaging in behaviors they would otherwise resist, a condition called **deindividuation**. The focus instead is on the present environment, as in mass looting or taunting or even physical aggression. The group setting offers anonymity, and deindividuated people may act in uncharacteristically hostile ways, quite different from their usual behavior.

☙

COMPLIANCE AND OBEDIENCE

As we turn now to compliance and obedience, the social influence changes. It is no longer unintentional. It is direct and purposeful. In **compliance,** people yield to pressure to think or behave in a certain way, responding to a direct request by someone else. One party does not have complete authority over the other, however. The relationship involves negotiation or persuasion.

When the three Americans on the first summit team began their trek toward the top of the world, Pasang Timba, the most experienced of three Sherpas, climbed with them. Two assistants, Appa and Pemba, each carrying an extra bottle of oxygen, brought up the rear, some 100 yards behind. But as the ascent continued across steep terrain, the gap grew larger and larger. Then, for the third or fourth time, Jim stopped to wait for them and, as he peered through the morning darkness, a stream of profanity erupted from his lips: Appa and Pemba

were *descending* the mountain. They had turned around; they were traveling down steadily and quickly, not like injured men, who would have moved more slowly. Money was no longer an issue; they were interested in safety (Allison, 1993).

For Appa and Pemba, compliance was out of the question. And the situation did not involve obedience, for Jim had no physical, legal, or even substantial financial control over them. So the three Americans watched most of their oxygen disappear down the mountainside.

This issue of compliance commonly occurs in small groups or one-to-one relationships, as between spouses, a salesperson and a potential customer, or among friends. In these situations, pressure toward compliance is often exerted in one of two ways, each with a sales-pitch emphasis: the foot-in-the-door and door-in-the face techniques.

OBTAINING COMPLIANCE. The idea behind the **foot-in-the-door technique** is that after complying with a smaller request, a person is more likely to comply with a larger one. The first step is to get your foot in the door—*then* ask for more.

In one study, homemakers were requested to support safe driving by signing a petition or placing a small sign in a window of their home. That was the small beginning. After two weeks, a different investigator asked all subjects to place a large, attention-getting sign on their lawns. As expected, compliance with this almost unreasonable request was related to prior compliance. Among householders who had agreed to the smaller request, 55% agreed to display the new sign. Among a control group, who had not been approached previously, only 20% agreed to do so (Freedman & Fraser, 1966).

After complying with the first request, people apparently regard themselves as "doing that sort of thing." Thus they continue, complying with the next request (Wagener & Laird, 1980).

A different technique begins with an unreasonably large request. Called the **door-in-the-face** technique, the person is confronted with a request that almost certainly will be refused; then, when the second and real request is made, the likelihood of acceptance is increased. When college students were asked to donate two hours per week for two years working with juvenile delinquents, none agreed to do so. But afterward, approximately 50% were willing to take juvenile delinquents to the zoo one afternoon for two hours. Among students who were asked merely to accompany juvenile delinquents to the zoo, only 17% complied (Cialdini, Vincent, Lewis, Catalan, Wheeler, & Danby, 1975).

Here again, speculation follows self-perception theory. The subjects who refused the first request perhaps viewed themselves as uncooperative and uncongenial. Thus, they complied more readily with the second opportunity, redeeming themselves and enhancing their self-image (Cialdini, 1993).

OBEDIENCE TO AUTHORITY. Obedience involves even more direct pressure than compliance. In **obedience,** people respond to a demand, not a request, and the conditions of the relationship are not negotiable. The power, through physical strength or circumstances, lies with one party, and the other is expected to be submissive and dutiful. The relationship between a salesperson and a customer raises the issue of compliance; the relationship between a boss and the salesperson involves obedience (Table 17–4).

One investigation of obedience became known as the *Milgram study,* owing to its controversial nature and the name of the chief investigator, Stanley Milgram. As explained in the chapter on research methods, each subject, serving as a teacher, was required to punish a learner's incorrect responses by administering electric shocks to that person. The learner made errors regularly, and the research question was: How much shock would the subject administer before refusing to follow the experimenter's requests?

When this experiment was completed with 40 subjects, the results were totally unexpected. Altogether, 65% of the subjects obeyed *all* of the experimenter's orders, punishing the learner with 450 volts, the maximum shock available. They did so even when the learner no longer responded to the task and therefore was being punished for doing nothing. In the remaining cases, the experiment was discontinued when the subject refused to administer a stronger shock, but *no one* refrained from administering 300 volts, labeled "intense shock," at which point the learner pounded on the wall and then became silent (Figure 17–10).

The learner, an accomplice of the experimenter, never received any shocks at all. He simply disconnected the generator.

Further studies with different subjects in different settings gave the same result, demonstrating the overwhelming significance of the social setting.

TYPE	DESCRIPTION	EXAMPLE
Conformity	Without direct pressure, people adopt the behavior or thoughts of others; there is no coercion.	All Everest expedition members carried a toy pink flamingo in their packs.
Compliance	In response to a direct request, people behave in a certain way; the conditions may be negotiable.	Appa and Pemba climbed with the first summit team, until they changed their minds.
Obedience	People respond to an order or command in the expected way; the conditions are not negotiable.	Expedition members followed Jim's order, building the lower route before making summit attempts.

TABLE 17–4 TYPES OF SOCIAL INFLUENCE. Social influence results in a range of specific responses. Conformity, compliance, and obedience are the most prominent outcomes.

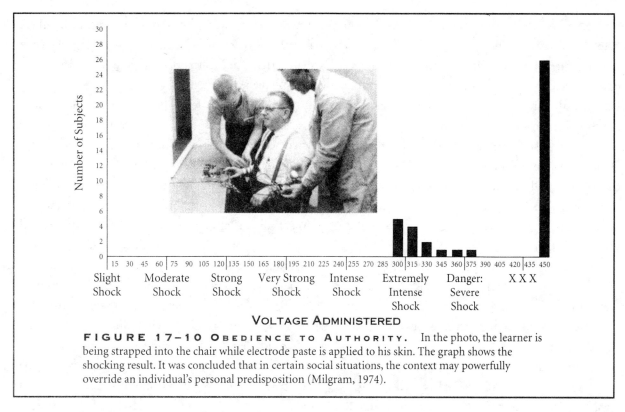

FIGURE 17–10 OBEDIENCE TO AUTHORITY. In the photo, the learner is being strapped into the chair while electrode paste is applied to his skin. The graph shows the shocking result. It was concluded that in certain social situations, the context may powerfully override an individual's personal predisposition (Milgram, 1974).

According to Milgram, the setting was *the* crucial factor in determining obedience (Milgram, 1974). Social pressure can be more influential than character and personality in determining behavior in certain situations (Blass, 1991). Looking back on this research, Milgram pointed out that people in daily life often must obey orders about which they have some doubt. The physician requests a certain medicine; a lieutenant orders a certain training procedure. The person receiving such an order typically obeys, but there may be moments when doubt or opposition should be expressed.

After the Everest expedition established camps high on the mountain, Jim asked Geoff to examine the eyes of each climber, searching for retinal hemorrhaging, often a symptom of more serious problems caused by high altitude. Then Jim said: "Don't tell anyone the results." Geoff resisted this order. He decided that his teammates deserved to know about the condition of their own bodies. Eventually Jim withdrew his order, but news of his plan swept through the camp, causing distrust and dis-

sension among the members. Geoff was lauded for his refusal to obey.

∾

ALTRUISTIC BEHAVIOR

Pasang and the three Americans struggled upward for two more hours, until the first morning light revealed their progress and the distance from the summit. At that point, Jim calculated their remaining oxygen and dejectedly shook his head. With a tone of finality, he announced: "That's it, then. We go back and try again tomorrow."

Stacy resisted. Noting the perfect weather, thinking of their enormous efforts, and well aware of commitments to other team members and people back home, she opposed the idea.

"Look," she insisted, gesturing to the clear skies. "One of us should go."

Steve immediately agreed, and then Jim did too. Thus, at that point, opportunities for altruism were open to all three climbers.

In the behavior known as **altruism,** for no obvi-

481

ous reward someone assists another person needing help. Altruism is a selfless act, a sacrifice for the welfare of others. Each of the climbers could have suggested that one of the others be allowed to achieve the goal all three of them so deeply desired. But none of them displayed this altruism.

Instead, Jim turned to Pasang and said, "Choose a number between one and ten." Pasang did so, not fully understanding the purpose, and the three American climbers guessed. Stacy announced, "Four." The number was *three*, and she was the winner.

Accepting this outcome and looking at the oxygen supply, Jim then said to Pasang: "You can come down with us if you want to."

"No," replied Pasang, perhaps displaying altruism. "I go up."

"You'll run out of oxygen," Jim countered.

"I go up," repeated Pasang, knowing his stronger lungs could function with distinctly less oxygen than that required by the Americans. Nevertheless, he was clearly placing himself in danger (Allison, 1993).

Altruism has long interested philosophers and scientists, for it appears to be a sacrificial act, performed as an end in itself, without any obvious gain to the helper. From an evolutionary perspective, this behavior promotes the species' genes. From a psychological perspective, altruism may satisfy personal motives. For many observers, therefore, the concept of altruism still lacks substantial evidence (Krebs, 1991; Sorrentino, 1991).

TEMPORARY STATES. In one early study, students in divinity school walked alone through a back alley, passing a slumping figure in a doorway. Shabbily dressed, he coughed and groaned as each student opened the door to the building. Some of the students were on their way to give a brief talk about the Good Samaritan, a tale of a good deed. Others were planning to speak on careers after divinity school. Some in each group were in a hurry; others were just about on time; still others had time to spare. Of all these people, less than half offered aid to the person slumped in the doorway. Which ones were they?

Those who offered help were not necessarily the students with the Good Samaritan in mind, and they were not those thinking about careers after graduation. The students most likely to help were those with a few minutes to spare. Those least likely to stop were in great haste. In later interviews, it was found that the hurried subjects experienced some emotional upset after their encounter in the alleyway, but to stop and help would have meant a delay in proceedings that other people had carefully arranged. Another loyalty, rather than insensitivity, seemed responsible for their failure to offer assistance (Darley & Batson, 1973).

Behavior is complex, however, and having time to spare is not the only facilitating state. Being in a good mood is also important (Isen & Levin, 1972).

SITUATIONAL FACTORS. In addition, situational factors can be influential. These findings have emerged from research studies and real-life incidents in which people have observed muggings or property damage without making any effort to assist. Collectively, they point to a **bystander intervention effect,** which states that the larger the group observing someone apparently needing help, the less likely it is that any one of them will offer aid. A lone bystander is more apt to help.

When several people are present, there is a perceived *diffusion of responsibility,* in which each bystander may decide that action can be taken or should be taken by others. For example, when college students overheard someone having an epileptic seizure, their efforts to help were decidedly slower and less frequent when they believed that another person also heard the victim's cries, although neither the victim nor anyone else was in sight. The innocent bystander apparently feels much more innocent when others are present too.

When a bystander is alone, the feeling of personal responsibility makes the person more likely to assist (Latané & Darley, 1968; Latané & Nida, 1981).

Another reason for lack of assistance is that among a crowd the situation sometimes is not regarded as an emergency. The result is *pluralistic ignorance*, in which many observers, well aware of one another but not fully understanding the situation, wait for someone else to make an interpretation. They think that the situation might be a prank or that the person can manage without assistance (Krebs, 1970).

Still another situational factor is the amount of *personal risk* to the helper. People are less inclined to intervene when they may incur harm themselves. In other words, the nature of the commitment is clearly a factor (Clary & Orenstein, 1991).

Whether people help depends significantly on how these situational factors interact with their temporary states at the time. What influenced Pasang on that desolate ridge of Mount Everest? Maybe it was the financial gain for assisting Stacy to the very top. Maybe it was his mood at the moment or a desire to reach the summit himself. Maybe it was all of those factors. And maybe it included altruism.

PERSONALITY FACTORS. We cannot dismiss personality completely. Other things being equal, some people are more likely to help than others. What can be said about these people?

In a field study of altruism, 34 people who had assisted victims of traffic accidents were assessed for personality. They were compared with 36 witnesses of accidents who had not provided assistance. The two groups were matched for age, sex, and socioeconomic status, and both groups completed a personality questionnaire. Compared to the witnesses, the altruistic subjects had a stronger belief in a just world, more concern for social responsibility, and greater empathy (Bierhoff, Klein,

& Kramp, 1991). They did not differ with respect to competence in administering first aid.

In summary, we can say that there seem to be few consistently all-around Good Samaritans among us (Gergen, Gergen, & Meter, 1972). Situational factors and temporary personal states play an important role in this behavior, but personal traits cannot be totally discounted (Bierhoff, Klein, & Kramp, 1991; Rushton, 1991).

• GROUP PROCESSES •

In social psychology, a **group** is two or more individuals who are united by some common characteristic and whose actions are interrelated. This relationship can be temporary and incidental, as strangers in an elevator, or relatively enduring and fundamental, as family members. Stacy and Pasang, standing high on that cold, steep mountain, were clearly a group, for they had climbed together, shared nourishment, and called out advice to one another.

Far below them, the University of Washington research team formed a very different group with different goals. They confronted this question: If climbers' memories are faulty at high altitudes, do the climbers know it? Are they aware of their deficits? Knowledge about one's knowledge, called *metacognition*, has vital implications throughout our lives, especially on mountain tops and in other dangerous situations (Nelson Dunlosky, White, Steinberg, Townes & Anderson, 1990). We now look more closely at the interactions among members of groups, referred to as group processes.

STATUS IN THE GROUP

In any group, each member has a **role,** which is a pattern of behavior expected of that member. A role typically is associated with a certain **status,** which is the respect or standing one has among the group members. On an Everest expedition, support climbers have the least experience, and therefore they are low in the hierarchy. The climber with the most experience is usually the expedition leader, at the top of the hierarchy.

Within a group, a person may have more than one role, and these roles may be formal or informal. In addtion, roles are often complementary. The role of a mother is defined with respect to the child. A team member has no role without other team members.

In the animal world, status and role seem to be functions of power, a condition called to scientific attention years ago by a Norwegian investigator who observed barnyard chickens. The most dominant chicken pecked all others and was pecked by none in return. Another chicken pecked all others except the most dominant one, which of course pecked it. This social order extended down to the bottom of the hierarchy, where one chicken was pecked by every other chicken and pecked none in return. This dominance hierarchy among members of a group, known as a **pecking order,** has been verified in many modern studies (Schjelderup-Ebbe, 1935). Research with mice, dogs, monkeys, and many other species shows dominance relations based on fighting, but the perfect, straight-line dominance seen in chickens is rare.

Usually a person's status is based on something other than physical domination, such as money, knowledge, social skills, verbal ability, or the interaction of many such characteristics.

Studies of two-person and three-person groups have shown that a dominance hierarchy begins to develop just seconds after strangers meet, evident in talking the most, successfully interrupting others, avoiding interruptions by others, receiving glances from others, and gesticulating in a dominant manner. Subtle nonverbal signals, such as the other person's appearance and level of activation, apparently serve as early cues for the assess-

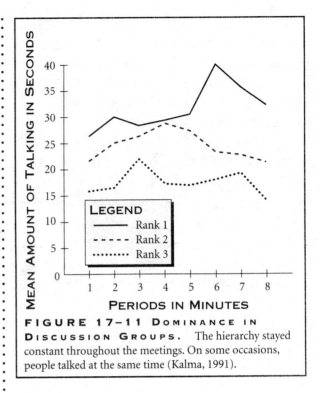

FIGURE 17–11 DOMINANCE IN DISCUSSION GROUPS. The hierarchy stayed constant throughout the meetings. On some occasions, people talked at the same time (Kalma, 1991).

ment of dominance in these discussions (Kalma, 1991; Figure 17-11).

On the basis of physical ability and knowledge of mountaineering, Stacy had moved to the top of the hierarchy of the Everest expedition, selected for the first summit team. Then, through luck in the lottery, she won first place on that summit team. And finally, through sheer determination, she and Pasang clambered across one icy wall after another, ridge upon ridge, until they reached a place where there was nowhere else to climb. They stood on the top of the world.

"We really did it," Stacy cried into the wind, which immediately swept her hat from her head. As she watched it sail down thousands of feet into Tibet, her eyes became hot and cloudy. She *was* the first American woman to climb Mount Everest, and she felt a blinding wave of emotion (Allison, 1993).

Pasang pumped his ice axe overhead, hooting and exulting with whatever air he had left in his lungs. After all, he was the first man, Sherpa or otherwise, to accompany an American woman to the peak of Chomolungma! And he did so without supplementary oxygen. Besides, Stacy might recognize his heroic effort with a very large tip.

~

COOPERATION
AND COMPETITION

As a rule, a group setting engenders a higher degree of responsiveness to a particular task than when the same individuals are alone, an outcome known as **social facilitation.** The necessary condition for social facilitation is the presence of someone else, or several people (Levine, Resnick, & Higgins, 1993). This increased activity—in working or eating or whatever—occurs even among animals, and the reason apparently lies in the increased arousal of the individual in the presence of others. Among human beings, for example, there is a strong positive correlation between the number of people present and the size of the meal consumed by each person (de Castro, 1991; Redd & de Castro, 1992).

When people are working in groups and told that their output will not be compared, the facilitating effect fails to appear. When they are working individually and told that they will be compared with others working in separate rooms, their performance is comparable to that in the group situation. Experiments of this sort, dating from the earliest days of social psychology, suggest that social facilitation is the result of some sort of rivalry or competitive effort, or perhaps simply an effort to keep pace rather than to outdo others (Dashiell, 1935; Levine, Resnick, & Higgins, 1993).

Human behavior is highly complex, however, and therefore we occasionally find almost the opposite response. People in groups sometimes engage in **social loafing,** expending less energy and producing less in the group than when by themselves.

In fact, the output of the individual seems to decrease in proportion to the size of the group (Geen, 1991; Levine, Resnick, & Higgins, 1993).

What causes this change in behavior or prompts such different behaviors in a group? The critical factor is *recognition.* If an individual's specific contribution probably will be noted or acknowledged, social facilitation is likely. Otherwise, social loafing will occur (Gabrenya, Wang, & Latané, 1985; Hardy & Latané, 1986).

Most group situations engender some form of striving to do well, with or against other group members. On Everest, all of the American summit teams were striving to reach the top of the mountain. Stacy and Diana vied to become the first American woman. And the international teams were competing for access to the lower routes or to win a "first" on the summit in some new category. One daredevil Frenchman wanted to become the first person to jump *off* Mount Everest, using a contraption that was partly a parachute, partly a hang glider. Another wanted to be the fastest person *on* the mountain, hoping to set a world speed record, climbing without supplemental oxygen.

Here we ask: What factors typically determine whether individuals or groups, striving to perform well, will become cooperative or competitive?

CHILDREARING PRACTICES. In daily life, two factors stand out as engendering cooperation or competition, one of which is childhood training. Earlier, we noted that cultural practices can mold aggressive or cooperative patterns.

In the United States, childrearing generally fosters competition and individuality, especially in school systems that stress high achievement. In certain other cultures, such as those of China and Israel, different habits are emphasized, and the child's identity is more involved with the group of which he or she is a member. Young children are taught to clean the table together or to calculate the

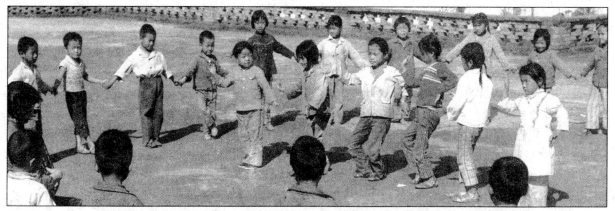

FIGURE 17–12 EDUCATION FOR COOPERATIVE BEHAVIOR. For children in elementary school in China, cooperating with classmates may be even more important than grades on examinations (Filstrup & Filstrup, 1983).

classroom budget together, an approach that fosters cooperative attitudes and behavior (Figure 17–12).

SUPERORDINATE GOALS. The second basic factor engendering cooperation or competition pertains to the setting, as illustrated in an investigation known as the *Robbers' Cave experiment,* so named for the state park in Oklahoma where it was conducted. At a summer camp, 12-year-old boys who did not know one another previously were separated into two groups. A tournament of games was then arranged between the two groups: touch football, tug of war, baseball, and a treasure hunt, and eventually what commenced as good sportsmanship became extremely rivalrous. The opposing groups began name calling, planned raids on opponents' territory, destroyed property, and engaged in scuffles.

The experimenters then attempted to change this situation, testing the hypothesis that pleasant social contacts would reduce the friction. When these contacts were provided, the procedure was sometimes successful, but at other times it merely provided greater opportunities for conflict. In the dining hall, individuals from the two groups shoved and pushed one another, called each other names, and threw food and utensils.

A second hypothesis was then tested. The experimenters created a series of problems producing **superordinate goals,** which are goals shared by all community members and having a higher priority than any others. Solutions would benefit both groups, but neither group could achieve them alone. A break in the water supply required close inspection of the terrain for one mile, and a breakdown in the truck that was to take both groups on a picnic required that everyone pull together on the same rope used previously in the tug of war. Eventually, new relationships developed to the point at which the boys sought opportunities to mingle with the other group, had best friends there, held a joint campfire, and went home together (Sherif, 1956).

It was more than proximity that reduced the tension; it was working together toward overriding goals, important to all concerned. Responding to an *outside* threat can make an enormous difference in overcoming rivalries.

Jim, as leader of the Everest expedition, made a concerted effort to establish *group* goals. Before leaving the United States, all expedition members agreed that no one would make a spontaneous summit bid, attempting a dash to the peak without regard for other members. The aim for all climbers and all backers in Seattle would be for the *expedition* to reach the summit. Stacy stressed this condition

486

in her detailed account of this adventure, *Beyond the Limits* (Allison, 1993).

A META-ANALYSIS. One group of psychologists decided to review all of this research on cooperation and competition by a procedure called meta-analysis. The aim of **meta-analysis** is not to contribute further empirical research but rather to examine carefully a large number of completed investigations, comparing their findings and thereby drawing some overall conclusion about the preponderance of evidence. In other words, meta-analysis is a technique for summarizing the results from many studies, viewing them as a population of subjects or items to be combined and analyzed (Lipsey & Wilson, 1993).

In this case, the meta-analysis was performed on the outcomes of research on cooperative, competitive, and individual efforts in groups. Altogether, 122 studies were compared, involving almost 300 separate findings. The results showed that cooperation is significantly more effective than competition or individual efforts in promoting achievement and productivity (Johnson, Maruyama, Johnson, Nelson, & Skon, 1981).

∾

MAKING DECISIONS

Eventually all groups with any sort of cohesion must make at least two fundamental decisions, explicitly or implicitly. A goal must be established—whether it is purely social, work-oriented, or both—and some means of pursuing that goal must be identified.

How do groups reach these decisions? What are the processes? In a dictatorship or other autocracy, these decisions are made by the leader, benevolent or malevolent. The group members do not participate; there is little group process. The following discussion concerns open, democratic groups, ones that encourage an exchange of ideas.

GROUPTHINK. An obviously critical factor in any group decision is the cohesiveness of the group—the extent to which it functions *as a group.* The stronger such ties among members, the more readily group decisions are reached, but sometimes agreement is reached too easily.

We cannot be certain what occurred among the members of the Czech summit team, but they reached a tragic decision. After three days seeking the summit, all without food, they decided to keep moving upward, rather than descend. By the fourth morning, Dusan and Jaroslav were losing their vision; Peter was dehydrated and starved; Josef was fatigued. Then, as darkness fell, a storm ripped the top of the mountain. The next day, the Czechs had vanished, presumably blown off the face of Chomolungma by the 150-mile-per-hour winds.

Perhaps the desire for group cohesion stifled individual challenges and critical thought. Perhaps the capacity to think had been diminished by the altitude, as suggested by the findings of the University of Washington research team. At higher and higher altitudes, with less and less oxygen, climbers become increasingly less certain about their intellectual capacities.

When all group members are reluctant to criticize or challenge one another, the group decision may not be the most effective response. The concept of **groupthink** occurs when a group places such a high value on cohesion and morale that decision-making ability is limited; the members suspend critical thinking to maintain group morale (Park, 1990).

Consider these presidential decisions in the last thirty years: Kennedy supported the disastrous invasion of Cuba at the Bay of Pigs; Johnson escalated the war in Vietnam; and Nixon and his advisors, when the Watergate break-in was discovered, attempted a cover-up. All of these decisions, according to the groupthink concept, arose because the effort to maintain group cohesion outstripped the concern for reaching a sound decision (Janis,

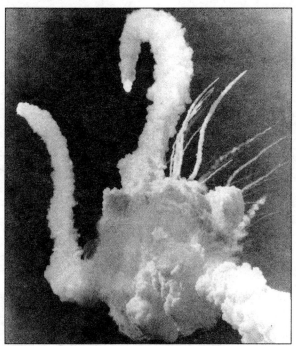

FIGURE 17–13 CONSEQUENCES OF GROUPTHINK. The Challenger explosion offers an example of the dangers of groupthink. In January 1986, a space engineer advised against the flight owing to hazards of subfreezing temperatures. To prevent groupthink outcomes, selected group members are sometimes assigned to play the role of gadfly or devil's advocate.

1982). Even in the Challenger explosion, one member of the group declared that the spaceship should not be launched. In the context of group solidarity and a certain leadership style, this sole dissenter was ignored, and the results were disastrous (Moorhead, Ference, & Neck, 1991; Figure 17-13).

How can we avoid groupthink? Some investigators claim there is not much to avoid, believing that the problem has been overemphasized in the public press and undersupported in the research laboratory (Aldag & Fuller, 1993). For others, the basic procedure is to point out the dangers in placing a high value on compatibility. Group members, instead, are urged to understand that dissenting opinions and a slower pace may be essential to long-term success (Neck & Moorhead, 1995).

GROUP SHIFTS. When problems are solved by a group, another outcome is likely besides the groupthink solution. The group decision may be more extreme than the average decision of all the individual members.

Early research showed that when college students solved problems in a group, they tended to reach riskier decisions than when working alone, an outcome called the *risky shift*. They took greater chances when companions shared the risk. Later, when other problems were used, a conservative shift was noted (Knox & Safford, 1976). In both cases, there was a shift away from moderation. On this basis, the concept of **group polarization** emerged, meaning that the group decision is frequently closer to one pole or the other than it is to the average position of the individuals. The reasons, still unclear, appear related to persuasive statements by group members holding extreme views and to the process of social comparison, in which we obtain guidance by observing what others do (Levine & Moreland, 1990).

BRAINSTORMING. Groupthink and group polarization are unexpected, potentially limited outcomes when groups make decisions. Positive outcomes can occur too, provided that group processes are held in check in the early momemts.

The aim in **brainstorming** is to generate as many creative ideas as possible, chiefly by suspending temporarily all criticism of these ideas. Each group member is first instructed to adopt a free-wheeling attitude toward the problem, thinking without restraint about *any possible solutions.* All members are encouraged to build on others' efforts, advancing any ideas in any way possible. Afterward, a critical attitude is adopted; all of these ideas are evaluated. Here the thought processes become more realistic and less fanciful than earlier. At the end, the group may vote on the most promising solutions that have emerged, perhaps ranking them in order of feasibility, cost, or related criteria.

When people engage in brainstorming in

an interactive group, the first person's suggestion often directs the thinking of the next person, and that member's response channels the thoughts of the next, and so forth. This interaction typically generates fewer and less creative ideas than those developed by people working separately (Paulus & Dzindolet, 1993).

The solution is relatively simple. The brainstorming session should begin with each person working alone, generating as many ideas as possible. Then, after this individual work, the group should assemble for brainstorming, using one another's ideas as springboards.

∾

GROUP LEADERSHIP

Even in an initially leaderless group, one or more people eventually assume a dominant role. This leadership, whether it is imposed from the outside or emerges through interactions among the members, of course can have a significant influence on the performance of the group.

On the Everest expedition, Jim was the leader, consulting occasionally with Don. His decisions seemed fair but sometimes unwise. For instance, he placed unwarranted trust in Karma as head of the Sherpas. His plan for the secret eye exams diminished morale. By choosing himself for the first summit team, he disrupted team spirit. And finally, Jim told news reporters that he and Steve *chose* Stacy to try for the summit with the last oxygen bottle. He suggested that they did so for the good of the team and to give her the chance to become the first American woman to scale Mount Everest.

Hearing this remark, Stacy objected, and Steve shook his head, smiling crookedly. They saw Jim, at that moment, trying to enhance his image as expedition leader. If he could not make the summit himself, then he would settle for the suggestion of altruism on his part and a superordinate goal held by the team, putting an American *woman* on top.

Jim was a capable leader on the mountain, but in making personnel decisions he showed less sagacity (Allison, 1993).

LEADERSHIP ROLES. What is leadership? It is persuasion; it is not domination. As defined in psychological research, leadership involves persuading people to ignore their individual concerns and devote themselves instead to a common goal, one that is important for the welfare of the group (Hogan, Curphy, & Hogan, 1994).

Just how and when a person is suited for leadership has been difficult to determine. For many years, investigators attempted to discover the essential traits of an effective leader.

Intelligence, flexibility, and strength of character were prominently mentioned, and it was assumed that the leader was the best-liked, most active, and most able member of the group, a view known as the *great-person theory* of leadership. The idea here is that each person has a single status, and an all-around great person is at the top.

As this research continued, the hope of discovering a highly prescriptive, invariant set of characteristics faded for two reasons. First, it was found that different situations usually require somewhat different traits in a leader. If a hierarchy could be established for one situation, it would have to be re-established for another, depending on the situation and the traits of the group members. Second, even within one situation, there seem to be at least two different leadership roles, each making its own contribution to the group process.

There is a **task specialist,** or *instrumental leader,* who is concerned with identifying the problem, discovering methods of dealing with it, and implementing the best solution. This person is oriented to a specific obstacle or threat in the group, and usually he or she ranks highest on activity and best ideas. In addition, there is a **social specialist,** or *expressive leader,* who is the central figure in maintaining group cohesion and morale (Bales, 1951). Also called the maintenance specialist, this person often has a good sense of humor, ranks highest on likability, and encourages others (Hogan, Curphy, & Hogan, 1994).

On rare occasions, the two roles are held by the same person. But especially as the group continues to function, different individuals emerge in these capacities.

LEADER–FOLLOWER INTERACTION. In most group situations, there are a few general characteristics of enduring leadership. The individual who assumes primary control is usually above average in intelligence, although not the most brilliant individual in the group. There is some truth in the old political maxim: The best-qualified person, in terms of ability, is not popular enough to be elected. Any enduring leader also must be close to the group members in attitudes and interests.

Certain situational factors also are influential. A task leader is more likely to be suitable if the morale of the group is unusually good or if the group has deteriorated almost to the point of disintegration. When conditions are neither extremely favorable nor extremely unfavorable, a social specialist may be more effective. The primary need here is to maintain solidarity (Fielder, 1964).

The study of leadership today therefore focuses on characteristics of the followers, as well as those of the leader, for followers certainly can influence leaders. In this sense, leadership is a shared and fluid process. Charisma, for example, is not simply a quality possessed by a leader—it is something accorded by followers, as part of the leadership process. Our understanding of leadership is incomplete if we fail to recognize leader–follower interactions (Wakefield, 1992).

As the group goals change, a leader may become a follower, especially in a very large group, such as a whole nation. Different situations require different leadership abilities, as illustrated by Jim's leadership, which was highly effective on the mountain but disparaged at base camp. Here again we encounter the interaction principle. The type of leadership that proves most effective depends on the followers, the situation, the level of development of the group, and its goals (Figure 17-14).

IN PERSPECTIVE. As we close this chapter, the reader may wonder about the other summit climbers. When it came time for her attempt, Diana's team was driven down the mountain by a severe storm, a bitter disappointment for her. Geoff reached the summit alone with great satisfaction, for it was his third attempt. The 209th person to climb to the top of Mount Everest, he celebrated by depositing there a pink flamingo and the American flag (Tabin, 1993). Peggy summited too, prompting admiration among some expedition members, animosity among others.

The admiration came from Jim and Don. As the least experienced climber on the expedition, Peggy fell twice, started to roll down the mountain, and stopped herself by digging her ice axe into the snow. Her success spoke for itself, as well as for Dawa Tsering, the Sherpa who accompanied her (Tabin, 1993).

Others had a very different view of Peggy's accomplishment. The American expedition, Steve pointed out, was based on teamwork and team goals. Members were to take only measured risks and to remain responsible for their own safety. By taking unnecessary risks, inexperienced Peggy had broken the agreement and been disloyal to everyone in the group. "And success in the face of stupidity," he declared, "is still stupidity" (Allison, 1993).

A few days earlier, Narayan Shrestha, a Sherpa in the Spanish expedition, had been swept to his death by an avalanche. Michel Parmentier, from the

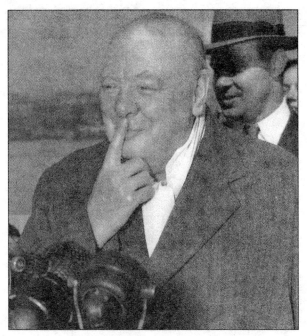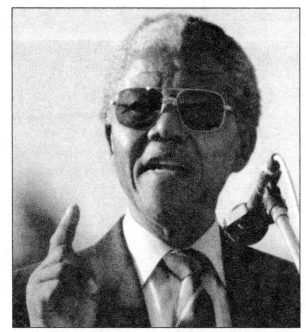

FIGURE 17–14 LEADERSHIP AND THE SITUATION. Winston Churchill was voted into the highest positions in England in times of war. When peace returned, he was twice immediately voted out of office. Even while in prison, Nelson Mandela maintained a powerful leadership in South Africa. Released from prison, he continues to maintain that role.

French team, was found frozen in the snow, apparently a victim of exhaustion and altitude sickness. They were among nine climbers who died on the slopes of Mount Everest during these three months. Only the American and Korean expeditions suffered no fatalities (Nelson et al., 1990). On the average, for every trek up Mount Everest, two people fail to survive (West, 1986).

Peggy was grateful to be alive, and she leaves us with several questions. Should her bold dash to the summit be explained by situational factors? Or might it be better explained by dispositional attributions? Or, more accurately, to what extent were each of these factors involved? In answering these questions, remember that people in Eastern cultures are often inclined to find the causes of behavior in the setting or situation. In Western societies, they are more likely to cite factors within the individual, as personal traits or dispositions (Lee, Hallahan, & Herzog, 1996).

Other things being equal, which they rarely are, we can sum up the cultural issue in this fashion. If we were to ask Dawa Tsering why Peggy sprinted to the summit, he would be likely to give reasons external to Peggy. She had fine weather, a prepared route, perfect timing, and even his presence as a support climber. If we were to ask Steve Ruoss, he would be more likely to explain Peggy's act on the basis of personal traits, including out-of-role behavior. In fact, he did, declaring that Peggy's dash to the peak, especially by a support climber, showed only ignorance and selfishness. Rescue efforts, if needed, would have endangered many members of the American expedition.

From a broader viewpoint, we must remember that we all have a cultural perspective, whether we look at the world from the top of Mount Everest or from a less lofty location. The contents of this book come largely from the Western world, and therefore the possible cultural bias of even this psychology is not to be taken lightly.

ATTITUDES

1. An attitude is defined as a tendency to make an evaluation, and it is considered to have three components: thinking, feeling, and acting. Attitudes are formed through direct instruction, modeling, and classical and operant conditioning, and the same processes are involved in changing attitudes.

2. Several theories of attitude formation and change are based on the principle that human beings try to avoid or eliminate inconsistencies. These approaches include: balance theory, which deals with harmony among attitudes in one or more individuals; congruity theory, concerned with attitude shifts; and cognitive-dissonance theory, which stresses that individuals can dispel inconsistency through rationalization, selective perception, and the acquisition of new information.

3. A most important factor in persuasion is the credibility of the communicator, who must be perceived as trustworthy and expert if the communication is to be persuasive. The use of fear depends on the initial level of fear in the audience and on the extent to which the message includes instructions on what to do, as well as what to avoid.

SOCIAL COGNITION

4. Person perception, which is part of social cognition, refers to the ways we understand another individual. In forming impressions of people, the warm–cold dimension often outweighs all other traits, partly because of the halo effect.

5. Stereotypes sometimes may facilitate first impressions, but it is extremely difficult to determine the accuracy of such generalizations. Many stereotypes are negative or ethnocentric, and they ignore individual differences. Prejudices are almost always harmful because the issue, by definition, has been prejudged.

6. Attribution theory is concerned with how people explain others' behavior, as well as their own. In general, they use a disposition attribution for others. Conversely, they use a situational attribution for themselves.

INTERPERSONAL ATTRACTION

7. Several factors seem influential in interpersonal attraction, but two are primary. These include similarity—of interests, intelligence, and even physical appearance—and familiarity with the other person.

8. In self-disclosure, one person communicates to another details of his or her personal life. Reciprocal self-disclosure is an important characteristic of a long-term relationship. In unsuccessful long-term relationships, a demand–withdraw pattern may develop in which one partner attempts to discuss a certain issue and the other withdraws from this interaction.

SOCIAL INFLUENCE

9. In conformity, an individual adopts the thoughts or behaviors of a social group without any direct pressure to do so. Individuals sometimes conform simply because they do not want to be different. Conformity also arises when people are uncertain about what to do.

10. In compliance, people are encouraged or induced to behave in certain ways; there is some direct pressure. Studies have shown two ways in which compliance can be obtained in negotiations: the foot-in-the-door technique and the door-in-the-face technique. In obedience, there is a demand, not a request. The Milgram study of obedience demonstrated that social pressure may be more influential than personality in determining behavior in certain situations.

11. Altruism seems generally less attributable to a particular type of personality than to the individual's temporary personal states, such as haste and mood, and to characteristics of the situation, especially the number of bystanders and degree of personal risk.

GROUP PROCESSES

12. A group member is usually assigned or adopts a role, which is a pattern of expected behavior. Status, which is closely related to role, refers to a person's position in the group hierarchy.

13. When people work in the presence of others, they often accomplish more than when working alone, an outcome called social facilitation. Two factors that seem important in inducing cooperation in natural settings are early childhood training and the existence of superordinate goals, which benefit all group members. According to a meta-analysis, cooperation is more effective than competition in promoting achievement and productivity.

14. In groupthink, a group places such a high value on cohesion and maintenance of morale that critical thinking is suspended and decision-making ability is thereby limited. The concept of group polarization indicates that a group decision is likely to be more extreme, in any direction, than the average decision of the individual members.

15. The emergence of a leader is dependent partly on intelligence and partly on congruence in leader–follower characteristics. Even within the same group, two prominent leadership styles may be required, one involving a task specialist and the other a social specialist. In any case, leadership is a process, a function of leader-follower interactions and the group context.

• WORKING WITH PSYCHOLOGY •

❧ REVIEW OF KEY CONCEPTS ❧

social psychology

Attitudes
attitude
balance theory
congruity theory
cognitive-dissonance
theory

Social Cognition
social cognition
central trait
halo effect
stereotype
prejudice
ethnocentrism
culture
multicultural awareness

attribution theory
dispositional attribution
situational attribution
overattribution effect

Interpersonal Attraction
interpersonal attraction
matching hypothesis
self-disclosure

Social Influence
social influence
conformity
social norms
deindividuation
compliance
foot-in-the-door technique
door-in-the-face technique

obedience
altruism
bystander intervention effect

Group Processes
group
role
status
pecking order
social facilitation
social loafing
superordinate goals
meta-analysis
groupthink
group polarization
brainstorming
task specialist
social specialist

❧ CLASS DISCUSSION/CRITICAL THINKING ❧

A NARRATIVE TWIST

The Sherpas assisted the Americans in reaching the peak of Mount Everest. Using the concepts of ethnocentrism and multicultural awareness, suggest some ways that each group might have perceived the other in seeking this goal. Then suppose that the conditions were reversed. The Americans assisted the Sherpas in achieving a goal, such as establishing and maintaining fast-food restaurants in Nepal. Show how the issues of ethnocentrism and multicultural awareness might arise in this context as well. ❧

TOPICAL QUESTIONS

• *Attitudes.* Ms. Zing takes a pro-life position on abortion. What position is she likely to take on capital punishment? Explain the reasons for your choice, referring to the consistency principle.

• *Social Cognition.* In the overattri-

493

bution effect, too much emphasis is placed on dispositional fa 's, too little on situational factors. If a friend and a stranger both observe a young man behaving in an unusual manner, such as wearing no shirt on a cold day, who is more likely to display this effect, the friend or the stranger? Why?

• *Interpersonal Attraction.* Ms. Able and Mr. Baker are single, live near each other, and share certain characteristics—such as high intelligence, a certain religious outlook, and financial concerns—and yet they have different careers, hobbies, physical appearances, and geographic backgrounds. Discuss the possibility that they will become longtime companions.

• *Social Influence.* The foot-in-the-door and door-in-the-face techniques are somewhat opposite approaches for obtaining compliance. For eliciting compliance from a small child, which technique seems more promising? To obtain a large donation to a charity, which technique appears more useful? Explain the reasons for your answers.

• *Group Processes.* Does groupthink occur more often in public life today than two centuries ago? Or are the media simply more adept at gaining details of incidents of groupthink? Explain your answer, using an example from politics or business.

❧ TOPICS OF RELATED INTEREST ❧

In many respects, psychotherapy is concerned with attitude formation and change (16). Interpersonal attraction, especially the development of intimate relationships, is viewed in the context of reinforcement theory (7) and emotion (11). The Milgram study was considered in the context of research methods (2).

16
EMOTION AND STRESS

DAWN AND STEPHEN ENJOYED ONE ANOTHER'S COM-
PANY, AND THEY SHARED SOME HAPPY TIMES IN
COLLEGE. THEY EVEN TOOK THE SAME PSYCHOLOGY
course and wrote their autobiographies as a class assignment. But they
came from very different backgrounds.

When she was just a little girl, living with her family in affluent circumstances, Dawn awoke one night to loud noises and the shuffling of feet.
This disturbance frightened her, for it formed no familiar pattern, such as
the sounds from someone making a late snack or using the bathroom.

She heard a voice amid the commotion and thought it was her mother.
Wriggling out of bed apprehensively, she opened the door a crack. Down
the hallway, she saw her mother's back in the kitchen. When her mother
turned around, she was a portrait of distress—biting her lower lip, her hair
in disarray, her clothes disheveled, her eyes half closed and mournful. She
began to shout in an incoherent jumble. "It was a raw scene," Dawn said
later. "A drunken, miserable mother and a rather tongue-tied child."

At this same time, in a distant city, a little boy named Stephen shared his bedroom with an older brother. For Stephen, it was hardly a bedroom. He slept in a low chair converted into a couch at night, an arrangement made necessary by his unplanned birth, seven years after one brother, eleven years after another.

Stephen pestered his brothers in small ways—stealing their cookies and hiding their stamp collections. Stephen's older brother laughed and joked about such deeds, which pleased the little boy enormously. Stephen felt very happy whenever that brother played with him.

For the other brother, sharing his room with a child, Stephen was a nuisance—much too noisy and wrong about everything. These reactions made Stephen angry, as did his mother's attitude. She was reluctant to let her youngest child grow up. He did anyway, asserting himself as a practical, rebellious adolescent (Goethals & Klos, 1976).

Living different lives in different parts of the country, Dawn and Stephen experienced moments of fear, joy, sadness, and anger, as well as the infinitely varied emotional states not so readily labeled. These diverse reactions, some from childhood, others in adulthood, provide a useful narrative for this chapter because they reflect the broad array of emotions we all experience with partners, family members, acquaintances, and even when alone.

This chapter begins with the basic components of emotion and then turns to theories of emotion. Afterward, we consider positive emotions, liking and loving, and then the negative side, anger and aggression. The chapter closes on a practical note, examining stress in daily life.

• COMPONENTS OF EMOTION •

After the encounter in the kitchen, Dawn found herself feeling afraid in almost every corner of their large house. Her heart pounded; she trembled; and her palms became moist. Sometimes she hid in her bedroom, out of harm's way, she hoped. In these events, we see the basic components of **emotion,** defined as a complex feeling state accompanied by physiological arousal and overt behaviors. Dawn felt afraid, the feeling component; her heart pounded and her palms became moist, the physiological component; and she hid in her room, the behavioral component.

Still another factor in emotion is the cognitive dimension. Merely thinking about an important event can make us emotional. Dawn explained later that just the thought of seeing her drunken mother caused her to become upset. Our thoughts often influence our feelings, but the other elements of emotion cannot be ignored.

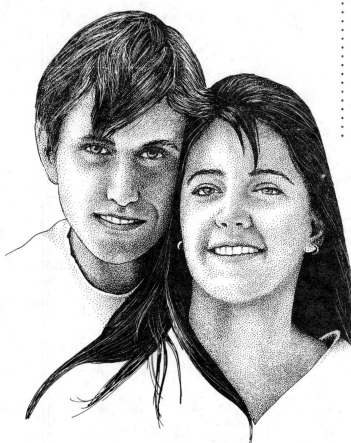

FEELINGS IN EMOTION

Both motivation and emotion imply motion, coming from the Latin verb *movere*, which means "to move." Motivation is typically purposeful; a motivated person moves toward some goal. Emotion is primarily expressive; an emotional person is moved. Emotion can be motivating, however, to the extent that feelings prompt activity toward a goal. Certainly this was the case in Dawn's fearful retreat from her mother's alcoholic condition and Stephen's joyful approach to his older brother's games. Whenever we try to attain or dispel happiness, anger, disgust, and so forth, there is no doubt about the motivational significance of our feelings.

CLASSIFICATION OF FEELINGS. Human feelings are also characterized by their diversity. Consider the term **anxiety,** defined as a general state of uneasiness or apprehension. It can involve timidity, mistrust, dread, alarm, suspicion, terror, diffidence, and many further shades of meaning. In addition, it has different meanings in the different systems of psychology, such as psychoanalysis, behaviorism, and the humanistic viewpoint.

In dealing with this diversity, psychologists have attempted to identify the most basic or fundamental human feelings. Some of these classifications include a half-dozen feelings, others 15 or more (Table 11–1). Each basic feeling is assumed to have its own properties, but all can occur in combination, thereby influencing one another and accounting for the diversity in human emotional experience (Izard, 1971; Lazarus, 1991, 1993).

FEELINGS IN OPPOSITION. If we approach feelings as positive or negative, rather than through multiple classifications, modern theory and research can offer further insight. In this perspective, it is understood that the human nervous system is designed to oppose deviations from

NEGATIVE	MIXED	POSITIVE
Anger	Hope	Happiness
Anxiety (fear)	Compassion	Pride
Guilt (shame)		Relief
Sadness		Love
Envy (jealousy)		
Disgust		

TABLE 11–1 BASIC EMOTIONS. Among many attempts to identify our fundamental feelings, anger and anxiety or fear are universally included first, making a statement about the human condition. Some expression of happiness is often the third entry (After Lazarus, 1993).

normal or neutral, just as the human body, through homeostasis, automatically mobilizes itself to counteract injury or disease. In the same way, according to **opponent-process theory,** one set of feelings automatically initiates arousal of the opposite feelings, which appear later. In other words, positive feelings inevitably set the stage for negative feelings, and negative feelings eventually set in motion positive feelings (Solomon, 1980; Solomon & Corbit, 1974).

In school, Dawn was anxious and unhappy, totally unable to make friends. "I was impossibly silent in classes," she said, "by far the shyest and most afraid student in the school" (Goethals & Klos, 1976). When the bell rang, signaling the end of class, she experienced a rapid decline in these negative feelings. Her fear disappeared, but her emotional state did not return directly to neutral. Instead, Dawn felt joyful for a while. Then, later, even her joyfulness disappeared. Everything became quite normal again.

These sequential deviations from normalcy represent the usual pattern in our lives, according to opponent-process theory, and they occur whether the initial feeling is positive or negative. The first feeling, *A,* is aroused by its adequate stimulus, but after this stimulation ceases, a second or *B* state appears, which is in opposition to *A* and has been indirectly activated by *A.* After persisting for a while, the second feeling also disappears, and then there is a return to normal (Figure 11–1).

For example, intense intimacy, sexual or otherwise, is usually a very pleasant feeling, after which the sensation gradually diminishes, all constituting state A. As time passes, the feeling eventually changes to a slightly aversive state, a let-down feeling, the B state. And finally, the normal state returns. In contrast, the novice parachutist is apprehensive or terrified in state A, before jumping, and looks stunned even during the descent. Then, after a safe landing, in state B, the chutist is relieved, perhaps joyful. It is this pleasant after-feeling that keeps chutists jumping, joggers running, and sauna lovers bathing. According to opponent-process theory, having a baby, consuming drugs, winning a lottery, and innumerable other experiences involve this automatic reversal of feeling. On leaving the dentist's office, you do not feel merely okay. Even with minor physical discomfort, you feel elated, at least for a while.

A second postulate of this theory states: With repeated stimulation, the first or A state grows weaker and the second or B state grows stronger. As our love for someone continues, year after year, we become adapted to this A state. The love becomes less intense. Moreover, as it continues, the loss of this love becomes more and more stressful. This B state, the absence of love, has grown steadily more powerful because its opposite, the A state, has been regarded more and more as a normal part of life. The loss of something that is increasingly expected, or taken for granted, becomes increasingly disruptive.

The same phenomenon occurs when the initial state is negative. After a person has become an habitual jogger, the negative A state, in which the runner feels stiff and cold during the warm-up, is increasingly regarded as just part of the daily routine. It becomes less and less aversive. With continued jogging, moreover, the addictive aftereffect, or B state, increases. Continuing to run, year after year, the jogger becomes more and more dependent on this regular exhilaration (Table 11–2).

Thus, human beings seek to maintain emotional experiences of both types, initially positive

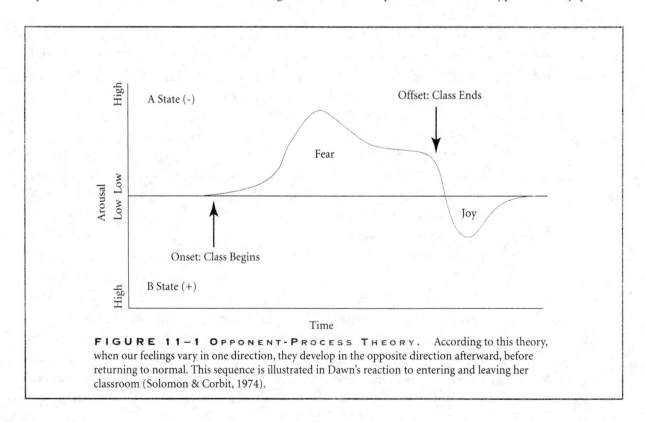

FIGURE 11–1 OPPONENT-PROCESS THEORY. According to this theory, when our feelings vary in one direction, they develop in the opposite direction afterward, before returning to normal. This sequence is illustrated in Dawn's reaction to entering and leaving her classroom (Solomon & Corbit, 1974).

498

EXAMPLE	EARLY STIMULATIONS		LATER STIMULATIONS	
	STATE A	STATE B	STATE A	STATE B
Parachutists	Terror, high arousal	Stunned, stony-faced	Tense, expectant	Jubilation
Persons in love	Ecstacy	Loneliness	Comfort	Grief
Dogs receiving shock	Terror, panic	Stealth, caution	Unhappiness	Joy
Drug users	Euphoria, rush pleasure	Craving	Normal feelings	Intense craving, agony

TABLE 11-2 CHANGES IN OPPONENT-PROCESS OUTCOMES.   In the early and later stimulations, the *A* state induces its opponent process, the opposite or *B* state. However, repeated stimulations weaken the *A* state and strenghten the *B* state. After many jumps, the parachutist becomes less terrified and enjoys it more. Similarly, the habitual drug user experiences less euphoria and more withdrawal symptoms (Solomon & Corbit, 1974).

and initially negative. The immediately pleasant ones, such as eating and drinking, may become addictive due to the prompt and positive *A* state. The mildly unpleasant ones, such as jogging and skydiving, become habitual due to the increasingly powerful aftereffect, or *B* state. This viewpoint has been applied to all sorts of activities, including blood donation, breast-feeding, and bicycling for long distances. So sayeth the theory of opponent processes, which emphasizes the costs of pleasure and the benefits of pain (Solomon, 1980).

PHYSIOLOGY OF EMOTION

Whether or not some sort of homeostatic condition underlies our feelings, it is clear that widespread physiological changes take place in emotion. Even when we try to control our emotions, we often give ourselves away with hand tremors, sweating, excessive blinking, and other signs of arousal. All of these reactions depend on a highly complex network of nerve pathways throughout the human body. Among them, the two most important in emotion are the central nervous system and the autonomic nervous system.

ACTIVITIES IN THE CENTRAL NERVOUS SYSTEM. The major communications network in the human body is the central nervous system, comprised of the brain and spinal cord. As

a coordinating system in emotion, it influences a wide variety of activities, directly or indirectly.

One region of the central nervous system, the **hypothalamus,** near the midbrain, plays a very large role in emotional and motivational behavior, including drinking, eating, fighting, fleeing, and sexual activity, as well as emotional expression. Impulses from the various receptors pass through or adjacent to the hypothalamus on their way to the upper brain regions. Impulses also come down into the hypothalamus from these regions, and the hypothalamus, in turn, relays them to the various muscles and viscera.

The outer covering and uppermost region of the brain, called the **cerebral cortex,** is instrumental in human thought and memory; therefore, it can influence emotion as well. We may become emotional or unemotional merely by the way we think about a particular situation. As Dawn explained, just thinking about the girl next door, who had many friends, made her feel lonely and upset (Goethals & Klos, 1976).

Recent experiments with animals suggest that fear can arise even without clear knowledge of the situation—that is, without the cerebral cortex. In these experiments, a tone or light was followed by a mild electric shock and eventually, through classical conditioning, rats learned to fear the tone alone. Whenever the tone was sounded, electrodes in the animals' brains showed complex neural activity in one particular brain site. A small almond-shaped region located close to the base of the brain, the **amygdala,** plays a significant role in motivation, emotion, and memory. In this case, the experiment went one step further. When the animals were deprived of information from the cortex by removal of that area, they nevertheless displayed the fear reaction. In other words, the animals were afraid without knowing the source of their fear (Le Doux, 1989). These findings may offer an explanation of those instances in which people react without really understanding the situation. Walking alone at night, you jump at the sound of footsteps behind you, and then afterwards you relax, realizing that a friend is running to catch up with you. Your initial fear perhaps arose through activities in the amygdala and then, moments later, the cortex had time to interpret the situation.

ACTIVITY IN THE AUTONOMIC NERVOUS SYSTEM.

Relatively independent of the central nervous system, the **autonomic nervous system** initiates and inhibits activities of diverse organs, thereby stimulating widespread, largely involuntary changes throughout the body during emotion.

The autonomic nervous system has two main branches, the sympathetic and parasympathetic divisions. As a rule, but not always, they work in opposition. If one division stimulates activity in an organ, the other inhibits it. The **sympathetic nervous system,** which plays the dominant role in emotion, accelerates the heart rate, increases the amount of adrenaline, inhibits activity in the intestines, activates the sweat glands, and prompts the pilomotor response—meaning goose bumps. The individual is emotionally aroused.

In fact, when a person is sufficiently aroused, one body part grows up to ten times its normal size. The enlargement of this organ, the pupil of the eye, is called dilation, and it has been known for centuries. It lies behind some familiar expressions:

"He became wide-eyed." "Her eyes grew big as saucers." In earlier days, women put a dilating fluid in their eyes, enlarging the pupils and thereby implying that their owner was emotionally aroused or at least attentive to the object of their gaze (Figure XI.I, Color).

When the event subsides the **parasympathetic nervous system** resumes control, for it becomes dominant in routine situations, reversing the changes that occur in an emergency. Heart rate and breathing become more normal, digestion begins again in the stomach, saliva reappears in the mouth, the pupils tend to constrict, and so forth. The individual begins functioning in a more routine fashion.

MEASURING PHYSIOLOGICAL ACTIVITIES.

Among the many measures of physiological activities in emotion, we have already considered the **electroencephalogram** (EEG), in which brain waves are recorded by a stylus on a moving sheet of paper. When the individual is resting a regular EEG rhythm appears, but in arousal other rhythms occur. For measuring the rate and rhythm of the heartbeat, electrodes are attached to the body and chest, and the tracings are called an **electrocardiogram** (EKG). The examiner looks for various patterns in this record, of which about a dozen have been established. Still another response of particular interest to psychologists is the activation of the sweat glands during emotional arousal. The resulting perspiration, especially on the palms of the hands, lowers the electrical resistance of the skin, called the **galvanic skin response** (GSR).

One instrument that measures several physiological responses simultaneously is the **polygraph,** a term that comes from *poly,* meaning "many," and *graph,* referring to writing. It records heart rate, breathing rate, blood pressure, and skin conductance, among other activities. It is called a *lie detector* because these responses change under arousal, and it is assumed that a person who is lying is highly aroused. Instead, it should be regarded as an emotion detector.

The subject is asked two types of questions, critical and neutral. The former concern the incident in doubt; the latter concern everyday events and are used to indicate the individual's typical or normal arousal level. The idea is that the guilty subject will show a higher emotional arousal to the critical questions (Figure XI.2).

But the body can be made to lie. Some subjects defeat the test by thinking about the same high-anxiety event in response to *every* question, critical and neutral, or they subtly tense their muscles as fully as possible, thereby portraying a uniformly high arousal level (Honts & Kircher, 1994). Others, accustomed to lying, can produce falsehoods with little anxiety. They may show uniformly low profiles. Still others, even when they have had no part whatsoever in the incident, may appear to be guilty simply because they are so worried about being found guilty. In one assessment of this device, polygraph experts studied 50 people known to be innocent and 50 who had confessed to a crime. Not knowing who was who, they made both types of errors—judging innocent people as guilty or guilty ones as innocent—in almost one-third of the cases (Kleinmuntz & Szucko, 1984; Saxe, Dougherty, & Cross, 1985).

. Most psychologists today have reservations about the use of polygraph tests. They feel that these tests, if permitted at all, should be employed only in narrowing a field of suspects (Steinbrook, 1992).

IDENTIFYING FEELINGS PHYSIOLOGI-CALLY. A question of theoretical interest has developed from the use of such instruments. Can our feelings be identified solely on the basis of these physiological conditions? By examining her physiological reactions, could we distinguish between Dawn's fear in school and her joy afterward? This capacity would have great significance for a theory of emotion, especially its physiological bases.

In a series of studies, records of heart activity and blood pressure were obtained from people exposed to various types of stress. Attempting to solve mental problems, they were criticized, given defective equipment, and administered mild electric shocks. Afterward, all subjects described their feelings, which were classified according to four categories: anxiety, anger directed toward the self, anger directed toward the experimenter, or no intense feeling. When these data were analyzed, physiological responses of low intensity were found to be associated with no intense feeling or with anger directed outward, toward the experimenter. Physiological responses of high intensity occurred with anxiety and anger directed inward, toward the self. In other words, the subjects with no anxiety or anger directed outward did not react physiologically in an emergency manner; the others responded physiologically as if there were in an emergency (Funkenstein, King, & Drolette, 1957; Schalling & Svensson, 1984).

However, a more convincing demonstration of physiological differences requires a prediction from one to the other. Knowing only a person's feelings, the investigator must be able to describe the pattern of physiological responses. Or knowing only the physiological reactions, the investigator must describe the person's feelings. Use of increasingly sophisticated equipment has facilitated progress toward this goal.

In one study, the subjects *imagined* past events in which they had become emotional—situations involving happiness, sadness, anger, or fear. Thinking about these situations reproduced the original feelings in abbreviated form. At the same time, the subjects' heart reactions were monitored by cardiovascular apparatus. Then it was discovered that certain cardiovascular patterns were associated with specific feelings (Schwartz, Weinberger, & Singer, 1981).

Studies with posed facial expressions also have yielded promising results. For this purpose, professional actors were videotaped as they produced emotional expressions and relived past emotional experiences. These contractions of facial muscles into the universal expressions of happiness, sadness, and so forth, perhaps combined with the cognitive arousal in reliving these states, generated specific changes in heart rate, stomach secretions, and other reactions. In the resulting autonomic nervous system activity, distinctions were made between positive and negative feeling states and, in several instances, among negative states (Ekman, Levenson, & Friesen, 1983). On such bases, there seems to be sufficient evidence for accepting the existence of physiological differences among emotions, however they may arise (Levenson, 1992).

EMOTIONAL BEHAVIOR

The emotional experience of another person is most readily evident in behavior. Fearful of her high school classmates, Dawn avoided them whenever possible. At a school dance, she was announced as the winner of the Most Studious Prize, but she did not dance. She stayed home, afraid to attend. Stephen became angry with his classmates, who taunted him with a derisive nickname. He responded by fighting and arguing.

All of us display our emotions on some occasions and try to hide them on others. To what extent do the behavioral aspects reveal the underlying emotion?

INTERPRETING EXPRESSIVE BEHAVIOR. Some emotional expressions are constant across different societies, and they provide cues about the emotion being experienced. Other emotional behaviors vary from culture to culture and even among people in the same culture. Sometimes we can identify the emotion; sometimes we are unsuccessful (Figure XI.3).

The universality of some facial expressions is evident when people turn the mouth up or down at the corners voluntarily, without some emotionally provoking event to stimulate them. These behaviors prompt subtle feelings of happiness and sadness, respectively. Such findings have increased speculation on the possible genetic bases of certain emotional expressions (Ekman, 1980).

Nevertheless, learning also plays a role—not only in when we express ourselves but also in how we do so. Among spectators at a European sporting event, whistling shows dissatisfaction with the performance. Among fans in the United States, whistling is more like cheering, a form of praise and encouragement. In some Asian societies, scratching the cheeks and ears is a sign of happiness. Clapping or rubbing the hands is a sign of happiness in this country.

When they win a lottery, some people clap, others cry, and still others show very little emotional expression. Therefore, we do not use just one set of cues in identifying an emotion in someone else. We consider what the person says, how the person looks and behaves, and also the circumstances, which can be very informative. We attempt to integrate all of these cues into one overall interpretation.

AROUSAL AND PERFORMANCE. When we speak of the magnitude of an emotional response, rather than the feeling involved, we are referring to the **arousal level,** which can be significantly related to behavior. If arousal is extremely high, the person may react wildly, as when Stephen, in a time of frustration about his tormentors in school, became rebellious and disruptive in class. Or the person may become unable to move at all. On that disturbing night when she discovered her mother's drunkenness, Dawn lay completely still in bed, hardly breathing (Goethals & Klos, 1976).

It has been suggested that maximum human performance is achieved with a moderate level of arousal. When arousal is very low, the individual is not sufficiently involved to perform successfully. When arousal is extremely high, the individual is too excited to maintain proper control, and again there is poor performance.

This statement about arousal level has been extended to include the nature of the task. According to the **Yerkes-Dodson law,** the optimal level of arousal depends on the complexity of the task to be performed. High arousal is appropriate for a relatively simple task, such as running away from something. Low arousal is appropriate when the task is more complex, such as learning a new computer program or writing poetry. This view seems reasonable and useful, but it has received only mixed support (Neiss, 1988; Teigen, 1994).

Studies of athletic contests offer impressive evidence that arousal can be too high. Common sense tells us, for example, that the home team usually has an advantage, which certainly is true in regular season games and even in early rounds of the World Series baseball and National Basketball Association playoffs. The home team wins more than 60% of the first games in a championship series. But in the *final* game of a seven-game playoff, when everything is on the line, the winning percentage of the home team drops to 39%. The speculated reason is that the home team performs in front of wildly cheering fans who expect and even demand a victory; these players experience more pressure than the visiting players and therefore do not perform up to their potential. Substantial evidence that the problem for the home team is choking under pressure appears in the fielding errors in baseball and the missed free throws in basketball, neither of which is significantly influenced by the play of the other team. In both sports these misplays by the home team are higher in game seven than in the earlier games (Baumeister & Steinhilber, 1984).

If a feeling of pressure is the critical factor, the same result should occur even when the home crowd is not demonstrative, as in golf championships. In one analysis of championship play, the performances of home-course favorites were compared with the performances of golfers from foreign courses. It was found that the play of the home golfers deteriorated more from the first to the last round than did the play of the visiting golfers (Wright, Jackson, Christie, McGuire, et al., 1991).

This finding, the home-field disadvantage, occurs only at the *end* of a long championship series, not at the beginning and not in a single-game championship. But do not bet on that.

COGNITION IN EMOTION

Among the diverse factors in emotion, the role of cognition is most widely debated. Feelings, physiological changes, and even behavior are inevitably involved, but is cognition also an inevitable component? Does it always play a role in emotion? According to some experts, the answer is "Yes." To experience an emotion, the individual must think about the stimulating circumstances. Why would Dawn lie frozen in bed without *any* understanding of the situation? The very different reactions of aroused animals also indicate some appraisal of the situation. According to the cognitive view, an evaluation of some sort is involved in *any* emotional reaction (Lazarus, 1993).

Other theorists argue that appraisal is not necessary. Different parts of the brain are involved in emotion and cognition, and everyday experience suggests that these responses are quite different. The alleged absence of cognition in extreme emotional states is indicated in familiar expressions: "I was so upset I couldn't think!" Cognition can cause emotion, and it can sustain emotion, but it is not a necessary or inevitable component of emotion (Plutchik, 1980; Weinrich, 1980).

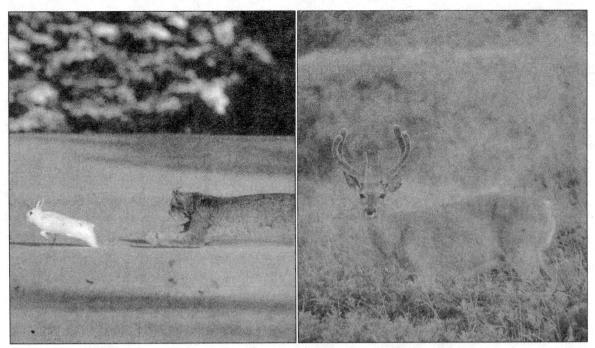

FIGURE 11–2 COGNITION IN EMOTION. Overt behavior is not a good index of emotional arousal. Both the rabbit and the deer have determined that they are in danger, though they attempt to escape their predators by using opposite reactions, running away and standing motionless.

Psychologists adopting this view argue that some emotional behaviors occur even *before* the individual has appraised the situation. A calm, peaceful person suddenly recoils from something without knowing why, discovering the dangerous element later. We noted already that experimental animals may display fear without appraisal of the situation, apparently through activities in the amygdala, before the cerebral cortex has become involved (Le Doux, 1989, 1995).

A speculative attempt to reconcile these different views emphasizes that the two hemispheres of the brain serve somewhat different functions. Many studies suggest that the right hemisphere is more responsive to emotional stimulation than the left hemisphere. Damage to the right hemisphere causes greater difficulties in assessing emotional information than does comparable injury to the left hemisphere (Leventhal & Tomarken, 1986). Clinical patients with depressive reactions also show greater

than normal right hemisphere activity (Schaffer, Davidson, & Saron, 1983).

This approach, then, postulates two types of cognition in emotion. One, referred to as *analytic cognition,* is associated with the type of thinking commonly ascribed to the left hemisphere: verbal and direct. This cognition is essentially a logical understanding of something. The other, called *syncretic cognition,* is mediated by activities more closely associated with the right hemisphere: nonverbal and more holistic. It is characterized by spontaneity rather than intent, and it is presumed to be less logical and less conscious than analytic cognition (Buck, 1985).

In any case, there is agreement that cognition plays an important role in precipitating and sustaining emotional experiences—in animals and people (Figure 11–2). Dawn felt delighted merely thinking about her acceptance by several colleges. Stephen too was pleased to be going away to col-

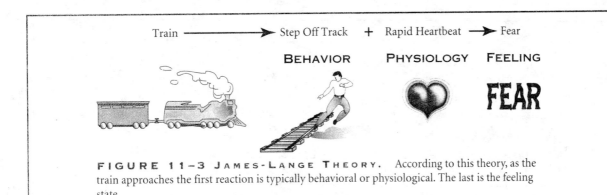

FIGURE 11-3 JAMES-LANGE THEORY. According to this theory, as the train approaches the first reaction is typically behavioral or physiological. The last is the feeling state.

lege. The prospect of escaping the confines of their hated schools made both of them happy indeed.

• THEORIES OF EMOTION •

In the fall of her junior year at college, Dawn gave a back-to-school party. Looking through a doorway, she saw Stephen for the first time, sitting on the stairs with friends, listening to someone's troubles. In her hostessing fervor, she did not have time to think more about that dark, appealing face.

Stephen remembered that first night differently. Sitting on the stairs, he met an old friend who was depressed. He felt a bit upset himself. Then he saw Dawn. She sat down next to him, waiting for his mood to change. It never did that night.

Later that week, Dawn and Stephen spent an evening together listening to music and discussing religion. The next day, they went to the beach. They swam, sat on the shore, and laughed a great deal. Dawn recalled, "I was truly happy for the first time in many months." Stephen thought to himself, "I have turned the corner and do not quite know where I am" (Goethals & Klos, 1976).

How would we attempt to explain these emotional reactions? What would we emphasize? Emotion is such a comprehensive concept that theories tend to focus on only one or two components, or they emphasize different components. Of all the major topics in psychology, understanding emotion seems to present the greatest challenge for an integrated approach (Oatley & Jenkins, 1992).

CLASSICAL VIEWS OF EMOTION

Among the major theoretical positions, the chief disagreement occurred between two classical viewpoints, the James-Lange and Cannon-Bard theories. At the time it appeared, the James-Lange theory promoted the opposite of what common sense suggests.

JAMES-LANGE THEORY. At the turn of this century, William James, in the United States, and Carl Lange, an eminent Danish scientist, came to a surprising conclusion. The behavioral and physiological reactions in emotion occur first, according to the **James-Lange theory,** and then they arouse the feelings. "We feel sorry because we cry, angry because we strike, afraid because we tremble," and not the other way around. Feelings are the result of feedback from bodily reactions, both muscular and glandular (James, 1890). Dawn felt happy that day at the beach because she smiled and laughed and because her heart palpitated.

James adopted this view largely on the basis of everyday situations. Standing in the path of an oncoming train, he claimed, you quickly step off the track and then you feel afraid (Figure 11–3). The feeling of fear is not truly experienced until you have retreated to the side and after the onset

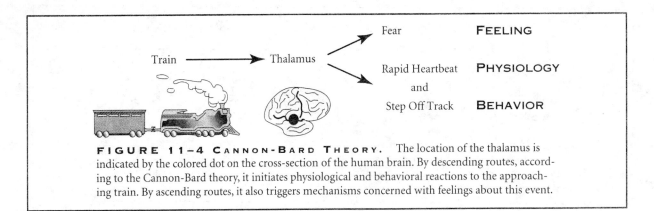

FIGURE 11–4 CANNON-BARD THEORY. The location of the thalamus is indicated by the colored dot on the cross-section of the human brain. By descending routes, according to the Cannon-Bard theory, it initiates physiological and behavioral reactions to the approaching train. By ascending routes, it also triggers mechanisms concerned with feelings about this event.

of physiological responses, such as rapid heartbeat, trembling, and increased breathing. When the results of this behavior and physiology reach the cerebral cortex, then you are truly afraid.

James's approach was the first modern theory of emotion and, despite its shortcoming, it set the direction for research for the next century (Mandler, 1990). In fact, one modern view reflects this position. The *facial feedback hypothesis* states that our facial expressions, through feedback from the controlling muscles, are partly responsible for the accompanying feelings (Izard, 1990).

In one test of this hypothesis, subjects were instructed to move their eyebrows down and together, raise their upper eyelids, narrow their lower lids, and press their lips together. This muscle-by-muscle instruction created the expression of anger in their faces, and physiological activities associated with anger occurred in the autonomic nervous system. Similar emotion-specific physiological reactions have been generated by using the instructions for expressions of fear, sadness, and disgust (Ekman, 1992).

Among the objections raised against the James-Lange theory, one concerns the timing of the events. Some physiological changes do not take place immediately, and yet our feelings appear rapidly. How can these feelings be explained on the basis of physiology? Our feelings sometimes continue even after the behavioral reaction has ceased. How can they be explained?

CANNON-BARD THEORY. One of those who took issue with the James-Lange theory was Walter Cannon, whose viewpoint was later extended by Philip Bard. Both physiologists, they produced the **Cannon-Bard theory**, sometimes called the *thalamic theory*, which emphasized that the thalamus plays a key role in stimulating the bodily arousal *and* the feelings of emotion. It sends signals to the autonomic nervous system, creating the bodily reactions, and also to the cerebral cortex, creating the feelings in emotion (Cannon, 1929).

According to this view, Dawn's happiness at the beach originated largely in the thalamus, which transmits *simultaneous* messages. The descending impulses, proceeding downward to the sympathetic division of the autonomic nervous system, activate the glands and skeletal muscles responsible for the physiology of emotion and the mechanisms for the behavioral reaction. Dawn's heart beat a bit faster, she laughed, and she danced around in a playful manner. The ascending impulses, relayed upward to the higher regions of the brain, initiate neural patterns responsible for the emotional experience. Dawn felt very happy. Through the thalamus, the sensations of bodily reactions and the feelings are combined almost simultaneously (Figure 11–4).

The Cannon-Bard theory was helpful in showing the importance of the thalamus, not considered in James's approach, but the neural anatomy of emotion is far more complicated. In the first place, the thalamus is not directly involved in activating

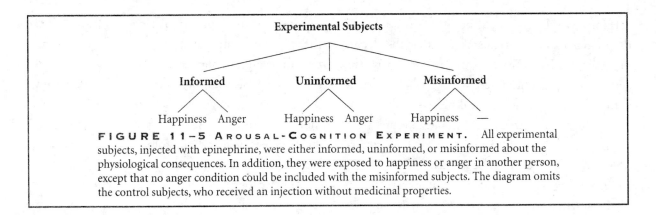

FIGURE 11–5 AROUSAL-COGNITION EXPERIMENT. All experimental subjects, injected with epinephrine, were either informed, uninformed, or misinformed about the physiological consequences. In addition, they were exposed to happiness or anger in another person, except that no anger condition could be included with the misinformed subjects. The diagram omits the control subjects, who received an injection without medicinal properties.

the muscles and glands. Second, the theory assumes that the thalamus, as a switchboard mechanism, prompts the emotional experience, but many other physiological structures are involved. Especially important is the hypothalamus, which plays a prominent role as a triggering mechanism. In addition, the limbic system and cerebral cortex are involved in emotion, as discussed earlier.

AROUSAL-COGNITION THEORY

The James-Lange theory ignored the role of the human brain in emotion, and the Cannon-Bard theory underestimated the role of the higher brain centers. Recent theorists have attempted to remedy these defects, focusing in particular on the cerebral cortex.

According to the **arousal-cognition theory**, emotional experience is a joint function of our degree of arousal, or physiological reactions, and our cognition, which is an interpretation of the situation. Initially, the arousal is simply nonspecific excitement; after cognition becomes involved, it is translated into a specific emotional experience. Aroused by a barking dog, a child interprets the condition as fear. Offended by a lack of consideration for the elderly, a senior citizen labels his aroused state as disgust. In these cases, the emotional experience arises through bodily feedback, and the reaction is brought into specific focus by an interpretation of the situation. Both factors, arousal *and* cognition, are important in the two-factor approach.

AROUSAL AND APPRAISAL. In an experiment by Stanley Schachter and associates, college students were injected with *epinephrine,* an adrenal hormone that induces an aroused state. The subjects in one treatment, called the informed subjects, were correctly informed that they would experience trembling hands, a pounding heart, and a flushed face. Others, the uninformed group, were told that they had received a vitamin compound with no immediate effects. The third group, the misinformed subjects, were led to expect symptoms that would not appear, such as numbness and itching. In addition, control subjects were injected with a saline solution that had no effect (Schachter & Singer, 1962).

All subjects were then exposed to one of two circumstances. In the euphoric or happy condition, they stayed in a waiting room with an accomplice of the experimenter who acted in a fun-loving, joking manner as he supposedly awaited his turn as a subject in the experiment. In the angry condition, the accomplice became highly irritated, complained about the questionnaire, made derisive comments, and stomped from the room. All subjects in both groups were observed through a one-way mirror and later were questioned about their feelings (Figure 11–5).

Schachter predicted that the misinformed and

uninformed subjects would be most susceptible to the mood in the environment and that the degree of susceptibility would be in proportion to the amount of epinephrine received. Having no explanation for their physiological arousal, which was readily apparent to them, they would interpret their feelings in terms of the circumstances. This prediction proved to be correct (Schachter, 1971).

According to this evidence, our interpretation of the situation determines the kind of feelings we experience, and the physiological changes determine the strength of this experience. In this view, also called *two-factor theory*, the cerebral cortex in particular plays a vital role in interpretation.

EVALUATION OF THE THEORY. A moment's introspection shows the powerful role of appraisal. Suppose you have just completed a term paper, and you are reviewing your accomplishment with joy and satisfaction. Suddenly you notice that you have used the wrong primary sources, and the paper is essentially worthless. Your ensuing response is disgust, fear, or shame. Your change in feeling has been produced solely by your reevaluation of your work.

The arousal-cognition view has focused attention on the role of cognition in emotional states, but it too has limitations. The subjects in the prior experiment, after being exposed to the different situations, were never asked to give their interpretation of those situations. We do not know about their cognitions. We only know that they were exposed to different stimulating conditions. Furthermore, our emotional reactions may be a function of cognition and physiological arousal, but all emotional states are not the same physiologically, differing *only* in cognitive factors. We need to know more about how the physiological factors are influential. Situational and physiological factors are relevant in all theories of emotion (Table 11–3).

This experiment has not been repeated with the same results, partly because there are now regulations against the use of epinephrine in this way (Leventhal & Tomarken, 1986). However, an experiment using incidental, unexpected exercise to induce arousal confirmed that people seek readily accessible explanations for their aroused states. When such cues are unavailable in the external environment, they look inward. By demonstrating the role of internal cues in emotional labeling, this research supported the arousal-cognition theory (Sinclair, Hoffman, Mark, Martin, & Pickering, 1994).

• LIKING AND LOVING •

"Stephen's entrance into my life was heralded by a joy . . . that quite surprised me," Dawn said. "I feel really protected and comforted by a PERSON."

"She is frank and open in what she wants and what she will give," Stephen said about Dawn. "Her smiling, which she has not shown before, makes me

THEORY	EXPLANATION	ILLUSTRATION
James-Lange	The behavioral and physiological reactions arouse the feeling.	Dawn became tongue-tied and trembled; which made her feel afraid.
Cannon-Bard	The thalamus stimulates bodily arousal and feelings.	Dawn became tongue-tied and trembled; simultaneously she felt afraid.
Arousal-cognition	The emotional experience depends on arousal *and* the interpretation of the situation.	Dawn interpreted her trembling as fear because she decided that the situation was dangerous.

TABLE 11–3 THEORIES OF EMOTION. A most important moment in Dawn's early life occurred when she encountered her drunken mother in the kitchen. These theories provide different interpretations of her emotional reaction.

feel like giving myself to her" (Goethals & Klos, 1976).

We often desire the company of someone *in particular*. We want to be with a specific person or group of people. Here we are speaking of liking and loving, topics that have aroused the poet and the philosopher, the cynic and the romantic. The feeling of *liking* someone involves enjoyment, appreciation, and common interests. It is not an abiding tie. In contrast, *loving* is a deep, enduring affection for another person, manifest in diverse ways.

One definition involves a love triangle—but not three people romantically inclined. Rather, the **triangular theory of love** describes three components, appearing in various amounts in any given love relationship: *intimacy*, which involves closeness and sharing; *commitment*, which is the devotion to the

relationship; and *passion*, referring to the intensity of the feeling, often sexual. Intimacy alone, for example, is essentially friendship or liking. Commitment alone appears in a caretaker relationship. And passion, by itself, often emerges as the first state of a romantic relationship. The presence of all three components is called *consummate love*, although the theory speculates that this condition is unlikely to be maintained for an extended period (Figure 11–6). As time passes and passion subsides, intimacy and commitment become more ascendant (Sternberg, 1986).

How do we explain the origins of liking and loving? More specifically, how do we understand the development of such a relationship outside the family? From an investment perspective, adults develop or maintain a relationship with a partner according to what is gained from the association.

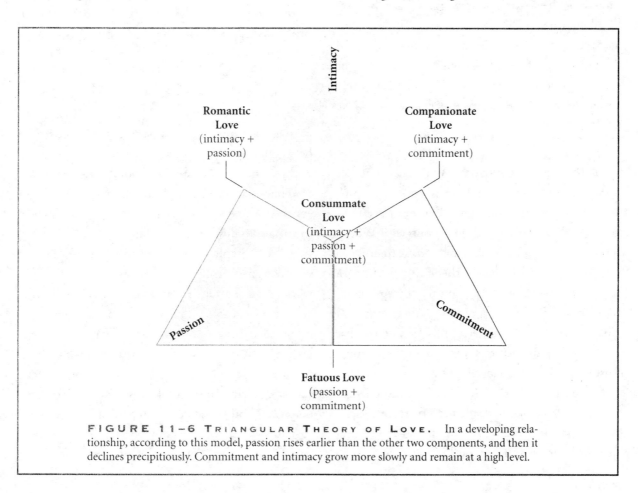

FIGURE 11–6 TRIANGULAR THEORY OF LOVE. In a developing relationship, according to this model, passion rises earlier than the other two components, and then it declines precipitously. Commitment and intimacy grow more slowly and remain at a high level.

DEVELOPING RELATIONSHIPS

The simplest explanation states that we like people associated with good times. Watching the ocean or enjoying a meal with someone can lead to liking that person. In the same way, through classical conditioning, a series of negative events with someone, such as shivering on a cold beach, becoming ill, or failing in school, can lead to an aversion.

Further, we prefer to be with people who support our actions, listen to our ideas, and provide physical comfort. Our response is a function of the outcome of our behavior, called the **reinforcement principle** in operant conditioning. In fact, B. F. Skinner has suggested that partnership love is simply mutual reinforcement. Each person gains something from the relationship. A man behaves in a humorous, playful style admired by his partner. He receives compliments; the partner enjoys the company of a light-hearted individual. The partner approaches the world in a practical, realistic manner that the man appreciates—and so forth.

EXCHANGE THEORY. Why then do people sometimes terminate a relationship from which they receive positive outcomes? During her sophomore year, Dawn stopped going out with Will, a handsome young man who was most attentive to her. According to **exchange theory,** maintaining a relationship depends not just on reinforcement but also on a gain that is greater than the overall expense. Crass as it may seem, this view states that an interpersonal relationship, like any other purchase or exchange, is judged in terms of profit and loss (Homans, 1974). Dawn's positive experiences with Will did not outweigh her effort and sacrifice—socializing only with Will's friends, tolerating his odd hours, and accepting his abuse. She broke off the relationship because the magnitude of the gain was not worth the cost.

Exchange theory is applicable even in abusive relationships and sexual harassment. An abused partner makes the decision to leave or remain on the basis of predictable decision rules regarding costs and benefits. The decision to stay may seem irrational to the outsider and may be irrational, but the decision process is not inherently abnormal or incompatible with exchange theory (Strube, 1991a).

In her emerging relationship with Stephen, Dawn was overjoyed by his attentiveness and willingness to help with her debts. These traits outweighed his tendency to drinking bouts and lack of academic focus. Stephen, in turn, found Dawn intellectually stimulating and physically attractive, characteristics more important to him than her emotional instability and financial problems. For both partners, the gain was greater than the cost.

EQUITY THEORY. According to another viewpoint, even relationships based on a gain greater than the cost are sometimes terminated, and here equity becomes the issue. Equity is concerned with fairness, and **equity theory** states that we maintain a relationship if the outcome is at least equal to what we feel we merit, weighing all of our social attributes against the norms of society. If Dawn and Stephen continued their relationship, it would be because each of them derived from it what he or she felt was merited, regardless of the cost–benefit margin. This viewpoint may seem even more calculating than exchange theory, but it has been demonstrated empirically that we tend to find partners of essentially our own social value, measured in terms of mental, physical, social, economic, and other indices. Mate selection, according to equity theory, is a compromise between our desire for an ideal partner and the realization that

THEORY	EXAMPLE
Conditioning: each partner gains something.	Dawn receives protection and comfort from a PERSON. Stephen gains the attention of someone who is open and smiling.
Exchange: each partner gains more than the relationship costs.	Dawn feels that Stephen's attentiveness and assistance with her debts outweigh his drinking bouts and lack of focus. Stephen finds Dawn's intellectual stimulation and physical attractiveness worth the problem of her emotional instability.
Equity: each partner gains what he or she feels is merited.	Dawn decides that Stephen, overall, is worth what she deserves. Stephen decides that Dawn is right for him, taking into account all their assets and limitations.

TABLE 11–4 MAINTAINING A RELATIONSHIP. The conditioning viewpoint merely considers the benefit. Exchange and equity theory consider the benefit in the context of cost and worth, respectively.

we probably must settle for what we seem to be worth (Walster & Walster, 1978; Table 11–4).

In one instance, support for equity theory was gathered from more than 300 college students, each engaged in a dating relationship. They were asked to make extensive observations about themselves, their partner, and the relationship. It was found that the students in the most equitable relationships were the most content with their partners and most committed to them (Winn, Crawford, & Fischer, 1991).

Equity theory does not maintain that all potential partners actively engage in a process of calculating their worth and then bartering for a mate on the open market, much as they might haggle over the purchase of an old picture frame at a garage sale. Rather, it states that an enduring relationship, within or outside marriage, often reflects some social assessment, intentionally or otherwise. As even the poet knows, "Everything must go to market." This search for equity has been found in physician–patient satisfactions and public interest transactions, as well as personal relationships (Koehler, Fottler, & Swan, 1992; Van Dijk & Wilke, 1993).

In contrast, the popular press strengthens a very different notion: romantic love, with its more idealized view of the participants and their alliance. Many partners regard their relationship in this manner. Their lives have been joined not through some vague assessment process but because they were destined for each other. According to this view, true love conquers all, even an assessment error.

LOVE RELATIONSHIPS

During her high school years, Dawn made a promise to herself. Looking at her parents' marital problems and at other unsuccessful marriages, she decided that she would marry someone who would simply find her comfortable and socially convenient, in return for his very definite economic assets. Dawn here espoused a form of equity theory, assuming that each partner receives what he or she is worth. She also implied that there are degrees of liking and loving.

The bond between Dawn and Stephen began as simple liking, and then it changed to love, at least for Stephen. "I am now a newer person," he said. "I feel myself glowing to the people around the dark room" (Goethals & Klos, 1976).

Love, the subject of ballads and the object of research, is very difficult to define—along with intelligence, adjustment, creativity, and many other psychological concepts. Nevertheless, one approach has identified six basic *styles* of love. The three primary styles include erotic love, game-playing love, and friendship love; the three secondary styles include practical love, possessive love, and selfless love (Lee, 1973; Table 11–5).

The love styles of women tend toward friendship and practical love. Men engage in more erotic and game-playing love (Hendrick, Hendrick, Foote, & Slapion-Foote, 1984).

Love also has been considered from the viewpoint of *stages* rather than styles, and here two stages have received special attention: passionate and companionate love. When compared with the styles just mentioned, they are closest to erotic love and friendship love, respectively.

PASSIONATE LOVE. The highly aroused, somewhat confused state Stephen described is known as passionate love, erotic love, or sometimes romantic love. In **passionate love**, the partner is perceived in an idealized form, often with the expectation of complete and lasting fulfillment, and sexual attraction is a potent factor. The relationship is intense, sometimes volatile, and viewed with high hopes.

Style	Attribute
Erotic	Instant physical attraction and passion
Game playing	Multiple partners, chasing and catching
Friendship	Long-standing relations, companionship
Practical	Careful assessment of specific traits
Possessive	Dependence on the relationship, lovesickness
Selfless	Spiritual, unselfish, concern for the partner

TABLE 11–5 STYLES OF LOVE. These styles also have Greek names. From top to bottom, they are: *eros, ludus, storge, pragma, mania,* and *agape* (Hendrick & Hendrick, 1986).

In this state of romantic love, Stephen proposed marriage. Dawn replied that she could not decide so quickly. A half hour later, she said simply: "Yes" (Goethals & Klos, 1976). In that interim, perhaps Dawn was pondering some dimension of equity theory. Stephen was having difficulty planning his life, and he came from a background quite different from hers. What were the long-range implications? What would her mother say?

In the United States, romantic or passionate love has been considered essential to a successful marriage and widely promoted in the mass media. Nevertheless, it is quite foreign to many contemporary cultures in which marriages are arranged, often early in life. Here the sexual aspects are considered less important than mutual interests and the exchange of ideas.

Passionate love is fleeting, despite the partners' fondest hopes. Inevitably, it must decline, not necessarily to end in pieces but at least in another form. One reason is that we cannot continue to receive increased pleasure from any form of stimulation, a phenomenon known as *adaptation*. Potato soup, a downhill ski run, and a partner's caresses all become less intensely satisfying with successive repetitions. A second reason concerns human development. We are always changing. Unless our partner, also changing, miraculously meets these new needs as well, we find that we are falling out of love, or in and out of love, or that our love is changing. It has been said that one difference between partners who decide to separate and those who stay together is the recognition of this fluctuating condition.

COMPANIONATE LOVE. If we stay in the relationship, this changed love often becomes **companionate love**, which is a deep affection for others with whom our lives are closely interwoven. It is less intense, more enduring, and more realistic than passionate love. In terms of the earlier triangular theory, companionate love can be considered a combination of intimacy and commitment. It is not true love any more than passionate love is true love. They are simply different forms of love.

Within long-term families there is companionate love between the spouses, between parents and children, and among brothers and sisters, but almost inevitably rivalries develop as well. Older people, as might be expected, place more emphasis on a companionate relationship, as opposed to a passionate one (Figure 11–7).

☙

EXPERIENCING SEX

And now for sex, a potent contributor to love at many ages, although far from indispensable. Sex can be involved at all stages of liking and loving, and it can be mixed with achievement and aggression.

Careful laboratory studies of the physiology of sex indicate two major changes in the body that underlie the great variety of sexual experiences in males and females alike. There is an increased flow of blood into the pelvic area, made possible by the dilation of the blood vessels. This extra blood supply, known as **vasocongestion,** has diverse repercussions, including engorgement of the sexual organs. In addition there is **myotonia,** which involves contractions of the muscles throughout the body, resulting in facial expressions, voluntary movements in the limbs, and involuntary spasms in the genital areas.

MALE SEXUAL RESPONSE. The reaction of the male is a continuous process best understood as four stages of a cycle: excitement, plateau, orgasm, and resolution. Physiological changes take place during each phase.

In the excitement phase, vasocongestion produces erection of the penis, possibly erection in the nipples, and perhaps reddening of the skin. There is a rise in pulse rate, respiration, and muscular tension until the plateau phase, during which the peak of sexual arousal is reached. The orgasm provides a release of this tension, and it occurs in two sub-

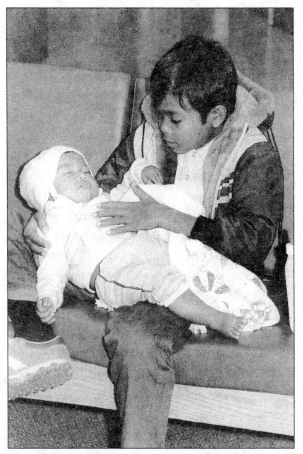

FIGURE 11–7 FAMILIAL LOVE.
Companionate love between siblings may be fostered by a significant age gap, enabling the older child to give and the younger to receive assistance. When children are closer in age, rivalries more often accompany familial affection.

stages. In the first, the inevitability of ejaculation is experienced in the contraction of the seminal vesicles, vas deferens, and prostate gland. The actual ejaculation, at intervals of .8 second, constitutes the second substage, and it is these contractions that are most closely associated with the pleasurable aspects of orgasm.

Following orgasm, there is a gradual return to the nonaroused state. This resolution phase, during which vasocongestion and myotonia disappear, involves a loss of sexual responsiveness. During this refractory period, the capacity for full sexual arousal, including erection, does not return immediately. The interval before its reappearance varies a great deal from one individual to another, lasting up to 24 hours or more in some instances.

FEMALE SEXUAL RESPONSE. Like the return of arousability in males, the whole cycle in females is highly variable from one person to another. Most females show the four-stage response, but in some women the excitement and orgasm stages are closely merged, as in a series of orgasms. In others there may be no discernible plateau. The four-step model is only representative of a typical sequence (Figure 11–8).

The important changes in the excitement phase include vasocongestion of the clitoris and seepage of vaginal fluid through the vaginal walls. This seepage, prompted by the blood engorgement of the genitals, furnishes the lubrication necessary for intercourse. It may be accompanied by the reddening sex flush and by swelling and erection of the nipples, resulting from vasocongestion and myotonia. These changes become intensified in the plateau phase, producing the tension necessary for orgasmic experience. Again, the rhyth-

mic contractions in orgasm occur at approximately .8-second intervals, but compared to the male's ejaculation, there is less external evidence of orgasm.

Afterward, there is no clear period of sexual inexcitability. With appropriate stimulation a woman can experience another orgasm during the resolution phase, but the reaction is diminished.

SEXUAL PROBLEMS. The chief sexual problems experienced by men are *erectile difficulties*, formerly known as impotence, and *premature ejaculation*, in which orgasm occurs too early. For women, the chief problems are *orgasmic difficulties*, traditionally known as frigidity. These newer terms reflect more tolerant attitudes toward sexual problems, including the view that they are often psychological. Many sexual problems reflect interpersonal factors *between* the partners, rather than the adjustment of one individual, and then they must be treated as such (Stravynski & Greenberg, 1990).

Sometimes there is no known physical or interpersonal problem, and then a straightforward pro-

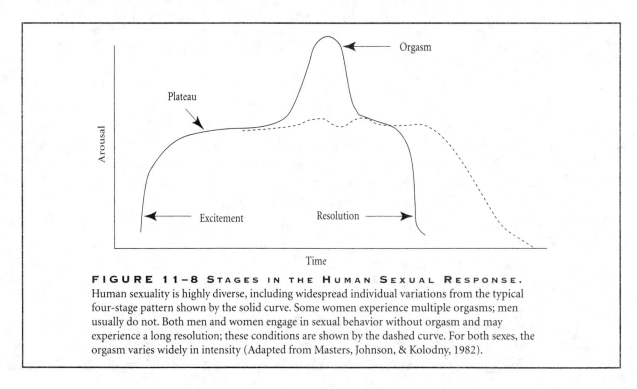

FIGURE 11–8 STAGES IN THE HUMAN SEXUAL RESPONSE. Human sexuality is highly diverse, including widespread individual variations from the typical four-stage pattern shown by the solid curve. Some women experience multiple orgasms; men usually do not. Both men and women engage in sexual behavior without orgasm and may experience a long resolution; these conditions are shown by the dashed curve. For both sexes, the orgasm varies widely in intensity (Adapted from Masters, Johnson, & Kolodny, 1982).

cedure may be used. It begins with the couple in counseling sessions, aimed at the identification of negative attitudes toward sex and common causes of sexual problems, including unexpressed anger and guilt feelings. Then, in private, the couple starts to practice sexual exercises. In these activities, called the **sensate focus,** the partners take turns being the giver and receiver of sensual touching and pleasure—exploring the contours, textures, and odors of the partner's body, with no demands for performance. Relaxed closeness is the goal. Eventually, the couple moves toward increased sexual contact.

SEXUAL BEHAVIOR

Superimposed on these bodily responses are countless psychological dimensions arising through opportunities for learning. They can be enormously influential in sexual behavior and preferences. During high school, Dawn found masturbation pleasurable, and she practiced it in the imagined company of others. Stephen's early experiences took place on a bus with a female partner two years older than he. To the extent that these experiences were successful and gratifying, they played an important role in subsequent sexual interests.

MASTURBATION. The most common approach to sexual activity among adolescents and young adults is *masturbation,* in which satisfaction is obtained from direct stimulation of the genitals, usually self-stimulation. Our changing attitudes toward this practice, which occurs throughout adult life, illustrate the potent role of social forces in sexual expression. During the first half of this century, masturbation was strongly discouraged in many parts of the United States. Children were told that it was sinful, would damage the nervous system, and would make them unfit for business careers. Physicians stated: "Masturbation is one of the causes of insanity. To ascertain this fact it is only necessary to look over the reports of any of the

insane asylums of the land" (Whitehead & Hoff, 1929).

Today, with greater understanding of problems of personal adjustment, masturbation has been suggested in some treatment plans for sexual dysfunction. In reputable therapies, these exercises are presented along with activities for developing social skills, self-confidence, and healthy attitudes toward other adjustment issues (Stravynski & Greenberg, 1990).

HETEROSEXUAL PARTNERS. The wide variety in sexual behavior has been evident ever since the groundbreaking Kinsey surveys in the middle of this century. These studies showed that both men and women engaged in more diverse sexual outlets inside and outside marriage than even the experts would have predicted (Kinsey, Pomeroy, & Martin, 1948; Kinsey, Pomeroy, & Gebhard, 1953). These included *heterosexuality,* in which the attraction is toward a person of the opposite sex, and *homosexuality,* an attraction toward a person of one's own sex. In the immediately succeeding decades, with more liberal attitudes toward parenting, education, and lifestyles, together with birth control devices and treatments for sexual diseases, attitudes toward sexual behavior became even more liberal. But rather suddenly, in the early 1980s, a condition arose that ran counter to this sexual revolution—acquired immune deficiency syndrome (AIDS). The ease with which this disease can be transmitted has prompted the need for restraint in sexual activity.

Under the threat of AIDS, to what extent have heterosexual individuals actually changed their sexual practices? In an extensive study in the Netherlands, 512 heterosexual adults with multiple sexual partners were interviewed. Follow-up interviews were arranged every four months over a period of two years, attended by 340 of the subjects, 60% female and 40% male. The results indicated little change in genital, oral, and anal practices between heterosexual *private partners*. However, both men and women considerably reduced the number of private partners. There has been no apparent decline in the number of *commercial partners*—prostitutes and clients—but condom use among these partners has increased considerably (Hooykaas, Van der Linden, Van Doornum, & Van der Velde, 1991).

In the United States, one study focused on 101 dating couples rather than individuals with multiple sexual partners. Within these apparently monogamous relationships there was little change in sexual behaviors, although women reported themselves as more cautious than men (Sprecher, 1990).

HOMOSEXUAL PARTNERS. Attitudes toward homosexuality also have changed markedly over the course of human history. Among the ancient Greeks, homosexuality was encouraged. Beginning in the 1700s, when all forms of sexuality were seen as medical issues, homosexuality became greatly suppressed in the Western world. By the mid-twentieth century, slightly more than one of every three males reportedly had experienced an orgasm by homosexual contact, a figure considerably higher than was expected despite a possible bias in the sample (Kinsey, Pomeroy, & Martin, 1948). More recently, the American Psychiatric Association decided that homosexuality is not a psychiatric disorder and classified it as a disturbance only if the individual is in conflict about it. To prevent or diminish this conflict, the homosexual community has made efforts to assist gay and lesbian adolescents in understanding their sexuality and gaining a positive identity (Schneider, 1991).

In many parts of the world, including this country, there are more homosexual men than women, and investigators have tried to explain this difference. One hypothesis stresses the time of onset of the sex drive. Females begin puberty around age 11, but the sex drive does not appear for another three or four years. In males, puberty and the sex drive both begin around age 13. Until the early teens, friendships in both sexes are typically with members of the same sex. Males experience the onset of the sex drive in this context, whereas females experience it after the initiation of heterosexual contacts. On this basis, it is reasonable to expect more eroticization of homosexual cues among males and, insofar as fantasy is a component of sexual orientation, more homosexuality also (Storms, 1981).

From a very different perspective, one investigator compared the development of the hypothalamus in 41 human adults, many of whom had died from AIDS. The subjects included 19 homosexual men, 16 heterosexual men, and 6 heterosexual women. Prior studies with animals had shown that certain regions of the hypothalamus are larger in males than females and that this development depends in part on hormones, specifically in utero exposure to androgens. Among the men, one area of the hypothalamus in the heterosexual group was found to be approximately twice the size of this area in the homosexual subjects. For the women and homosexual men, the hypothalamic regions were approximately the same size. When comparisons were made between people who died of AIDS and those who died of other causes, no differences were found (Le Vay, 1991). Thus, it appeared that the cause of death probably was not a factor in the different sizes of the hypothalamus.

These results may be viewed in various ways. First, are they reliable? If so, does sexual orientation influence brain development or vice versa? Is there an interaction between sexual preference and development of the hypothalamus? To what extent, if any, are these differences related to hormonal conditions prior to birth? Whatever the outcome, these findings certainly do not rule out social factors, and again, the central message in the first chapter of this book is relevant: the multiple bases of behavior. Homosexuality, like creativity, alcoholism, heterosexuality, and artistic success, appears to be stimulated by a complex interplay of social, psychological, and physiological interactions, perhaps varying widely from one individual to another (Money, 1988).

SEX WITH AN OBJECT. Individuals are sometimes motivated to engage in sexual behavior in connection with a particular object. When this attachment is so strong that the presence of the object is essential for sexual gratification, the condition is called **fetishism.** Clothing, especially shoes, gloves, beads, and underwear, often becomes involved in fetishes. It is believed that the attachment is acquired through learning experiences in the early years, perhaps related to a neurological readiness for the conditioning of certain stimuli.

Within and across cultures, all sorts of objects and events are intended to augment sexual interest. These range from perfumes and cosmetics used in everyday life to hardware and apparel employed behind closed doors. The latter activities are discussed more fully in the chapter on adjustment.

• ANGER AND AGGRESSION •

Dawn was worried. Her mother opposed her approaching marriage for all sorts of reasons. In the first place, the bride and groom were too young. Worse yet, Stephen espoused a different religion, was an underachiever, and showed no clear job prospects. And Dawn had a promising career in arts and letters if she devoted herself extensively to those pursuits.

Dawn was worried because anger and aggression had been recurrent problems in their family; she argued loudly with her mother over the phone; and she wondered what would happen at the wedding. "There was always a battle," she said about her parents, who lived in bitterness on separate floors at opposite ends of the house.

Matters were little better for Stephen. His parents accepted the forthcoming marriage, but that was one of the few topics on which they agreed. Stephen's mother often insulted his father, and

eventually they became divorced. There was anger on both sides and actual aggression by his mother (Goethals & Klos, 1976).

Anger and aggression both involve hostility, but there is an important difference. In **anger,** *feelings* of hostility and displeasure are the chief characteristic. There may be angry behavior too, but there is no significant attack. In **aggression,** the *behavior* is dominant; there is an assault on another person or some object. However, angry feelings often underlie aggressive behavior.

ORIGINS OF AGGRESSION

American society is an aggressive society. Football is not a contact sport—but a collision sport. Our television thrives on shootouts, war stories, and murder mysteries. The press widely publicizes crime and aggravated assault. With this problem so extremely prevalent, not just in the United States but elsewhere as well, the origins of aggression have become a controversial issue (Figure 11–9).

PREDISPOSITIONAL VIEW. According to some experts, human beings may have an inherited

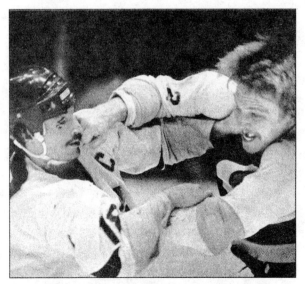

FIGURE 11–9 AN ENVIRONMENT OF AGGRESSION. Aggressive acts dominate sports, films, and newspapers in the United States. Without doubt, a great deal of aggressive behavior is learned through these displays.

517

predisposition for aggressive behavior. These experts, typically from backgrounds in ethology and animal behavior, note the aggression in the animal kingdom. Iguanas butt heads; howler monkeys battle with deafening vocalizations; spiders and praying mantises eat their own kind. Animals fight to obtain food or a mate, to establish a territory, and to gain a position in a social hierarchy. Human beings have all of these concerns. Territorial rights, in particular, have been an object of warfare throughout human history (Lorenz, 1963; Morris, 1967).

Another view of aggression as innate comes from psychoanalysis and the work of Sigmund Freud, widely recognized for postulating two human instincts. One of these, the **life instinct,** or *eros*, motivates us to self-preservation, love, and sexual urges that result in the preservation of the species. The other, the **death instinct,** or *thanatos*, impels us toward the cessation of life's tensions. The ultimate aim of life, in this sense, is death, which is brought about partly by our destructive tendencies toward ourselves and others. Freud arrived at this conclusion through studies in evolutionary biology, experiences in World War I, and the military buildup before World War II. For him, the life and death instincts were constantly at odds, but the eventual winner was always the death instinct (Freud, 1915).

The chief objection to Freud's view is that there is no solid evidence in biology that a fundamental instinct in life aims to abolish all tension. This concept contradicts biological principles (Brun, 1953). However, the term *instinct* here reflects a lack of precision in translation from the German. Freud was not intending our modern definition of instinct—a complex, unlearned behavior pattern—but rather a broad urge, a *drive*, a motivational disposition. It is reasonable to postulate an aggressive drive much as one might postulate a sex drive, as a reservoir of energy to behave in a certain fashion. The two basic Freudian drives, sex and aggression, are regarded by many modern psycho-analysts and others as underlying a wide variety of behaviors, ranging from striving for power to conquests in love.

Both drives appear to be involved in **rape,** a violent sexual act based on physical assault or threats of harm. Rape is far more frequent than the crime statistics suggest, chiefly because many cases go unreported for fear of reprisal, embarrassment, or both. One form of rape, called *date rape*, involves acquaintances, not strangers, and in one large survey almost 10% of college women reported that they had been forced into sexual intercourse in this way (Koss, Gidycz, & Wisniewski, 1987). Sexual and aggressive elements are intertwined in rape of all kinds, making this behavior a highly complex problem.

ROLE OF LEARNING. For other investigators more compelling evidence on the origins of aggression is found in the environment. Learning theorists contend, for example, that if guns were more restricted, there would be less violence, and most studies favor this position—that aggressive behavior is increased by the presence of stimuli related to aggression. In typical research, subjects who experience frustration in the context of guns, clubs, and so forth show more aggressive reactions than do those who experience the same frustration in neutral circumstances (Berkowitz & LePage, 1967; Cahoon & Edmunds, 1984).

In addition to stimuli directly related to aggression, less obvious environmental conditions also are associated with aggressive behavior, such as crowdedness and even the weather. In one experiment with four rat colonies, conditions were arranged so that the first and last pens had only one entrance each. A dominant male controlled each of these pens, and the population stabilized at the expected level. The other two pens had two entrances each, and these colonies soon became extremely crowded. Social organization was markedly disrupted, with fighting and cannibalism among the males, neglect of the young by females, and aberrant sexual behavior in both sexes. The outcome in this environment was called a *behavioral sink,* referring to the destructive, pathological reaction that developed in the overcrowded conditions (Calhoun, 1962).

Still another factor involves observational learning. Children who are controlled by aggression become aggressive themselves (Bandura, 1986). There is some humor but no consolation in the cartoon showing an angry father spanking his child and saying: "There! That'll teach you not to hit your little brother!" There is, in fact, research evidence indicating that harsh parenting is transmitted across generations in this way (Simons, Whitbeck, Conger, & Wu, 1991). Investigations of televised aggression support this viewpoint. Most of the thousands of studies, reviewed in a massive report by the National Institute of Mental Health, indicate that watching aggression on television is a likely *cause* of aggression in children and adolescents (Figure 11–10).

REDUCING AGGRESSION

The argument over innate and learned factors in aggression arises partly because different definitions are involved. Sometimes aggression is defined as a vigorous pursuit of self-preservation, as when dispassionate animals kill merely for food. On this basis almost all organisms are potentially aggressive, for all of us have an innate desire to satisfy physiological needs. Aggression is also defined as the desire to inflict harm on another individual or object, even when there is no obvious gain. This behavior certainly seems learned, for it does not appear in animals or even in most human beings.

Regardless of the difficulties in definition, the important issue is this underlying question: How can we diminish whatever destructive predispositions exist among us?

CATHARSIS HYPOTHESIS. One view involves catharsis, which is a release of pent-up emotion. According to the **catharsis hypothesis,** the expression of anger, anxiety, or other feelings reduces

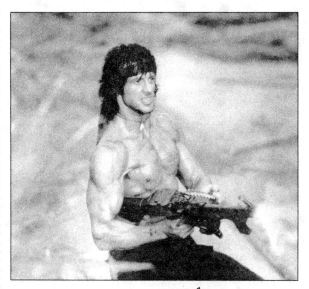

FIGURE 11–10 VIOLENCE IN FILMS. For most psychologists, the burden of proof has shifted. It now stands for film makers to demonstrate that the portrayal of violence does not stimulate aggression in viewers (Hoberman, 1990; Rubinstein, 1983).

the underlying drive, just as eating reduces the hunger drive. In this view, Dawn's ranting and raving after a disruptive phone conversation with her mother decreased her tendency to behave aggressively. Similarly, Stephen's expressions of anger diminished his inclination to behave aggressively against the furniture. However, the research points to a different conclusion. Opportunities for crying do not necessarily reduce depressive feelings (Kraemer & Hastrup, 1988). Opportunities for expressing anger have even sustained this feeling (Averill, 1982). Overall, the evidence is against the catharsis hypothesis (Bennett, 1991; Lewis & Bucher, 1992).

A variety of studies from the laboratory and clinic indicate another approach: talking and writing about the problem. This procedure can be helpful—up to a point. Reviewing what happened often brings a sense of completion. The person needs to confront the anger directly, make a confession, and then try to view it as a resolved matter.

FRUSTRATION-AGGRESSION HYPOTHESIS. A very different hypothesis points to the role of frustrating circumstances in the origins of aggression and therefore has implications for reducing it. In this view, called the **frustration-aggression hypothesis,** aggressive behavior always presupposes frustration, and frustration inevitably leads to some form of aggression. When the boss fails to negotiate a business deal, we are not surprised if she is a bit nasty (Dollard, Miller, Doob, Mowrer, & Sears, 1939).

Dawn was very happy with Stephen, unless her new world was ruptured by a phone call from her mother. After yelling over the telephone, frustrated by their inability to communicate, Dawn sometimes became aggressive with Stephen too. More respectful of his partner, Stephen bashed the furniture when he felt frustrated about his schoolwork (Goethals & Klos, 1976). The frustration-aggression hypothesis seems to be supported in these everyday examples.

The role of frustration in aggression also has been demonstrated in laboratory and field studies. In young children, the single best predictor of physical aggression is language immaturity—that is, an inability to express oneself well in words, clearly a source of frustration (Piel, 1990).

However, aggression sometimes occurs without frustration, and frustration does not always lead to aggression. A frustrated person may cry, complain, or withdraw instead. On these bases, the hypothesis has been revised: Frustration leads to a *readiness* to behave in an aggressive fashion. Then the appearance of aggressive behavior is significantly determined by environmental factors (Berkowitz, 1988, 1989). Even in this revised form, the hypothesis has implications for reducing aggression. These efforts must begin in the home, teaching children to deal more effectively with frustration, and they must include programs of assistance for underprivileged people who face overwhelming frustration daily.

This view, sometimes called the *cultural hypothesis,* states that aggression is learned through social or cultural patterns. The Zuni in North America have long been a pastoral, peaceful people. The Comanche, in earlier years, had a tradition of aggressiveness and self-assertion. In New Guinea, the Arapesh regarded self-assertion and aggressiveness as abnormal. The Mundugumor fostered these behaviors and used aggressive methods to prepare the young for survival (Mead, 1939). It is clear that social conditions can mold aggressive, aggression-prone, or basically peaceful individuals, almost regardless of the ways their needs are satisfied.

• STRESS IN DAILY LIFE •

All cultures involve restrictions of some sort, and all of us are faced with the problem of satisfying physiological needs, as well as psychological motives. To the extent that we encounter difficulties in these respects, we experience stress. The condition of **stress** is a state of tension, strain, or conflict within an individual that has the potential to disrupt physical, mental, and behavioral functions. The person's normal balance or stability is threatened, requiring compensatory reactions or readjustments.

For Dawn, Stephen, and their families, the impending wedding brought forth various forms of stress and efforts at readjustment. Dawn's mother ordered the invitations and, in a moment of tension, forgot the RSVP cards. Aunts and uncles tried to find suitable gifts and make appropriate travel plans. The wedding couple faced last-minute chores and doubts. And both families made efforts to adjust to future in-laws.

☙

STRESSFUL EVENTS

Stressful events can be chronic or fleeting, physical or psychological. Winning a scholarship, having a baby, and taking a vacation all require readjustment, as do divorce, loans, and retirement. In short, stressful events are changes of all sorts, positive or negative.

LIFE CHANGES. A popular approach to the measurement of stress emphasizes these changes in routines. Barriers and choices underlie many of them, but the chief issue in *life changes* is the extent to which they require readjustment by the individual. An instrument called the *Social Readjustment Rating Scale* presents 43 life changes in decreasing order of the readjustments they typically require. The sequence and numerical values assigned to these events were determined by asking many subjects to rate them for the degree of readjustment involved, regardless of its desirability. On this basis, death of a spouse and divorce were the most stressful events; Christmas and vacation were toward the bottom of the scale (Holmes & Rahe, 1967).

With their marriage, Dawn and Stephen would commence the life change ranked seventh on the scale. Both partners had already experienced trouble with their prospective in-laws, a problem ranked in the middle of the scale. With school over for the year, they were beginning a vacation, a mildly stressful occasion. As for their parents, they were having a son or daughter leave home, an event also ranked in the middle of the scale. For both families, the wedding was stressful beyond any bumbling or personal animosities that occurred (Table 11–6).

The wedding day also proved stressful. It rained the whole time. Dawn forgot her lines; the couple kissed too early in the ceremony; the reception was anything but jovial; and the crowd dwindled early. "The day . . . bestowed heroism on us all," observed Stephen wryly (Goethals & Klos, 1976).

CRITIQUE OF THE SCALE. People with high scores on the readjustment scale are considered to be under greater stress than those with low scores, especially if these scores are generated by negative events. The scale is not without its limitations, however. It omits events that may be highly significant for certain individuals, such as crime in the city and loneliness in the country. It also ignores how the person *feels* about that event. Earthquakes, surgical operations, and bankruptcy may be regarded very differently by different people.

RANK	LIFE EVENT	SCORE
1	Death of spouse	100
2	Divorce	73
3	Marital separation	65
4	Jail term	63
5	Death of close family member	63
6	Personal injury or illness	53
7	✓ Marriage	50
8	Fired at work	47
9	Marital reconciliation	45
10	Retirement	45
11	Change in health of family member	44
12	Pregnancy	40
13	Sex difficulties	39
14	Gain of new family member	39
15	Business readjustment	39
16	Change in financial state	38
17	Death of close friend	37
18	Change to different line of work	36
19	Change in number of arguments with spouse	35
20	Mortgage over $10,000	31
21	Foreclosure of mortgage or loan	30
22	Change in responsibilities at work	29
23	Son or daughter leaving home	29
24	✓ Trouble with in-laws	29
25	Outstanding personal achievement	28
26	Wife begin or stop work	26
27	Begin or end school	26
28	✓ Change in living conditions	25
29	Revision of personal habits	24
30	Trouble with boss	23
31	Change in work hours or conditions	20
32	Change in residence	20
33	Change in schools	20
34	Change in recreation	19
35	Change in church activities	19
36	Change in social activities	18
37	Mortgage or loan less than $10,000	17
38	Change in sleeping habits	16
39	Change in number of family get-togethers	15
40	Change in eating habits	15
41	✓ Vacation	13
42	Christmas	12
43	Minor violations of the law	11

TABLE 11–6 SOCIAL READJUSTMENT RATING SCALE. To determine the amount of stress someone is experiencing, the scores for all applicable events are summed. The checkmarks indicate events experienced by Dawn and Stephen at the time of their wedding. Note that the mortgage in item 20 depicts economic conditions 30 years ago (Holmes & Rahe, 1967).

Also, people who have suffered the death of a spouse or some other recent tragedy are especially vulnerable to other sources of stress. In fact, several of the life changes indicated on the stress scale may be the *result of stress,* rather than its cause. Divorce, disease, and dissatisfaction at work all may be exacerbated, if not caused, by the individual's reaction to some other major stressful event.

The readjustment scale also ignores hassles and minor problems, such as the late arrival of the mail, waiting lines for the bathroom, and poor service at the bus station. There is also routine but subtle stress in many jobs: the vigilance of the air traffic controller, the strain of the keyboard operator, and conflict with coworkers. In combination with other minor adversities, these events may be more stressful than some of those on the scale (De Longis, Coyne, Dekaf, Folkman, & Lazarus, 1982).

TYPES OF CONFLICT. Other stressful situations do not necessarily involve a life change but rather making a choice. In this circumstance, called a **conflict,** one choice or motive is opposed by one or more alternatives; all outcomes cannot be achieved. The conflict may be minor, as in selecting music for a wedding, or major, as in deciding whether or not to get married in the first place or choosing between two parents in a custody case. The latter conflicts clearly precede a life change.

Conflicts have been viewed in several categories. In the first, the **approach-approach conflict,** two or more equally attractive alternatives are incompatible. The fabled donkey, flanked by equally enticing and distant bales of hay, is said to have starved in the midst of plenty, a highly unlikely outcome. In contrast, two or more alternatives may be equally repellent, resulting in an **avoidance-avoidance conflict.** A man must work for a nasty boss or search for other employment.

Sometimes, rather than two or more alternatives, there is a single possibility with both positive and negative aspects, which is the **approach-avoidance conflict.** The use of alcohol is often a complex approach-avoidance conflict for college students (Schall, Kemeny, & Maltzman, 1992). Here we speak of *ambivalence,* meaning that the individual has positive and negative feelings about the same event. Sometimes, however, there are several possibilities, each with positive and negative features, resulting in a multiple approach-avoidance conflict. Contemplating a vacation, a woman wants to please her husband by visiting his family, but she finds them boring. She also wants to go to a conference on mountaineering, but it will be very expensive. One reason decisions are so difficult is that we experience opposed feelings about so many things (Lewin, 1935).

OUTCOMES OF CONFLICT. Compared to other conflicts, the approach-approach situation is easily resolved. When faced with two equally attractive choices, human beings will find a reason to select one of them. After all, they are *attractive.* A hungry man who likes lobster and steak will not let himself starve because he cannot make a choice. Even donkeys make choices, overcoming approach-approach dilemmas.

The avoidance-avoidance conflict presents more complications because the individual does not want to make any choice at all. A man must pay a large debt or run the risk of a lawsuit. Trying to avoid these *unattractive* alternatives, he may take a business trip, obtain another legal opinion, or decide that he must file for bankruptcy. In daily life, people often seek some escape from the whole situation.

Now what would happen if someone needing surgery, for example, viewed the hospital as having both positive and negative implications? That person would be in an approach-avoidance conflict, a troublesome situation because it involves ambivalence. This decision is made all the more difficult because, as shown in various experiments, when viewed from afar, the positive features of an approach-avoidance conflict often seem to outweigh the negative features. Viewed up close, the negative features seem more prominent. Thus, the person is brought into the conflict by the positive features, readily evident at a distance, and driven away by the negative features, more apparent at close range. For these reasons, the person vacillates, back and forth, and the approach-avoidance conflict may be prolonged.

Sitting in his living room, the prospective patient may have comforting thoughts about a clean and caring hospital with a friendly physician at his bedside. When he arrives at the hospital door, smells the medicinal odors, and hears the screeching ambulance at the emergency dock, he may promptly reject the idea of hospitalization. The approach-avoidance conflict often ends when another factor becomes involved, upsetting the balance between the approach and avoidance tendencies. A friend accompanies the patient to the hospital, and with this new element the balance is shifted and a decision is reached (Figure 11–11).

In resolving these conflicts, flexibility is most important. Nevertheless, it is difficult to inculcate flexibility—inducing chronic "avoiders" to approach a problem and chronic "approachers" to ignore some situations (Roth & Cohen, 1986).

BODILY REACTIONS TO STRESS

Response to stress involves all of the basic dimensions of emotion previously noted: feelings, physiological processes, behavior, and cognitive factors. Each of these topics is considered later in the chapter on adjustment, but certain physiological reactions should be noted here as well.

GENERAL ADAPTATION SYNDROME. Whether it arises from a wedding, an infection, or bankruptcy, stress can produce bodily changes. These physiological reactions to stress, known as the **general adaptation syndrome,** are characterized by three phases: alarm, resistance, and exhaustion. A syndrome is a pattern or organization of symptoms, and here they occur in a sequence (Selye, 1976).

The first phase is the **alarm reaction,** which is the organism's initial defense, an overall bodily

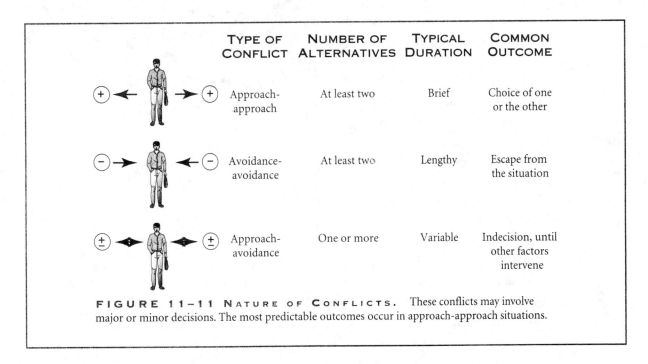

	TYPE OF CONFLICT	NUMBER OF ALTERNATIVES	TYPICAL DURATION	COMMON OUTCOME
	Approach-approach	At least two	Brief	Choice of one or the other
	Avoidance-avoidance	At least two	Lengthy	Escape from the situation
	Approach-avoidance	One or more	Variable	Indecision, until other factors intervene

FIGURE 11–11 NATURE OF CONFLICTS. These conflicts may involve major or minor decisions. The most predictable outcomes occur in approach-approach situations.

response to any stress. Among these defensive forces are increased secretions from the pituitary and adrenal glands, producing the adrenocorticotropic hormone and cortisone. Combined with other stress-reducing changes, these responses enable the organism to sustain the second stage, called **resistance,** which is an emergency reaction requiring much energy. However, the individual's psychological and physiological resources cannot cope endlessly with constant tension; they gradually become depleted, and the person runs the risk of illness. With no diminution of stress, the third and final stage is reached, called **exhaustion,** for the organism's earlier reactions have been repeated until they are no longer possible. If the stress continues, death occurs.

On other occasions, the stress may be brief and beneficial for the individual, facilitating completion of a difficult task, and then it is called **eustress.** In all forms of human existence, stress is inevitable and a certain amount of eustress enhances our lives. The purpose of life is not to avoid all stress; some stress makes us feel good and enables us to engage in athletic competitions, climb mountains, and write term papers.

PSYCHOPHYSIOLOGICAL DISORDERS.

Extended, adverse stress contributes to headaches, sinus problems, skin disorders, allergies, kidney damage, high blood pressure, and many other malfunctions in the individual. Stephen believed that several puzzling physical ailments experienced by his parents were influenced by the stress in their lives. Some years ago these problems were called *psychosomatic disorders,* for they involved psychological influences on the body, or *soma,* but this term was misunderstood. People erroneously decided that there was no bodily problem in a psychosomatic reaction. Today when physical illness or disease is caused or increased by psychological stress, the reaction is known as a **psychophysiological disorder.**

The first clear evidence that ulcers in human beings can be influenced by emotional stress came from observations of a man whose stomach was partially exposed because of injury. While it was being repaired through surgery, it was possible to observe the gastric activities directly and to collect samples of the stomach's contents. When the subject was under stress, his stomach became red and turgid and the production of acid increased sharply. This sequence of events seemed to illustrate the origin of peptic ulcers in human beings (Wolf & Wolff, 1943; Figure 11–12).

Earlier, we noted the relationship between the type A personality and vulnerability to coronary heart disease. The **type A personality** is character-

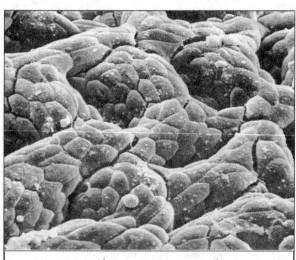

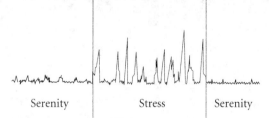

Serenity   Stress   Serenity

FIGURE 11–12 EMOTION AND THE STOMACH. The photo shows the lining of the stomach enlarged 500 diameters. During a period of stress, the patient's stomach activities increased markedly. Amid this overactivity, the stomach tried to digest itself, resulting in hemorrhaging and perforation of ulcers (Wolf & Wolff, 1943; Davenport, 1972).

ized by a sense of urgency, time pressure, and often hostility. Over a period of eight years, the Framingham Heart Study, in Massachusetts, examined more than 1,500 adults classified as type A or as *type B personality*, more relaxed and dispassionate. The incidence of heart disease among type A men was found to be almost triple the incidence among type B men. Among women, the incidence was twice as high for the type A personality (Haynes, Feinleib, & Kannel, 1980).

Related studies have shown the role of extended stress in infectious diseases (Barker, 1987), heart disorders (Taylor, 1991), asthma and arthritis (Friedman & Booth-Kewley, 1987), and even the common cold. In the last study, approximately 400 subjects were administered a cold virus and then, during a seven-day quarantine, they were assessed for cold symptoms. It was discovered that subjects experiencing high levels of stress displayed a rate of cold symptoms twice that of subjects experiencing low levels of stress (Cohen, Tyrrell, & Smith, 1991).

COPING WITH STRESS

Whatever the problem and the physical reaction to it, the individual usually has available a variety of potential coping responses. These have been depicted in several categories, based on the reports of many people coping with stressful events over a period of several weeks (Stone & Neale, 1984). They can be usefully considered with respect to the stressor, stress reaction, and outside assistance.

DEALING WITH THE STRESSOR. In approaching any stressful situation, the first task is to identify the source of the problem. If the problem can be resolved, then the action should deal with the **stressor,** the event in the environment most directly responsible for the stress. After the wedding, Dawn took direct action against an event that could be changed. She asked her mother to stop calling her with problems, making it quite clear that she had new priorities and that Stephen was at the top of the list. "I have my own family now," she said, and her mother responded with silence (Goethals & Klos, 1976).

Sometimes the problem cannot be resolved directly or the cost is too great. Then the best plan may involve a less direct approach. Two such strategies, at times quite effective, include reframing and distraction. In **reframing,** the person thinks about the problem in a new way, viewing it as more tolerable, as a temporary disruption, or perhaps even as a good learning experience. Also known as *restructuring,* the procedure basically involves a transformation of meaning (Bandler & Grinder, 1982).

In counseling situations, reframing has been used with all sorts of personal problems, including divorce. For women in midlife, divorce can mean the loss of social contacts, a small remarriage pool, and possibly discriminatory practices in the labor market, as well as the stresses of aging. In the reframing technique, divorced people are encouraged to regard the experience differently—as an opportunity for growth, independence, and perhaps renewed contacts with their adult children (Bogolub, 1991). Evidence for the beneficial effects of positive thinking has been mounting steadily. A hopeful outlook is good for people (Scheier & Carver, 1993).

The other strategy, **distraction,** focuses attention on some other activity instead. It is commonly useful with children, for they have a short attention span and therefore are readily distracted.

Following the stress of the wedding, Dawn and Stephen left for the seashore and found themselves booked with a middle-aged tour group with whom they were not compatible. They solved the problem by reframing. After all, they *were* at the beach and Dawn's mother had paid for the trip. They also used distraction, making friends with a couple on the islands—who gave Dawn the feeling that a responsive, open-minded marriage was possible.

Another prominent method, hardly a coping strategy, is to accept the situation. In fact, the survey on coping with stress showed acceptance to be the second-most common coping response. Here the individual takes no significant action, direct or indirect, to decrease the stress. Presumably, it seems that nothing can be done, that no action is worth the effort, or that any action would only make matters worse.

After the honeymoon, Stephen went looking for work and found it impossible to obtain any respectable job. "So I turned my sights toward the less respectable," he reported, and his new boss precipitated another problem. The man phoned Dawn and invited her to dinner—secretly. When Stephen found out, he made no secret of his displeasure. "We never got along very well after that," he confided about his boss. But he accepted the situation, working every day for an employer he actively disliked (Goethals & Klos, 1976).

MODIFYING THE STRESS REACTION.
Other approaches involve the physical dimension, rather than the cognitive, and the focus is on the stress reaction, not the stressor. The aim here is to reduce bodily tension which, if chronic, might lead to ulcers, backache, or other psychophysiological disorders. Now widely recognized, these methods include biofeedback and meditation, discussed in earlier chapters, and also systematic desensitization, considered later in the context of therapy.

In addition, modern *relaxation techniques* include methods for control of breathing, muscle relaxation, and visualization. Some people employ this method before going to work or even on the job, using long, slow exhalations, progressively relaxing the muscles from head to toe, and imagining themselves in a green forest or beside a gentle stream, warm and quiet. At the other end of the continuum, vigorous *physical exercise* includes running, aerobics, weight training, and other activities. Among people experiencing stress and then assigned to various exercise programs, including a no-exercise condition, numerous studies show the value of physical exercise for reducing the stress reaction (Folkins & Sime, 1981).

SEEKING OUTSIDE ASSISTANCE.
Eventually, like all couples, Dawn and Stephen began to experience some problems with each other. She decided that Stephen's interest in sex had diminished distinctly during the summer. "A point of great delicacy between us," she noted. She tried not to be demanding, but her requests made them both uneasy.

Stephen quit his job in September, pleased to be finished, but then there were school problems. By this time his "lazy way of life," as he called it, apparently had exerted an undesirable effect on Dawn, diminishing her sense of control and energy. She found herself unable to work around the house and lost a writing routine that previously had produced publishable poetry and prose (Goethals & Klos, 1976).

In coping with these problems, the couple might have sought outside assistance—specifically *support from friends or peers*, obtaining advice or encouragement. As an alternative, they might have sought *support from experts*, consulting a marriage counselor, career counselor, or other professional person. Rejecting both approaches, they might have done nothing significant and the problems might have diminished or vanished. Problems sometimes disappear as spontaneously as they have arisen.

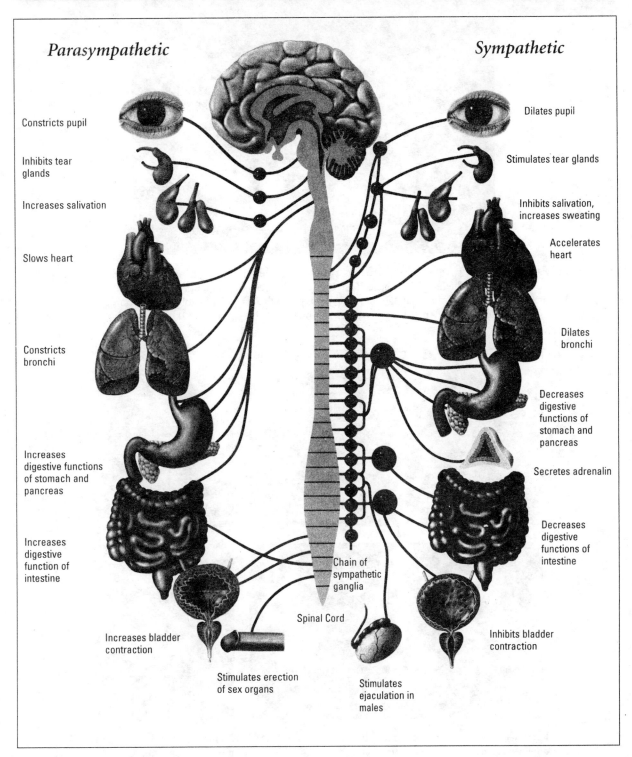

Parasympathetic

Constricts pupil

Inhibits tear glands

Increases salivation

Slows heart

Constricts bronchi

Increases digestive functions of stomach and pancreas

Increases digestive function of intestine

Increases bladder contraction

Stimulates erection of sex organs

Sympathetic

Dilates pupil

Stimulates tear glands

Inhibits salivation, increases sweating

Accelerates heart

Dilates bronchi

Decreases digestive functions of stomach and pancreas

Secretes adrenalin

Decreases digestive functions of intestine

Inhibits bladder contraction

Stimulates ejaculation in males

Chain of sympathetic ganglia

Spinal Cord

FIGURE XI.1 SYMPATHETIC AND PARASYMPATHETIC SYSTEMS. As shown, the sympathetic and parasympathetic systems may influence the same organs, but they do so in different ways. The sympathetic system serves for the release of energy; the parasympathetic serves for its restoration.

527

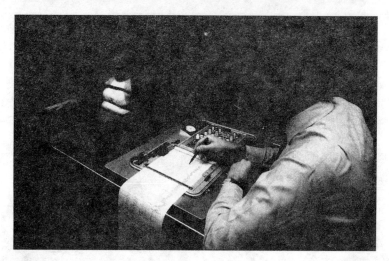

FIGURE **XI.2** USE OF THE POLYGRAPH. The examination begins with neutral questions, establishing the individual's general level of arousal. Then critical questions are intermittently included, and the examiner searches for sudden changes in the person's physiological reactions. Even with current safeguards, this procedure is not highly reliable (Lykken, 1991).

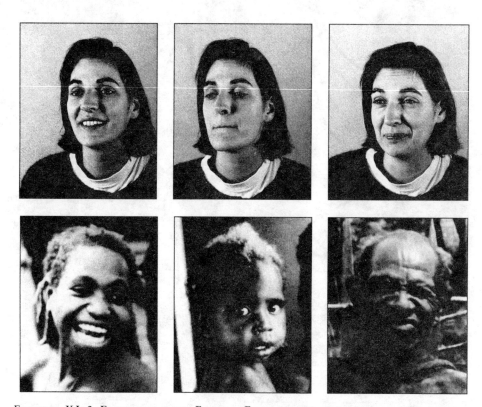

FIGURE **XI.3** FEELINGS AND FACIAL EXPRESSIONS. In most cases, the pleasant-unpleasant dimension is readily discernible. It is more difficult to determine which photographs show fear, happiness, and disgust. Try to do so with these photos. Answers: for the woman, these reactions were elicited by the arrival of a friend, a sharp reprimand, and a raw egg dropped in her hand. For the man and boys, they were elicited a friend, by a stranger from another culture, and the sight of someone eating canned food, respectively (Ekman, 1980).

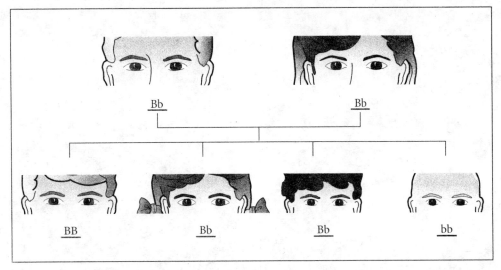

FIGURE **XII.1** DOMINANT AND RECESSIVE GENES. The child receives one member of each pair of genes from each parent. With these parents, brown eyes will be more prevalent than blue because *B* is dominant over *b*. In this case, the ratio is 3:1. While this example illustrates the transmission process, physical and behavioral traits typically are determined in a far more complex manner.

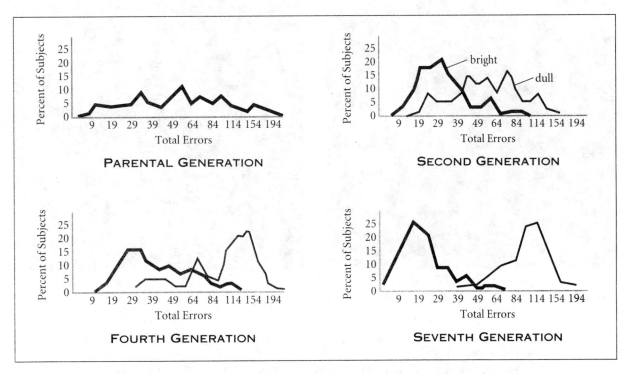

FIGURE **XII.2** POLYGENIC TRAIT. Beginning with a normal population, shown in black, the brightest rats were bred with the brightest rats and the dullest with the dullest rats. In the second generation, two separate groups began to appear, shown in red and green. By the seventh generation, the difference in error scores between the bright-bred and dull-bred groups was indeed marked (Tryon, 1940).

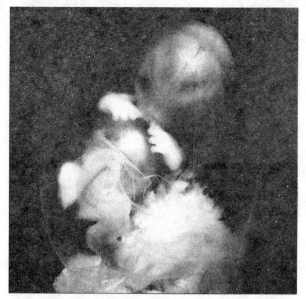

THREE-MONTH-OLD FETUS

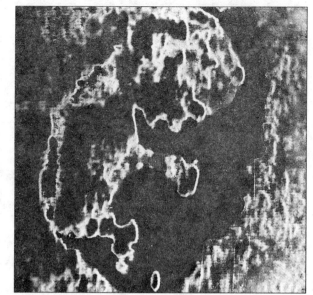

THREE-MONTH-OLD FETUS

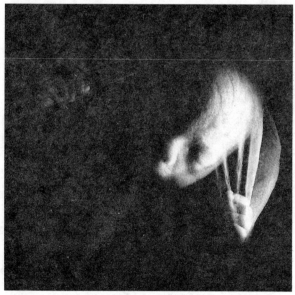

FOUR-MONTH-OLD FETUS

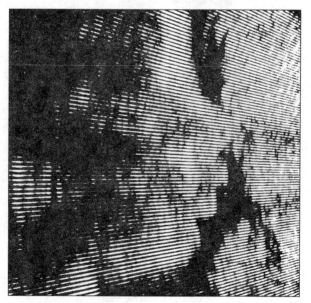

SIX-MONTH-OLD FETUS

FIGURE XII.3 THE HUMAN FETUS. In the upper row, on the left, a three-month-old fetus is shown from above by using a very fine, plastic viewing fiber; on the right, it is shown from the side in an ultrasound image. In the lower row, a four-month-old fetus is seen from above through fiberoptics; a six-month-old fetus is seen from the side by ultrasound.

Instead, they wrote about their problems, each composing an autobiography during their senior year. Writing these reports may have been therapeutic—a way of coping. They were published under the title *Experiencing Youth: First-Person Accounts* (Goethals & Klos, 1976).

IN PERSPECTIVE. These methods of coping with stress are often combined. In dealing with school, Stephen used family support, obtaining assistance from his new wife, as well as a tutor, and reframing, comparing school with his summer job, which left him working for a disagreeable boss with questionable ethics. He *could* have taken direct action by going to the library a few hours each day.

For both Dawn and Stephen, relaxation became most important. "Laughing is what makes us happy," said Stephen. "We are incredibly foolish with each other" (Goethals & Klos, 1976).

Looking at her new life, Dawn felt optimistic. "It makes me feel very lucky," she said. Perhaps she was thinking about how much she had changed since the time of her resolution in high school—to marry only for comfort and money.

Amid this optimism, certain facts must be recognized. Dawn was the daughter of separated parents, Stephen the son of divorced parents. Dawn and Stephen both experienced considerable family strife during their childhoods, and they married immediately after adolescence. People coming from these circumstances—family strife in childhood, parental unions terminated by law or choice, and youthful marriages of their own—tend to become divorced or separated themselves (Amato & Keith, 1991).

We know nothing more of Dawn and Stephen. Their separate autobiographies conclude at this point, leaving the reader to decide whether they reached the next phase of their relationship—the stage of companionate love.

• SUMMARY •

COMPONENTS OF EMOTION

1. The basic components of emotion are feelings, physiological reactions, behavior, and cognitive factors. For the individual, the most obvious aspect of emotion is the feeling. According to opponent-process theory, the onset of a positive or negative feeling automatically sets in motion the opposite feeling before there is a return to the normal state.

2. The physiological components of emotion include widespread excitatory and inhibitory reactions that occur through stimulation of the hypothalamus and cerebral cortex in the central nervous system and subsequent arousal of the sympathetic division of the autonomic nervous system. There has been some success in differentiating feelings on the basis of physiological reactions alone.

3. Emotional experience in others is most evident in the behavioral component. Efforts to identify feelings through behavior, focusing on facial expression and postural-gestural reactions, have indicated similarities and differences across cultures.

4. In emotion, the role of cognition is most widely debated. According to some experts, an emotional reaction cannot occur without some appraisal of the situation. According to others, an evaluation of the situation may produce an emotional state, but it is not a necessary component of emotion.

THEORIES OF EMOTION

5. The James-Lange theory states that feelings are the result of bodily responses and behavior. The Cannon-Bard theory emphasizes the role of lower brain centers, especially the thalamus, which activates the various dimensions of emotion simultaneously.

6. According to the arousal-cognition view, also called two-factor theory, physiological changes determine the strength of the feelings, and our interpretation of the circumstances determines what kinds of feelings we experience.

LIKING AND LOVING

7. The reinforcement principle, in operant conditioning, states that a relationship is maintained if it leads to positive outcomes for both parties. According to exchange theory, maintaining a relationship depends on achieving a gain greater than the overall expense. According to equity theory, the partners maintain the relationship if they feel they are deriving from it what they merit or deserve.

8. Compared to liking, love is more intense and appears in two basic forms. Passionate or romantic love often involves fantasy, is likely to be negative as well as positive, grows weaker with the passage of time, and includes sexual involvement. Companionate love is affection among people whose lives are deeply intertwined; it is friendlier, less intense, and more stable than passionate love.

9. The basic physiological changes in sexual behavior in males and females include vasocongestion, which is dilation of the blood vessels, and myotonia, which involves muscle contractions throughout the body. The associated psychological processes in both sexes occur in four stages: excitement, plateau, orgasm, and resolution.

10. Sexual behavior among human beings is significantly influenced by learning. The origins of sexual orientation, toward a homosexual or heterosexual preference, are still unknown, but there is potential evidence for both biological and social factors.

ANGER AND AGGRESSION

11. Aggression has been considered by some experts as universal among human beings. This view arises chiefly from research on aggressiveness in the animal kingdom and from psychoanalysis, which postulates a human predisposition for destructive tendencies. According to another view, the environment plays a crucial role, providing opportunities for learning aggressive or peaceful behavior.

12. The catharsis hypothesis, that the expression of anger reduces the underlying drive, has not been impressively supported. The frustration-aggression hypothesis, in revised form, states that frustration leads to a readiness to behave aggressively. The cultural hypothesis states that different cultures can mold people into aggressive, aggression-prone, or peaceful peoples.

STRESS IN DAILY LIFE

13. Stress is produced by life events, positive and negative, requiring readjustment. These events have different meanings for different individuals, and therefore subcultural and individual norms must be considered. There are three general types of conflicts: approach-approach, avoidance-avoidance and approach-avoidance.

14. The general adaptation syndrome, a pattern of symptoms in response to chronic stress, is characterized by three broad phases: the alarm reaction, resistance, and exhaustion. These processes also may contribute to psychophysiological disorders.

15. In managing stress, if the problem cannot be solved directly or if the cost is too great, then indirect coping strategies may be useful: reframing, distraction, relaxation, exercise, and outside assistance.

❧ REVIEW OF KEY CONCEPTS ❧

Components of Emotion
  emotion
  anxiety
  opponent-process theory
  hypothalamus
  cerebral cortex
  amygdala
  autonomic nervous system
  sympathetic nervous system
  parasympathetic nervous system
  electroencephalogram (EEG)
  electrocardiogram (EKG)
  galvanic skin response (GSR)
  polygraph
  arousal level
  Yerkes-Dodson law

Theories of Emotion
  James-Lange theory
  Cannon-Bard theory

arousal-cognition theory

Liking and Loving
  triangular theory of love
  reinforcement principle
  exchange theory
  equity theory
  passionate love
  companionate love
  vasocongestion
  myotonia
  sensate focus
  fetishism

Anger and Aggression
  anger
  aggression
  life instinct
  death instinct
  rape

catharsis hypothesis
frustration-aggression hypothesis

Stress in Daily Life
  stress
  conflict
  approach-approach conflict
  avoidance-avoidance conflict
  approach-avoidance conflict
  general adaptation syndrome
  alarm reaction
  resistance
  exhaustion
  eustress
  psychophysiological disorder
  type A personality
  stressor
  reframing
  distraction

❧ CLASS DISCUSSION/CRITICAL THINKING ❧

A NARRATIVE TWIST

Consider the relationship between Dawn and Stephen from a social assessment perspective. Stephen embraced a religion different from Dawn's and, while she achieved academic success easily, he was doing poorly in school. From Dawn's viewpoint, were these characteristics of Stephen costs or benefits for her? Argue both sides of the case. Imagine that Stephen became a prominent political figure on the campus. Would this development have been a cost or benefit, or both, for Dawn? Why? ❧

TOPICAL QUESTIONS

• *Components of Emotion.* Does identifying the components of emotion through modern research diminish romance today? Or does it incite romance by teaching people what they are feeling and how to manage their feelings? Explain.

• *Theories of Emotion.* Using the arousal-cognition theory, explain one onlooker's rescue of a child from a burning building and another onlooker's immobility at the scene. Compare them in terms of both arousal and cognition.

• *Liking and Loving.* You must choose whether to live on an island where there is only passionate love or only companionate love. Which would you select? Why? What personal consequences does your choice involve? How would you compensate for unfilled needs?

• *Anger and Aggression.* What would you do to reduce aggressive behavior in prisons?

• *Stress in Daily Life.* To what degree is our culture responsible for our personal level of stress? Would changes in American society significantly alleviate your own stress? Is stress largely a matter of the ways in which you think about things? Present your view.

Physiological mechanisms in emotional arousal and relaxation are discussed in the context of the biological bases of behavior (3). In psychoanalytic theory, aggression is an expression of the id (14). Violence on television is an issue in observational learning (7).

FAILURE TO ESCAPE TRAUMATIC SHOCK[1]

Martin E. P. Seligman[2] and Steven F. Maier[3]

Dogs which had first learned to panel press in a harness in order to escape shock subsequently showed normal acquisition of escape/avoidance behavior in a shuttle box. In contrast, yoked, inescapable shock in the harness produced profound interference with subsequent escape responding in the shuttle box. Initial experience with escape in the shuttle box led to enhanced panel pressing during inescapable shock in the harness and prevented interference with later responding in the shuttle box. Inescapable shock in the harness and failure to escape in the shuttle box produced interference with escape responding after a 7-day rest. These results were interpreted as supporting a learned "helplessness" explanation of interference with escape responding: Ss failed to escape shock in the shuttle box following inescapable shock in the harness because they had learned that shock termination was independent of responding.

Overmier and Seligman (1967) have shown that the prior exposure of dogs to inescapable shock in a Pavlovian harness reliably results in interference with subsequent escape/avoidance learning in a shuttle box. Typically, these dogs do not even escape from shock in the shuttle box. They initially show normal reactivity to shock, but after a few trials, they passively "accept" shock and fail to make escape movements. Moreover, if an escape or avoidance response does occur, it does not reliably predict future escapes or avoidances, as it does in normal dogs.

This pattern of effects is probably not the result of incompatible skeletal responses reinforced during the inescapable shocks, because it can be shown even when the inescapable shocks are delivered while the dogs are paralyzed by curare. This behavior is also probably not the result of adaptation to shock, because it occurs even when escape/avoidance shocks are intensified. However, the fact that interference does not occur if 48 hr. elapse between exposure to inescapable shock in the harness and escape/ avoidance training, suggests that the phenomenon may be partially dependent upon some other temporary process.

Overmier and Seligman (1967) suggested that the degree of control over shock allowed to the animal in the harness may be an important determinant of this interference effect. According to this hypothesis, if shock is terminated independently of S's responses during its initial experience with shock, interference with subsequent escape/avoidance responding should occur. If, however, S's responses terminate shock during its initial experience with shock, normal escape/avoidance responding should subsequently occur. Experiment I investigates the effects of escapable as compared with inescapable shock on subsequent escape/ avoidance responding.

EXPERIMENT I

METHOD. *SUBJECTS.* The Ss were 30 experimentally naive, mongrel dogs, 15–19 in. high at the shoulder, and weighing between 25 and 29 lb. They were maintained on ad lib food and water in individual cages. Three dogs were discarded from the Escape group, two because they failed to learn to escape shock in the harness (see procedure), and one because of a procedural error. Three dogs were discarded for the "Yoked" control group, two because they were too small at the neck to be adequately restrained in the harness; the third died during treatment. This left 24 Ss, eight in each group.

APPARATUS. The apparatus was the same as that described in Overmier and Seligman (1967). It consisted of two distinctively different units, one for escapable/ inescapable shock sessions and the other for escape/avoidance training. The unit in which *Ss* were exposed to escapable/inescapable shock consisted of a rubberized, cloth hammock located inside a shielded, white, sound-at-tenuating cubicle. The hammock was constructed so that *S*'s legs hung down below its body through four holes. The *S*'s legs were secured in this position, and *S* was strapped into the hammock. In addition, *S*'s head was held in position by panels placed on either side and a yoke between the panels across *S*'s neck. The *S* could press the panels with its head. For the Escape group pressing the panels terminated shock, while for the "Yoked" control group, panel presses did not effect the preprogrammed shock. The shock source for this unit consisted of 500 v. ac transformer and a parallel voltage divider, with the current applied through a fixed resistance of 20,000 ohms. The shock was applied to *S* through brass plate electrodes coated with commercial electrode paste and taped to the footpads of *S*'s hind feet. The shock intensity was 6.0 ma. Shock presentations were controlled by automatic relay circuitry located outside the cubicle.

Escape/avoidance training was conducted in a two-way shuttle box with two black compartments separated by an adjustable barrier (described in Solomon & Waynne, 1953). The barrier height was adjusted to *S*'s shoulder height. Each shuttle-box compartment was illuminated by two 50-w. and one 7 1/2-w. lamps. The CS consisted of turning off the four 50-w. lamps. The US, electric shock, was administered through the grid floor. A commutator shifted the polarity of the grid bars four times per second. The shock was 550 v. ac applied through a variable current limiting resistor in series with *S*. The shock was continually regulated by E at 4.5 ma. Whenever *S* crossed the barrier, photocell beams were interrupted, a response was automatically recorded, and the trial terminated. Latencies of barrier jumping were measured from CS onset to the nearest .01 sec. by an electric clock. Stimulus presentations and temporal contingencies were controlled by automatic relay circuitry in a nearby room.

White masking noise at approximately 79-db. SPL was presented in both units.

PROCEDURE. The Escape group received escape training in the harness. Sixty-four unsignaled 6.0 ma. shocks were presented at a mean interval of 90 sec. (range, 60–120 sec.). If the dog pressed either panel with its head during shock, shock terminated. If the dog failed to press a panel during shock, shock terminated automatically after 30 sec. Two dogs were discarded for failing to escape 18 of the last 20 shocks.[4]

Twenty-four hours later dogs in the Escape group were given 10 trials of escape/avoidance training in the shuttle box; *S* was placed in the shuttle box and given 5 min. to adapt before any treatment was begun. Presentation of the CS began each trial. The CS–US interval was 10 sec. If *S* jumped the barrier during this interval, the CS terminated and no shock was presented. Failure to jump the barrier during the CS-US interval led to shock which remained on until *S* did jump the barrier. If no response occurred within 60 sec. after CS onset, the trial was automatically terminated and a 60-sec. latency recorded. The average intertrial interval was 90 sec. with a range of 60–120 sec. If *S* failed to cross the barrier on all of the first five trials, it was removed, placed on the other side of the shuttle box, and training then continued. At the end of the tenth trial, *S* was removed from the shuttle box and returned to its home cage.

The Normal control group received only 10 escape/avoidance trials in the shuttle box as described above.

The "Yoked" control group received the same exposure to shock in the harness as did the Escape group, except that panel pressing did not terminate shock. The duration of shock on any given trial was determined by the mean duration of the corresponding trial in the Escape group. Thus each *S* in the "Yoked" control group received a series of shocks of decreasing duration totaling to 226 sec.

Twenty-four hours later, *Ss* in the "Yoked" control group received 10 escape/avoidance trials in the shuttle box as described for the Escape group. Seven days later, those *Ss* in this group which showed the interference effect received 10 more trials in the shuttle box.

RESULTS[5]. The Escape group learned to panel press to terminate shock in the harness. Each *S* in this group showed decreasing latencies of panel pressing over the course of the session ($p = .008$, sign test, Trials 1–8 vs. Trials 57–64). Individual records revealed that each *S* learned to escape shock by emitting a single,

Group	Mean Latency (in sec.)	% Ss Failing to Escape Shock on 9 or More of the 10 Trials	Means No Failures to Escape Shock[a]
Escape	27.00	0	2.63
Normal Control	25.93	12.5	2.25
"Yoked" Control	48.22	75	7.25

[a] Out of 10 trials.

TABLE 1 INDEXES OF SHUTTLE BOX ESCAPE/AVOIDANCE RESPONDING: EXP. 1

discrete panel press following shock onset. The Ss in the "Yoked" control group typically ceased panel pressing altogether after about 30 trials.

Table 1 presents the mean latency of shuttle box responding, the mean number of failures to escape shock, and the percentage of Ss which failed to escape nine or more of the 10 trials during escape/avoidance training n the shuttle box for each group. The "Yoked" control group showed marked interference with escape responding in the shuttle box. It differed significantly from the Escape group and from the Normal control group on mean latency and mean number of failures to escape (in both cases, p< 05, Duncan's multiple-range test). The Escape group and the Normal control group did not differ on these indexes.

Six Ss in the "Yoked" control group failed to escape shock on 9 or more of the 10 trials in the shuttle box. Seven days after the first shuttle-box treatment, these six Ss received 10 further trials in the shuttle box. Five of them continued to fail to escape shock on every trial.

DISCUSSION. The degree of control over shock allowed a dog during its initial exposure to shock was a determinant of whether or not interference occurred with subsequent escape/avoidance learning. Dogs which learned to escape shock by panel pressing in the harness did not differ from untreated dogs in subsequent escape/avoidance learning in the shuttle box. Dogs for which shock termination was independent of responding in the harness showed interference with subsequent escape learning.

Because the Escape group differed from the "Yoked" control group during their initial exposure to shock only in their control over shock termination, we suggest that differential learning about their control over shock occurred in these two groups. This learning may have acted in the following way: (a) Shock initially elicited active responding in the harness in both groups. (b) Ss in the "Yoked" control group learned that shock termination was independent of their responding, i.e., that the conditional probability of shock termination in the presence of any given response did not differ from the conditional probability of shock termination in the absence of that response. (c) The incentive for the initiation of active responding in the presence of electric shock is the expectation that responding will increase the probability of shock termination. In the absence of such incentive, the probability that responding will be initiated decreases. (d) Shock in the shuttle box mediated the generalization of b to the new situation for the "Yoked" control group, thus decreasing the probability of escape response initiation in the shuttle box.

Escapable shock in the harness (Escape group) did not produce interference, because Ss learned that their responding was correlated with shock termination. The incentive for the maintenance of responding was thus present, and escape response initiation occurred normally in the shuttle box.

Learning that shock termination is independent of responding seems related to the concept of learned "helplessness" or "hopelessness" advanced by Richter (1957), Mowrer (1960, p. 197), Cofer and Appley (1964, p. 452), and to the concept of external control of reinforcement discussed by Lefcourt (1966).

In untreated Ss the occurrence of an escape or avoidance response is a reliable predictor of future escape and avoidance responding. Dogs in the "Yoked" control group and in the groups which showed the interference effect in Overmier and Seligman (1967) occasionally made an escape or avoidance response and then reverted to "passively" accepting shock. These dogs did not appear to benefit from the barrier-jumping—shock-termination contingency. A possible interpretation of this finding is that the prior learning that shock termination was independent of responding inhibited the formation of barrier-jumping—shock-terminated association.

The Ss in the "Yoked" control group which showed the interference effect 24 hr. after inescapable shock in the harness again failed to escape from shock after a further 7-day interval. In contrast, Overmier and Seligman (1967) found that no interference occurred when 48 hr. elapsed between inescapable shock in the harness and shuttle-box training. This time course could result from a temporary state of emotional depletion (Brush, Myer, & Palmer, 1963), which was produced by experience with inescapable shock, and which could be prolonged by being conditioned to the cues of the shuttle box. Such a state might be related to the parasympathetic death which Richter's (1957) "hopeless" rats died. Further research is needed to clarify the relationship between the learning factor, which appears to cause the initial occurrence of the interference effect, and an emotional factor, which may be responsible for the time course of the effect.

The results of Exp. I provide a further disconfirmation of the adaptation explanation of the interference effect. If Ss in the "Yoked" control group had adapted to shock and, therefore, were not sufficiently motivated to respond in the shuttle box, Ss in the Escape group should also have adapted to shock. Further, the Escape and the "Yoked" control groups were equated for the possibility of adventitious punishment for active responding by shock onset in the harness. Thus it seems unlikely that the "Yoked" control group failed to escape in the shuttle box because it had been adventitiously punished for active responding in the harness.

∾

EXPERIMENT II

Experiment I provided support for the hypothesis that S learned that shock termination was independent of its responding in the harness and that this learning inhibited subsequent escape responding in the shuttle box. Experiment II investigates whether prior experience with *escapable* shock in the shuttle box will mitigate the effects of inescapable shock in the harness on subsequent escape/avoidance behavior. Such prior experience might be expected (*a*) to inhibit S's learning in the harness that its responding is not correlated with shock termination and (*b*) to allow S to discriminate between the escapability of shock in the shuttle box and the inescapability of shock in the harness.

METHOD. *SUBJECTS.* The Ss were 30 experimentally naive, mongrel dogs, weight, height and housing as above. Three dogs were discarded: two because of procedural errors and one because of illness. The remaining 27 dogs were randomly assigned to three groups of nine Ss each.

APPARATUS. The two units described for Exp. I were used.

PROCEDURE. The Preescape group received 3 days of treatment. On Day 1, each S received 10 escape/avoidance trials in the shuttle box as described in Exp. I. On Day 2, approximately 24 hr. after the shuttle-box treatment, each S in this group received an inescapable shock session in the harness. All inescapable shocks were unsignaled. The inescapable shock session consisted of 64, 5-sec. shocks, each of 6.0 ma. The average intershock interval was 90 sec. with a range of 60–120 sec. On Day 3, approximately 24 hr. after the inescapable shock, S was returned to the shuttle box and given 30 more escape/avoidance trials, as described for Day 1.

The No Pregroup received no experience in the shuttle box prior to receiving inescapable shock. On the first treatment day for this group, each S was placed in the harness and exposed to an inescapable shock session as described for the Preescape group, Day 2. Approximately 24 hr. later, S was placed in the shuttle box and given 40 trials of escape/avoidance training as described above. If S failed to respond on all of the first five trials, S was moved to the other side of the shuttle box. If S continued to fail to respond on all trials, it was put back on the original side after the twenty-fifth trial. Thus, if S failed to escape on every trial, it received a total of 2,000 sec. of shock.

The No Inescapable group was treated exactly as the Preescape group except that it received no shock in the harness. On Day 1, S received 10 escape/avoidance trials in the shuttle box. On Day 2, it was strapped in the harness for 90 min., but received no shock. On Day 3, it was returned to the shuttle box and given 30 more escape/avoidance trials.

RESULTS. The No Pregroup showed significant interference with escape/avoidance responding in the shuttle box on Day 3. The Preescape and the No Inescapable groups did not show such interference. Figure 1 presents the mean median latency of jumping responses for the three groups (and a posterior control group, see below) over the four blocks of 10 trials. Analysis of variance on the three groups revealed that the effect of groups, $F (2, 24) = (3.55, p < .05,$ and the effect of trial blocks, $F (3, 72) = 6.84, p < .01$, were significant. Duncan's multiple-range test indicated that the No Pregroup differed from the other two groups across all 40 trials both $p < .05$. The Preescape and the No Inescapable groups did not differ from each other. Similar results held for the mean of mean latencies. A small, transitory disruption of improvement in shuttle-box performance following inescapable shock in the harness occurred in the Preescape group relative to the No Inescapable group. Difference scores for latencies between consecutive blocks of trials measure improvement in performance. A comparison of the Preescape group with No

Inescapable group on the difference between the mean latency on Trials 1–10 and the mean latency on Trials 11–20 revealed that the No Inescapable group showed significantly more improvement than the Preescape group, Mann-Whitney U test, $U = 15, p < .05$. No significant differences were found on difference scores for any subsequent blocks of trials.

Figure 2 presents the mean number of failures to escape shock for the three groups across the four blocks of trials. Analysis of variance revealed a significant overall effect of blocks, $F (3, 72) = 5.94, p < .01$, and a significant Groups × Blocks interaction, $F (6, 72) = 17.82, p < .01$. Duncan's tests indicated that the No Pregroup showed significantly more failures to escape than the other two groups across the 40 trials, both $p < .05$. The Preescape and the No Inescapable groups did not differ.

Figure 3 presents the total number of avoidance responses for the groups across the blocks of trials. Only the blocks effect was significant in the overall analysis of variance, $F (3, 72) = 27.90, p < .01$. No other effects were significant.

Panel presses made in the harness during the escapable shock session were counted. On either side of S's head were panels which S could press; panel pressing had no effect on the shock, but merely indicated attempts to response and/or struggling in the harness. The Preescape group, having received 10 trials with *escapable* shock in the shuttle box the previous day, made more panel presses during the

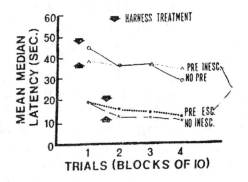

FIGURE 1 Mean median latency of escape/avoidance responding. (The position of the arrow denotes whether the harness treatment occurred 24 hr. before the first or second block of trials.

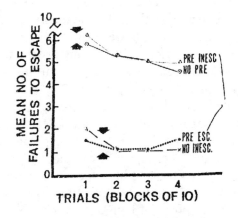

FIGURE 2 Mean number of failures to escape shock. (The position of the arrow denotes whether the harness treatment occurred 24 hr. before the first or second block of trials.)

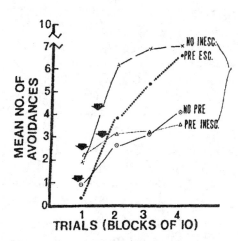

FIGURE 3 Mean number of avoidances. (The position of the arrow denotes whether the harness treatment occurred 24 hr. before the first or second block of trials.)

inescapable shock session that did the No Pregroup, the group for which the inescapable shock in the harness was first experimental treatment, Mann-Whitney U test, U = 9, p < .02.

POSTERIOR CONTROL GROUP. Subsequent to this experiment, a control group was run to determine if the *escapability* of shock in the shuttle box on Day 1 for the Preescape group was responsible for its enhanced panel pressing the harness and lack of interference with responding in the shuttle box. Or would the mere occurrence of inescapable shock for a free-moving animal in the shuttle box have produced these results? Nine naive dogs received the following treatment: On Day 1, Ss were placed in shuttle box and given 10 trials as for the Preescape and the No Inescapable groups. Unlike these groups, however, S's barrier jumping did not (except adventitiously) terminate the shock and CS, because trial durations were programmed independently of S's behavior. The duration of each of the 10 trials for the Preinescapable group corresponded to the mean trial duration for the Preescape and the No Inescapable groups on that trial. On Day 2, Ss received 64 trials of inescapable shock in the harness. On Day 3 Ss received 40 escape/avoidance trials in the shuttle box.

Figures 1, 2, and 3 presents the escape/avoidance performance of the Preinescapable group on Day 3. In general this group performed like the No Pregroup. This impression was borne bout by statistical tests. The

Preinescapable group showed significantly slower median latency of barrier jumping than the Preescape and the No Inescapable groups across all 40 trials, both p < .05, Duncan's test. The Preinescapable group did not differ from the No Pregroup. Similar results held for the other indexes.

Analysis of the panel press data showed that the Preinescapable group made significantly fewer panel processes in the harness than the Preescape group, Mann-Whitney U test, U = 14, p < .05. The Preinescapable group did not differ significantly from the No Pregroup, U = 26.

DISCUSSION. Three main findings emerged from Exp. II: (a) Ss (Preescape), which first received escapable shock in the shuttle box, then inescapable shock in the harness, did not react passively to subsequent shock in the shuttle box, as did Ss which either first received inescapable shock in the shuttle box (Preinescapable) or no treatment prior to shock in the harness (No Pre). (b) The Preescape group, having received experience with escapable shock in the shuttle box, showed enhanced panel pressing when exposed to inescapable shock in the harness, relative to naive Ss given inescapable shock in the harness. Such enhanced panel pressing was specifically the result of the *escapability* of shock in the shuttle box: The Preinescapable group did not show enhanced panel pressing. (c) The interference effect persisted for 40 trials.

The Ss which have had prior experience with *escapable* shock in the shuttle box showed, more energetic behavior in response to *inescapable* shock in the harness. This contrasts with the interference effect produced by inescapable shock in Ss which have had no prior experience with shock or in Ss which have had prior experience with inescapable shock. Thus, if an animal first learns that is responding produces shock termination and then faces a situation in which reinforcement is independent of its responding, it is more persistent in its attempts to escape shock than is an naive animal.

∾

GENERAL DISCUSSION

We have proposed that S learned as a consequence of inescapable should that its responding was independent of shock termination, and therefore the probability of response initiation during shock decreased. Alternative explanations might be offered: (a) Inactivity, somehow, reduces the aversiveness of shock. Thus S failed to escape shock in the shuttle box because it had been reinforced for inactivity in the harness. Since the interference effect occurred in Ss which had been curarized during inescapable shock, such an aversiveness-reducing mechanism would have to be located inward of the neuro-myal junction. (b) S failed to escape in the shuttle box because certain responses which facilitate barrier jumping were extinguished in the harness during inescapable shock. In conventional extinction procedures, some response is first explicitly reinforced by correlation with shock termination, and then that response is extinguished by removing shock altogether for the situation. Responding during extinction is conventionally not *uncorrelated* with shock termination; rather, responding is correlated with the total absence of shock. In our harness situation, no response was first explicitly reinforced, and shock was presented throughout the session. A broader concept of extinction, however, might be tenable. On this view, any procedure which decreases the probability of a response by eliminating the incentive to respond is an extinction procedure. If the independence of shock termination and responding eliminates the incentive to respond (as assumed), then our harness procedure could be thought of as an extinction procedure. Such an explanation seems only semantically different for the one we have advanced, since both entail that the probability of responding during shock has decreased because S learned that shock termination was independent of its responses.

Learning that one's own responding and reinforcement are independent might be expected to play a role in appetitive situations. If S received extensive pretraining and rewarding brain stimulation delivered independently of its operant responding, would the subsequent acquisition of a bar press to obtain this reward be retarded? Further, might learned "helplessness" transfer from aversive to appetitive situations or vice versa?

If dogs learn in one situation that their active responding is to no avail, and then trans-

fer this training to another shock situation, the opposite type of transfer (avoidance learning sets) might be possible: If a dog first learned a barrier-hurdling response which avoided shock in the shuttle box, would that dog be facilitated in learning to panel press to avoid shock in the harness (to a different CS)? Our finding, that dogs which first successfully escape shock in the shuttle box later showed enhanced panel pressing in the harness, is consonant with this prediction.

Does learning about response—reinforcement contingencies have its analogs in classical conditioning? If S experienced two stimuli randomly interspersed with each other (adventitious pairings possible), would it be retarded in forming an association between the two stimuli once true pairing was begun? Conversely, pretraining in which one stimulus is correlated with a US might facilitate the acquisition of the CR to a new CS. Pavlov (1927, p. 75) remarked that the first establishment of a conditioned inhibitor took longer than any succeeding one.

In conclusion, learning theory has stressed that the two operations, explicit contiguity between events (acquisition) and explicit non-contiguity (extinction), produce learning. A third operaton that is proposed, independence between events, also produces learning, and such learning may have effects upon behavior that differ from the effects of explicit pairing and explicit nonpairing. Such learning may produce an S who does not attempt to escape electric shock; an S who, even if he does respond, may not benefit from instrumental contingencies.

∾

REFERENCES

Brush, F. R. Myer, J. S., & Palmer, M. E. Effects of kind of prior training and intersession interval upon subsequent avoidance learning. *J. comp. physiol. Psychol.*, 1963, 56, 539–545.

Cofer, C. N., & Appley, M.H. Motivation: *Theory and research.* New York: Wiley, 1964.

Lefcourt, H. M. Internal vs. external control of reinforcement: A review. *Psychol. Bull.,* 1966, 65, 206–221.

Mowrer, O. H. *Learning theory and behavior.* New York: Wiley, 1960

Overmier, J. B., & Seligman, M. E. P. Effects of inescapable shock on subsequent escape and avoidance learning. *J. comp. physiol. Psychol.* 1967, 63, 28–33.

Pavlov, I. P. *Conditioned reflexes.* New York: Dove, 1927.

Richter, C. On the phenomenon of sudden death in animals and man. *Psychosom. Med.,* 1957, 19, 191–198.

Solomon, R. L., & Wynne, I. C. Traumatic avoidance learning: Acquisition in normal dogs. *Psychol. Monogr.,* 1953, 67 (4, Whole No 354).

NOTES

1. This research was supported by grants to R. L. Solomon from the National Science Foundation (GB-2428) and the National Institute of Mental Health (MH-04202). The authors are grateful to R. L. Solomon, J. Aronfreed, J. Geer, H. Gleitman, F. Irwin, D. Williams, and J. Wishner for their advice in the conduct and reporting of these experiments. The authors also thank J. Bruce Overmier with whom Exp. I was begun.

2. National Science Foundation predoctoral fellow.

3. National Institute of Mental Health predoctoral fellow.

4. It might be argued that eliminating these two dogs would bias the data. Thus naive dogs which failed to learn the panel-press escape response in the harness might also be expected to be unable to learn shuttle box escape/avoidance. Once of these dogs was run 48 hr. later in the shuttle box. It escaped and avoided normally. The other dog was too ill to be run in the shuttle box 48 hr. after it received shock in the harness.

5. All *p* values are based upon two-tailed tests.

JOURNAL ARTICLE REVIEW FORM

Name _____ Date _____

Article Name: _____

Article Authors: _____

1. Why did the authors perform this study? (What question(s) did the authors want to answer?)

2. Identify the IV(s) and the DV(s) used in this study (Note: there may be more than one of each).

3. How was the welfare of human subjects or animal subjects safeguarded?

4. What were the major findings of this study?

5. Why were these results significant?

6. What would be a good follow-up to this study? (What study should be done next?)

1. Which of the following groups of mental health professionals can prescribe drugs to treat psychological disorders:
   a. psychiatrists
   b. clinical psychologists
   c. counseling psychologists
   d. psychiatric social workers

2. In diagnosing psychopathology, psychologists use the DSM system which, following the medical model, classifies behavioral disorders according to:
   a. root causes
   b. proximal causes
   c. clinical symptoms
   d. recommended therapy

3. The cause of schizophrenia is almost surely
   a. abnormal functioning of the serotonin and dopamine neurotransmitters systems.
   b. a childhood environment in which parents are withdrawn and their behavior toward the child is inconsistent.
   c. exposure to a traumatic event in early adulthood.
   d. learned maladaptive thinking processes.

4. The most common age of onset for both schizophrenia and depression is:
   a. early childhood
   b. late teens or early twenties
   c. middle age
   d. after 60 years of age

5. Drugs used to treat schizophrenia and depression typically:
   a. control the symptoms of severe mental disorders but do not cure those disorders
   b. cure moderate disorders but are no use with severe disorders
   c. are generally more successful than insight therapies with various forms of disorders
   d. do not really work well with any of the disorders

6. Drugs in which of the following classes are most likely to produce true physiological addiction?
   a. stimulants
   b. depressants
   c. hallucinogens
   d. none produce true addiction

7. The current view on the drug "problem" is that:
   a. only depressant drugs produce true addiction.
   b. few drugs produce addiction, many can produce abusive patterns of drug use.
   c. cocaine is responsible for more deaths than all the other illegal drugs combined.
   d. genetics are responsible for most drug abuse.
   e. All of the above.

8. A friend proclaims the virtues of a smaller government that does not interfere with our behaviors, yet, he also is pro-life and frequently pickets "abortion" clinics. We can assume our friend would experience the social psychology principle of :
   a. disparity
   b. resistance
   c. rationalization
   d. cognitive dissonance
   e. attribution

9. Which of the following is true of friendship?
   a. Friendship takes time to develop.
   b. We make friends with people who are similar to ourselves.
   c. Friendship is a relationship that involves mutual rewards.
   d. All of the above are true of friendship.

10. The romantic or passionate component of love usually lasts _____.
    a. 6 months
    b. 30 months
    c. 5 years
    d. none of the above
11. Milgram's studies of obedience showed that most people will do what a legitimate authority figure tells them _____.
    a. only if they like the authority figure
    b. only if the authority figure's demands are reasonable
    c. even if it means harming or killing another human being
    d. only in emergency situations
12. Attribution is the process by which people:
    a. assign motives for behavior to other people to respond appropriately to them.
    b. judge the attitudes of other people's behavior based on a set of personal ethical principles.
    c. attempt to remove cognitive dissonance so they can move toward a more rational cognitive state.
    d. attempt to reconcile their emotional reactions to the behavior of others with their own cognitions.
13. Which of the following is an important part of the General Adaptation Syndrome?
    a. it includes the stages alarm, resistance, and exhaustion
    b. it is a normal response system for acute stress but leads to deterioration of body systems when chronic or long-term stress is present
    c. it produces the same pattern of response to both physiological and psychological stress
    d. all of the above
14. There is current evidence that PTSD (post traumatic stress disorder) has clear _____ symptoms?
    a. psychological
    b. physiological
    c. hormonal
    d. all of the above
15. Match the anti-schizophrenic and anti-depressant drug to the neurotransmitter system that is (are) primarily affected. Note that answers may be used more than once or not at all.
    _____ Prozac
    _____ Haldol
    _____ Thorazine
    _____ Marplan (an MAOI)
    _____ Clozaril
    a. dopamine
    b. serotonin
    c. norepinephrine
    d. both dopamine and serotonin
    e. all 3 neurotransmitters

PART FIVE:
HUMAN BRAIN–
BEHAVIOR
INTERACTIONS

That the 1990s have been designated as The Decade of the Brain gives an inkling to the importance of Part Five. After years of research with experimental animals, we now have accumulated substantial data on the way the brain determines behavior, as well as ways behavior can influence workings of the brain. Moreover, new techniques available to examine the working human brain have opened a world of study unimaginable to psychologists of old. Now, psychology has the opportunity to become a true partner in the brain research field, a field known as "neuroscience." The chapter on Biological Foundations provides an overview of neuroscience, with emphasis on those issues of special interest to those of us interested in behavioral *neuroscience. The other, shorter chapters are included as in-depth coverage of topics of interest to both students and behavioral neuroscientists. The first topic is perception, how individuals gather, sort and organize the information coming into the nervous system from the environment. Next is a description of the EEG measurements of brain waves that have provided most of what is known about sleeping and dreaming. Finally, there is the chapter describing what is known about hunger and eating that determine body weights. You will recognize much of the terminology and some of the concepts in these chapters because they have been introduced in one form or another in previous parts of the course. Hopefully, all of it will come together after reading these chapters and you will end Part Five, and the course, with the same conviction as your instructors. A solid understanding of the brain is a fundamental requirement for the next century of psychology.*

∾ ∾ ∾ ∾ ∾ ∾

17

BIOLOGICAL FOUNDATIONS

THE DRUMMER'S SOUL MATE SAT AMONG THE AUDI-
ENCE, AWAITING THE BEGINNING OF THE NIGHT'S
CONCERT. WE SHALL CALL HER SACHA, WHICH MEANS
"helper of humanity," for she was indeed loyal to Ray, supporting him
in all sorts of circumstances.

Imagine the scene. Out on the floor, the bass player flexed his fingers,
his mind seemingly elsewhere. Ray bent over the snare drum, lightly
tapped its head, listened, and tightened a lug. He repeated the process
at the next lug, and the next, moving slowly around the head of the
drum. Reaching the last lug, he banged the drum, jerked his head up,
and swore loudly. The vocalist turned in Ray's direction; the bass player
turned a bit rosy; and Ray turned the last lug on his drum. Sacha did
not change her expression; she simply looked on intently.

As the musicians tuned up for another night of jazz, miraculous activity
was taking place inside their heads. Among the tens of billions of microscopic cells in each brain, with its millions of threadlike connections, innu-

merable nerve networks were transmitting and receiving messages. Traveling faster than 100 miles per hour, they prompted Ray to smile at his audience, to strike the drum again, and to drink a bit of soda, wriggling his tongue to move the residue around in his mouth.

The human brain, capable of mediating all of these activities, can also study itself, as yours is about to do. Referred to as the most intricate mechanism on this planet, it is the only structure sufficiently complex to turn on itself in this extraordinary way. If it were much simpler, making it easier to understand, our thinking probably would be too simple to conduct this inquiry.

In many respects, Ray was just a normal, fun-loving young man who happened to be a very talented musician. He was also athletic, witty, loyal, and persevering, characteristics that raise a vital question. What are the underlying mechanisms that enabled him to respond in these ways? Modern answers to this question form the basis for this

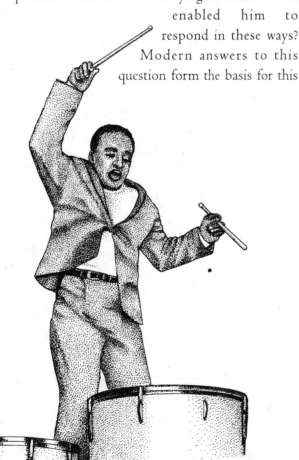

chapter. Indeed, Ray's story is appropriate for this purpose because, due to a specific, rare neurological disorder, addressed later, he provides an excellent example not only of the functions but also of the dysfunctions of these underlying mechanisms. His case is of particular interest in neurospsychology, physiological psychology, and clinical psychology (Sacks, 1987).

With a focus largely on neural structures, we begin this chapter with an overview of the body. Then we examine neural communication, specifically the pathways that connect the chief organs. Afterward, we concentrate on our major integrating organ, the human brain. Finally, we emphasize that the body is composed of interlocking systems.

• OVERVIEW OF THE BODY •

Throughout the animal kingdom, biological mechanisms are studied in terms of organs and systems. The focus is on structures and their relationships.

ORGANS AND SYSTEMS

In the biological sense, an **organ** is a distinct and specific body part specialized to perform a particular function. The ears receive auditory information; the stomach digests food; the brain prompts thoughts about an enjoyable night of jazz. A **system,** in biology, refers to a series of interacting organs and connecting links, making a functional whole. We speak of the auditory, gastrointestinal, and respiratory systems, referring to the interrelated organs that result in hearing, digestion, and breathing, respectively.

BASIC ORGANS. Awaiting her husband's moment to begin, Sacha's sense organs were attuned to incoming cues from the band leader, his fellow musicians, and even the audience. In all of us, some organs are concerned with the intake of information; others are concerned with the management of information; still others are concerned with output.

Within the eyes, ears, nose, and other sense organs are the **receptors,** nerve cells specialized for receiving information and transmitting it to adjacent nerve tissue. They receive information about the external environment: musical sounds, bright lights, and the odor of food. They also receive information about the internal environment: the action of the muscles, condition of the stomach and heart, and so forth. When receptors are acted on by appropriate stimuli, they transmit that information to the brain via the nervous system.

Ray smiled, hunched his shoulders, leaned forward in his chair, and began a light drum roll, signaling the start of the concert. The **effectors** are the muscles and glands that enable the organism to do something, to take some action—that is, to have an effect on the environment. Ray lifted his head and swore again, this time more softly.

Still other organs do not receive information from the environment or take direct action in the environment. They are primarily concerned with activities within the body, especially maintenance and integration functions. Again, the brain is foremost among them. Other vital organs include the heart, lungs, stomach, and so forth.

INTEGRATED SYSTEMS. The complex interactions among these different sorts of organs, for input and output and maintenance, could not occur without intricate, highly differentiated body systems. In human beings, these systems play a central role in communication; foremost among them are the *nerve networks,* also called the *nervous system.*

In the jellyfish, the nerve network is extremely simple, shaped much like a wheel with a hub, an outer rim, and a few spokes. The jellyfish moves in a slow, repetitive fashion, without much variation. The earthworm, at a higher level, has a nervous system with two symmetrical halves, both divided into parts, much like a ladder in appearance. The earth-

worm can move its different segments separately, allowing it to inch along, extending one part of its body and then another in sequential fashion.

In contrast, vertebrates have extensive concentrations of nerve cells along the backbone and especially in the head. This central pattern, with its countless interconnections, permits a wide variety of specific and distinct actions. An impressive example occurs in human beings, who can execute a roll on the snare drum and simultaneously wink at a friend, performing with a versatility and complexity not found in any other organism.

GENETIC BACKGROUND. The growth of these organs and systems is directed by a code passed on to all of us at the moment of conception. The basic principles of this genetic unfolding, known for some time, are discussed in a later chapter on human development. However, recent investigations with animals suggest that the expression of the genetic code may be more variable than was once thought.

Among a species of African cichlid, a few male fish control virtually all of the feeding territories and access to most of the female fish. These aggressive males are bigger and more brightly colored than their more submissive counterparts. However, once a dominant fish has been displaced by combat or a predator, the newly ascendant fish not only becomes domineering but also develops a bigger body, becomes more brightly colored, and experiences marked growth in its brain and testicles. The brain increase occurs in the hypothalamus, which plays a vital role in feeding, fighting, and mating. Certain cells may grow to six or seven times the size of those in the subordinate fish (Davis & Fernald, 1990).

After its defeat, the displaced male fish swims away and remains largely by itself. Within a few days, its hypothalamus diminishes in size; its bright colors disappear; and even its testicles become reduced in mass. In other words, the social position of the male African cichlid, which is part of its external environment, influences the structure and function of its brain and other organs (Bond, Francis, Fernald, & Adelman, 1991; Davis & Fernald, 1990).

Internal influences on the genetic code were demonstrated when 100 different viruses, easily distinguished from one another, were injected into the developing brains of the fetuses of pregnant rats. This procedure gave the injected cells an unmistakable virus "tag" without influencing the brain development of the fetus. The pregnant rats gave normal births; the newborn pups developed normally; and after an appropriate period, the brains of these young rats were examined to determine the locations of the various tagged cells.

The brain cells produced by the division of a parent cell, or progenitor, had extended in various directions, eventually migrating to very different parts of the brain. Offspring nerve cells from the same parent cell were found in many *different locations* in the upper brain regions and performed *different functions,* relevant to the particular site in which they had become established: vision, hearing, taste, and so forth, depending on the activity in that region of the brain. In other words, the genetic code in a parent cell did not instruct all offspring cells to perform the same task. Their final performance was also influenced by their neighbors' functions (Walsh & Cepko, 1992).

Collectively, these experiments suggest that the development of nerve cells is under the influence of the genes, the external environment, *and* a particular internal environment. Genes certainly do influence development but perhaps not in the rigid manner suggested by earlier studies.

∾

HUMAN NERVOUS SYSTEM

The consequences of inheriting a certain physical structure are most readily observed in the nervous system, which accounts for so much diversity in behavior. At the human level,

for example, it enabled Ray to become a highly accomplished musician, a drummer of real virtuosity. When he played in a weekend jazz band, his wild extemporizations never failed to delight the audience. His unpredictable swearing also attracted an audience from time to time. Over the years, Sacha had learned somewhat to tolerate these unexpected bursts of coarse language. From her perspective as his wife, Ray was just that way.

Ray was also quick in conversation. "Tell me how long drum rolls should be played," an admirer might ask. "The same as short ones" was a likely reply.

Integrating all such activity, the **nervous system** is a coordinating network that regulates internal responses and reacts to external and internal stimulation, transmitting information throughout the body. It is the major integrating system in many animals and human beings, consisting of the brain, spinal cord, and numerous related nerve pathways.

PERIPHERAL NERVOUS SYSTEM. *Peripheral* means "outlying," and the **peripheral nervous system** includes essentially all the nerves of the body lying outside the brain and spinal cord. It transmits messages to and from the brain and the spinal cord. Some of these nerves may be quite long. Nerve structures not found within the brain and spinal cord generally belong to the peripheral nervous system (Figure 3–1).

The peripheral nervous system makes connections with two types of organs. The largely involuntary organs include the heart, lungs, stomach, and adrenal glands, and they are controlled by a part of the peripheral nervous system called the **autonomic nervous system.** This subsystem, in turn, has two divisions, the sympathetic and parasympathetic, considered later in this chapter and elsewhere. Suffice it to note here that the sympathetic division prepares the body for emergencies; the parasympathetic division maintains the body in more routine situations. The other part of the peripheral nervous system, the **somatic nervous system,** involves the striated mus-

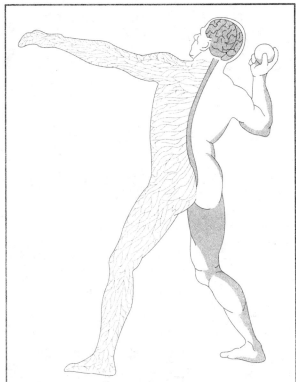

FIGURE 3-1 PERIPHERAL AND CENTRAL NERVOUS SYSTEMS. The peripheral system, extending to and from the body's extremities, is represented in color. The central nervous system, which includes the brain and spinal cord, is shown in black. Neither system is fully depicted here.

cles and sense organs and therefore is responsible for the regulation of most voluntary behavior, providing control and also feeling in diverse parts of the body. It enables students to walk to class, drummers to play their instruments, and professors to write textbooks.

CENTRAL NERVOUS SYSTEM. The brain and spinal cord are the two basic elements of the **central nervous system,** the primary integrating and control center in the human body, receiving impulses from the peripheral nervous system and from its own subdivisions. Integrations of greatest complexity occur in the human **brain,** an exquisitely intricate concentration of nerve tissue enclosed within the skull.

A ropelike structure with the diameter of the little finger, the **spinal cord** is an intricate bundle of nerve fibers extending down the spinal column of organisms with a backbone, serving two purposes. It contains the nerve fibers for reflexes, our most primitive and automatic responses. Through these pathways, it also conveys messages to and from the brain, providing the basis for much more complex reactions.

The ascending and descending pathways to and from the brain form definite spinal tracts, most of which cross over near the brain from one side of the body to the other. Ascending pathways from the left side of the body, for example, cross over to the right side of the brain. Descending pathways from the left side of the brain eventually reach the right side of the body. When a drummer uses his right hand, impulses for this action originate in the left side of his brain—the left cerebral hemisphere—and vice versa.

In the brain, the ascending impulses, in addition to serving involuntary functions, activate the so-called higher mental processes, which include perceiving, remembering, reasoning, and other forms of thinking. After examining the transmission of information throughout the nervous system, we shall consider various parts of the human brain in further detail.

• NEURAL COMMUNICATION •

While Ray was thumping his drums in weekend concerts, a physician in New York City was engaged in more sedentary activity. Dr. Oliver Sacks was studying neurological disorders, defects in the nervous system that disrupt behavior. Interested in diseases and people, he wrote numerous articles on his work, one of which was published in the *Washington Post* (Sacks, 1987). This newspaper account, of course, reached far beyond the scientific community. Sacks thought about the thousands of citizens who might be exposed to it.

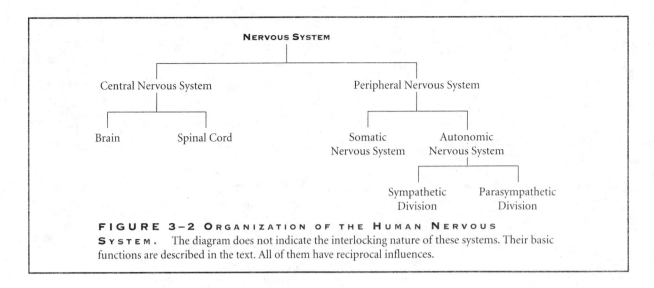

FIGURE 3–2 ORGANIZATION OF THE HUMAN NERVOUS SYSTEM. The diagram does not indicate the interlocking nature of these systems. Their basic functions are described in the text. All of them have reciprocal influences.

THE NEURON

Whether we are thumping drums, writing articles, or thinking about other people, underlying all of our behavior is the **neuron,** a cell specialized for electrochemical communication. The fundamental unit of all nerve tissue, it typically appears in bundles with other neurons. A nerve is a bundle of neurons; collectively, these bundles make up the human nervous system (Figure 3–2).

STRUCTURE OF THE NEURON. Basically, a neuron is composed of three parts. The **cell body** is the central part, containing the nucleus; there are also two types of fibers, slender threadlike structures known as dendrites and axons. The **dendrite,** typically the shorter of these fibers but with innumerable branches, receives impulses and carries them toward its own cell body. The neuron also receives impulses directly at its cell body and sometimes even at the axon. The **axon,** often a very long fiber, characteristically carries impulses away from its cell body toward other neurons. Each neuron has only one axon, which follows the *law of forward conduction,* meaning that it carries impulses only in one direction, away *from* the cell body *to* the dendrites

and cell bodies of other neurons, thereby making connections with those neurons (Figure 3–3).

In many cases, the axon is covered by a substance called the **myelin sheath,** which serves chiefly to insulate one axon from the electrical activities of other axons. It prevents interference among adjacent neurons and speeds the transmission of the impulse. A white, fatty substance, myelin basically covers the gray matter of the neuron itself.

TYPES OF NEURONS. There are three widely recognized types of neurons. The **sensory neuron** transmits messages from the sense organs, such as the ears, tongue, and skin. When such a message reaches the brain, where it is integrated with other messages, we hear, taste, or have other experiences. These neurons are also known as *afferent neurons,* which means "carrying toward" or "input," for they bring information into the central nervous system.

The **motor neuron** transmits impulses away from the central nervous system to the muscles and glands. These neurons initiate actions and create effects, as in striking the drums. Hence, they are also called *efferent neurons,* which means "carrying away" or "output." Both sensory and motor neurons are part of the peripheral nervous system.

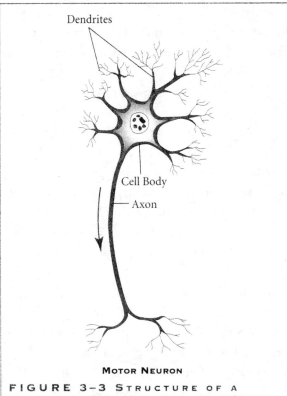

Dendrites

Cell Body

Axon

MOTOR NEURON

FIGURE 3-3 STRUCTURE OF A NEURON. Although neurons have a typical structure, they differ enormously in shape and size. The arrow shows the direction of impulse. Tiny knobs at the ends of the axon make connections with other neurons.

Some nerve impulses entering the spinal cord remain confined to that particular region. These may result in a *reflex*, a relatively simple, automatic response, typically integrated within the spinal cord. If you prick yourself with a pin, you withdraw your hand immediately. You feel pain from the pinprick only afterward, when the message reaches your brain; a reflex occurs faster than the brain can respond. This connection between sensory and motor nerves, known as the simple **reflex arc,** is the basic pattern of the spinal reflex.

Most nerve impulses entering the spinal cord ascend to the brain, and in both locations a third type of neuron is involved. The **interneuron** transmits messages from sensory neurons to motor neurons and also to other interneurons (Figure 3–4). Interneurons not only complete certain reflex arcs; they enable most impulses to ascend the spinal cord, stimulate innumerable circuits within the brain, and eventually prompt other impulses that descend the spinal cord through efferent neurons. Interneurons are thousands of times more common than the other types. When Ray heard about the concert, he did not

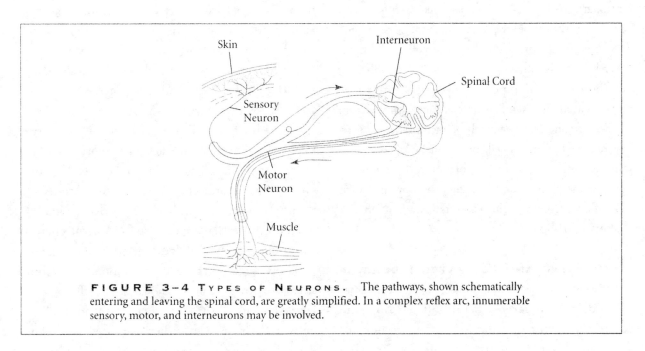

Skin

Interneuron

Spinal Cord

Sensory Neuron

Motor Neuron

Muscle

FIGURE 3-4 TYPES OF NEURONS. The pathways, shown schematically entering and leaving the spinal cord, are greatly simplified. In a complex reflex arc, innumerable sensory, motor, and interneurons may be involved.

respond in an automatic way. Instead, chiefly through interneurons, several brain circuits were aroused as he thought about the opportunity.

✍ NATURE OF THE MESSAGE

The neural message is an electrochemical impulse. It travels along the nerve fiber chiefly by means of its electrical properties—through an exchange of electrical charges known as *ions.* This exchange can occur because the covering of each fiber is porous.

The nerve fiber, in effect, is a very tiny but lengthy battery. In its resting state, without stimulation, the fiber carries no message or current. The battery is not in operation. The membrane has positively charged sodium ions outside and positively charged potassium ions inside, but the overall charge is less positive inside than outside. Thus, relatively speaking, the charge inside is negative whenever the fiber is at rest.

In recent years, the passage of charged ions across the cell membrane has been studied by a revolutionary method. The *patch clamp technique* employs an extremely thin tube or pipette made of glass, which can be very tightly sealed to the cell membrane, thereby establishing a small area, or patch, adhering to the tip of the pipette, and this patch can be investigated by chemical or electrical stimulation. With a strong seal, the patch of membrane can even be removed from its cell, or it can be opened into the cell, offering further opportunities for stimulating the membrane and deducing the ways in which ions flow across it, influencing its voltage (Neher & Sakmann, 1992).

RESTING AND ACTIVATED FIBERS. In its resting state, without stimulation, the nerve fiber is said to be **polarized** because it has opposite poles, or charges, on either side of the membrane. This unactivated state is also called the **resting** potential of the nerve fiber as it awaits a stimulus of a certain minimum intensity. A stimulus must be above a certain level of intensity, or threshold, to activate the fiber.

When the resting fiber has been sufficiently stimulated, either by an impulse from a receptor or by activity in adjacent fibers, the membrane becomes more permeable or porous in the region of stimulation. Some closed "sodium gates" of the membrane open very briefly, permitting positively charged sodium ions to flow in for an instant. This part of the nerve fiber, where the positively charged particles have moved inside, is momentarily **depolarized,** or activated. This change prompts positively charged potassium ions to flow out, causing the inside of the fiber to become increasingly negative. Then tiny ionic pumps in the cell restore the normal balance within a few milliseconds, returning that part of the fiber to its original resting state.

This change in voltage passes successively along the length of the neuron, constituting the nerve impulse. In a crude way, the traveling impulse is like a burning fuse on a firecracker. It produces a similar increase in permeability, or depolarization, in the immediately adjacent part of the neuron, causing an influx of sodium particles there, and so on, until the depolarization has traveled the length of the fiber. Its maximum speed in human nervous tissue is 240 miles per hour, and it is fastest in the relatively thick fibers (Figure 3–5).

This brief shift in electrical energy, the nerve impulse, is also called the **action potential,** and all impulses traveling along a particular neuron have the same energy, regardless of the nature or intensity of the activating stimulus. The reason is that a stimulus does no more than release the electrical energy already in the fiber; it does not contribute energy. This property of the neuron, responding at full strength or not at all, is known as the **all-or-none law,** which is illustrated whenever a doorbell is pressed. If you press it hard enough, the bell sounds; if you press harder, it does not sound any louder.

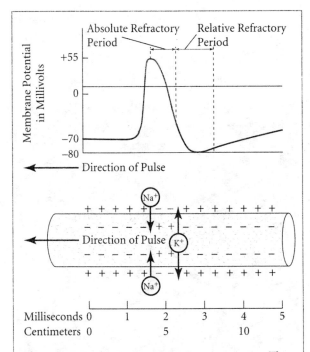

FIGURE 3–5 NERVE IMPULSE. The top of this figure shows the electrical changes in the action potential as it moves along the neuron. The bottom of the figure shows the corresponding chemical changes. Sodium ions (Na) enter the neuron, causing potassium ions (K) to flow outward. This successive release of energy along the neuron constitutes the nerve impulse.

The nerve fiber is like a doorbell in another sense. Most doorbells cannot be reused until the button pops out again. A waiting or recovery period, known as the **refractory period,** is also necessary with the nerve fiber as the sodium and potassium particles return to their original positions, ready for another firing. This refractory period has two phases. Immediately after activation, during the *absolute refractory phase,* no stimulus of any strength can start a nerve impulse. This phase differs from fiber to fiber but it is very brief, usually only about 1/1,000th of a second.

After this phase, there is a progressive increase in sensitivity. During this period, a stimulus that is stronger than normal can produce another response. This interval between the absolute refractory phase and restoration of the normal resting state is known as the *relative refractory phase,* and it lasts a few thousandths of a second.

If a nerve, when it does fire, responds only on an all-or-none basis, how are we able to experience different levels of stimulus intensity? How can we discriminate, for example, between a dim pocket light and the glare of a bright neon sign? The answer lies in the arrangements of nerve fibers, which typically occur in bundles, allowing thousands of fibers to be activated simultaneously, depending on the intensity of the stimulus. The optic nerve, for example, has an estimated 400,000 fibers, and increasing the stimulus intensity can have two effects. It can increase the frequency of discharge in each fiber that responds during the relative refractory phase, and it can activate more and more receptors and fibers.

INTERACTIONS AT THE SYNAPSE. Musical ability, the capacity for conversation, and all other manifestations of human flexibility are due to a vital feature of the human nervous system. Unlike the jellyfish, in which each fiber is welded to another fiber, and the worm, in which fibers in certain segments are welded together, the ends of nerve fibers in human beings do not make direct contact with each other to form fixed connections. Rather, their endings are simply very close together.

The small space between all adjacent neurons, where the nerve impulse passes from one neuron to another, is called a **synapse.** It is the site at the end of an axon where the stimulation is transmitted to the dendrite or cell body of the adjacent neuron, and it occupies a central position in our understanding of the flexibility of mammalian behavior. At some synapses, nerve impulses are inhibited and go no further. At others, they converge and activate one or many other fibers in the spinal cord and brain. Hence the behavioral outcomes are indeed innumerable.

Here, at the synapse, where several impulses converge, the all-or-none law no longer prevails. Instead, small changes in polarization may occur in the membrane of the receiving cell. A change of this sort is known as a **graded potential** because the size of the shift can vary, depending on the amount and type of information in the incoming message. One shift may be slight, too small to activate the fiber. Another may be larger. Amid this interplay of numerous influences, the graded potential may reach a certain level of intensity. It then stimulates the nerve to fire, producing an action potential.

In other words, transmission of the impulse *along the neuron* follows the all-or-none law. Transmission *from neuron to neuron* follows the principle of the graded potential.

How does the graded potential reach the necessary intensity to fire the neuron? It does so in two ways. Sometimes impulses from several different axons converge at adjacent points on a receiving membrane, causing it to fire, an outcome known as *spatial summation.* Sometimes, as the axons continue to fire in very quick succession, collectively they cause the nerve to fire, a phenomenon known as *temporal summation.*

CHEMICAL FOUNDATIONS

But how does the nerve impulse cross the synapse? It does not jump across, like a spark, as once was thought (Figure 3–6). Instead, the chemical bases of this electrochemical impulse become more significant. They convey the impulse across the synapse to adjacent neurons. In the final analysis, the diversity of human behavior is significantly dependent on these chemical substances.

Consider the diversity in Ray's behavior. At one moment, he reached a frenzied high in a musical improvisation. At another, he enjoyed table tennis, taking much pleasure in his swift reactions. Even opponents agreed that his successful play was marked by very sudden, unexpected shots. *"Frivolous* shots," Ray called them (Sacks, 1987). On still other occasions, he accepted the enticing challenge of revolving doors. For him, they made the world go round. He gleefully dodged in and out of them with lightning speed and a ready quip, spinning a tale about his fancy footwork. This broad range of activity, from beating drums to beating doors, was made possible by chemical substances in the synaptic spaces.

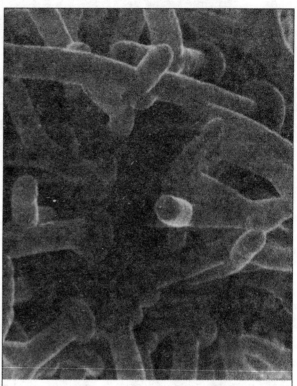

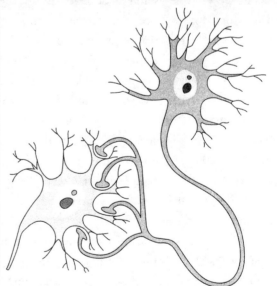

FIGURE 3–6 THE SYNAPSE. A small space, known as the synaptic space, lies between the transmitting axon and the receiving dendrite or cell body, as shown in the drawing and magnified in the photograph.

**OPERATION OF NEUROTRANSMIT-
TERS.** These chemicals are contained in small sacs or vesicles in the knobs at the ends of axons. Each of them is called a **neurotransmitter substance,** meaning a chemical that, when discharged into a synapse, travels across the space to act on the membrane of the adjacent nerve fiber. One chemical may depolarize the receiving membrane, causing activity in that membrane, contributing to an *excitatory reaction.* Another may make the receiving membrane more polarized and therefore more resistant to firing, contributing to an *inhibitory reaction.* In a broad sense, there are two kinds of reactions at synapses, excitation or inhibition, depending partly on which receptor sites are activated.

More specifically, in traveling across the synapse, the neurotransmitter substance encounters a neurotransmitter receptor, which is a site on the receiving neuron with a specific molecular structure. If the shape or structure of the transmitter substance matches that of the receptor site, then the receiving neuron can accommodate that transmitter. Since different neurotransmitters have different molecular structures, some fit a particular site, initiating a reaction or amplifying an effect; others, at the same site, block the transmission, preventing further stimulation. Still others do not fit the site at all. Thus, arousal of a receiving neuron depends not only on the neurotransmitter chemical but also on the nature and structure of that receptor site.

This interpretation of synaptic transmission has been known as the *lock-and-key hypothesis,* meaning that the shape of the neurotransmitter substance, the key, must fit the structure of the receiving membrane, the "lock." And, of course, the key needs to work in the lock, either through summation or on its own, initiating an excitatory or inhibitory reaction in the receiving cell membrane.

This release of chemicals into the synapse occurs in a fraction of a second, with thousands of neurons firing, resulting in a deluge of neurotransmitters into the synaptic space. Between firings,

those neurotransmitters that remain in the synapse are drawn back into their sacs once again or otherwise rendered ineffective by various clean-up chemicals also in the system. The whole process is designed to produce an infinite variety of activating and inhibiting forces, depending on the chemical structures of the transmitter substances and receptor sites (Figure 3–7).

Alcohol consumption, for example, blocks certain neurotransmitters responsible for brain activity, eventually inducing sleep. But it also disrupts the work of other neurotransmitters, awakening the person earlier than usual. Certain mind-altering drugs that cause distortion in perception and consciousness appear to have these pronounced effects because their chemical structures are similar to

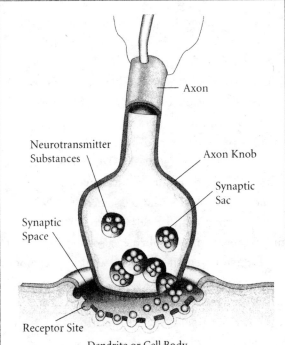

**FIGURE 3–7 TRANSMISSION IN
SYNAPTIC SPACE.** Upon reaching the knob at the end of the axon, the nerve impulse releases chemical messengers from small sacs, and these neurotransmitter substances travel into the synaptic space. If they fit the molecular structure of the receptor site in a receiving dendrite or cell body, they cause a voltage change in that cell, exciting or inhibiting a nerve impulse. If they do not fit into that molecular structure, they are removed by other chemicals or return to the original axon.

those of natural neurotransmitters found in the brain. In other words, there are critical differences among the neurotransmitters released in the brain.

The number of different transmitters in the human body is not known at this time, for proposed substances must meet several stringent criteria. Nevertheless, experts have identified 50 or more, and a few have been studied extensively.

PROMINENT NEUROTRANSMITTERS.
Perhaps the most thoroughly studied neurotransmitter is **acetylcholine,** which plays a prominent role in muscular activity. It can be either excitatory or inhibitory. It is excitatory at motor synapses in the peripheral nervous system, important in such activities as making music, playing table tennis, and dodging revolving doors. Certain gases and poisons that produce convulsions or seizures apparently do so by prolonging the action of acetylcholine.

A decrease of acetylcholine in the central nervous system is prominent in **Alzheimer's disease,** a rapid deterioration of brain functions, especially in the elderly. It involves memory loss and disorientation in time and place. The decrease in acetylcholine associated with Alzheimer's disease is well documented, and it correlates with the severity of the disease (McDonald & Nemeroff, 1991).

Operating in a diffuse fashion, the neurotransmitter called **norepinephrine,** also known as *noradrenaline,* is influential in general arousal and mood, as well as in learning and memory. Exerting excitatory influences at synapses for the heart, blood vessels, and genitals, it can result in a highly pleasurable reaction. Amphetamines, stimulating its release, promote an alert, active state.

Another neurotransmitter, apparently related to norepinephrine, acts without such widespread effects. Thus **dopamine** influences emotional reactions, rather than general wakefulness, as well as learning and memory. It too is influenced by amphetamines and reserpine, and it may be a factor in severe behavior disorders, including schizo-

phrenic reactions (Goteborgs, 1990). Blocking the transmission of dopamine at synapses, by the administration of chlorpromazine and other drugs, has proved useful in the treatment of psychosis and related mental disorders.

The operation of dopamine illustrates the exquisite complexities among and within neurotransmitters, for it also influences the control of voluntary movements. If dopamine is depleted in motor neurons, the result is slowness and inability to move, as in **Parkinson's disease,** characterized by muscular tremors, rigidity, and loss of voluntary control. This disease occurs primarily in men in later life and may be related to depression (Guze & Barrio, 1991; Oles, 1992). These patients need additional dopamine to become aroused. Sometimes their disease is combated with the administration of L-dopa, called a *dopamine precursor* because it is converted into dopamine.

Some people who are frenetic and highly aroused may profit from lower levels of dopamine, enabling them to act in a more stable, normal fashion. This outcome is achieved by administering a medication that is *antagonistic* to dopamine, meaning that it blocks or impedes the action of dopamine. In contrast, a drug or other substance that triggers or increases the action of a neurotransmitter is said to be *agonistic* to that neurotransmitter.

A light snack before bedtime can lead to increased production of **serotonin,** a neurotransmitter associated with drowsiness, sleep, and food metabolism. It plays a role in food intake and appetite, especially the ingestion of protein, carbohydrates, and even alcohol (Tollefson, 1991). Foods high in carbohydrates, such as spaghetti and bread, enhance the production of serotonin. Turkey also is high in the precursors of serotonin. If you must be an after-dinner speaker, do so only if you can choose the menu: no spaghetti, no turkey, no bread, and so forth. Serotonin operates in several areas of the brain and is known to be related to depression and hypertension, as well as to appetite and sleep (Bonate, 1991).

NEUROTRANSMITTER	GENERAL INFLUENCES	FUNCTIONS AND DISORDERS
Acetylcholine	Excitatory	Muscle movement, emotion, memory, cognitive functions.
Norepinephrine	Excitatory	Arousal, cognitive functions. Excess: mania. Deficit: depression.
Serotonin	Inhibitory	Sleep, appetite, awareness. Deficit: depression.
Dopamine	Inhibitory	Movement, emotional arousal, memory. Excess: schizophrenia.
GABA	Inhibitory	Deficit: seizures
Endorphins	Inhibitory	Suppression of pain.

TABLE 3–1 PROMINENT NEUROTRANSMITTERS. These functions are constantly being confirmed or revised. Additional functions and neurotransmitters are regularly being identified.

In normal functioning, there is an extraordinarily delicate balance among these neurotransmitter influences. One condition in which this balance goes awry is *epilepsy*, a neurological disorder characterized by attacks of convulsive movements, mental malfunction, and sometimes loss of consciousness. One important neurotransmitter in this disorder is **GABA**, an acronym for *gamma amino butyric acid*, recognized as the most widespread inhibitory transmitter.

Given the literally countless neurons in the central nervous system and their innumerable synapses, it is not surprising that the great majority of synaptic events in the brain are inhibitory. Without this inhibition, we would be overwhelmed by torrents of competing and unwanted messages. One might speculate about Ray in this regard. In his sudden, impulsive swearing, and even in other activities, did he sometimes experience a failure to inhibit?

COMPLEXITY OF NEURAL COMMUNICATION. As the delicate chemical messengers of the nervous system, neurotransmitters have produced several unexpected research findings. Early investigators reported that serotonin is associated with sleep; others found that it has no such role. Gradually, it was understood that any given neurotransmitter can serve in diverse ways. Moreover, different neurotransmitters have similar functions.

Serotonin and norepinephrine are both associated with depression; norepinephrine and dopamine influence arousal; acetylcholine and dopamine both play a role in memory and emotion; and so forth (Table 3–I).

Further evidence for the complexity of neural communication comes from the brain chemicals called **endorphins,** so named because they are endogenous, meaning produced in the body, and yet possess properties of morphine, an addictive opiate compound that reduces pain. In short, "endogenous morphines" are natural anesthetics apparently secreted by certain brain cells. They regulate pain by blocking pain signals from the peripheral nervous system. Their production may be stimulated during acupuncture, for example, thereby suppressing the experience of more painful medical procedures. They may operate locally in some situations, as in acupuncture, and more generally in others, when athletes or people in emergencies perform at high levels under otherwise painful circumstances, seemingly unaware of their injuries. These bodily changes have survival value, enabling animals and human beings to escape the immediate danger and then, afterward, tend to their wounds.

There has been some debate over the classification of endorphins as neurotransmitters. Some investigators simply regard them as endogenous opiate compounds produced in greater quantities under conditions of pain or stress. Others believe that they meet the basic requirements for neurotransmitters: chemical substances produced in the presynaptic neuron, released by the nerve impulse, and resulting in excitation or inhibition at the receptor site.

• THE HUMAN BRAIN •

Ray's quick wit and considerable strength of character enabled him to complete school and college. Afterward, he enjoyed a successful marriage, maintained friendships, and held several jobs. When not at work, he succeeded in all sorts of physical endeavors requiring quickness and accuracy. In sports, games, and physical challenges, his timing seemed almost unnatural, beyond the normal range.

Ray also engaged in various mental activities, including reading and writing. One day he read an article in the *Washington Post* that described some unusual behaviors he had experienced himself, and he decided to write to its author. He thought Dr. Oliver Sacks would receive hundreds of such letters, far more than he might answer, but he wrote anyway.

Ray was right. Sacks received many letters, and he gave all but one to appropriate colleagues. He intended to answer that one letter, thinking its author might profit from his assistance.

All of these diverse responses—playing games, reading, writing, thinking, and endless others—are related to developments in the human brain. Variously described as a wrinkled boxing glove, a head of cauliflower and its stalk, and a thick sack crumpled into a small space, the human brain is three pounds of moist rubberiness usefully studied from several viewpoints.

BRAIN AND EVOLUTION

From an evolutionary perspective, study of the human brain is usually considered in terms of its three major divisions: the hindbrain, midbrain, and forebrain. Approaching the brain in this way allows the discussion to proceed from the biological processes we share with other creatures to the mental capacities that uniquely characterize the human condition.

HINDBRAIN. Closest to the spinal cord and oldest of the three divisions in an evolutionary sense is the hindbrain, so named because it appears at the rear of the brain. The **hindbrain** plays a significant role in *vital functions*, such as waking, sleeping, balance, and coordination. One part, the **medulla,** controls digestion, breathing, and blood circulation. An adjacent organ, the *pons*, meaning "bridge," consists chiefly of motor neurons; it connects several structures serving underlying functions in waking and sleeping states, including dreams.

The largest structure of the hindbrain is the **cerebellum,** or "little brain," a major mechanism in maintaining posture and coordinating body movements. Impulses from receptors in the muscles, tendons, and joints provide it with information about movements throughout the body. Integrated in the cerebellum and associated structures, this information prompts return impulses to the muscles, tendons, and joints, initiating the proper adjustive actions. In this manner, when coupled with other organs, the cerebellum plays a role in our capacity to repeat well-practiced motor movements.

Some parts of the cerebellum appear to control movements of the whole body; others concern specific regions. Thus, damage to the central area may cause difficulty in posture and locomotion; damage in more lateral areas may disrupt arm and leg motions and rapidly alternating hand and finger movements. When Ray surprised the members of the band with his unexpected improvisations, the cerebellum played a key role in controlling these movements.

MIDBRAIN. A short segment between the hindbrain and upper brain regions is called the **midbrain,** serving a vital role in *processing information*

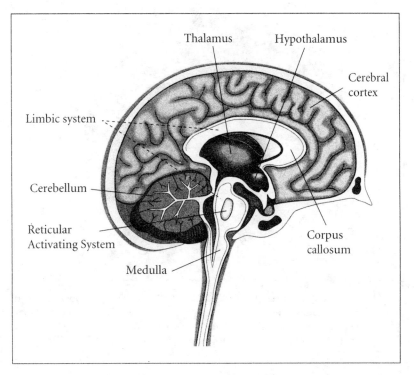

HINDBRAIN

Medulla: controls digestion and breathing. Example: Bodily processes convert Ray's dinner into assimilable substances.

Cerebellum: coordinates balance and muscle movements. Example: Ray plays a drum roll.

MIDBRAIN

Reticular Activating System: influences the onset of sleep and arousal. Example: Ray dozes off during intermission.

FOREBRAIN

Thalamus: relays incoming and outgoing messages. Example: Sounds of a bass fiddle and guitar are integrated and transmitted elsewhere in Ray's brain.

Hypothalamus: regulates biological activities, including eating, drinking, and many others. Example: Ray begins to feel hungry.

Limbic System: plays a key role in emotion and motivation. Example: On hearing familiar music, Ray feels sentimental.

Cerebral Cortex: guides perceiving, learning, memory, thinking, and voluntary behavior. Example: Ray thinks about meeting Sacha after the concert.

FIGURE III.1 BRAIN STRUCTURES AND FUNCTIONS. This cross-section shows the human brain from the right, indicating its major structures and functions. No one structure is solely responsible for any function; the brain operates in an integrated manner. The loosely defined limbic system, not clearly depicted here, is a group of interconnected structures lying deep beneath the cerebral cortex. The corpus callosum is discussed later.

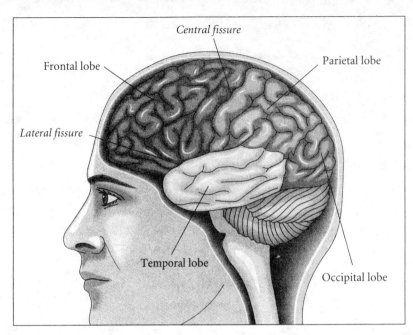

FIGURE III.2 LOBES OF THE CEREBRAL CORTEX. The four lobes, seen here from the left, are divided in some cases by a major crevice or fissure. The frontal and parietal lobes are separated by the central fissure. The temporal lobe is largely separated from them by the lateral fissure. The occipital lobe is not clearly delineated from either of its neighbors.

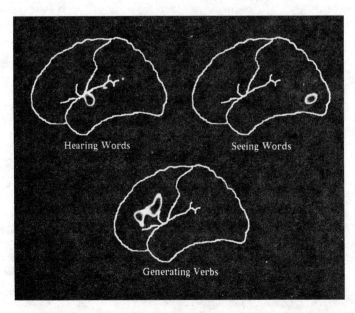

FIGURE III.3 PET SCANS. Different uses of language involve activities in different brain areas, as shown when a person is hearing, reading, or saying words. In these PET images, the red depicts the areas of most activitiy, followed in decreasing order by yellow, green, and then blue.

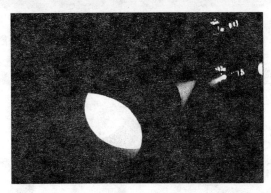

FIGURE IV.1 ADDITIVE COLOR MIXTURE. Combining lights of different colors adds wavelengths to the mixture. The result is some new color or, when all colors are combined, white light.

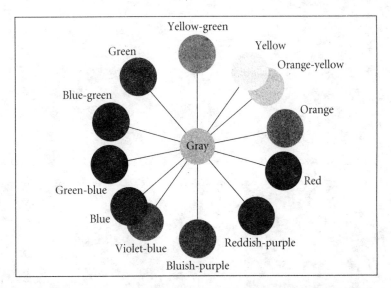

FIGURE IV.2 THE COLOR CIRCLE. The circle represents the color spectrum plus various shades of purple created by mixing red and blue. Mixing complementary colors, opposite one another on the circle, gives gray, but mixing any other pair produced an intermediate hue.

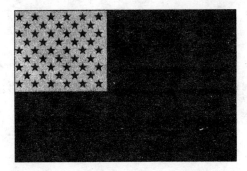

FIGURE IV.3 NEGATIVE AFTERIMAGE. Under bright illumination, gaze steadily for about one minute at the lower right corner of the yellow field of stars. Then look immediately at any white space above or beside the flag. The "Old Glory" you experience is composed of the complementary colors in your visual system, apparently due to receptor adaptation.

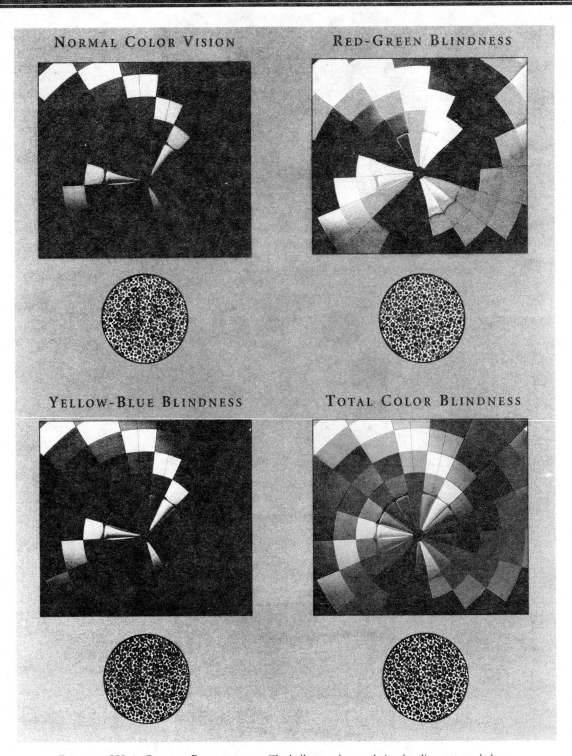

FIGURE IV.4 COLOR BLINDNESS. The balloon colors and circular disc patterns below each photograph are shown as they would appear to people with normal color vision, red-green blindness, yellow-blue blindness, and total color blindness. The discs illustrate a test for color blindness. A person with normal color vision would readily perceive the red 48 against the green background, as would a person with yellow-blue blindness. People with red-green or total color blindness would not perceive the number at all.

for the upper brain regions, especially information coming from the eyes and ears. Sometimes the midbrain and hindbrain together are called the *brain stem.* In any case, they share many fibers that have a diffuse, netlike appearance and therefore are called the *reticular formation.* These shared netlike connections are also known as the **reticular activating system,** for they influence the arousal of the whole organism, acting like gates. When you fall asleep suddenly, the reticular activating system has abruptly stopped sending impulses to the many cortical synapses with which it has connections. When you are unable to fall asleep, the reticular system is still active.

The neurons in the reticular activating system vary widely in size. They also have long dendrites with diffuse branches, creating innumerable synaptic pathways, and axons that apparently make connections with their own cell bodies. Poorly designed for transmitting specific information, they appear to be well constructed for arousal and nonarousal.

Chiefly because he was so readily aroused, Ray was successful at table tennis, revolving doors, and repartee, but he also suffered a great deal. At work, he had been fired several times, not for incompetence, but for lack of restraint. At home, his emotional outbursts occasionally unsettled his wife. According to Ray, they were completely involuntary.

Worse yet, Ray was plagued by tics. A *tic* is a sudden, involuntary muscle twitch appearing habitually, usually in the face or extremities. In Ray, they appeared every few seconds, causing him to be severely stigmatized in public (Sacks, 1987).

Recognizing his condition as both a gift and a curse, he called himself "Witty Ticcy Ray." He was the "ticcer of Broadway," prone to "ticcy witticisms and witty ticcicisms" (Sacks, 1987).

All of these reactions—Ray's quickness, tics, and uncontrollable swearing—were influenced by elements of the hindbrain and midbrain. To the knowledgeable person, they suggested a possible disturbance in the midbrain, especially in those parts involved with the emotional aspects of personality. Ray was free from tics, tension, and uncontrollable outbursts only when completely at rest or working in some evenly paced, melodic fashion (Sacks, 1987).

FOREBRAIN. From an evolutionary viewpoint, the **forebrain**—the upper and most recently developed of the three major brain areas—most clearly separates the human brain from those of other animals, for it is fundamentally involved in *perceiving, remembering, and thinking.* The olfactory bulb, concerned with smell, is relatively smaller and less important in human beings than in many other animals, but other structures become larger and more elaborate as we ascend the evolutionary order.

These include, in particular, the *cerebral cortex*—the large, rounded structure at the top of the forebrain, divided into two nearly symmetrical hemispheres. This structure, to which we shall return shortly, allows human beings to recall the past and to ruminate on forthcoming events in ways apparently impossible for other species (Figure 3–8).

Of these three brain divisions, the human forebrain constitutes our greatest advance over all other

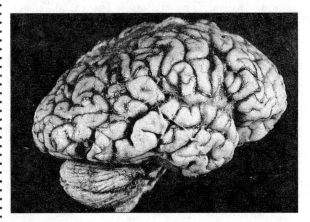

FIGURE 3–8 BRAIN AND EVOLUTION.
Shown from the right side, the forebrain is the large oval mass occupying most of the photo. The midbrain, in the interior, is not shown. The hindbrain is chiefly the lower, smaller oval-shaped region.

species, including other primates. The midbrain, prominent in biological motivation and emotion, is found in all mammalian species. And the hindbrain represents what human beings have in common with even the most primitive aquatic creatures: reflexes and other involuntary functions.

SUBCORTICAL STRUCTURES

In further study of the human brain, we turn from the evolutionary perspective to a somewhat simpler distinction between the lower and upper brain regions. The lower regions, at the very center of the brain, are often referred to as **subcortical structures,** for they lie beneath the outer covering, or cerebral cortex, occupying a region just above the spinal cord. These structures, for the most part, are found in the lower part of the forebrain. They play an important role in regulating basic bodily functions, including eating, sexual behavior, and emotional reactions.

RELAY ROLE OF THE THALAMUS. Among the major subcortical structures, the thalamus, hypothalamus, and limbic system are especially important in emotional behavior and general arousal. The **thalamus,** meaning "inner room," is situated at the very center of the brain, serving as a prominent switchboard for various brain regions. It is, according to many, the brain's finest relay station. With the exception of impulses for smell, which go more directly from the olfactory bulb to the olfactory cortex, the thalamus manages the input from sensory systems throughout the body. It is justifiably called a fundamental link between the external environment and the various parts of the nervous system, especially the cerebral cortex.

The axons of the optic nerve, for example, connect largely with the thalamus, which integrates these visual signals with information already in the system. The thalamus also receives auditory, tactile, and related information from other sensory systems. Then it relays this information to appropriate regions in the central nervous system, especially the cerebral cortex. At the same time, the thalamus is responsive to feedback *from* the cortex, for it has both ascending and descending connections. Especially in the context of sensory input, it deserves its reputation as a relay station.

In addition, the thalamus plays a role in the formation of memories, particularly the reception of new information. It is not evident, however, that it has any significant function in the consolidation and retention of these memories.

REGULATION BY THE HYPOTHALAMUS. If there is any significance in the old aphorism about not judging a package by its size, then in brain regions it certainly applies to the hypothalamus. The prefix *hypo* means "under" or "lower," and the **hypothalamus,** a very small structure situated just below the thalamus, has a major role in regulating all sorts of biological and psychological activities. It is often said to be critically involved in four fundamental functions: feeding, fighting, fleeing, and—making love. It maintains this pervasive control partly through its influence over the autonomic and endocrine systems, considered at the close of this chapter.

The role of the hypothalamus in eating is evident with damage to its central area, which results in overeating. In contrast, damage to its peripheral regions causes self-imposed starvation. Injury or disease in still other areas can disturb thirst, sexual behavior, and emotional expression.

Not solely responsible for full emotional experience, the hypothalamus is nevertheless a central organ in emotional reactions. Numerous experiments have verified this integrative role of the hypothalamus in emotional behavior.

Overwhelmed by his uncontrollable emotional reactions, Ray was delighted to receive a letter from

Oliver Sacks, author of the article in the *Washington Post* and world-renowned neurologist. Especially interested in disorders of the subcortical structures, including the hypothalamus, Sacks had decided that Ray perhaps was afflicted with an unusual disorder and invited him for a consultation. This disorder, *Tourette's syndrome*, is characterized by tics—repetitive movements or nonword noises—and often by unprovoked swearing, as well (Berecz, 1992). In addition, there may be an impulsive tendency to repeat the words or phrases of other people, or even their gestures (Table 3–2).

The causes of Tourette's syndrome are unknown, but it seems that people with this disorder have an excess of certain neurotransmitters in subcortical regions, particularly dopamine. Just as lethargic patients with Parkinson's disease can be aroused to more normal action by the administration of L-dopa, with its dopamine derivatives, patients with Tourette's syndrome can achieve more normal functioning by blocking this neurotransmitter through administration of haloperidol, known under the brand name Haldol, which is antagonistic to dopamine. When Ray met with Dr. Sacks, the diagnosis of Tourette's syndrome was confirmed. Ray was then tested for responsiveness to Haldol and proved extraordinarily sensitive. He received a prescription for three very small doses daily. Initially this treatment seemed satisfactory, suppressing both the tics and the unpredictable emotional episodes.

LIMBIC SYSTEM. Certain portions of the thalamus and hypothalamus, along with several other organs lying in a circuit along the brain stem, constitute the **limbic system,** which plays a key role in emotion and motivation. The term *limbic* means "border" or "outlying," and this system of organs represents the inner or under border of the cerebral hemispheres. There is still some controversy, however, about just which subcortical organs should be included in this system.

The basic point here is that emotion is not the exclusive function of any specific brain center but rather is the result of an activated circuitry of organs called the limbic system. Within this system our sensory experiences take on an emotional tone. The thalamus, with sensory input, and the hypothalamus, with regulatory functions, are natural contributors to this system. Overall, the limbic system plays an important role in the integration of emotional behavior. Generally, it is slow to turn on, but once turned on, it is slow to turn off.

The *amygdala*, a limbic organ that looks like a large almond, is situated between the thalamus and hypothalamus. It also mediates emotional behavior, and it plays an important role in the emotional aspects of memory. Stimulation with a needle microelectrode implanted in this area has produced aggressive attacks and apparently unpleasant emotions in animals. Electrodes in adjacent areas prompt only a momentary disruption, not a prolonged reaction.

SYMPTOM	DESCRIPTION	ROLE IN DIAGNOSIS	RAY'S CASE
Tics	Involuntary, repetitive movements or noises	Essential	Present
Swearing	Unprovoked foul language	Not essential	Present
Echolalia	Involuntary repetition of someone's words	Not essential	Absent
Onset of illness	Prior to 21 years of age	Essential	Present

TABLE 3–2 DIAGNOSIS OF TOURETTE'S SYNDROME. Swearing and echolalia are not essential for the diagnosis. In severe Tourette's syndrome, there may be imitation of gestures (Comings, 1990).

Oliver Sacks had decided that Ray's uncontrollable outbursts were related to disturbances in the limbic system, including the hypothalamus and amygdala, where the basic emotional determinants of personality are lodged (Sacks, 1987). Ray's symptoms disappeared and reappeared with the presence and absence of a slight amount of medication, which apparently had its strongest impact in this region. Nevertheless, the limbic system is concerned with more than emotion and motivation. It also plays a complex role in learning and memory.

Another area of the limbic system, the *septal area*, was accidentally discovered to play a role in pleasurable emotional experience. Around midcentury, a young psychologist named James Olds, bent on replicating some earlier studies with needle electrodes, apparently used a bent needle, positioning it slightly in the wrong part of the brain. To his surprise, a rat with the improperly implanted electrode, allowed to stimulate itself in the septal area by pressing a bar, eventually did so at the rate of 500 to 5,000 times per hour. Other animals also behaved as if they were experiencing pleasure, some stimulating themselves 2,000 times per hour for a full day, prompting Olds to call this particular brain region the "pleasure center" (Olds, 1956).

Today we know that it is the neurochemical system in the septal area, not the septum itself, that supports this phenomenon. The prominent substances appear to be norepinephrine and dopamine. We also know that human beings examined in a clinical setting apparently do not respond with the same emotional intensity as do animals studied experimentally in a laboratory (Valenstein, 1973).

The nature of these limbic regions is indeed puzzling. Unlike such obviously motivated behaviors as eating and sexual activity, electrical self-stimulation is sometimes not marked by temporary diminution of interest for extended periods. Still further, alcohol and other drugs seem to have a stronger effect in this area than in other brain regions. Thus, it has been hypothesized that its motivating effects may involve some sort of physiological addiction; successive stimulations may increase the craving.

This topic has developed into a broad research field now called *intracranial self-stimulation* (Olds & Forbes, 1981). The most promising findings to date suggest that dopamine may play a critical role (Wise & Rompre, 1989). Overall, this research provides an excellent example of a basic theme of this book: the role of empiricism in modern psychology. Investigators have tried one approach, then another, and another, all based on stimulation of specific areas and direct observation of the behavioral reactions.

CEREBRAL CORTEX

The largest and most obvious aspects of the human brain are structures of the forebrain or upper brain regions, the two cerebral hemispheres. They are vital in learning, memory, and other high-level thought processes. The term *cerebrum*, often applied to the brain as a whole, refers to these two hemispheres. Each hemisphere, for the most part, pertains to the opposite side of the body. The left hemisphere serves the right side; the right hemisphere serves the left.

Our special interest lies in the outer covering, or bark, of the cerebral hemispheres, known as the **cerebral cortex,** which has a smooth surface in most lower animals but contains many folds, or convolutions, in human beings, providing a large neural surface. The significance of these folds becomes readily evident when you imagine trying to place a large piece of thin tissue paper into a small cup. When crumpled, it readily fits. Owing to its important role in higher mental processes, the cerebral cortex is sometimes called our "thinking cap." Much of it is also called the neocortex, meaning "new covering," for it covers other parts of the cortex that are older in an evolutionary sense (Figure III.I Color).

Structurally, the two hemispheres are separated by the longitudinal fissure, a large crevice that runs from front to rear. In addition, each hemisphere is less obviously divided into four sections or lobes: **frontal lobes,** over the eyes, involved in motor control, as well as cognitive functions; **temporal lobes,** near the ears, for processing of auditory information; **occipital lobes,** at the extreme back of the head, where visual information is processed; and **parietal lobes,** at the top and back of the brain, concerned with body feeling, especially sensitivity in the skin, muscles, and body cavity (Figure III.2).

STUDYING THE CORTEX. There are several ways of studying the subcortical and cortical regions of the brain. Some have been mentioned already, including clinical studies of brain damage in human beings, experimental studies of brain lesions in animals, and electrical brain stimulation. Additional methods permit non-invasive studies of the intact living brain. One of these, called the **electroencephalograph** (EEG), is a device for recording the spontaneous electrical patterns of the brain, sometimes called *brain waves.* Regular and irregular patterns can be detected. This procedure is described more fully in a later chapter on consciousness.

Newer, more dramatic methods use powerful electronic devices that produce photograph-like images of the living brain. These successive images are called *brain scans,* and the device is known as a *brain scanner.* The basic technique is evident in the term *tomography,* which comes from two Greek words. *Tome* means "cutting," for these images cut across different regions of the brain. *Graphein* means "recording." Thus, a *tomograph* is a device that records a series of brain images.

The most common brain scan is *computerized tomography,* called the **CT scan,** or *CAT scan,* produced by successive X-rays of a given location in the head, each from a slightly different angle, fed into a computer. There they are synthesized, giving an in-depth computerized image of the structure of the brain. By combining successive images, each depicting a different slice of the brain, large areas of the brain can be portrayed, thereby revealing evidence of damage from injury or disease.

Another promising method which shows the brain's structure is *magnetic resonance imaging,* called the **MRI scan** because it uses an intense magnetic field to generate these images. When the magnetic field is turned on and off, each brain element has its own particular response, and when these different resonances are combined and analyzed by a computer, they show normal and abnormal brain conditions. These pictures are extraordinarily sensitive and more detailed than those available in the CT scan, and there is no danger from radiation. However, they are also more expensive at this time.

Another tomographic method, the **PET scan,** meaning *positron emission tomography,* requires the subject to ingest a glucose compound that is utilized in the brain. Then the subject engages in various activities, such as talking, solving problems, or relaxing. The brain areas most activated utilize the most glucose and thus reveal the function with which they are most closely associated. This technique receives its name because it shows *positively* charged particles *emitted* from the *tomogram,* or cross section, of the brain. Extremely useful in brain research, it reveals activities in the brain, not just its structure. In other words, the PET scan shows the brain *at work* (Figure III.3).

One review over a five-year period reported the CT, MRI, and PET techniques as equally effective in detecting moderately to severely impaired patients with Alzheimer's disease, often with 100% accuracy. However, with mildly impaired patients, the PET and CT techniques were most accurate (Albert & Lafleche, 1991). In contrast, studies of patients with head injuries showed MRI to be more sensitive than the CT scan for detecting organically based neuropsychological deficits (Wilson, 1990). Thus, the different techniques can serve similar and also different functions.

MOTOR CORTEX. We know that the primary area for controlling body movements is a narrow strip of cortical tissue at the rear of the frontal lobe directly in front of the central fissure, known as the **motor cortex**. Here, the degree of control required for specific body parts is closely related to the size of the brain area involved. The finer and more coordinated the movements, the larger is the cortical region devoted to these movements. The fingers, hands, lips, and tongue occupy large parts of the motor cortex; the arms and legs occupy lesser areas; and the hips and shoulders, which involve the least precision, occupy the smallest areas.

Furthermore, control of the body parts is represented in an inverted sequence with reference to an upright human being. Control of the toes, feet, and legs appears near the top of each hemisphere; the trunk is toward the middle; and the arms, hands, neck, and head are near the bottom.

When Ray moved his feet, dashing through a doorway, impulses occurred at the top of his motor cortex. Impulses were emitted lower down the side when he smiled and boasted about his success. In both cases, the locations were just forward of the central fissure (Figure 3–9).

Within a week after beginning his medication, which was less than 1 milligram daily, Ray returned to the clinic with a black eye, a broken nose, and several disparaging remarks about the medication. "So much for your f——— Haldol," he growled. As it turned out, even these very small doses so interfered with his neural transmission and motor coordination that he had been bashed by a revolving door. His tics, rather than disappearing, simply became slow and extended.

Ray wanted to give up the medication. If there were only two alternatives, he much preferred to be his quicker, sharper "old self," dashing through doorways and winning at table tennis, suffering his accustomed tics and obscenities. Others, however, had higher hopes. Most important, Ray's physician decided that the medication, to be successful, required a new psychological outlook on the part of the patient (Sacks, 1987). Learning perhaps played a role in Ray's behavior.

SENSORY CORTEX. Research on the **sensory cortex**, which receives incoming information, has shown that the primary visual areas are in the occipital lobes and that each eye sends nerve impulses to both lobes. Impulses for auditory experiences are received chiefly in the temporal lobes. Reception by each ear is also represented in both lobes.

The primary cortical area for body feeling is the front part of the parietal lobes. This specialized area is called the *somatosensory cortex* because it mediates feeling within the body. Body feeling, also called **somesthesis,** has two divisions: external or *cutaneous sensitivity*, involving sensitivity to pressure, temperature, and pain on the skin; and internal, including *kinesthesis*, which is the feeling in muscles, tendons, and joints, and also *visceral sensitivity*, the feeling in internal organs and glands. Receptors for these forms of stimulation are located throughout much of the body. Again, the body is represented in an inverted sequence. When Ray felt something underfoot, impulses arrived at the top of his cortex. When the revolving door bashed his nose, messages were sent to the lower portions of his somatosensory area. And again, there is a relationship between the degree of cortical specialization and the performance of the body. The larger the relevant brain area, the greater is the sensitivity in the corresponding body part. In this region of the brain, human beings are largely fingers and palms, lips and tongue (Figure 3–9).

ASSOCIATION CORTEX. As suggested previously, these cortical areas are not the exclusive seat of any movement or experience. Despite our need to discuss them separately, no one area completely controls any complex human reaction. The control is inevitably shared by other areas as well.

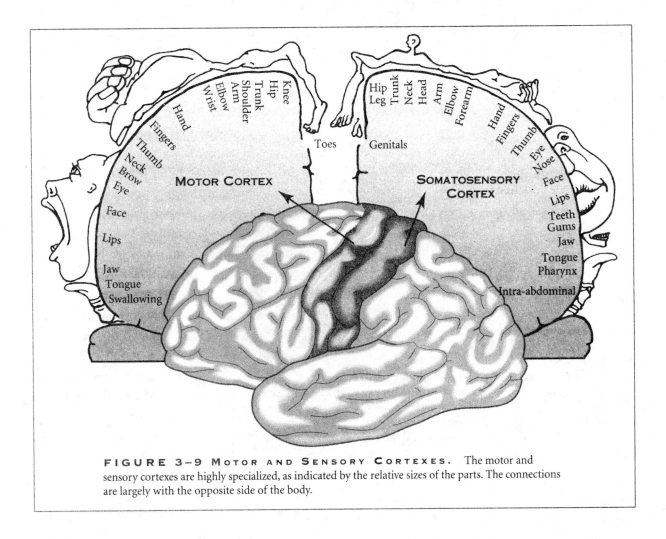

FIGURE 3–9 MOTOR AND SENSORY CORTEXES. The motor and sensory cortexes are highly specialized, as indicated by the relative sizes of the parts. The connections are largely with the opposite side of the body.

Occupying large sections of the human brain around the motor and sensory areas is the **association cortex,** so called because it seems to be involved in the integration of information. It does not receive information directly from the sense organs; instead, data are brought together and presumably analyzed here. Not surprisingly, the association cortex seems to be most significantly involved in memory, language, and other complex mental processes. Knowing a certain piece of music, Ray nevertheless introduced variations. The association cortex was intimately involved in these improvisations.

The significance of the association areas for touch can be illustrated by reference to a disease known as *astereognosis,* literally meaning "without tac-

tual knowledge of space." Normally, a blindfolded person asked to handle a small cube has no difficulty identifying this object. But a person with seriously impaired association areas for touch is unable to recognize it by touch alone. Loss of the association tissue causes impressions of touch to lose their meaning. Differences in sharpness and smoothness can be experienced, assuming that the sensory areas remain intact, but they cannot be identified.

When brain disorders involve language functions, we speak of **aphasia,** meaning "without language." This disruption is most likely if the damage is in the left cerebral hemisphere, for language is managed by that hemisphere in most of us. A portion of the frontal lobe, called *Broca's area,* plays a central role in *producing* speech. An afflicted individual makes sense but talks very slowly and with difficulty.

A region in the left temporal lobe, known as *Wernicke's area,* is involved in *understanding* speech and making it meaningful. An afflicted individual cannot comprehend language. Or this person may speak fluently but utter statements that are nonsense, completely lacking in meaning. The separate words may be intelligible, but they are used in a jumbled sequence, showing no meaningful relation to each other.

HEMISPHERIC SPECIALIZATION

When playing the drums, Ray used both hands simultaneously, rapidly and rhythmically. In more routine activities, such as taking his medication, one hand held the container while the other unscrewed the top. How did Ray coordinate such movements?

The key organ here is the **corpus callosum,** a large bundle of nerve fibers between the two cerebral hemispheres, joining them at the lower areas of the association cortex. Although it was considered for years to be merely a structural connection, researchers eventually showed that the corpus callosum plays a very important role in coordinating functions in both sides of the body, enabling the hemispheres to cooperate by sending visual, auditory, and other information back and forth (Figure 3–10). Later, they showed that what happens in one side of the brain does not necessarily take place in the other. This condition, referred to as **hemispheric specialization,** means that the two hemispheres do not perform exactly the same functions; they have somewhat different but largely overlapping capacities.

SPLIT-BRAIN RESEARCH. A surgical procedure in which the corpus callosum is completely cut, leaving the two hemispheres joined only at subcortical levels, is called the *split-brain technique.* This unusual procedure eventually led to an impor-

tant discovery: that the two hemispheres do not handle the same information in the same way. This condition was suddenly brought to public attention in the 1960s by Roger Sperry and his colleagues, who conducted studies with human subjects after they had under-gone split-brain surgery for severe epilepsy. Afterward, the epileptic activity did not spread to the other hemisphere; there were decreased attacks in the initiating hemisphere; and previously hopeless epileptic cases went for years without seizures (Gazzaniga, Bogen, & Sperry, 1965; Sperry, 1968). Moreover, people with this operation appeared to be essentially normal.

Later, Sperry noted that with the midconnections destroyed, each hemisphere has its own style, storing its own memories and functioning adequately alone. Thus a strong case can be made for two consciousnesses or two minds housed in the same skull (Sperry, 1968, 1984). This finding has led to an enormous upsurge of interest in similarities and differences in information processing between the two hemispheres (Hellige, 1990).

In one study, split-brain patients were compared with normal people for attention to visual stimuli. Different patterns were positioned simultaneously on each side of the head, and each subject engaged in a visual search task, scanning these patterns as rapidly as possible. Split-brain patients performed the task faster than normal people, suggesting that each of the surgically separated hemispheres maintained an independent focus of attention during the visual search (Luck, Hillyard, & Mangun, 1989).

NORMAL DIFFERENCES. This research showed that even if the right hemisphere knows the answer in a simple test involving two objects, the split-brain patient cannot *say* the correct answer. The person will reply that he or she does not know or did not see the test objects. The reason is that for most people the *left hemisphere* is more dominant in using words, numbers, and reasoning,

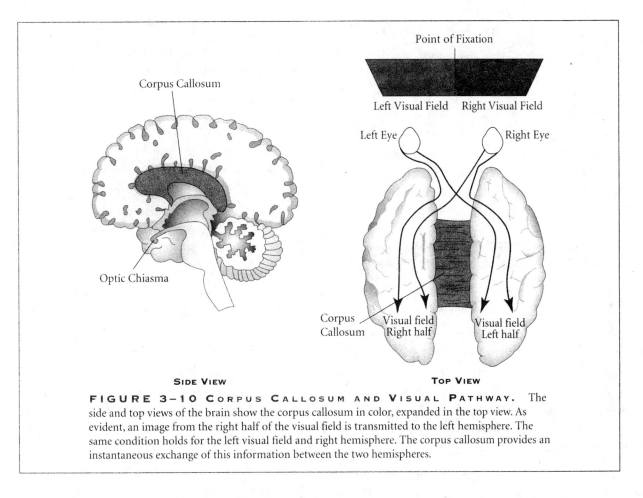

Corpus Callosum

Optic Chiasma

Point of Fixation

Left Visual Field   Right Visual Field

Left Eye   Right Eye

Corpus
Callosum

Visual field
Right half

Visual field
Left half

SIDE VIEW   **TOP VIEW**

FIGURE 3–10 CORPUS CALLOSUM AND VISUAL PATHWAY. The side and top views of the brain show the corpus callosum in color, expanded in the top view. As evident, an image from the right half of the visual field is transmitted to the left hemisphere. The same condition holds for the left visual field and right hemisphere. The corpus callosum provides an instantaneous exchange of this information between the two hemispheres.

especially spoken language. If you ask the individual to grasp the correct object or point to the correct word instead, the person can do so with the left hand, using the right hemisphere.

The right hemisphere, although generally subordinate in the use of language, also has special capabilities. It can manage only simple numerical problems but, for example, it exceeds the left hemisphere in recognizing faces, important for social responsiveness; in assembling objects, such as blocks and puzzles; and in drawing three-dimensional objects. Split-brain people using the left hand and therefore the right hemisphere assemble objects more readily than when using the right hand and left hemisphere, even when they are naturally right-handed. Thus the *right hemisphere* appears to be the locus of control for synthesizing and utilizing spatial information.

Evidence for this specialization has been obtained in a variety of ways. With split-brain patients, electrical impulses in the left hemisphere increased during language problems and those in the right hemisphere increased during spatial relations problems (McCallum & Glynn, 1979). Among subjects who underwent diverse forms of brain surgery, recognition of the words for songs was related to activity in the left hemisphere; recognition of the melodies was related to activity in the right or both hemispheres (Samson & Zatorre, 1991).

In general terms, the left hemisphere tends to be analytical and logical, concerned with words. The right hemisphere seems more holistic and intuitive, concerned with spatial processes. On this basis, creativity perhaps involves contributions from both hemispheres. In fact, both hemispheres have some competence for many tasks, but they seem to process the information in qualitatively different ways (Hellige, 1990).

Again, a reminder is appropriate. The terms "right-brained" and "left-brained" are grossly inaccurate when used in the same way that we speak of handedness. The cerebral hemispheres are *integrated*. They are separate but complementary information processing subsystems (Hellige, 1993).

• INTERLOCKING SYSTEMS •

Integration is further emphasized when we consider the context in which the nervous system must operate. Directly or indirectly, it becomes involved in routine activities, emergency situations, and maintenance functions, such as growth, conservation of energy, and reproductive reactions. In short, the nervous system has interlocking associations with many other systems of the body. The story of Witty Ticcy Ray emphasizes this point: The biological mechanisms that underlie human behavior and experience are interconnected in exquisitely complex and balanced ways. This integration is also readily evident in the autonomic nervous system and endocrine system, to which we now turn.

And here, a further word about Ray is in order. His physician had decided that Ray's problem was no longer exclusively one of brain malfunction. Over the years, it had become *partly* psychological, as well. There was an interaction between Ray's physiological and psychological conditions; one could not be readjusted without the other.

Ray had a different view. "Suppose you *could* take away the tics," he said. "What would be left? I consist of tics—there is nothing else." Partly joking because he was obviously very skillful in many ways, Ray and his physician struck a bargain. For 3 months Ray would go off the medication, during which time they would make a deep and patient exploration of Ray's thoughts about himself, his tics and emotional upheavals, and what life might offer without Tourette's syndrome. After this intensive insight therapy, Ray would try the medication once again, taking the same small doses prescribed previously.

Ray proved adept at this self-scrutiny; later, when he began taking the medication again, the result was remarkable. Prepared to understand its effects, he found himself released from a problem that had dominated his life since he was 4 years old. With a freedom from tics he never imagined, he became loved not as a clown but as a valued member of society, joking less but certainly pleasing Sacha and his coworkers more. For nine years, Ray lived with no tics and no emotional outbursts.

These and further details of Ray's life were reported by Sacks in a series of clinical cases with an odd title, *The Man Who Mistook His Wife for a Hat* (1987). This title had nothing to do with Ray. The narrative about Ray, however, was supplemented by a brief conversation with the author, who kept all identities confidential.

∽

AUTONOMIC FUNCTIONS

Regrettably, this more settled life that Ray experienced came at a high cost, at least for him. The drug eliminated his emotional crises and tics, but it also reduced him to an average, competent individual in music, conversation, and sports. His sudden, wild musical improvisations, which formerly arose from a tic or after compulsively striking the drum, no longer appeared. For someone of his earlier talents, life had become routine—too routine and even a bit discouraging (Sacks, 1987).

To experience a stable, routine life, we all depend on several interconnected systems of the body, devoted to respiration, circulation, digestion, urination, and so forth. They provide an appropriate internal environment within which the central and peripheral nervous systems operate, and they also influence behavior. The system chiefly responsible for regulating these involuntary actions, both in routine and emergency situations, is called the *autonomic nervous system* because it was once thought to be completely independent of voluntary control. As the name indicates, it is part of the nervous system and, as the research shows, this earlier conception of total autonomy has changed.

OPPOSITIONAL DIVISIONS.

The autonomic nervous system, as noted earlier, is composed of two divisions that operate essentially but not completely in opposition to one another. The **sympathetic nervous system** plays a dominant role in emotion. The heart pounds, gastric and salivary secretions are checked, and adrenaline flows, all in an integrated fashion because the sympathetic division has assumed control. It causes blood vessels of the intestine and stomach to constrict, inhibiting the digestive process. At the same time, it permits more blood to flow to the arms and legs in anticipation of "fight or flight." Indeed, the sympathetic division acts as an *emergency system*, significantly influenced by the hypothalamus.

When the crisis subsides, the **parasympathetic nervous system** resumes control, and the activity of the related organs returns to its usual level. Heartbeat becomes more normal, saliva appears in the mouth, and blood flows more readily in the stomach. This division serves as a *routine system*, providing for normal body functioning.

When Ray was fleeing from revolving doors, the sympathetic division was dominant. When he was resting from these labors, the parasympathetic division became ascendant.

The traditional conception of the sympathetic and parasympathetic divisions as completely involuntary has been brought into question on two

bases. First, there are numerous reports of voluntary control of blood circulation and breathing, brought about through forms of meditation, and they have been at least partially verified. Second, similar control has been achieved by subjects in experiments on biofeedback (Wallace & Benson, 1972). Together, these findings show that the autonomic nervous system, which is part of the peripheral nervous system, is partly under the control of the central nervous system.

AUTONOMIC FUNCTIONS AND BIOFEEDBACK.

Biofeedback is not a system in which some chemical or electrical impulse is delivered to the body. Instead **biofeedback** occurs when information about body functions is made available to the brain. Typically, an electronic monitoring device is used that, for example, indicates the heart rate or blood pressure. The question is this: Can people who receive feedback about their biological processes thereby control these processes?

The sympathetic nervous system, for example, initiates blood flow in certain parts of the body, including the brain. When an individual is constantly tense, the blood supply to the brain may become extreme, contributing to migraine headaches. For this reason, some patients susceptible to these headaches receive training in biofeedback. Monitoring devices sound a tone whenever the blood flow decreases by a certain amount, enabling subjects to become more aware of this relaxed state. With this procedure, some subjects achieve lowered cerebral blood flow and report fewer migraine headaches (Sturgis, Tollison, & Adams, 1978).

Nevertheless, the daily human environment is infinitely more varied than a medical setting. Patients sometimes cannot maintain control in the home (Engel, 1972). Furthermore, the patient's expectation about the therapist or the treatment may play a significant role in the outcome of biofeedback procedures (Borgeat, Elie, & Castonguay, 1991). For many problems, such as heart disease and cancer, the biofeedback procedure is not clearly superior to more traditional treatments, especially relaxation and cognitive therapy (Johnston, 1991; Figure 3–11).

When used for a very different specific purpose—problems of muscular control—biofeedback has been quite successful, comparing very favorably with other treatments. For example, after sustaining severe head injuries, five patients displayed both fecal and urinary incontinence. Following a biofeedback program of neuromuscular re-education, all of them developed complete continence, voiding normally and regularly (Tries, 1990).

〜

THE ENDOCRINE SYSTEM

The second great communication network within the body, after the nervous system, is the **endocrine system,** composed of a series of interlocking glands that secrete fluids directly into the bloodstream. Both systems are feedback systems, both involve contact with the environment, and both are critical for adaptation (Drickamer & Vessey, 1992). Among the differences between them, speed of reaction and breadth of distribution are most important. The nerve impulse travels rapidly and must stay within the limits of the axons and dendrites. The endocrine system generally has a slower and broader influence. Its secretions, carried by the blood, travel to various parts of the body, where they typically have a maintenance function pertaining to growth, general vigor, and other long-range developments.

While at least a dozen endocrine glands have been identified, eight are well known today, including the placenta, which appears only in the pregnant female. Four have special significance for physiological psychology: the pituitary, thyroid, gonads, and adrenals. These tiny glands have incred-

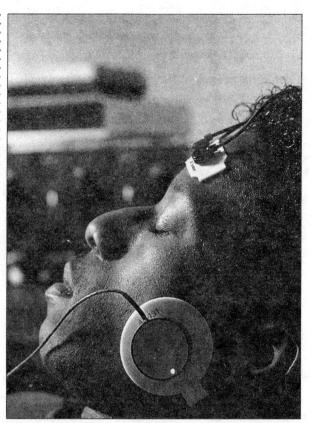

FIGURE 3–11 BIOFEEDBACK.
In treating headaches, electrodes attached to the facial muscles sound a tone when muscle tension decreases in that area.

ibly small secretions, yet they form an interlocking system to the extent that disturbance in any one of them may lead to malfunctioning of the others. These glandular secretions, called **hormones,** ensure fundamental chemical activities within the whole organism. For example, they influence body growth, the utilization of food, energy expenditure, and reproductive reactions. They are involved in almost every aspect of body functioning.

ENDOCRINE GLANDS. The most important gland, in the sense of influencing others, is the **pituitary gland,** a small structure located just below the center of the brain. It is attached to the hypothalamus and sometimes considered part of the brain. Its location is not surprising, for in many ways it is regulated by hypothalamic activities. Often called the *master gland,* its front, or anterior, portion influences the secretions of several other endocrine glands, including those for sexual behavior and physical growth. The dwarf may have an underactive and the giant an overactive pituitary gland. The rear, or posterior, portion of this gland, through hormones exchanged with the hypothalamus, maintains a complex interaction with the central nervous system (Figure 3–12).

General body vigor is affected by the pituitary and also by the **thyroid gland,** lying at the base of the neck. The thyroid hormone is thyroxin. Lack of this hormone early in life can result in inactivity and cretinism, a condition of various bodily defects and low intelligence. Undersecretion at later ages often produces lethargy. Both conditions can be corrected by injection of thyroxin. In contrast, oversecretion seems to result in tension, which can be diminished through surgery.

The testes in men and the ovaries in women, situated in the genital area and collectively known as the **gonads,** are key factors in sexual behavior. They produce hormones responsible for the major physiological changes that occur at puberty; they contribute significantly to accompanying psychological development; and they continue to influence sexual responsiveness throughout adulthood. Normal adult sexual behavior can occur in their absence, although typically at a reduced rate.

Still another hormone from the pituitary, the adrenocorticotropic hormone or ACTH, stimulates the **adrenal glands,** which are located in the back of the abdomen below the rib cage, immediately above the kidneys. They have two basic parts. The adrenal medulla, inside the gland, secretes *adrenaline,* another name for **epinephrine,** which serves to increase energy in emergencies and other emotional situations. The adrenal cortex, on the outside, has diverse influences. When there is inadequate secretion in the adrenal cortex, there may be widespread changes in personality. The individual often becomes weak

and lethargic, loses the appetite for food and sexual activity, and suffers a widespread breakdown of physiological functions. In contrast, overactivity in this part of the adrenal gland may produce sexual maturity at an unusually early age.

HORMONAL AND NEURAL COMMUNICATION. The major communication networks in the human body involve both hormonal *and* neural messages. In fact, certain chemical substances act as both hormones and neurotransmitters. Endocrine and neural tissues are connected by multiple bidirectional pathways (Daruna & Morgan, 1990).

The pituitary gland, through the discharge of ACTH, stimulates the adrenal gland, which in turn discharges several additional hormones. The pituitary also secretes the gonadotropic hormone, act-

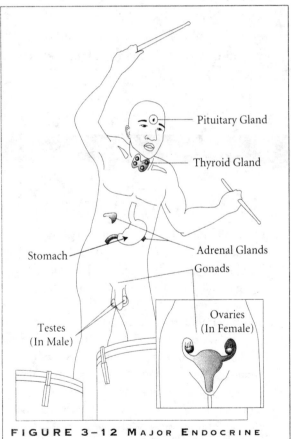

FIGURE 3–12 MAJOR ENDOCRINE GLANDS. These four glands, with vital implications for behavior, are interconnected in various ways.

ing on the gonads, which release their own hormones, regulating male and female sexual behavior. In both cases, the pituitary gland, part of the endocrine system, is activated by the hypothalamus, considered part of both the endocrine and nervous systems. The chief but not exclusive control of these interlocking systems lies in the brain, sending messages based on feedback it receives from other parts of the systems.

For Ray, this concept of interlocking systems was all too apparent. Medication made him a more normal citizen. "Sober, solid, square," he said of himself. It also made him a dull musician and a dim wit. With the drug, the favorable and unfavorable components could not be separated (Sacks, 1987).

One day Ray came to a momentous two-part decision. He would stay on medication throughout the working week. He thereby remained calm and deliberate Monday through Friday, making life easier for Sacha, himself, and his colleagues at work. Slower and more deliberate in thought and action, he experienced no emotional crises.

Especially costly in this decision was his loss of musical talent, both as a means of economic support and as a mode of self-expression. Without full freedom in his music, Ray forfeited his soul, his energy, and his enthusiasm for life. Hence, Ray made another decision—to avoid the Haldol on weekends. He "let fly" instead, becoming witty, ticcy, and inspired. At these times, Ray delighted himself and his companions with improvisations on the drums and bold shots at table tennis.

In looking at his double life, Ray noted that neither of his selves was completely free. One was controlled by the disorder, the other by its treatment. Normal people, he said, have a natural balance; he had to be content with an artificial balance (Sacks, 1987).

However, Ray had achieved a balance of a different sort, a balanced outlook on life. In his admirable, jocular style, he realized that sometimes he had to suffer his adversity, and sometimes he could put his "bold biological intruder" to advantage, using it for sudden, brilliant excursions into the worlds of music and conversation and also, of course, through revolving doors.

· SUMMARY ·

OVERVIEW OF THE BODY

1. Organs perform specific functions; systems involve interacting organs. Genes, the basic determiners of heredity, are largely but not entirely responsible for our physical characteristics and contribute to other characteristics.

2. The chief integrating system of the body is the nervous system One part, the peripheral nervous system, is essentially a transmitting system; it sends impulses to and from the central nervous system. It includes the autonomic nervous system and the somatic nervous system. The central nervous system consists of the spinal cord and brain. The spinal cord is responsible for sending impulses to and receiving impulses from the brain.

NEURAL COMMUNICATION

3. There are various types of neurons in the human body. Some are sensory; they enable us to become aware of our environment and the condition of our own bodies. Others are motor; they enable us to respond, to take some action. In addition, the nervous system includes countless interneurons, which make other connections that can result in a wide range of behavior.

4. The nerve impulse is an electrochemical change in the nerve fiber, and it operates on an all-or-none principle. The synapse, which is the junction between neurons, plays a most important role in the flexibility of human behavior. Conditions at

the synapse operate according to a graded potential.

5. At the synapse, the action potential, or nerve impulse, releases a chemical substance into the synaptic space. This substance, a neurotransmitter, exerts an excitatory or inhibitory influence on the adjacent neuron. The action of these neurotransmitters—acetylcholine, norepinephrine, dopamine, serotonin, GABA, and others—can be influenced in many ways by internally produced and externally administered chemical substances.

THE HUMAN BRAIN

6. From an evolutionary perspective, the human brain can be considered in three sections. The hindbrain plays a central role in many vital functions: digestion, breathing, blood circulation, posture, and coordination. The midbrain processes sensory information and is also designed for arousal of the whole organism. The forebrain, the newest of the three major sections, clearly separates the human brain from those of other animals.

7. Portions of the brain near the spinal cord and midbrain are called the lower brain centers, or subcortical structures, for they lie beneath the cortex. The thalamus, at the center of the brain, serves as a relay station, especially for sensory impulses. The hypothalamus plays an important role in regulating all sorts of behaviors, including eating, fighting, fear reactions, and sexual behavior.

8. The cerebral cortex has specialized areas in each of four lobes. Visual areas are located in the occipital lobes, auditory areas in the temporal lobes, and areas for body feeling in the front part of the parietal lobes. Voluntary motor activities are mediated in the back part of the frontal lobes. These lobes also have association functions relating especially to the higher mental processes, including language.

9. In split-brain research, the cerebral hemispheres are separated by cutting the corpus callosum. The results suggest some important differences between these consciousnesses. These differences involve analytical and logical functions in the left hemisphere and holistic and perhaps intuitive functions in the right hemisphere.

INTERLOCKING SYSTEMS

10. The interlocking nature of human physiology is illustrated in the autonomic nervous system, which has connections with the endocrine system, the central nervous system, and the peripheral nervous system. It has two divisions: the sympathetic operates in emergencies, and the parasympathetic is dominant in routine functioning.

11. The endocrine system communicates by secreting hormones. It regulates growth, helps control the body's energy, and plays an important integrative function. Disturbances in any one of the endocrine glands may have widespread repercussions in physical structure and behavior.

• WORKING WITH PSYCHOLOGY •

REVIEW OF KEY CONCEPTS

Overview of the Body
organ
system
receptors
effectors
genes
nervous system
peripheral nervous system
autonomic nervous system
somatic nervous system
central nervous system

brain
spinal cord

Neural Communication
neuron
cell body
dendrite
axon
myelin sheath
sensory neuron
motor neuron

reflex arc
interneuron
polarized
resting potential
depolarized
action potential
all-or-none law
refractory period
synapse
graded potential
neurotransmitter substance

acetylcholine
Alzheimer's disease
norepinephrine
dopamine
Parkinson's disease
serotonin
GABA
endorphins

The Human Brain
hindbrain
medulla
cerebellum
midbrain
reticular activating system
forebrain

subcortical structures
thalamus
hypothalamus
limbic system
cerebral cortex
frontal lobes
temporal lobes
occipital lobes
parietal lobes
electroencephalograph (EEG)
CT scan
MRI scan
PET scan
motor cortex
sensory cortex
somesthesis

association cortex
aphasia
corpus callosum
hemispheric specialization

Interlocking Systems
sympathetic nervous system
parasympathetic nervous system
biofeedback
endocrine system
hormones
pituitary gland
thyroid gland
gonads
adrenal glands
epinephrine

❧ CLASS DISCUSSION/CRITICAL THINKING ❧

A NARRATIVE TWIST

When Witty Ticcy Ray began using Haldol, his extraordinary quickness and fine muscular coordination disappeared. Dr. Sacks then requested him to undergo several months of insight therapy, and thereafter Ray achieved an improved adjustment to the medication. Suppose that Ray had refused the insight therapy but continued taking Haldol. Simply by attempting each day to cope with his altered physical condition, would he eventually have adapted in essentially the same way? Might some other experience have promoted this adaptation? Defend your view. ❧

TOPICAL QUESTIONS

• *Overview of the Body.* Investigators often use studies with animals as windows to the human condition. Cite an instance in which this procedure might be useful, referring to a specific animal or a specific organ or system.
• *Neural Communication.* Consider our national telephone system as an analogy to neural communication in human beings. Indicate the assets and limitations of this analogy.

• *The Human Brain.* Does it seem possible that the CT, PET, or MRI scan will yield further understanding of intracranial self-stimulation? If not, why? If so, which technique may prove most useful? Why?
• *Interlocking Systems.* Complete this analogy: The pituitary gland is to the endocrine system as the ——— is to the central nervous system. Select one alternative and defend your answer: reticular activating system, thalamus, hypothalamus, cerebral cortex.

❧ TOPICS OF RELATED INTEREST ❧

Numerous references to the biological bases of behavior appear throughout this text. The chief discussions occur with respect to sensation (4), interpretation of dreams (6), the memory trace (8), motivation (10), emotion (11), and human development (12).

18

PERCEPTION

GROUP OF FRENCH HUNTERS IN THE CAUNE WOODS OF AVEYRON, FRANCE, FINALLY CLOSED IN ON THEIR PREY, A WILD BOY WHO HAD BEEN RUNNING FREE and naked in the forest for some years. After pulling him from a tree he had climbed to evade their pursuit, they assigned him to the care of a neighboring widow. He escaped within a week. Wandering through the country-side in the most rigorous weather, he was captured again and this time transferred to Paris. Ministers and scholars in the capital city had requested a scientific study of this savage, thinking it would shed some light on the development of the human mind.

He was called the "Wild Boy of Aveyron," and his arrival along the banks of the Seine in 1800 aroused two quite different expectations. Some people were anticipating Rousseau's noble savage in all his dignity. After a few months' education, he would give a most interesting account of life in the wilds. Others looked forward to the boy's astonishment at the wonders of Paris. He would be profoundly impressed with modern clothing, furniture, buildings, and modes of transportation.

Both groups were disappointed.

Visitors to the Wild Boy encountered instead a dirty, frightened creature who crawled and trotted like a wild beast. About 12 years old, he spent most of his time rocking back and forth like an animal in the zoo. No sound left his mouth except for an infrequent growl from the back of his throat. Finding a dead bird, he stripped off its feathers, opened it with his fingernail, smelled it, and then threw it away. He scratched and bit those who opposed him but otherwise was largely indifferent to everything and everyone in his new environment (Itard, 1807).

The famous French physician Phillippe Pinel, renowned for developing positive attitudes towards mental illness, was the first to examine the boy thoroughly. Dr. Pinel thereupon declared that the Wild Boy was an incurable idiot and that his wildness was probably overestimated. In Pinel's opinion, the poor creature was the product of a decidedly subnormal mentality. He was a man-animal or perhaps a man-plant, for his only development beyond that of the flower was locomotion. His behavioral deficiencies lay in his defective intelligence.

A much younger physician, Jean-Marc-Gaspard Itard, requested a meeting with the boy, an historic occasion in the Luxembourg Gardens. The boy wore only a gray, loose-fitting robe like a nightshirt, which he tore from his body at the first unguarded moment. He said nothing, appeared deaf, and gazed distantly across the gardens. Sitting across from him in a long coat and tie, with ruffles and cuff links, Itard looked kindly on the boy. At age 26, he had just come to Paris in search of a career, and the boy's condition aroused his interest. Little did either of them know that they had, at that moment, joined their lives in a long and difficult search (Lane, 1979).

And little did writers and observers of that day appreciate the unflagging efforts of a third person in this joint venture. Today, with greater understanding of the contribution of the daily caregiver, we pay special tribute in this instance to Madame Guerin, who became the boy's guardian and daily companion.

After examining the boy briefly, Itard took a bold view, quite different from that of the renowned Pinel. The Wild Boy's subnormality, he declared, was due to his lack of experience in

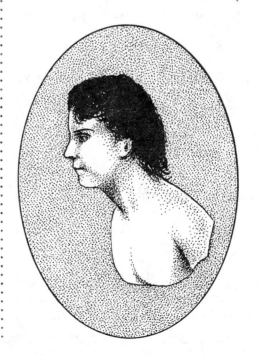

human civilization. If carefully trained in a normal environment, the boy would show corresponding gains in mental life. Itard staked his youthful reputation on this opinion and sought permission from the Ministry of Interior to begin a treatment that would produce a normal child.

According to Itard, the Wild Boy was a *feral child*, meaning that he was totally uncivilized from living in the wilds, perhaps in the company of animals. Approximately 50 such cases have been recorded, most in scant detail, some apparently as hoaxes (Malson, 1972). Among them, the story of this boy from France is the most widely accepted as scientifically sound (Table 5–1).

Specifically, Itard planned to increase the boy's perceptual, intellectual, and emotional responsiveness, thereby enabling him to take his rightful place in human society. The starting point would be perception, the gateway to knowledge, the portal of the mind, the avenue to a fuller intellectual and emotional life. Permission was granted, and Itard began his treatment. As it turned out, this treatment formed the roots of modern educational and behavioral psychology, as well as psychological testing.

Our concern in this chapter is with **perception,** the process by which we select, organize, and interpret stimuli, thereby gaining an understanding of ourselves and our environment. In doing so, we combine sensory information with information already stored in the nervous system, as memory.

Name	Date	Age
Hesse wolf-child	1344	7
First Lithuanian bear-boy	1661	12
Irish sheep-child	1672	16
Wild Boy of Aveyron	1799	11
Amala of Midnapore	1920	2
Kamala of Midnapore	1920	8

TABLE 5–1 CASES OF FERAL CHILDREN This partial list shows the date and estimated age of each child at the time of capture (Malson, 1972).

The term **sensation,** as we saw in the previous chapter, refers to a more basic condition; it is raw experience, direct from the sense organs. Sensation and perception overlap considerably, but the process of perception involves more cognitive activities. In perception, we derive some meaning based on sensation *and* prior experience.

The citizens of Paris expected the young boy to perceive the excitement and nuances in their sophisticated environment, but such was not the case, at least initially. The Wild Boy saw and heard the city, but these events were little more than sensations for him. He had insufficient prior experience to find meaning in the colors, shapes, odors, and sounds. Itard's attempt to train him therefore provides a useful narrative, illustrating the contributions of innate and acquired factors in human perception.

Three phases of perception are considered in this chapter: attending to stimulation, organizing the perceptual field, and interpreting perceptual information. At the end of the chapter, we note that, among all of the influences on perception, learning plays a central role. It helps us to find meaning in this "blooming, buzzing confusion," as William James once called the infant's environment.

• ATTENDING TO STIMULATION •

Less than five feet tall, with straight brown hair and a round face, the Wild Boy looked at the world with deep, dark eyes. His well-tanned skin showed numerous scars on his arms and legs, neck and face. Outdoors, he trotted barefoot, restrained by a leash. Inside, he roamed the house like a prisoner. At mealtimes, he dragged his food into a corner, kneaded it, and chewed only with his incisors. Otherwise, the Wild Boy paid little attention to human civilization .

OBJECT/EVENT	RESPONSE
Food	Avoided all prepared foods
Drink	Rejected all liquids except water
Clothing	Resisted clothes, including shoes
Furniture	Ignored beds; slept on the floor
Speech	Paid no attention to words
Music	Insensitive to all melodies

TABLE 5–2 THE WILD BOY'S RESPONSE TO HUMAN SOCIETY

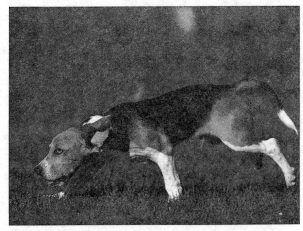

FIGURE 5–1 SELECTIVE ATTENTION. If one neural channel becomes prominent—as when a particular odor arouses a dog, the responsiveness of other channels may be diminished. Impulses from the primary stimulation appear to activate the reticular formation in such a manner as to block irrelevant sensory input.

Itard thus began to increase the range of stimuli to which the boy attended. The process of **attending** involves a readiness to perceive. It is an active process, an orientation toward certain stimulation, often involving an adjustment of the sense organs. To respond properly to human civilization, the boy needed to attend properly to all sorts of events (Table 5–2). For the most part, we perceive only those aspects of the environment to which we attend.

∾

SELECTIVE ATTENTION

Attending is based significantly on interests and motivation; we attend to stimuli relevant to our needs and desires. When Itard began his lessons, the Wild Boy paid no attention at all to the shrillest human cries or words of any sort, even with sharp differences in intonation. They meant nothing to him. Owing to the importance of speech in daily life, improved attention to these sounds was considered indispensable.

Giving exclusive attention to something, focusing on one aspect of the environment and shutting out others, is called **selective attention.** This term may seem redundant, but shortly we shall turn to divided attention, in which we try to focus simultaneously on two or more events (Figure 5–I).

ADJUSTMENTS IN ATTENDING. In the first weeks of training, Itard used the simplest objects and colors, but still the Wild Boy attended only to stimuli associated with his earlier life in the forests. Spying a large earthen plate with many foods, he grasped only the potatoes, which he had eaten previously. At the sound of a walnut cracked behind him, he immediately turned around, and he invariably tried to smell anything that was given to him, even objects we would consider without odor. In the streets of Paris, he constantly picked up pebbles and pieces of dry wood, discarding them only after holding them to his nose.

The process of attending involves adjustments in the brain, muscles, and sense organs in exquisitely complex and reciprocal fashion, each modifying the other. Adjustments in the brain, for example, require cooperative activity among millions of neurons, especially in the cortex.

When a person sniffs an odor, the molecules carrying this scent are detected by receptor neurons in the upper passages of the nose. The intensity of the stimulation is indicated by the number of receptors activated and the nature of the odor by the specific site stimulated. This pattern of receptor activity is then transmitted to a lower region of the brain known as the *olfactory bulb*, which synthesizes the information. The bulb then sends its own messages up to the *olfactory cortex*, which disperses signals throughout other brain areas, including the *frontal cortex*. Some of these go by way of the *thalamus*, a relay center and switchboard. Others go to the *limbic system*, which contributes elements of memory and emotion and combines this mass of information with incoming messages from other sensory systems. On the basis of these intricate interconnections, the odor may be recognized, the brain may send a message to sniff again, or it may initiate some other message (Figure 5–2).

The outcome, a meaning-laden perception, is based on what seems to be chaos in the brain—activity so complex that it appears random. Of course, it has a hidden order, demonstrated in the capacity of massive groups of neurons to shift simultaneously and abruptly from one complex pattern of activity to another in reaction to seemingly insignificant changes in stimulation (Freeman, 1991).

Adjustments in the muscles, in response to any signal from the brain, are especially evident when someone stoops to look at something on the ground or leans forward to listen more carefully. The Wild Boy holding a pebble to his nose, the dog pointing, and the cat crouching to pounce on its prey all illustrate sustained attentive postures.

Obvious adjustments of the sense organs occur when someone displays tracking movements of the eyes while watching a ball game. In tasting, we sometimes move a substance around in the mouth so that it falls on different parts of the tongue. Other changes in the sense organs are not learned, and some are too subtle to be readily observed. These include, for example, dilation of the pupils and changes in the skin's electrical activity.

Despite all of these adjustments, we can attend to only a few of the many stimuli to which we are regularly exposed. To which stimuli, therefore, do we attend?

STIMULUS CHARACTERISTICS. A stimulus catches our attention partly because it is relevant to conditions within us, such as biological motives and personal interests. It also catches attention through its own special characteristics. Advertisers use high-intensity stimuli to catch attention. For this reason, we see full-page ads, billboards, and

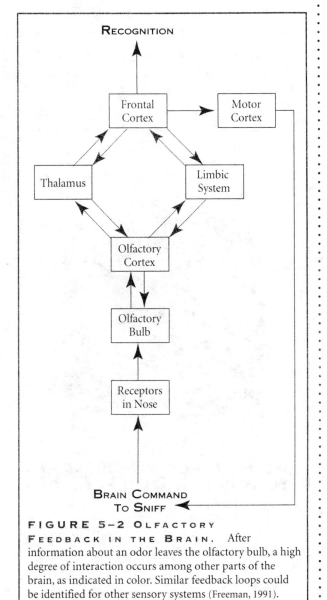

FIGURE 5–2 OLFACTORY FEEDBACK IN THE BRAIN. After information about an odor leaves the olfactory bulb, a high degree of interaction occurs among other parts of the brain, as indicated in color. Similar feedback loops could be identified for other sensory systems (Freeman, 1991).

skywriting. Among all of these factors, however, prior experience exerts a profound impact. It influences both our selective exposure to certain stimuli and our interpretation of them (Cohen & Chakravarti, 1990).

The best location for a visual stimulus, when not directly in front of the eyes, is the upper portion of a page or screen. That part receives more attention than the lower part, and the left side receives more attention than the right, at least in the Western world, where people read from left to right and top to bottom.

Color attracts more attention than black and white, and movement attracts more attention than a stationary stimulus. In addition, the novelty of a stimulus is important. A familiar item in unexpected surroundings or an unfamiliar item in common surroundings usually catches attention.

EMBEDDED MESSAGES. Is it possible for advertisers to catch our attention without any obvious stimulus at all? One alleged procedure is called *subliminal advertising* because the message or stimulus is presumably below awareness yet somehow influential. This possibility, received with much excitement in midcentury, has little research support, partly because each of us has a different threshold, or limen, and all of us vary from day to day. Flashing on a screen an advertisement that would be both subliminal and effective on a large scale appears highly unlikely, and evidence has been negative (Moore, 1985). There is no need to fear these hidden persuaders, at least at this point.

In another procedure, advertisers presumably influence us by messages skillfully obscured in a visual display. These stimuli are called **embedded messages,** for they are purposely indistinct or hidden in some larger context, allegedly influential without the viewer's awareness. A photographic ad for a certain brand of beer, for example, shows a rumpled napkin or discarded vest. Within the folds of the cloth, if you look carefully—or possess a

vivid imagination—there may be a sexual symbol, promoting your interest in the advertised product. If you look carefully enough, then the merchants have achieved their purpose. You have attended to the advertisement, although the presumably potent stimuli, if present at all, certainly are not subliminal. They are above threshold, and you have taken the time to find them (Figure 5–3).

One study tested the claim that the word *sex*, when embedded in a pictorial advertisement, increases viewers' memory for that ad. In a set of slides depicting vacation scenes, the word *sex* was embedded several times in each slide. Nonsense syllables, such as *vib* and *res*, were embedded in another

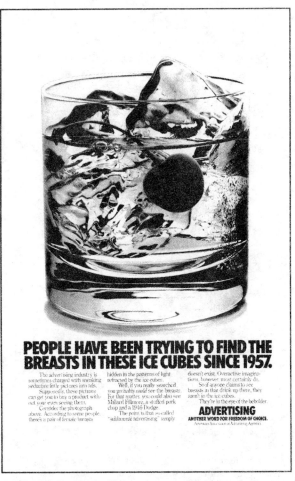

FIGURE 5–3 EMBEDDED FIGURES. Viewers are prompted to make this search not only by the challenge but also by the alleged image.

590

set of the same slides, using the same locations, and the control slides contained no embedded messages. The subjects observed these slides and then, two days later, observed them again, along with completely new slides. The subjects were asked to indicate which slides they had seen previously, and they showed no greater recognition for the *sex*-embedded slides than for the slides with nonsense syllables or no message at all. None of the subjects reported anything unusual about the slides, although they could detect the embedded messages after they were pointed out (Vokey & Read, 1985).

Instead of worrying about subliminal or embedded messages, our concern should be with the obvious, sometimes obnoxious, advertisements, which are all too detectable. These overt persuaders prompt most of us to buy far more goods than we can afford or use or store or even discard (Zanot, Pincus, & Lamp, 1983).

DIVIDED ATTENTION

Sometimes attention is not so concentrated. The Wild Boy always noticed the weather, and his appetite never abated. A sudden gust of wind and a bowl of potatoes competed for his attention. Similarly, a modern partygoer, engaged in a boring dialogue, at the same time tries to eaves-drop on a nearby conversation. This process of attending simultaneously to two or more events is called **divided attention**. To what extent is it possible? Can we really do two things at once? Everyday experience suggests that most people can indeed walk and chew gum at the same time.

TASKS IN THE SAME MODALITY. In one instance, subjects were asked to listen to two different messages simultaneously, one in each ear. To ensure that they attended to one of the messages, they were required to repeat it word for word as it appeared. After performing this task, they did not even know whether the other message had

included nonsense syllables or a foreign language (Cherry, 1953). In a variation of this experiment, the subjects watched two films presented simultaneously on the same screen, one superimposed over the other. In one film, people were slapping hands; in the other, they were playing ball. The subjects were instructed to attend to one of the games by indicating each occurrence of a given event. Again, it was found that they had essentially no memory of the other events (Neisser & Becklen, 1975).

Except for the basic features of the nonattended communication, such as the sex of a speaker or the number of players, the subjects could not simultaneously monitor two sequences in the same sensory modality. That level of comprehension, involving *what occurred* in each situation, was simply too difficult.

TASKS IN DIFFERENT MODALITIES. Two factors facilitate divided attention. While listening to a caller on the telephone, you can simultaneously admire a painting or taste a pudding. Dual attention is most readily achieved when different sensory modalities are involved (Pashler, 1990).

The other factor is the extent to which one stimulus can be responded to routinely. While playing some very well remembered tunes, the pianist can also attend to the decor of the room and perhaps even nearby conversation. But as one habit increases in strength, the case for divided attention weakens. Attention simply shifts to the novel task. When full attention is required for both tasks, lapses occur for one or the other on the order of milliseconds, but they go unnoticed. The conversation, game, or business is resumed as memory smoothly bridges the gap (Pashler, 1992).

Studies of asymmetry in the cerebral hemispheres add to the complexity of this issue. Each hemisphere has a processing capacity partly independent of the other, one more analytic, the other more holistic. To the extent that they involve separate processing, it may be inappropriate to think of attention as a single, undifferentiated response (Hellige, 1990).

PERCEPTION AND THE UNCONSCIOUS. Studies of divided attention have prompted a new perspective on unconscious mental life. Focused on attention and perception, it contrasts with an older, more theoretical perspective prominent in studies of motivation and personality.

The older focus is called the psychoanalytic or *motivational unconscious*, for it is concerned with past events that have emotional or motivational significance for an individual. These experiences arouse anxiety, and therefore they have been pushed out of awareness and into the realm of the unconscious. In contemporary terms, the motivational unconscious has been wryly described as "hot and wet" because its contents appear in expressions of lust, anger, fear, competition, and related manifestations (Kihlstrom, Barnhardt, & Tataryn, 1992).

From a very different perspective, some psychologists today speak of a *cognitive unconscious*, referring to the apparent role of nonconscious processes in perception and learning. This form of the unconscious is not concerned with long-forgotten events but rather with current stimulation, especially events that are barely perceptible or perceptible but unnoticed. Compared with the motivational unconscious, the cognitive unconscious is "cold and dry" because it is more rational and more closely bound to reality (Kihlstrom, Barnhardt, & Tataryn, 1992). Some of the evidence for it has been mentioned already in connection with the absolute threshold, which includes a region of uncertainty, and certain ambiguities in divided attention. The cognitive unconscious seems to be simpler intellectually and more severely limited than the motivational unconscious portrayed in psychoanalysis (Greenwald, 1992).

Speculated to be at the edge of consciousness, the cognitive unconscious has not yet generated impressive research support. (Holyoak & Spellman, 1993). It does, however, continue to intrigue some investigators and fuel the imagination of an interested public.

• ORGANIZING THE PERCEPTUAL FIELD •

Gradually, the Wild Boy became more receptive to his new environment. Still without modesty or manners, he no longer tore off his nightshirt, which covered most of his scars, variously counted at 23 to 26. Taken for walks, or rather scampers, he no longer needed a leash. Beside the measured gait of Madame Guerin, his scurrying mode of locomotion was an obvious remnant of his life in the wild.

Perceptually, he had made progress too, attending to human objects and recognizing patterns among them. In one series of training tasks, with a bandage over his eyes, the boy was induced to give a signal on each occasion that a sound differed from the preceding one. Striking diverse objects and using his own voice in varied ways, Itard eventually enabled the boy to take genuine pleasure in discriminating these sounds. In fact, the boy, still completely mute, began to come to Itard with the bandage in hand, his way of requesting further training (Figure 5–4).

Some forms of stimulation require no such training. Instead, they automatically arouse similar perceptual experiences in all of us. They appear to be independent of previous experience. In a word, they seem largely innate. We now turn to the first of these fundamentals of perception.

PRIMITIVE ORGANIZATION

Something that is primitive is not readily reducible to something else. It is, instead, original, basic, or primary. Hence, the concept of **primitive**

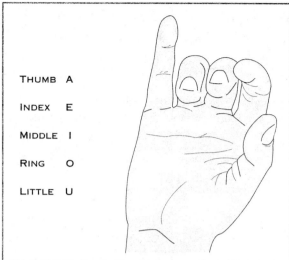

THUMB	A
INDEX	E
MIDDLE	I
RING	O
LITTLE	U

FIGURE 5-4 TRAINING THE WILD BOY. Without language, the Wild Boy needed a way to indicate which sound he had heard. Itard trained him to raise a specific finger for each vowel.

organization refers to aspects of perception that are determined by the fundamental, inborn characteristics of the sense organs and nervous system. It would be difficult, perhaps impossible, to prove that these perceptual tendencies are inborn, but animals, children, and preliterate people, which would include the Wild Boy, behave as if the stimulating properties were the same for them as for normal adults.

Even in these primitive stages, however, perception is not simply the act of recording a stimulus. It is a dynamic event. The brain obtains information through the sense organs, delves into its own environment—its store of memories and motivations—and then modifies the incoming message to suit its particular purposes (Freeman, 1991).

PERCEIVING FIGURES. In our simplest perceptions a figure, or pattern, is perceived as having a certain contour, and it stands out against a background, or ground. There is a certain theme and its surroundings, which comprise a **figure–ground relationship.** The sound of a trombone is heard as a figure against a background of conversations; a bird is seen as a figure against the clouds. Figure–ground discrimination is so basic that it is usually considered the starting point in organized perceptual experience.

Figure–ground relationships are determined partly by the intensity of the stimulus. A sudden, loud clap of thunder or flash of lightning inevitably becomes the figure for a moment, not the background. Figure–ground relationships are also influenced by the process of attending. If you are attending to conversations, then the voices become the figure and the trombone music is the background. If you focus on the clouds, you may not even notice the bird at all.

Eagerly shelling kidney beans with Madame Guerin, the Wild Boy tossed each bean into a pot, and occasionally one fell to the floor. He watched it, retrieved it, and then placed it with the others to be cooked. For him, the fallen bean was a figure, standing out against a background of the floor.

As you read this page, you focus on the black print, not the white paper. The separation of figure from ground is accomplished readily, apparently as an unlearned response.

More important for understanding perceptual processes are the *impossible figures* in which figure–ground relations are altered (Figure 5–5). These outcomes can be induced by clever drawings in which part of the visual image appears to be *both*

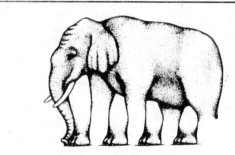

FIGURE 5-5 IMPOSSIBLE FIGURE. The legs of the elephant at times appear to be the figure, at times the ground. The outcome depends on the viewer's point of fixation—at the shoulders or feet of the elephant.

the figure and the ground. They can also be observed in *reversible figures,* in which part of the visual image is viewed as *either* the figure or the ground. After viewing such an image for a few moments, it shifts automatically from one interpretation to the other (Figure 5–6).

According to one explanation, these unintentional shifts are the result of stimulus satiation in the central nervous system. With prolonged observation the neural mechanisms become progressively more fatigued, and the shifts to new stimulation take place more frequently. Human beings confined to an unchanging environment seek sensory variation, which is perhaps imposed on them in these automatic shifts. A different explanation focuses on the activity of the sense organs, which do not passively receive stimulation. The regular reversals, according to this viewpoint, are the efforts of our visual apparatus to make sense of the data. We are asking ourselves: "Is it this? Or this?" We actively seek to understand our environment.

To test the second hypothesis, the ambiguity of the reversible figure was reduced. With no other change, the reversals presumably would be less frequent, for the pattern would be more readily interpreted. This result was obtained when subjects touched a potentially reversible three-dimensional cube, thereby gaining assurance about which corner was closest and which was most distant. The reversals immediately decreased, suggesting that the influential factor was not fatigue but rather a proper understanding of the environment (Shopland & Gregory, 1964).

These demonstrations and this research with impossible and reversible figures show a fundamental characteristic of our perceptual systems: They attempt to construct *meaningful* images out of whatever information becomes available to them.

GROUPING PRINCIPLES. Stimulation usually has several parts, and therefore the next ques-

tion concerns their organization. Here the relevant principles are known as **perceptual grouping,** in which the parts are perceived according to various patterns, depending on their specific properties. These principles are also called *Gestalt* principles, after the German word for "shape" or "configuration." Emerging from Gestalt psychology, they emphasize the perception of whole patterns or whole situations, regarded as greater than or different from the sum of their parts. A Wagnerian opera is much more than the tones of the separate instruments, available to any composer. The beauty and meaning come from their interactions.

In Gestalt terms, these interactions are called *emergent properties* because they are not inherent in the parts of the figure. Rather, they arise through the relationships among the parts.

According to the **principle of similarity,** stimuli that are alike tend to be grouped together. When Itard trained the Wild Boy's sense of touch, he used this principle. He put a mixture of chestnuts, acorns, and coins into an opaque vase and made the boy bring forth all items of a similar shape, which he did readily, even when Itard added metal letters (Figure 5–7).

The **principle of proximity** refers to the tendency to perceive stimuli near one another as

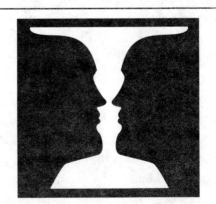

FIGURE 5-6 REVERSIBLE FIGURE.
Sometimes you see a white vase against a dark background; sometimes you see two dark faces against a white background.

GROUPING PRINCIPLES

Similarity. The dark and light squares are grouped together on the basis of shading.

Proximity. The triangles comprise four groups. They are not seen as one scattered group.

Closure. The drawings are generally perceived as five incomplete rectangles, although no figure is a rectangle.

Good Continuity. The crossing pattern appears as two gently curving and bisected lines, not as a pair of half-oval, pointed figures just touching one another.

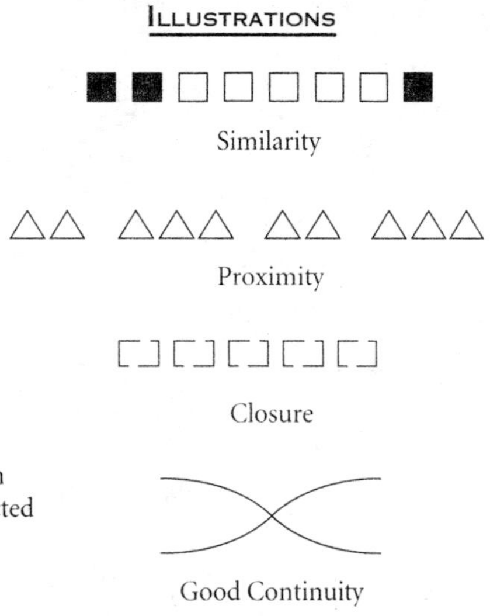

ILLUSTRATIONS

Similarity

Proximity

Closure

Good Continuity

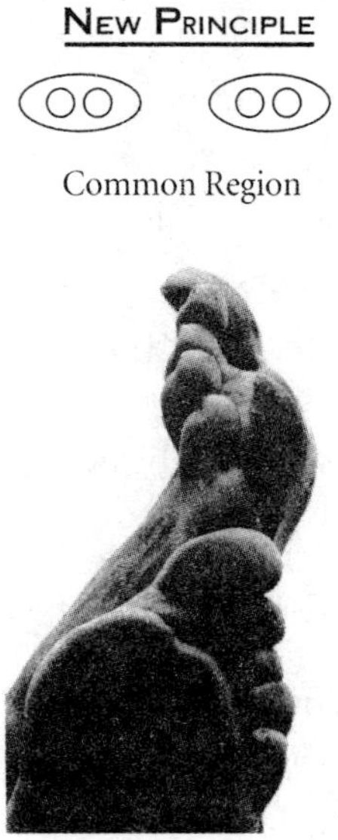

NEW PRINCIPLE

Common Region

FIGURE 5–7 PRINCIPLES OF GROUPING. Four original principles, illustrated in the drawings, are present but less evident in the photo of the feet. One newly proposed principle, common region, is illustrated by the toes on each foot (From Freeman, 1990).

belonging together. Ask a friend to listen while you tap twice in rapid succession, wait a while, and tap twice again. When asked how many taps he or she has heard, your listener probably will report two pairs of taps, rather than four altogether.

In teaching the alphabet, Itard used both of these principles, one pitted against the other. He drew on the blackboard two equal circles, one in front of himself and one facing the boy. At six or eight points on the circumference of each circle he wrote a different letter, and then within the circles he wrote the same letters but placed them differently in the two circles. Next, Itard drew lines connecting each letter on the circumference of his circle with its counterpart in the interior of that same circle, obviously following the principle of similarity. Then he requested the Wild Boy to do likewise for the other circle. At first this task was too challenging for the boy,

who wanted to connect the letters on the basis of proximity. Later he used the principle of similarity, no longer influenced by the arrangement of the letters.

The third principle occurs when we cannot perceive the whole figure. Following the **principle of closure,** we make assumptions about the undetected parts, ignoring their absence. A person partly hidden behind a tree is still perceived as a human being, provided that enough of the person is visible. When a band strikes up in the distance, the music is heard only intermittently, but the song is often recognized.

In the last principle, called the **principle of good continuity** or *good form,* any stimulus tends to be perceived as continuing in its established direction. Stimuli that form a continuous pattern are perceived as a whole; they make an obvious or "good" figure (Saariluoma, 1992). If several balloons are clustered together, we decide which contours belong to which balloons on the basis of the natural continuity of the lines.

There are other principles of grouping as well. These principles are used intentionally to render objects less visible, a result known as camouflage. Soldiers in battle, a thief at a cocktail party, and unprepared students who fear being called on in class all try to blend in with their surroundings.

༄

FORM PERCEPTION

Perception is not merely active but, more accurately, interactive. It is influenced on one side by sensory input and on the other side by memories and thoughts about the incoming stimulation. Many cognitive psychologists therefore emphasize **information processing,** meaning the fundamental operations used by the human mind in understanding our world. These studies attempt to describe the interactive mental operations by which incoming information influences human behavior and experience (Massaro & Cowan, 1993). In particular, they stress today the concept of **parallel distributed processing,** which states that the brain can manipulate different kinds of information at the same moment. It can engage in simultaneous processing even when the information is distributed in different brain regions.

What takes place in our brains as we seek this information, trying to make sense of a given figure, its ground, or some combination of these events? How do we go about deciding that something has this or that form? In this process, called **form perception,** the task is to determine *what* is being observed.

Invariably, the object has some familiar qualities. Therefore, we typically speak instead of *pattern recognition,* in which the task is to compare incoming information with stored information, determining the similarities and differences. Decisions about incoming information arise from two perspectives, the bottom and top.

BOTTOM-UP APPROACH. Consider the Wild Boy's task in matching the letters in Itard's circles. Or consider your own task in reading this book. In both cases, the problem is letter recognition. In addressing this problem, the **bottom-up approach** begins at the most fundamental level of perception, close to the receptors, attempting to analyze the basic features of the incoming message. This approach to information processing is sometimes referred to as the *direct perspective,* for it *begins with* what is "out there."

The bottom-up approach is illustrated in the role of feature detectors, discussed in the previous chapter. A feature detector is a cell in the organism's visual system that is highly responsive to a specific stimulus. These detectors react to certain visual forms in the environment—a straight edge, brightness, a dark point, and so forth. In reading or identifying letters, the bottom-up approach involves the same sort of analysis, postulating the role of *horizontal detectors* and *curve detectors.* If Itard wrote the letter T on the edge of the circle and the Wild Boy searched for its mate within, the horizontal detector would be activated by the letters E, L, and A, all of which include horizontal lines, but not X and Y, which contain only diagonal and vertical lines.

Then, according to the theory, these horizontal, diagonal, and vertical detectors combine with each other in stimulating what might be called *letter detectors.* Recognition of the letter L would be aroused by a configuration of horizontal and vertical detectors and inhibited by diagonal detectors. The letter A would be aroused by a pattern of horizontal and diagonal detectors and inhibited by vertical and curved detectors. The French word LA would be recognized through stimulation of these two sets of letter detectors, combined in this sequence, and so forth. As evident from this description, approaching the problem this way means that the ultimate conception of the solution becomes extremely complex, based on countless combinations of single, highly specific responses to the original stimulation.

TOP-DOWN APPROACH. From the other direction, the **top-down approach** emphasizes the brain activity in the higher-level thought processes, including expectancy, motivation, and set. This approach is referred to as an *indirect perspective*, for it embodies a constructivist view of the world, stressing that we *impose our perception* on the world out there. In a very general sense, bottom-up processing begins closer to characteristics of the stimulus; top-down processing begins closer to the state of the perceiver.

The top-down perspective is readily illustrated by comparing the pattern recognition of the Wild Boy and Itard. The boy, laboriously studying one letter and then the next, did not use the top-down approach effectively. Seeing the combination LAI, for example, he had no idea about what letter might come next. With no overall sense of these patterns of black and white, he did not anticipate the word for his favorite food.

Itard, in contrast, used rules derived from his experience with the French language. A set of expectancies guided his processing of information. If he saw LAI, he would read LAIT, making an assumption about the fourth letter, for in French LAIT means "milk." A great deal of efficiency presumably is added in the top-down approach.

COMBINED APPROACHES. Both approaches have been used in electronic solutions to everyday problems, such as sorting mail. A bottom-up analysis begins with specific details, such as straight lines and curved lines, parts of the digits in the zip code. A top-down analysis begins with computer recognition of the global features of the item in the mail: envelope, stamp, and address. The process of using television images with bottom-up and/or top-down analysis is called *visual pattern recognition* or *computer vision.* An interdisciplinary field with contributions from neuropsychology and computer science, it has enormous potential for solving practical problems and providing further understanding of visual processes (Banks & Krajicek, 1991).

It seems most likely that human pattern recognition involves both approaches, solving the problem up from the bottom, near the receptors, and down from the top, beginning with the brain. In fact, it can be argued that our high speed of pattern recognition *requires* this parallel distributed processing. With so much information available to us, we need both avenues to understand our world.

Sometimes the bottom-up approach is called *data-driven,* for it begins with the stimulus. Similarly, the top-down approach is said to be *knowledge-driven,* for it commences in the brain. Sometimes we cannot use either direction. The context is ambiguous, inhibiting top-down analysis, and the printed letters are unclear, preventing bottom-up analysis: consider PAPIS. If the third letter were complete, facilitating a bottom-up approach, you could have read the word. If you knew we were referring to the city where Itard trained the Wild Boy, enhancing a top-down approach, you also could have read it.

∾

PERCEPTUAL CONSTANCY

The Wild Boy recognized Itard when the physician was far out in the fields, when he was below a window, and at dusk when he sat in his study enjoying a drink from his favorite decanter. Yet on the boy's retinas the image of Itard was different at these different moments. When he was distant, the image was small. When he was directly below, the

Wild Boy saw little more than a hat. In the dusk, the image was faint. Even when stimuli represent the same object, they can change a great deal as the observer moves about and as conditions of the environment change.

In the midst of all this change and potential ambiguity, it is remarkable that we achieve a stable perception of the world. This capacity for recognizing objects under conditions of different stimulation is known as **perceptual constancy,** of which there are several types. Imagine the domestic crises that might arise if you did not recognize your spouse or significant other when viewing that person in different positions.

TYPES OF PERCEPTUAL CONSTANCY. The hallway door in the home of Madame Guerin appeared rectangular, regardless of the position from which it was viewed. This condition is an example of **shape constancy,** meaning that something is perceived as having the same shape regardless of the perceiver's vantage point. Similarly, the opening in Itard's decanter appeared circular, even though the image was oval when viewed at an angle. This phenomenon occurs whenever an object appears to maintain its form or shape despite marked changes in the retinal image (Figure 5–8).

When you hold a familiar object close to your eyes and then gradually move it away, the retinal image becomes smaller. But the perceived size of the object does not change greatly under different viewing conditions, demonstrating **size constancy.** Similarly, people far away have a smaller image than those closer to you, but they look about the same size.

A white rabbit in the setting sun reflects orange rays, but it is perceived as white. When the normal hue is perceived, despite changes in lighting, **color constancy** has occurred. Actually, some compromise takes place in all cases. The rabbit appears a little less white than usual, just as people far away, especially if they are unfamiliar, look a bit smaller than their actual stature. All of the constancies involve some degree of compromise between perceiving something as constant and perceiving it as somehow altered due to its place in the visual scene.

Turn a light from high to low while looking at some familiar object. The brightness of the object does not change appreciably with the change in illumination, a phenomenon known as **brightness con-**

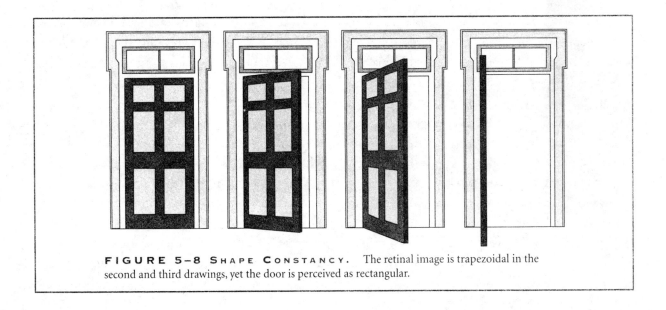

FIGURE 5–8 SHAPE CONSTANCY. The retinal image is trapezoidal in the second and third drawings, yet the door is perceived as rectangular.

stancy. A black belt can be illuminated until the amount of light entering the eye is greater than that received from a white shirt, and yet the belt will still appear black and the shirt white.

All constancy phenomena depend on environmental cues. When these cues are removed, a person far away, for example, appears smaller than is really the case. In the maintenance of constancies, prior experience and knowledge of the context are most important (Figure 5-9).

DISTAL AND PROXIMAL STIMULI. In discussions of perceptual constancy, the term **distal stimulus** refers to the properties of the stimulus out there in the world. It is physical energy at its source, such as the light waves emanating from the figure of Itard at dusk. The term **proximal stimulus** refers to the stimulation at the receptor, the light waves impinging on the Wild Boy's retinas. The difference between these stimuli is created not only by molecules of air as the light waves are scattered but also by the lens of the viewer's eyes, which refocuses the light, and by the humors and other eye mechanisms as the light passes to the retinas. The paradox, and also the essence of the constancy phenomena, is that the perceived stimulus, influenced by the viewer's expectancy as he or she looks at the world, corresponds not so much to the proximal stimulus, on which it is based, as to the distal stimulus out there. In visual judgments of size, for example, the brain somehow performs a transformation on the proximal stimulus at the retina, thereby recovering the original distal size. This transformation, as expressed in mathematical theory, depends on the angle of the stimulus, its distance, and its orientation (Baird & Wagner, 1991).

The relative constancy of perceived objects is essential in achieving a stable perception of the world. Think of the confusion that would exist if we responded to every aspect of our world in terms of mental images alone. Even the simplest routines of daily life would be almost impossible to accomplish.

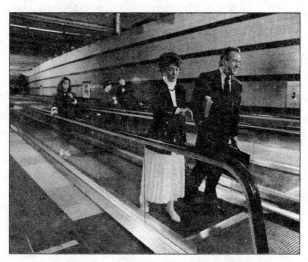

FIGURE 5-9 SIZE CONSTANCY. The retinal image of the woman in the white skirt is twice the size of that cast by the woman in the background holding onto the railing. Yet owing to distance cues, the two women are perceived as essentially the same size.

• INTERPRETING PERCEPTUAL INFORMATION •

As the months passed, the Wild Boy's progress was unmistakable. He was not the same lad who had paid little attention to household objects or human speech. At mealtime, he sat at the table with Madame Guerin and ate quite a range of foods. He managed common utensils and certainly knew the meaning of his wooden bowl. Still without speech of any sort, he asked for milk by bringing it to her.

Whenever Madame Guerin's food preparation reached a certain stage, he went to the cupboard, pulled out the tablecloth, and began setting places for the meal. When curious visitors overstayed their leave, he offered them, without mistake, their hats, gloves, and canes and pushed them gently toward the doorway. Itard submitted a report on these early developments, the first of two classic papers, entitling it *De l'Education d'un Homme Sauvage* (1801).

We too have made progress. Perception begins, as we have seen, with the process of attending. Next, there is the problem of organizing these stimuli. Distinctions must be made among the various figures and grounds as we attempt to discover what is being perceived. We now turn more fully to the interpretation of this information, considering such issues as where the object is, whether it is moving, the accuracy of the perception, and so forth.

• SUMMARY •

ATTENDING TO STIMULATION

1. Attending is a readiness to perceive, based on internal states and characteristics of the stimulus. The subtle physiological adjustments in attending include activities in the brain, muscles, and sense organs.

2. The process of attending to two or more stimuli simultaneously is called divided attention. As a rule, human beings are not highly successful in this endeavor unless one of the tasks is simple, the tasks involve different sensory modes, or one of the tasks is habitual.

ORGANIZING THE PERCEPTUAL FIELD

3. Discrimination of figure–ground relationships seems to be the starting point in organized perceptual experience. According to Gestalt principles of perceptual grouping, the parts of a figure, or several figures, are grouped on the basis of similarity, proximity, closure, and good continuity.

4. Form perception concerns detection of the shape of the object being observed. The bottom-up approach begins at the most fundamental level of perception, close to the receptors; the top-down approach emphasizes the brain activity in higher-level processes, including expectancy, motivation, and thinking.

5. Stable perception of the world is also based on perceptual constancy, which is the tendency to perceive any given object as the same, even though it stimulates us in a variety of ways. Important types of perceptual constancy include shape, size, color, and brightness constancy.

19

CONSCIOUSNESS

WORKING INTERMITTENTLY AS A WAITRESS, ON HER FEET SIX TO TEN HOURS EACH EVENINGS, PETRA WAS FATIGUED BY HER schedule, even as a young woman of 24 years. She did have the daylight hours for painting, and she tried to recuperate through an irregular pattern of eating and resting.

Like most of us, Petra also devoted about one-third of her life to a distinctly diminished state of consciousness—sleep. Think of it: The average person of 60 has spent about 20 years in bed. However, human beings are not the sleepiest species. The cat spends more than half of its life in that mode of consciousness (Figure 6–I).

Prolonged deprivation of sleep can be devastating to our mental functions. It can produce perceptual distortions, depression, anxiety, and even extreme elation. In other words, going without sleep seriously disrupts normal consciousness. Talkathon contestants who stayed awake for 88 consecutive hours became irritable and withdrawn and then developed an intense concern about their mental health (Cappon & Banks, 1960). After a 146-hour tennis match, allowing less than 4 hours of sleep each night, the competitors displayed pronounced intellectual and emotional deficits, although they differed sharply in overt signs of sleepiness and endurance (Edinger, Marsh, McCall, & Erwin, 1990).

❧ WAKE-SLEEP CYCLE

For most people, the daily wake-sleep pattern includes about 16 hours of wakefulness and eight of sleep, but there are marked differences among us. To become fully refreshed, some people require nine or ten hours of uninterrupted sleep. Older people are often rejuvenated after only five or six hours of sleep each night. In contrast, some college students seem to get along very well on just a few hours of wakefulness each day.

This tendency for regular alternation between greater and lesser activity in physiology and behavior is known as the **circadian rhythm,** especially when it refers to a 24-hour period. This term comes from the Latin *circa*, meaning "around," and *diem*, meaning "day." Such rhythms occur in insects, plants, and animals, as well as in people. In human beings, they bring out subtle differences in body temperature, heart rate, and hormonal secretion, as well as the obvious differences in energy expended (Figure 6–2).

The importance of these biological rhythms is evident when light-dark schedules are altered. Variations in periods of illumination, or in the intensity of light, influence the length, type, and duration of sleep in many species, as well as the level of energy. Under constant illumination, laboratory rats sleep an hour longer each day, but cats and fish sleep less under the same condition (Campbell & Tobler, 1984). When human beings are in an isolated environment, without clocks or sunlight, their natural rhythm often drifts toward a 25-hour cycle (Webb & Agnew, 1974).

Flying into space or into another time zone partway around the world produces a change in this rhythm in human beings, resulting in a mental syndrome called *jet lag*, involving slower reaction time, poorer problem-solving capacity, and less concentra-

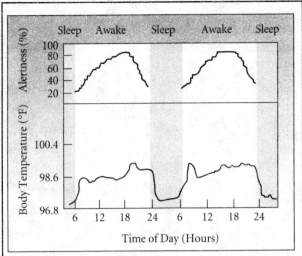

FIGURE 6–2 CIRCADIAN RHYTHM. Alertness and temperature increase and decrease together (Coleman, 1986).

tion. The term is not precise, however. These same reactions appear among people who change their work schedule every few weeks—from daytime hours to the evening shift and then to early morning hours. There is still debate on the rate at which these schedules should be rotated forward in order for workers to become most effective (Wedderburn, 1992; Wilkinson, 1992).

In passing, it should be noted that there is some validity in "Early to bed, early to rise makes one healthy . . ." Body temperature, hormones, and energy rise in the morning. When a person sleeps late into the day, metabolic processes may be depressed, resulting in a groggy, "blah" feeling.

❧ THE SLEEPING STATE

Almost no matter when they go to bed, some people fall asleep immediately. Other need a half hour or more. Petra often needed more, partly because she was worried about her daughter. Her recurrent nightmare involving her baby always woke her, leaving her extremely frightened. Afterward, unable to sleep again right away, she watched late night television or stayed awake making small pieces of jewelry that she enjoyed giving away. She often hung these little gifts on people's doors or draped them over her African fertility goddess.

Regardless of how fast people fall asleep, the pattern for everyone is much the same. Gross body movements and postural changes occur first. These are followed by twitching in the limbs, heavier breathing, and slow rolling of the eyes. At this point, the gentle journey toward sleep has taken the individual into the **hypnagogic state,** which is the interval of drowsiness between waking and sleeping. Special interest has been attached to this state because it includes vivid images, particularly before falling asleep. These images are not dreams; they lack the narrative, unfolding quality of dreams, and they are generally not bizarre.

During the hypnagogic state, a person may experience a pronounced muscle spasm, much more than a twitch. This shocklike reaction, known as the *hypnagogic jerk* or, more formally, **nocturnal myoclonia,** is sometimes so violent that it awakens the individual for a brief, painful instant. Purely physiological, it is apparently unrelated to the mattress, dinner, bedclothes, or even the sleeping partner. It is perhaps stimulated by dream images and motor commands from the lower brain centers, reflecting the ways in which the brain manages the process of entering and leaving the various stages of sleep (Chase & Morales, 1990).

SLEEPING BRAIN. Contrary to popular thought, the sleeping part of the wake-sleep cycle is not necessarily passive. Muscle tension, blood pressure, and heartbeat all decrease during sleep, but we cannot dismiss sleep as a passive, unchanging state.

Several brain mechanisms are actively involved in producing sleep. The thalamus, lower brain centers, and cortex are all part of our sleep system. In particular, a subcortical arousal mechanism called the **reticular activating system** (RAS) plays a prominent role, influencing sleep by ending the transmission of impulses to many cortical synapses. Electrical stimulation of the reticular activating system in animals awakens them immediately, and when this mechanism is inoperative through surgery, the animal remains in a sleepy or drowsy state.

The arousal state of the brain is also influenced by chemical factors called *neurotransmitters,* discussed previously. These substances include acetylcholine, norepinephrine, and serotonin, all of which are secreted in waking life by lower brain centers, and they have ramifications throughout the brain. At sleep onset, the output of acetylcholine and norepinephrine declines. Although it is only vaguely understood, the neurotransmitter **serotonin** may play a special role in drowsiness and sleep, for it is involved in brain circuits that can be inhibitory or excitatory, thus influencing arousal.

Another reason that sleep cannot be considered merely a passive state in the wake-sleep cycle is found in its different stages. One of these, in which dreaming occurs, involves considerable physiological activity.

STAGES OF SLEEP. In investigating these stages, psychologists have employed several electronic devices, including the electroencephalograph, used to detect the spontaneous electrical activity of the brain. These patterns, or brain waves, are detected by electrodes placed on the scalp and recorded by a writing stylus on a moving paper tape. This record of the brain waves is known as an **electroencephalogram** (EEG), in which regular and irregular patterns may be observed (Figure 6–3).

Before entering sleep, when the person is just resting or relaxed, a regular EEG rhythm appears, called *alpha waves.* These waves occur at a rate of 8–12 cycles per second. The individual is awake but relaxed, and then, in a series of gradual transitions, moves into the various stages of sleep, numbered at four or five. In stage I, drowsiness, the EEG becomes a somewhat disorganized pattern of fast

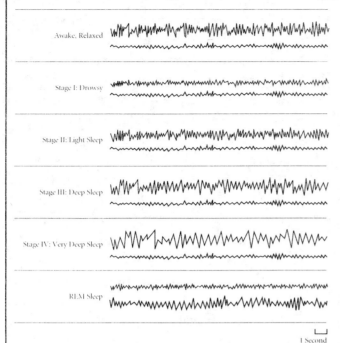

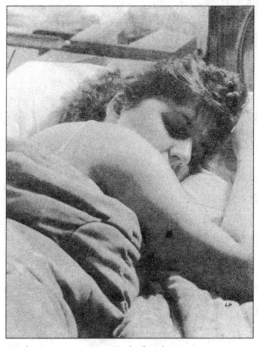

FIGURE 6-3 STAGES OF SLEEP. Certain brain waves are typical of each stage, though they may appear throughout the night. Overall, the waves become slower and deeper from stages I through IV. Stage I sleep and REM sleep are much alike in EEG patterns, but REM sleep is also characterized by rapid eye movements, dreams, and difficulty in waking the sleeper. The EEG tracings are shown in red; the REMs appear in black.

waves of low voltage; the regular alpha rhythm largely disappears. The onset of stage II, light sleep, is marked by occasional spindles, which are brief, rhythmic patterns of approximately 15 cycles per second. In stage III, these spindles become mixed with very slow waves of high voltage occurring at the rate of three cycles per second. These slow, deep waves, called *delta waves*, are indicative of deep sleep. In stage IV, also called deep sleep, the delta waves become predominant, appearing in at least 50% and sometimes in 100% of the EEG pattern (Hobson, 1988).

All of these stages reappear predictably, but often in reverse order, from IV back to III and then to II and so forth. One full cycle lasts for approximately 90 minutes, sometimes longer. Then, when stage I should recur, a new phenomenon appears. At this time, the slow, rolling movements of the eyes quicken considerably. They become **rapid eye movements** (REMs) as the eyes dart in one direction and then in another, in coordinated fashion, under the closed lids. Breathing becomes heavy and irregular, blood pressure increases, and muscles begin twitching. Most surprising, the EEG pattern in this state shows a level of brain activity much like that of someone poised and alert. High-frequency, low-amplitude waves dominate the pattern. This wide-awake profile appears to be incompatible with a sleeping brain, and therefore this REM state is sometimes called *paradoxical sleep.* This expression is also appropriate because a person in the REM state is difficult to awaken.

These characteristics of sleep, which occur in the second and subsequent cycles, are sometimes called stage V, but many investigators simply refer to this sleep as *REM sleep* and to all other stages as *non-REM (NREM) sleep.* Altogether, REM sleep

604

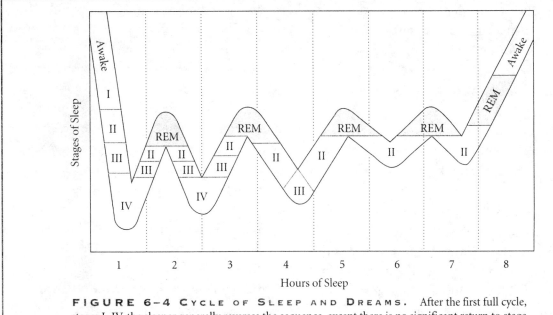

FIGURE 6–4 CYCLE OF SLEEP AND DREAMS. After the first full cycle, stages I–IV, the sleeper generally reverses the sequence, except there is no significant return to stage I. The sleeper enters REM sleep instead, presumably dreaming. As the graph indicates, the deepest sleep, stages III and IV, occur early in the night; the longest periods of dreaming occur toward morning.

appears four or five times during the night, constituting about 25% of the total time spent in sleep. During the first cycle it lasts for about 10 minutes, but this stage grows longer during the night. Toward the end of sleep, it becomes more prominent, sometimes lasting for a half hour or even an hour (Figure 6–4).

DISCOVERY OF REM SLEEP. In the early 1950s, while Eugene Aserinsky was collecting basic facts about sleeping infants, he noted twitches of the arms and legs as each child went to sleep. He also noted the slow, rolling movements of their eyes under the lids, which investigators knew to be prominent just prior to sleep. During one cribside visit, after the slow, uncoordinated, drifting eye movements, his attention suddenly was caught by something else—the rapid, jerky, but coordinated movements in both eyes, similar to those of someone watching a spirited game of table tennis in waking life.

Aserinsky's first reaction was one of disbelief

and surprise that no one had reported these rapid eye movements previously. Immediately, he and a colleague, Nathaniel Kleitman, went to their laboratory and confirmed these movements, painting sleepers' eyelids black and using a flashlight to observe them more carefully. Later, they performed a controlled investigation, using ten subjects who were awakened sometimes during REMs and sometimes when there were no REMs. In each case, the subject was asked to report what he or she had just been experiencing while asleep.

Among 27 awakenings during these movements, 20 revealed detailed memories of dreams, including visual imagery; the other seven produced only the feeling of having dreamed or no dreams at all. Among the 23 awakenings in the absence of these movements, 19 indicated no dreams and four included only a few details. Altogether, almost 80% of the REM subjects reported dreams compared to only 20% of the non-REM subjects. This procedure of awakening people during REM sleep provided the first means for determining accurately and efficiently the incidence and duration of dreams, and it inaugurated widespread research (Aserinsky & Kleitman, 1953).

NATURE OF REM SLEEP. Several characteristics of the REM state distinguish it from the other stages of sleep. In addition to REMs and the alert, high-frequency EEG pattern, breathing becomes irregular and heavy. There is also a loss of normal muscle tension, currently used in some research laboratories as a sign of the onset of the REM period. This limpness of the muscles, even in the face, particularly under the chin, stands in sharp contrast to their condition in the other sleep stages. It appears to serve a protective function, preventing sleepers from acting out their dreams.

There is much evidence for similar physiological activity in animals. Using the REM state as an indicator, psychologists have discovered that pigeons dream, sea turtles do not, and elephants stand up to sleep but lie down to dream. However, dreams and REMs are not perfectly correlated. We can only assume that animals in the REM state are dreaming (Hartmann, Bernstein, & Wilson, 1967; Hobson, 1988).

Among human beings, another physiological reaction suggests that we constantly dream about sex. Changes in blood flow cause erections in men and engorgement of vaginal regions in women, but these reactions occur with any dream content— even when the dreamer is simply conjugating Latin verbs or weeding the garden. The only notable exception to these physiological changes occurs in cases of extreme fatigue. Brain chemistry also may change in REM sleep. The release of acetylcholine and norepinephrine appears to decline to levels even lower than those in non-REM sleep.

The physiological activities during dreaming are so marked that investigators have examined the results of preventing them. This outcome is achieved simply by waking subjects when the REM pattern occurs and then permitting them to fall asleep again.

Cats, rabbits, and other animals deprived of REM sleep, as well as human subjects, immediately spend considerable time in REM sleep when allowed to do so. They make up for the deficit by increasing the REM state from 60% to 160% above normal. This outcome has led researchers to speak of the **REM rebound effect,** meaning that people deprived of REM sleep or dreams must compensate later by dreaming more than usual. There seems to be a *need* for dreaming. People awakened during the REM state show signs of personality disorder and anxiety; those awakened for comparable intervals at other times show fewer adverse effects (Dement, 1960, 1992; Tolaas, 1980).

Different sleep stages may serve different purposes. Deep, slow-wave, non-REM sleep apparently has a restorative function. It allows the body to replace energy diminished during the previous day. REM sleep, in contrast, appears to be more related to circadian rhythms, regulating or reflecting the wake-sleep cycle. Deprivation of REM sleep may interfere with the conservation of energy rather than its restoration. Our stages of sleep each night may be triggered by both sources, the homeostatic mechanisms of restoration and the circadian mechanisms of rhythm and conservation (Borbely, Achermann, Trachsel, & Tobler, 1989).

SLEEP DISORDERS. We have all gone to bed and been unable to sleep. Usually the problem is temporary. The chief causes include stressful daytime activities, mental effort just before retiring, too much coffee or another stimulant, or simply insufficient fatigue. The chief feature in **insomnia** is *chronic* inability to go to sleep or to remain asleep. Young people are more likely to find that they cannot fall asleep within a reasonable period, a condition known as *initial insomnia.* Older people have the other complaint. They awaken too early or too frequently, a sleep disturbance known as *terminal insomnia.* People of all ages complain at times that they have not had restful sleep, and sleeplessness is often overestimated by the alleged insomniac. The condition is considered insomnia only if it continues for at least a month (American Psychiatric Association, 1994).

Petra experienced both types of insomnia. Sometimes she could not fall asleep because she was worried about her daughter; often she could not sleep because she had consumed too much coffee. On other occasions, she found herself wide awake after sleeping for just a few hours, frightened by her nightmare. Unknown to her, consumption of alcohol is also a factor in terminal insomnia. Alcohol blocks certain neurotransmitters responsible for brain activity, thus inducing relaxation and promoting sleep (Sudzak, Glowa, Crawley, Swartz, et al., 1986). At the same time, it disrupts the work of other neurotransmitters, thereby awakening the person earlier than normal.

In particular, alcohol suppresses REM sleep, which is why alcoholics in a detoxification center experience such frequent and terrifying dreams. They are undergoing the REM rebound effect, dreaming more to make up for the earlier dream loss. Drugs, including alcohol, are responsible for numerous sleep disturbances (Table 6–1).

The recommended treatments for insomnia are well known. Avoid concerted mental effort before going to bed. Do not use drugs under the impression that they induce relaxation, for they too interfere with the sleep pattern. Many people adapt to sleeping pills, and in the long run these substances

may even disrupt sleep (Figure 6–5). Instead, exercise as much as possible during the day; start relaxing a couple of hours before bedtime; and do not go to bed with a completely empty stomach. Consume a warm nonalcoholic drink.

The opposite of insomnia, *hypersomnia*, is the inability to stay awake. The wake-sleep cycle is again disrupted, but the disturbance is in the opposite direction. In a severe case, called **narcolepsy,** the individual experiences sudden, uncontrollable episodes of falling asleep. These recurrent states are usually of short duration, and mild cases may even pass almost unnoticed, as though the individual were simply in a daze or inattentive for a moment. More serious cases can jeopardize the safety of the individual and others. The underlying causes remain unknown, although there is evidence for an inherited predisposition (Dement, 1992).

Some people go to sleep easily and normally but awake tired the next morning, not realizing that they have awakened briefly several times during the night. This condition, **sleep apnea,** arises because breathing is interrupted during sleep, and waking for a moment restores breathing. Most common among overweight men, this disorder occurs because the muscles controlling the air passages become relaxed during sleep. Then the passages may become temporarily blocked by the surrounding tissues. Surgery, certain medications, and weight loss are recommended treatments.

Sometimes people get out of bed after going to sleep and move around without awakening. This disturbance, **sleepwalking,** includes all sorts of activities—eating, dressing, and going to the bathroom, as well as walking around and climbing stairs. It typically does *not* occur during dreams, but rather in stages III and IV, and it continues for no longer than a half hour. At its outset, the person may sit up in bed and engage in some simple, repetitive activity, such as picking at the bedclothes. Then, with a blank look, the person leaves the bed and walks around, typically avoiding obstacles while still asleep.

√   Chronic stress: family, health, work, finances
√   Consumption of alcohol, coffee, tea
     Endocrine disorders
√   Concern about insomnia
     New work or school setting
     Temporary anxiety over minor matters
     Consumption of psychoactive drugs
     Jet lag or shift work

TABLE 6–1 DISRUPTION OF SLEEP. The chief factors, listed in order of their importance for the general public, vary considerably from individual to individual. Those most disruptive for Petra are indicated by the checkmarks (Larson, 1990).

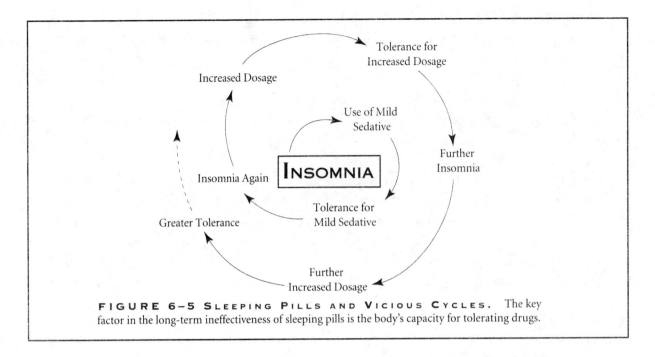

FIGURE 6–5 SLEEPING PILLS AND VICIOUS CYCLES. The key factor in the long-term ineffectiveness of sleeping pills is the body's capacity for tolerating drugs.

THE DREAMING STATE

By waking people during REMs, we now know that nearly everyone has **dreams,** which are images, thoughts, and feelings experienced during sleep. They occur about four or five times during the night and, contrary to belief, do not take place in a momentary flash. They may last a half hour or more, corresponding somewhat to the time required for the activities during waking life, and they grow longer toward morning, which is why, when awakened at that time, you are likely to find that you have just been dreaming. Babies are in REM sleep almost one-third of their lives, although we cannot be certain that they are dreaming. Adults spend one-twelfth of their lives dreaming. In other words, we dream, on the average, two hours each night.

Dreams during the REM state are especially vivid, although the rapid eye movements do not necessarily correspond to what is being dreamed. Dreams also occur in non-REM sleep. These are less frequent and contain less imagery, both visual and auditory.

CONTENTS OF DREAMS. Since discovery of the REM state, dreams are no longer considered completely inaccessible. People keep dream logs, go to dream seminars, and serve as subjects in dream laboratories. One investigator collected thousands of dreams from hundreds of college students. Among the numerous findings, one was quite clear. We dream mostly about the familiar in our lives, the fabric of our existence—an old couch cover, a recent dinner, fences that need to be mended. We dream about ourselves, our family, and our friends, not about famous people or historic events. The settings are our homes, neighborhoods, and schools, not faraway places with strange-sounding names (Hall & Van de Castle, 1966).

Petra's recurrent nightmare about her baby illustrates this tendency to dream about ourselves and our surroundings. Actually, the nightmare had two parts, the first of which took place in an adoption agency. In the dream, Petra brought her baby to the agency and handed her to the adoption nurse. Then she turned around and began walking away. As she did so, the baby began crying and pushed and struggled to escape from the nurse. Still crying, the baby reached out for Petra's soothing

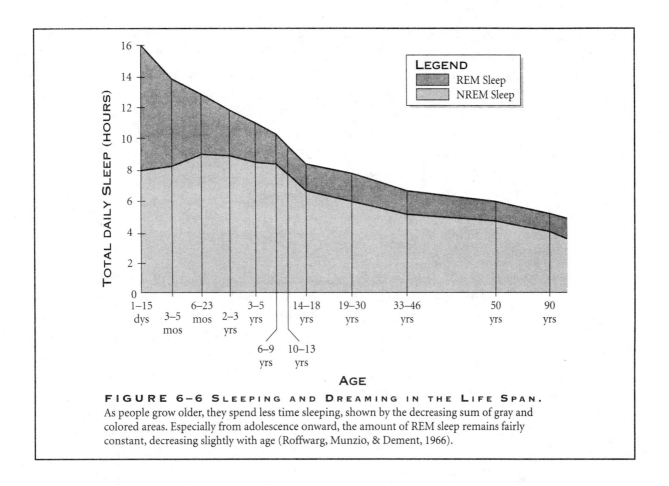

FIGURE 6-6 SLEEPING AND DREAMING IN THE LIFE SPAN.
As people grow older, they spend less time sleeping, shown by the decreasing sum of gray and colored areas. Especially from adolescence onward, the amount of REM sleep remains fairly constant, decreasing slightly with age (Roffwarg, Munzio, & Dement, 1966).

embrace. As the dream ended, Petra ignored the baby and left forever (O'Neill, 1990).

A *nightmare* is a vivid, detailed, frightening dream experience, often characterized by an inability to move, usually awakening the dreamer. It typically occurs late at night, associated with the REM state. A *night terror*, in contrast, is a very sudden awakening, often with a scream, but without vivid imagery. It is not a dream; it is not associated with REM sleep; and, not surprisingly, it occurs in the early hours of sleep (Oswald, 1987).

Petra was terrified by her nightmare because she had never wanted to give her baby up for adoption in the first place. Eight years earlier, at age 16, she had been an honors student in high school, doing very well, and then she became pregnant. Her father forced her to place the baby for adoption, a scene she felt was re-enacted in her recurrent night-

mare. A short time later, her father forced her to leave the home too (O'Neill, 1990).

The chief characters in Petra's dream are herself and her baby. The setting is familiar, the local adoption agency, and the nurse is a minor character, perhaps a stranger. In most of our dreams, even strangers are more common than public figures. If you want to know who is dreaming about you, think of the people who appear in your own dreams. On these bases, it is postulated that waking and dream thoughts blend in some fashion. Our lifestyles influence our dreams, and dreams somehow become part of our daily thoughts. Dreams are a constant element in adult mental life (Figure 6–6).

INFLUENCES ON DREAMS. It is sometimes thought that dreams are influenced by events that occur while we are sleeping. The sleeper

609

dreams about the event instead of being awakened by it. The first recorded experimental studies of this hypothesis occurred in 1861, when a Frenchman named Alfred Maury had simple experiments performed on himself. When the sleeping Maury was pinched, he reported the next morning that he dreamed about receiving medical treatment. When exposed to a heated iron, he dreamed about people with their feet on hot coals (Maury, 1861).

Maury's work prompted a cause-and-effect conclusion: Dream contents are caused by external factors. However, this work suffered from serious defects. Maury set up these experiments himself. He perhaps went to bed thinking about being pinched or exposed to heat.

In fact, Maury's view has not been confirmed by more recent experiments using more precise laboratory techniques. When a sleeper is sprayed with water or exposed to a tone, that person may or may not dream about being wet or listening to music. The dream includes a wide variety of contents not evident in the external stimulation (Dement & Wolpert, 1958; Webb & Cartwright, 1978).

Most investigators agree instead that people dream about recent events that are important to them. To test this hypothesis, the experimental method was used again, but rather than stimulating sleeping people, the investigators exposed the subjects to several types of stimulation *before* they went to sleep. The subjects viewed films that were likely to be stimulating and personal—erotic, violent, athletic, and so forth. Then, awakened at appropriate times, they recorded their dreams. The overall finding was that these stimuli did influence the content of their dreams (Tolaas, 1980).

To what extent are dreamers aware that they are dreaming? The answer to this question varies considerably, not only among individuals but also at different times during an individual's dreams. If no one is present in the dream, then the person may not realize that he or she is having a dream. In contrast, a person dreaming about himself or herself is likely to be aware that dreaming is occurring. Whenever someone is sound asleep and also aware of being in the dreaming state, the condition is called **lucid dreaming,** a concept that is widely debated. The individual presumably possesses a conscious mind in a sleeping brain (Gackenbach & LaBerge, 1988; Walsh & Vaughn, 1992).

THEORIES OF DREAMING

Questions about the reasons for our dreams are still far from answered, and they can be approached in at least two different ways, as physiological or psychological issues. From the physiological perspective, the question concerns the origins of dreams. How do they arise? From the psychological viewpoint, the main issue seems to be function. What purpose do dreams serve?

PHYSIOLOGICAL VIEWPOINT. One approach to the physiology of dreams stresses the human brain as a dynamic whole, a self-sustaining system capable of generating and then analyzing its own information. Specifically, the **activation-synthesis hypothesis** proposes that the brain activates itself through neural activity in the lower brain centers and that these random pieces of information are then combined with memories in the upper brain regions (Hobson, 1988).

In the activation stage, the sleeping brain must somehow turn itself on. It is proposed that this internal activation occurs automatically after a period of sleep of 90 minutes or so. The responsible neurons are presumed to be part of the *reticular activating system*, the basic arousal system in the human brain. In the synthesis stage, the auto-activated brain processes these random signals by interpreting them in terms of information already in storage. The *cerebral cortex* thus becomes the critical brain region during synthesis but, disconnected from the outside world, it lacks the opportunity to test its activities against external realities. It takes the spurts of random signals and weaves them into the best possible story by using information in preexisting memories.

In Petra's dream about the adoption agency, the activation of these impulses came from the lower brain regions, as her brain was turned "on" every 90 minutes or so. This jumble of impulses included images of her baby, the agency, crying, and so forth. Simultaneously, the reticular activating system blocked out other messages, external and internal, which might have disrupted the dream. Then the synthesis of these messages took place in the cerebral cortex, responsible for higher-level symbolic activities. It constructed from this disorganized mass of information a reasonably coherent story or whole, which was the dream Petra experienced.

The activation-synthesis hypothesis does not indicate in any detail how certain neurons are turned on, perhaps by acetylcholine, and the synthesis of the brain stem impulses and cortical memories, if it even occurs, certainly is not understood. The purpose of theory is to guide research; the activation-synthesis hypothesis may prove fruitful in this regard.

FREUDIAN VIEW. Interpretations of dreams from a psychological perspective are much older than the physiological theories, dating to the earliest recorded history. This speculation was enormously augmented by the publication of Sigmund Freud's book *The Interpretation of Dreams* (1900), regarded with some skepticism today. It states that the obvious dream story, known as the **manifest content,** is relatively unimportant. A mask for something more significant, beyond the dreamer's awareness, it reflects unfinished business or events that the dreamer has dealt with in waking life, a view supported by modern research.

The manifest content of Petra's recurrent nightmare concerned her baby, even in the second part, an imaginary scene years after the adoption. In this part of the nightmare, the rejected baby had become a young woman, searching for Petra, her natural mother. Petra's dream depicted their reunion. When they encountered each other, the young woman, screaming wildly, rushed toward Petra in anger because of her abandonment years earlier. She was furious, and her anger was growing stronger and stronger. At this point, Petra inevitably awoke in a state of anxiety (O'Neill, 1990). She reported this dream to the psychologist who assisted her at the clinic.

How would Freud regard this dream?

Freud argued that the manifest content protects the dreamer from threatening thoughts and memories lying beneath its surface. These traumatic experiences, typically from childhood, have become unconscious through the process of *repression,* a form of motivated forgetting. The resulting collection of unconscious, forbidden memories from earlier years forms the **latent content** of the dream, which is its underlying significance. It is a symbolic representation of an earlier problem in the dreamer's life, presumably an unconscious wish.

To ensure that this latent content is kept out of awareness while we are asleep, repression is aided by the dreamwork, which generates a disguise, transforming the threatening latent content into the dream story, or manifest content, using universal and private symbols of all sorts.

The effort to understand the psychological significance of a dream, called **dream interpretation,** is a highly complex and speculative process requiring skill, experience, and a broad fund of knowledge. Moreover, Freud was emphatic on one point: The dream must be understood in the context of the *dreamer's* spontaneous thoughts about it, not in terms of someone else's ideas. Otherwise, the interpretation presumably reveals more about the interpreter than it does about the dreamer.

After his interviews with Petra, the clinical psychologist, using psychoanalysis, speculated that Petra's two-part nightmare depicts the abandonment theme through three generations—from the parents to Petra to her daughter. The first-generation rejection occurred when the parents forced Petra to leave their home. The second-generation rejection occurred when Petra left her child to be adopted. According to psychoanalytic theory, the disguise in these dreams is that the parents, who were the real source of the problem, do not appear at all. At the same time, this omission is a most revealing element of the dreamwork (O'Neill, 1990).

The third rejection occurred only in the dream. Here the daughter, after finally finding her mother, spurns her, further intensifying Petra's concerns about abandonment and loneliness.

These details about Petra's dreams, and other facts in her life, were reported in a research journal under the title *Case Study* (O'Neill, 1990). Additional information was obtained through an interview with the author, who asked that Petra's true identity be concealed in various ways.

JUNGIAN VIEW. A colleague who eventually left Freud's circle, Carl Gustav Jung developed his own brand of psychoanalysis and took a very different view of dreaming. The manifest content, in his opinion, is a mirror, not a mask. It reflects the dreamer's current concerns, often rather openly. The dream is concerned with here-and-now issues, although elements of the past may be evoked.

For Jung, the basic approach to understanding dreams is to expand the contents in any way possible, a process called **amplification of dreams**. For this purpose, he urged the use of an *interior dialogue*, meaning that the dreamer holds an imaginary conversation with the elements in the dream, including people, animals, and even objects and events. During this dialogue, the dreamer plays any and all parts, behaving and speaking in ways that seem appropriate for each element (Jung, 1963, 1964).

In amplifying the nightmares about leaving her baby, Petra might carry out an interior dialogue, expressing to herself the anguish she experienced. She could also include the baby's part, struggling and crying, protesting against the abandonment. The aim would be to discover, in any way possible, what each of the dream images and ideas might mean to her. These amplifications might show that Petra *herself* felt abandoned, just as she had abandoned her baby.

DREAMS AS INFORMATION PROCESSING. A more recent approach continues somewhat along Jungian lines. The **information processing viewpoint** regards dreaming as a process of sorting and sifting, storing and dumping recently acquired information. This review and rehearsal may serve three functions. First, dreams may assist in *problem solving* by playing an active role in the elaboration of current information. Dreaming somehow enables us to organize recent thoughts into coherent forms and perhaps to consolidate previously acquired information (Table 6–2).

When they encountered one another, the young woman, screaming wildly, rushed toward Petra in anger because of her abandonment years earlier. She was furious, and her anger was growing stronger and stronger...

THEORY	EXPLANATION
Activation-synthesis	This dream is the best possible narrative sequence of random messages from the lower brain centers, mixed with information already stored in memory.
Freudian	The nightmare is a disguised expression of aggression against her parents, for Petra is the young woman in this dream, screaming about her own abandonment.
Jungian	Petra's dream rather directly reveals the anxiety she experienced in abandoning her child; here she imagines the child's response to this abandonment.
Information processing	Dreaming plays a role in organizing, remembering, and forgetting information; Petra, perhaps stimulated by the sudden departure of a friend, is sifting and sorting recent experiences for later use.

TABLE 6–2 THEORIES OF DREAMING. The second part of Petra's nightmare is shown at the top of the table. Each theory offers a somewhat different explanation.

Taken at face value, both of Petra's nightmares are attempts to work through her adolescent pregnancy, her abandonment of the baby, and her fears of the child's reaction. The manifest content tells this story.

Second, dreams may play a role in *remembering*, serving as a means of assessing new and old information and deciding whether new information needs to be stored. Redundant information is discarded, and the remainder is processed for storage (Hobson, 1988). It is known that sleep has a beneficial effect on certain memories, possibly because our dreams early in the night seem to be a review of the day's events.

A third possibility goes one step further, arguing that the most basic purpose of dreams lies in *discharging information*—that is, to forget. The idea here is that the brain is a highly complex mechanism, the most intricate structure on earth, managing truly remarkable amounts of information daily, but it needs an opportunity to discharge itself. In this view, dreaming is an unwinding process, releasing superfluous or unwanted information from potential storage (Crick & Mitchison, 1983).

20
MOTIVATION

IN TURNING TO SURVIVAL MOTIVES, WE BEGIN WITH *INDIVIDUAL SURVIVAL*, WHICH IS THE CAPACITY OF AN ORGANISM TO REACH A normal life span for its species. At the human level, the chief concerns, apart from respiration and safety, are obtaining adequate food, drink, and sleep. Sailing slowly among the hundreds of islands in the South Pacific, Robin had no problem here. In his leisurely travels, he found clams and squid, bought limes and papayas, and slept in the warm sun. He also met Patti Ratterree. They swam and sailed together and enjoyed the native foods.

Afterward, we turn to *species survival*, which is the preservation and continuation of a whole class or category of organisms. This survival is made possible by sexual and parental motivation, but if the species is to survive, the individual survival motives of course are essential too.

HUNGER AND THIRST

"A man seldom thinks of anything with more earnestness," said Samuel Johnson, "than he does of his dinner." What we want for dinner varies widely, however, showing the role of environmental factors in eating. The French and Arabs consume whole birds; Australian aborigines devour ants; and certain Indian societies consider cow urine in milk delectable. In the South Seas, Robin Graham sampled octopus in the Tonga Islands, spider conchs in the Yasawa Islands, and in the Viti Levu Islands he heard stories about the consumption of boiled human flesh.

REGULATION OF EATING. Some of the clearest signs of hunger are pangs in the stomach. Therefore, in early experiments, one subject swallowed a small balloon that could be inflated through an attached tube. When the tube was connected with appropriate apparatus, it gave indications of changes in pressure within the stomach. Contractions of the stomach were found to coincide with the gnawing feeling reported by the subject. On this basis, stomach contractions appeared to be the critical issue in the experience of hunger (Cannon & Washburn, 1912).

Later studies found that both stomach contractions and hunger pangs ceased with the administration of dextrose, a substance that raises the blood sugar level. Thus, the next research step was to examine the relationship between blood sugar level and hunger. Investigators injected blood from a starved dog into a normal dog and observed the contractions sometimes found in hunger. Injection of blood from a well-fed animal stopped these contractions (Luckhardt & Carlson, 1915). Such experiments supported the idea that blood sugar level is closely related to hunger, but again the answer is more complex. Blood sugar level is monitored by the brain.

Electrical stimulation of the side of the hypothalamus, called the **lateral hypothalamus**, activates and sustains eating in animals, even those presumably satiated. When this area is damaged or removed, experimental animals cease eating despite the availability of food, even though their normal needs have not been satisfied. Apparently they do not know when to start eating (Keesey, Corbett, Hirvonen, & Kaufman, 1984). Stimulation in the middle of this area, the **ventromedial nucleus** of

DEALING WITH OBESITY. In *obesity,* a person's body weight is at least 20–25% greater than the ideal weight, as determined by the height–weight ratio for that person, using tables for the two genders, different races, and various ages. The influential physical factors fall into two categories: food intake, by which we gain energy; and physical activity, metabolism, and thermogenesis, by which we spend it. In food intake, the amount of fat in the diet can be most important, contributing significantly to body weight. In spending energy, physical activity accounts for about 15–20% among average people. Metabolism usually accounts for 65–75% of our energy expenditure. A low metabolic rate is clearly a predisposing factor for obesity, apparently complicated by a deficiency in serotonin. Finally, thermogenesis is the process of producing heat in the body. Usually 10–15% of the body's total energy is spent in this manner, and even less may be required in obese individuals (Shah & Jeffery, 1991).

If a change is desirable, and the aim is to lose weight, the next steps emerge—more readily enumerated than followed. Collectively, they illustrate the multiple bases of behavior. First, it is useful to know the nutritional value of foods. An excess of blood sugar, also known as *glucose,* is stored as body fat. The chances of becoming overweight are increased by the consumption of foods high in glucose, such as cake and cookies, rather than those low in glucose but equivalent in caloric content, such as spinach and fish. Second, lasting weight loss is accompanied by a change in bodily processes related to metabolism; therefore, adequate exercise is essential. Twenty minutes may be the minimum to break a sweat, but a longer workout may be more useful for most people. Third, external conditions, such as watching television, prompt needless eating. The issue is partly mind over platter (Figure 10–4).

And finally, eat very s–l–o–w–l–y—for both physiological and psychological reasons. Physiologi-

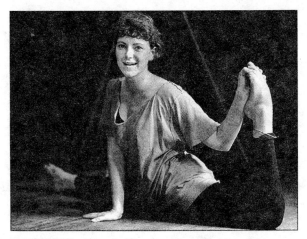

FIGURE 10-4 DUAL VALUE OF EXERCISE. The potential weight gain from a chocolate sundae can be diminished or eliminated by exercise, which consumes calories. In addition, regular exercise can increase the normal metabolic rate. Thus, the body consumes calories at a faster rate even when the person is not exercising vigorously.

cally, a person begins to feel satisfied when food reaches the digestive tract, bloodstream, brain, and so forth. A person eating slowly will have consumed less food when that point is reached. On the psychological side, a person eating slowly will savor the food more and therefore consume less just for the taste.

ANOREXIA AND BULIMIA NERVOSA. Other eating disorders are almost the opposite of obesity. In **anorexia nervosa** a person eats barely enough to stay alive, producing physiological and psychological conditions associated with starvation: weakness, disruption of systemic functions, dizziness, and even hallucinations. Losses of 25% of the normal body weight are not uncommon. The most obvious precipitating cause of this disorder, almost ten times more prevalent in women than in men, is excessive dieting, prompted by a distorted body image. No matter how thin the person becomes, she still feels she is overweight and continues a semistarvation diet. In a seemingly related condition, **bulimia nervosa,** the individual eats regularly or even voraciously but then regurgitates the food. Some bulimic people eat constantly;

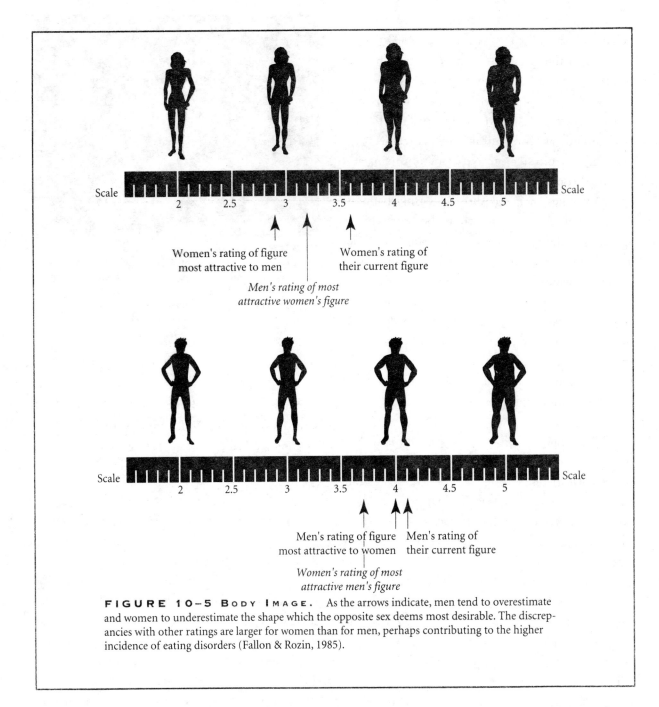

FIGURE 10-5 BODY IMAGE. As the arrows indicate, men tend to overestimate and women to underestimate the shape which the opposite sex deems most desirable. The discrepancies with other ratings are larger for women than for men, perhaps contributing to the higher incidence of eating disorders (Fallon & Rozin, 1985).

others engage in binges. If self-induced vomiting is not employed, laxatives may be used. People suffering from this disorder may be of normal weight and appear normal, if they can keep the regurgitation undetected (Varnado, Williamson, & Netemeyer, 1995).

Overall, for problems of body weight, health maintenance and, to some degree, body image, the preferred solution seems to lie in a program of regular, reasonable exercise.

With these conditions in mind, one key principle emerges for approaching the problem of body image. Determine whether it is a real or imagined problem. In the social context, studies show that both men and women hold misconceptions about the most desirable body shape (Figure 10–5). Men typically are trying to bulk up and women to slim down to reach what they feel is the ideal body image. And yet they are often wrong (Fallon & Rozin, 1985).

THIRST AND THE BRAIN. To survive, the human body also needs a constant supply of water. In fact, extreme thirst is more agonizing than extreme hunger—and more dangerous to health. Human beings can live without food for more than a week, but just a few days without water may be fatal. The depleted condition is called **cellular dehydration,** meaning loss of water in the cells of the body, which occurs constantly because the normal human being excretes about a quart of water each day through urination, exhalation, perspiration, and elimination.

Robin needed pure water at sea. Consuming sea water does not restore the body's water supply. It depletes it instead because sea water is almost 4% salt, much too salty for human consumption. To eliminate from the body the waste from one pint of sea water requires approximately one quart of body fluids—clearly a losing proposition. At sea, Robin caught rainwater in buckets and used it for showers only when he was certain that his physiological needs would be met.

The most obvious internal symptom of the need for water is dryness of the mouth and throat. But when people are subjected to different degrees of water deprivation, they drink water in proportion to the deficit. This accurate estimation is difficult to explain in terms of dryness of the mouth and throat because the first mouthful wets these areas, removing the condition that might provide a guide to the amount needed. To be effective in satisfying the body's need, water must enter tissue in other regions.

Parts of the hypothalamus are sensitive to a chemical agent in the blood called *angiotensin*, which indicates cellular dehydration. Angiotensin appears in greater quantities as the volume of blood decreases, and the volume of blood depends partly on the volume of water in the body. These cells of the hypothalamus have been called **osmoreceptors,** meaning that they signal the passage of fluids through membranes, a process known as *osmosis.* Injections of salt solutions into osmoreceptors of the hypothalamus prompt dehydration and elicit drinking. Injections of plain water stop drinking only when they are placed in the anterior portion. Hence the anterior hypothalamus appears to be most closely related to drinking.

Environmental factors also influence the amount of drinking, as well as the types of beverages consumed. In the Vavau Islands, Robin drank kava, a slightly narcotic drink from shrub root, which made his lips and tongue feel as if he had just received a novocaine injection. "Kava is drunk by customers and staff," he said, speaking of the local shops, "the way that Americans use office water fountains" (Graham, 1972).

NEED FOR SLEEP

Twelve days after leaving the Solomon Islands, the sea churned up 20-foot swells and water poured into the cockpit as the tail of a hurricane kept Robin awake for 48 hours at a time, struggling for survival. When the winds finally subsided, Robin was completely exhausted. This extreme fatigue, he explained later, had a strange effect on him. At one point he had a spurt of energy, and then, a moment later, he felt totally unable to move at all—even to perform the simplest tasks (Graham, 1972).

Staying awake for long periods results in depression, extreme elation, anxiety, and other disorders. In an extensive two-year study, military personnel remained sleepless for 40, 65, or 90 hours; afterward, they showed hallucinations, loss of emotional control, and diminished intellectual functioning (Morris & Singer, 1961). Earlier, we noted similar deficits in sleep-deprived contestants in a tennis match (Edinger, Marsh, McCall, & Erwin, 1990).

Our need for sleep has been viewed from two theoretical positions, the first of which is a popular public view. According to the **restoration theory,** sleep replaces in the body biochemical and other factors depleted by the day's activities. During sleep we are repairing and recharging ourselves. Evidence for this view comes largely from studies of sleep deprivation (Horne, 1988).

From a different perspective, **adaptation theory** states that sleep evolved as an adjustment to a hostile environment, enabling human beings and other animals to avoid predators and, at the same time, to avoid expending useless energy. To serve both purposes, individuals went to sleep in safe places (Webb, 1974, 1983). For example, bats sleep in hiding places during the day, and they remain awake during the night, when their poor vision is not such a hazard. Most of their predators have poor night vision, too.

As so often is the case, the two theories are not incompatible. We need to recharge and repair ourselves periodically, as the restoration theory states. At the same time, adaptation theory recognizes the survival value of different patterns of sleep among the species. The human pattern is currently being subjected to modification by shift work, jet lag, artificial lighting, and the global economy. As noted earlier, these changes can lead to disruptions of normal physical and mental functioning.

∾

SEXUALITY AND PARENTING

The survival of the species depends not only on individual survival but also on propagation. Here the limits of behavior among human beings, and even among apes, are so broad that no complex universal pattern can be identified. Survival of the species also depends on parental care, and again, the limits expand as one ascends the evolutionary scale.

SEXUAL MOTIVATION. There is little variation in sexual activity among rats and guinea pigs because this behavior depends chiefly, but not exclusively, on hormonal secretions, described earlier as androgens and estrogens in the male and female, respectively. Withdrawal of androgenic hormones in males distinctly alters sexual activity, as well as aggressive and scent-making behavior. When newborn and even prenatal males are deprived of these hormones, their sexual behavior in adulthood is like that of females (Drickamer & Vessey, 1992). The genetic constitution of young mammals is highly susceptible to early hormonal influences (Figure 10–6).

In human beings, the sex hormones are secreted by the **testes** in the male and **ovaries** in the female, collectively known as the *sex glands,* or *gonads.* If the testes are removed before puberty, sexual development is commonly disrupted. The effects of removing the ovaries before puberty are more difficult to predict, partly because the adrenal glands also secrete sex hormones. Castration after puberty usually does not result in complete cessation of sexual behavior in men or women, showing the influence of learning, although sexual behavior may appear at a reduced rate. In any case, the results are not nearly as significant as in lower animals.

Both men and women whose sex glands have degenerated late in life may continue to participate in sexual activities. Some women who have passed through menopause actually increase their sexual activity. When responsiveness does decrease in healthy, aging men, it appears to be related to diminished function in the pituitary gland as well as in the testes (Schiavi, Schreiner-Engel, White, & Mandeli, 1991).

Sexual behavior among human beings clearly illustrates the relationship between inborn and acquired factors in motivation. While there is no human sexual instinct, in the sense of a complex behavior pattern shared by all, there are genetically

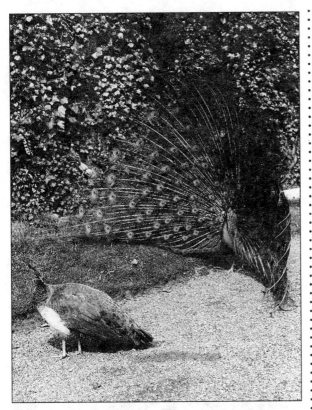

FIGURE 10-6 SEXUAL BEHAVIOR IN ANIMALS. Mating patterns are much the same among members of the same species and same sex. Highly elaborate rituals are determined largely by hormonal and other inborn factors. Here the male peacock attempts to attract the female by an elaborate display of feathers.

driven sexual urges and various reflexes prompted by hormonal secretions. In addition, the pervasive influence of learning is evident in the wide variety of sexual behaviors of interest to some people but not to others. Even mouth kissing is learned. Once, after Robin was pulled from the surf by rescuers, he showed his interest in this activity (Graham, 1972). "And now," he gasped, turning to Patti, "what about some mouth-to-mouth resuscitation?"

SEXUALITY AND EVOLUTIONARY THEORY. A broad evolutionary perspective has implications for human sexuality. The aim in **evolutionary psychology** is to understand the ways in which human beings have developed solutions to their two overriding adaptive problems—survival and reproduction. The individuals who were successful at these tasks are our ancestors. Today, the subtasks for survival include learning a language, making friends, gaining competence at work, and so forth. The subtasks for reproduction include obtaining a mate, engaging in sex, offering parental care to offspring, and so forth.

Men and women are rather differently prepared for the reproduction task—at least in a biological sense. Healthy men have millions of sperm, readily available. Healthy women have a limited number of eggs, available only during periods of fertility. Furthermore, women who want to bear children must find a mate who will furnish the extensive resources necessary for this extremely demanding task. A promising candidate would be loyal, industrious, and assertive, a man capable of gaining status in the group. In contrast, men who want to rear children must find a mate capable of giving birth. Women who show this reproductive promise will be young, and they will be physically attractive to men. As a rule, women in our society generally prefer to marry successful, somewhat older, experienced men. Men are prompted to seek younger, sexually attractive women. These different mating preferences are presumably evolutionary outcomes of the different requirements for men and women in solving the reproduction problem (Buss, 1995; Simpson, 1995).

According to evolutionary psychology, sex differences in jealousy are also part of our biological inheritance. Among men, jealousy is elicited chiefly by evidence of sexual infidelity. Among women, it is also evoked by loss of attention and resources in the mating relationship (White & Mullen, 1989). In the same way, aggression in men and empathy in women may have their origins in the different reproductive tasks that confronted our male and female ancestors. These responses may be the evolved solutions of

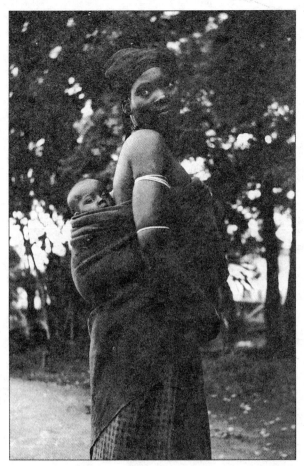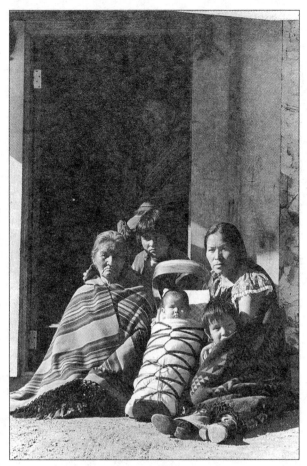

FIGURE 10–7 MATERNAL BEHAVIOR. Patterns of mothering vary widely, showing the influence of learning. Some babies are bundled up in a procedure called swaddling, leaving them unable to reach, sit up, or crawl, yet they show no handicap in motor development.

the two genders for the task of reproduction (Buss, 1995).

Differences in sexual motivation appear to be related to these different reproductive tasks. For men, the dominant aim seems to be physical satisfaction; for women, it is more likely to involve love and a sense of personal commitment (Carroll, Volk, & Hyde, 1985). On these bases, it is not surprising that men's interest in sex is stimulated by direct, explicit communication, as in pornography; women are more motivated by the overall mood, style, and setting of the scene (Masters, Johnson, & Kolodny, 1982).

PARENTAL MOTIVATION. In many species, parental care is significantly influenced by hormonal factors. Especially among animals, prolactin is the most basic condition for **maternal behavior,** meaning care of the young by the mother. Secreted by the pituitary gland, prolactin is also influential in sexual development. Guided somehow by these secretions, maternal behavior in lower animals is highly stereotyped. Without such influences, **paternal behavior,** care of the young by the father, is distinctly less predictable.

At the human level, despite the presence of prolactin, there is no worldwide pattern of mothering, unless it is feeding the child at the breast. Even breast-feeding is not universal, and in different cultures there are marked differences in weaning, both of which indicate the central role of learning (Figure 10–7). Hence, we cannot speak of a human maternal instinct, although this expression often appears, even in professional journals. The countless books and magazines on raising children show the overwhelming role of learning in human parental care.

Among human beings, a time comes when the offspring is ready to leave the parents. If kept too long under parental protection, children may never develop an adequate sense of independence and self-worth. If forced or permitted to leave too soon, they may encounter dangers that they cannot handle or may fail to develop certain skills. But when should a child, moving from infancy through adolescence, be allowed to do what? This question, the *universal parental dilemma*, can be answered only in terms of the readiness of the individual and the demands of the specific environment.

When Robin sailed from California, his parents received so much criticism that Robin's father published a letter explaining his view. It would have been easier to keep him home, he said, but he felt Robin could meet the challenges ahead.

• STIMULATION MOTIVES •

For Robin, sailing across the Coral Sea to New Guinea proved surprisingly difficult. Here he reached the doldrums, regions of the ocean near the equator where it is almost always calm, with only light winds.

Exposed to little more than the sky, the sea, and the sounds of his boat for days and days at a time, Robin began to "hate the bloody boat . . . her every creak, every bubble of her blistered paint." He decided that he would rather face hungry piranhas than go to sea alone again. "The calm began to get to me," he said. "I wanted to keep moving so I wouldn't go crazy."

The motivation for stimulation is typically considered in two categories, both essential for normal survival and development. First, there is the need for sensory variation, meaning that human beings need changes in stimulation. Second, there is the need, early in life, for affectional stimulation, meaning physical and emotional contact with other members of the species. Thus, **stimulation motives** appear to be biologically determined needs for excitation of some sort, not directly related to immediate survival. As yet, the underlying bases for such motives have not been established.

BOREDOM AND CURIOSITY

The need for sensory variation is particularly acute among solo, long-distance travelers. Especially on the high seas or in the skies, where there is little change in the surroundings, the traveler's mind can wander from the task at hand and even play tricks, apparently in an attempt to deal with the monotony.

Charles Lindbergh, flying the Atlantic alone, kept alert by singing, solving riddles, and doing mental exercises, but he still found himself upside down at one point, just a few feet above the water. Admiral Byrd, surrounded only by the wind, snow, and Antarctic darkness, imagined himself in a world of sunlight, full of green and growing things, surrounded by peaceful, kind people. Joshua Slocum, first to sail alone around the world, deliriously imagined a phantom helper who managed the helm while he was asleep, an experience that is common in such environments and perhaps an adaptive reaction (Suedfeld & Mocellin, 1987).

At the same time, these travelers undertook their trips to have new experiences, accomplish new feats, and try new procedures. The **sensory variation motive** includes both concerns, boredom *and* the need for a new form of stimulation, beyond that available in our normally changing environment.

PROBLEM OF SENSORY CONSTANCY.
In one study, human adults in a completely dark room were immersed in a tank of water, almost in a

suspended position. They could hear only their own breathing and some faint sounds from the piping; they later reported that this environment was the most even and monotonous they had ever experienced. After an hour or two, a tension developed that was described as desire for stimulation. Their muscles twitched at an increasing rate, and they used methods of self-stimulation, such as swimming slowly and stroking their fingers against one another. Longer periods in this environment brought intense concentration on a single aspect of the situation, such as slight noises, reveries, or visual hallucinations (Lilly, 1956).

The problem for these subjects was not lack of stimulation, which was admittedly low, but rather the constancy of the situation. Lying quietly in a tepid tub is not aversive initially, but after a while the subject seeks some change. Human beings, as noted in the earlier chapter on sensation, are responsive to *changes* in stimulation. In this aspect of the sensory variation motive, the **problem of sensory constancy,** people become disturbed due to lack of stimulus change. Basically, they are bored. There is no variety, no significant variation in their sensory experience. This problem is most common among people who are confined, such as the elderly, prisoners, and hospitalized patients (Corbin & Nelson, 1980; Grassian & Friedman, 1986; Rothblum, 1990).

Restricted to his 24-foot *Dove*, Robin tried various methods of gaining increased stimulation. Sometimes he made extra work out of daily chores. Sometimes he used his tape recorder extensively, speaking into it, recording other sounds, and then replaying what he had just heard. And sometimes Robin simply indulged in fantasies, which included thoughts of a reunion in Australia with Patti, who was making her own way through that part of the world (Graham, 1972).

DESIRE FOR NOVEL STIMULATION. The motivation for sensory variation also includes the need for *new forms* of stimulation.

In the **desire for novel stimulation,** there is a high degree of curiosity, an interest in exploration and manipulation in a normally changing environment. Human beings expend considerable effort simply trying to find out about things, as Robin's trip illustrates.

The problem here is not sensory constancy. Even if our surroundings change regularly in some way, at times we want to visit different restaurants, try new foods, and meet new people. City workers want a holiday in the country, and country folk want to visit the city. Robin wanted to visit foreign cultures and to test his skill as a sailor.

Monkeys are notorious for their curiosity. They stare endlessly at each other; they sniff and taste things constantly; and when a new object is presented, they investigate it thoroughly. When interest is satiated, another object prompts further manipulation and exploration (Van Lawick-Goodall, 1971).

There is an irony in Robin Graham's voyage. Ashore, he found much novel stimulation; at sea, he was sometimes bored to the point of becoming delirious. Illustrating many issues in motivation, his voyage shows that the human being is a "continually wanting animal."

AFFECTIONAL STIMULATION

The desire for early physical and emotional contact with other members of the species and stimulation by them is called the motivation for **affectional stimulation.** It has been studied experimentally with animals and through observations of human infants. Like sensory variation, the satisfaction of this motive is not necessary for life, but apparently it is necessary for the full development of one's natural endowments. It too appears rooted in the organism's biological inheritance, although no clear physiological basis has been identified.

In one series of studies at the University of Wisconsin, Harry Harlow and his associates observed infant monkeys deprived of their mothers. Instead, the monkeys were provided with mechanical substitutes. One substitute consisted of a piece of wood covered with sponge rubber and terry cloth; the other substitute was made of wire mesh, thus lacking warmth and softness. Both models were the same size and shape, but the babies demonstrated a clear preference for the soft one, which provided contact comfort. In times of stress, they ran and clung to it as monkeys normally do to their real mothers, and when strange stimuli suddenly appeared, they were calmer with the soft model present (Figure 10–8).

The infants also preferred a rocking mother to one that was stationary and a warm one to a cool one. But *contact comfort*, consisting of touching, cuddling, and hugging, was clearly the most crucial maternal factor for infants. Even the features of the mother's face were unimportant. Further studies indicated that infant monkeys not only preferred cuddliness, warmth, rocking, and hugging but also *needed* such stimulation for normal development. Without it, they displayed deviant behavior. Infants reared with wire mothers eventually showed inadequate social, sexual, and even intellectual development in adulthood. Those reared with cloth-sponge mothers were better adjusted as adults (Harlow & Suomi, 1970).

A CELLULAR MECHANISM OF CLASSICAL CONDITIONING IN *APLYSIA*: ACTIVITY-DEPENDENT AMPLIFICATION OF PRESYNAPTIC FACILITATION

R.D. Hawkins, T. W. Abrams,
T.J. Carew and E.R. Kandel

Abstract. *A training procedure analogous to differential classical conditioning produces differential facilitation of excitatory postsynaptic potentials (EPSPs) in the neuronal circuit for the siphon withdrawal reflex in Aplysia.* Thus, tail shock (the unconditioned stimulus) produces greater facilitation of the monosynaptic EPSP from a siphon sensory neuron to a siphon motor neuron if the shock is preceded by spike activity in the sensory neuron than if the shock and spike activity occur in a specifically unpaired pattern or if the shock occurs alone. Further experiments indicate that this activity-dependent amplification of facilitation is presynaptic in origin and involves a differential increase in spike duration and thus in Ca^{2+} influx in paired versus unpaired sensory neurons. The results of these cellular experiments are quantitatively similar to the results of behavioral experiments with the same protocol and parameters, suggesting that activity-dependent amplification of presynaptic facilitation may make a significant contribution to classical conditioning of the withdrawal reflex.*

One of the major goals of neurosocience has been to specify the cellular mechanisms of asso-ciative learning. Although cellular correlates and analogs of associative learning have been observed in several vertebrate species (*1, 2*), it has been difficult to study these events with intracellular techniques, and it has been impossible to establish a causal relationship between the cellular events and behavior. In the last decade, neural correlates of associative learning have been investigated in a number of invertebrate species in which intracellular analysis is more feasible, but the behaviors studied have generally been complex (*3, 4*). It has therefore not been possible, even in these cases, to specify a minimal neuronal circuit for the learned behavior, making a complete analysis of the cellular mechanisms of the learning difficult. Recently, classical conditioning of a very simple behavior, the gill and siphon withdrawal reflex of *Aplysia*, was demonstrated with weak tactile stimulation of the siphon as the conditioned stimulus (CS) and electric shock to the tail as the unconditioned stimulus (US) (*5*). Carew *et al.* (*6*) extended this finding by demonstrating differential conditioning of the siphon withdrawal reflex. Thus, if stimulation of one site on the siphon or mantle shelf was temporally paired with tail shock (the US) while stimulation of another site was specifically unpaired with the tail shock, the withdrawal response to the unpaired CS. The neuronal circuit for the withdrawal reflex has been described; identified siphon mechanoreceptor neurons make monosynaptic excitatory synaptic connections onto both gill and siphon motor neurons as well as onto interneurons that contribute to the reflex (*7–9*). Sensory neurons that mediate input from the tail have also been identified (*10*).

In addition to classical conditioning, the gill and siphon withdrawal reflex also exhibits sensitization, a nonassociative form of learning, when tail shock is presented either alone or unpaired with siphon stimulation (*5, 11*). The biophysical and molecular mechanisms of sensitization have been explored in some detail. Tail shock excites a group of facilitator neurons that are thought to be serotonergic, the L29 cells, that produce presynaptic facilitation of the siphon sensory neurons (*12, 13*). This facilitation is due to adenosine 3',5'-monophos-phate (cyclic AMP)–dependent protein phosphorylation (14), which produces a decrease in K^+ conductance, leading to an increase in the duration of action potentials in the sensory neurons. The increase in spike duration in turn leads to an increase in Ca^{2+} influx and increased transmitter release (15, 16). Because sensitization and classical conditioning both involve an increase in the response to one stimulus as a result of presentation of a second stimulus, it is attractive to think that classical conditioning might also involve presynaptic facilitation as a mechanism for strengthening the CS pathway. Conditioning and sensitization differ, however, in that conditioning requires that the two stimuli be presented in a temporally paired fashion, whereas sensitization does not. One mechanism that might confer temporal specificity on presynaptic facilitation would be enhancement or amplification of the facilitation by preceding spike activity in the facilitated neurons, as proposed by Kandel and Tauc (17). To examine whether this mechanism contributes to differential conditioning of the withdrawal reflex, we investigated whether an experimental protocol based on the one used in the conditioning experiments would produce differential facilitation of excitatory postsynaptic potentials (EPSPs) in the circuit for the withdrawal reflex. The experimental protocol and parameters were the same as in the behavior experiments (6), except that we substituted intracellularly produced spike activity in two individual siphon sensory neurons for cutaneous stimulation of the siphon, and we measured the size of the EPSPs in a siphon motor neuron instead of siphon withdrawal. As in the behavioral experiments, we used a differential training procedure. Thus, spike activity in one sensory neuron was paired with the US, while spike activity in a second sensory neuron was specifically unpaired with the US. This procedure allowed us to subtract any nonspecific effects from the effect of temporal pairing in each experiment.

The preparation we used was the isolated central nervous system attached to the tail by the posterior pedal nerves (18). We measured the amplitudes of the monosynaptic EPSPs produced in a common postsynaptic neuron by intracellular stimulation of each of two siphon sensory neurons both before and after training (19) Fig. 1, A_1 and B). The two sensory neurons were chosen arbitrarily from an homogeneous cluster of siphon mechanoreceptor cells (7). In most experiments, the postsynaptic neuron was one of a group of recently identified siphon motor neurons (20), but in a few experiments it was L7, a gill and siphon motor neuron. During training each sensory neuron was stimulated intracellularly, causing it to fire a train of five action potentials once every 5 minutes. Stimulation of one of the sensory neurons immediately preceded shock to the tail or posterior pedal nerve, while stimulation of the other (unpaired) neuron followed tail shock by 2.5 minutes (21) (Fig. $1A_2$). On average, the EPSPs from both sensory neurons were facilitated during training, but facilitation of the EPSP from the paired neuron was greater than that of the EPSP from the unpaired neuron (Fig. 1C). In fact, while the EPSP from the unpaired neuron was usually facilitated early in training, it often began to decrease in amplitude toward the end of training, probably as a result of the dominance of homosynaptic depression caused by repeated firing of the sensory neuron (7). When tested either 5 or 15 minutes after a series of five training trials, the EPSP from the paired neuron was significantly facilitated compared to its pretraining amplitude, whereas the EPSP from the unpaired neuron was not significantly facilitated. In 23 experiments, the mean ± standard error of the mean (S.E.M.) was 161 ± 27 percent of pretraining control for the paired neurons ($t_{22} = 2.25$, $P < .05$) and 86 ± 11 percent for the unpaired neurons (22). Moreover, the percent change in the amplitude of the EPSP from the paired neuron was significantly greater than that for the EPSP from the unpaired neuron ($t_{22} = 2.77$, $P < .02$). This differential facilitation of EPSPs was maintained for at least 45 minutes after training in the six experiments in which all three neurons were held that long (Fig. 1B).

The EPSPs from both the paired and the unpaired neurons probably undergo a combination of facilitation (caused by the US) and synaptic depression (caused by the repeated firing of the sensory neurons, compared to those from the unpaired neurons. To distinguish between these possibilities, we carried out

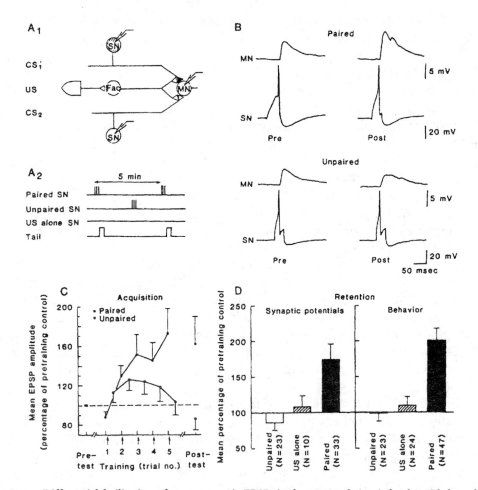

FIGURE 1 Differential facilitation of monosynaptic EPSPs in the neuronal circuit for the withdrawal reflex. (A₁) Experimental arrangement and (A₂) training protocol. The US also excites the motor neurons through pathways that are not shown. Shading indicates that activity in the neuron is paired with the US. See text for details. (B) Examples of the EPSPs produced in a common postsynaptic siphon motor neuron (*MN*) by action potentials in a paired and an unpaired sensory neuron (*SN*) before (*Pre*) and 1 hour after training (*Post*). Facilitation of the EPSP from the paired sensory neuron is greater than that of the EPSP from the unpaired sensory neuron in the same experiment. (C) Average acquisition of differential facilitation in 23 experiments similar to the one shown in (B). Bars indicate S.E.M. Arrows show times at which the US (tail shock) was delivered. (D) Comparison of cellular data showing differential facilitation of EPSPs and behavioral data showing differential conditioning of the withdrawal reflex. PSP data are pooled form two types of experiments: paired versus unpaired (23 experiments) and paired versus US alone (ten experiments). Behavioral data are from experiments on conditioning of the withdrawal reflex with the same experimental and protocol and parameters(6).

another series of experiments in which stimulation of one sensory neuron was paired with the US as before, but the other sensory neuron was not stimulated during training (it received US alone or sensitization training). Fifteen minutes after the end of training, facilitation of the EPSP from the paired sensory neuron was significantly greater than that of the EPSP from the sensory neuron receiving US-alone training. In ten experiments, the mean ± S.E.M. was 204 ± 36 percent of pretraining control for the paired neurons and 108 ± 16 percent for the US-alone neurons ($t_9 = 3.45$, $P < .01$). Since the EPSPs from neurons receiving US alone do not undergo synaptic depression during training, this differential effect can not be due to differential depression of the EPSPs. Rather, these results demonstrate that facilitation of the EPSP from a sensory neuron to a postsynaptic neuron is enhanced if the sensory neuron is active just before the facilitating stimulus (the US) is presented. The amplitude of this effect suggests that it can completely account for the differential facilitation of EPSPs from paired and unpaired sensory neurons shown in Fig. 1, B and C, although we cannot rule out the possibility that differential protection from synaptic depression might also contribute to those results.

These experiments demonstrate activity-dependent amplification of facilitation of the EPSPs from sensory neurons to motor neurons in the circuit for the siphon withdrawal reflex. The protocol and parameters used in these experiments are the same as those that have been used in behavioral experiments demonstrating differential conditioning of the withdrawal reflex (6). A comparison of the results of our cellular experiments with results from the behavioral experiments shows that they are similar quantitatively as well as qualitatively (Fig. 1D). This fit between the cellular and behavioral results and the fact that the sensory and motor neurons examined in this study mediate the withdrawal reflex suggest that activity-dependent amplification of facilitation may contribute to behavioral conditioning of the reflex (23).

Activity-dependent amplification of facilitation could result from either a presynaptic or a postsynaptic mechanism. Facilitation at these synapses underlying behavioral sensitization is presynaptic in origin (12) and is due to broadening of the action potentials, which leads to an increase in Ca^{2+} influx in the sensory neurons (15). We therefore investigated the possibility that this presynaptic mechanism might also be involved in the activity-dependent amplification of facilitation described above. We examined the durations of the action potentials in the sensory neurons in the presence of tetraethylammonium (TEA), which decreases K^+ current and thus broadens the action potential, making any changes in spike duration more apparent. Moreover, in the presence of TEA the late inward current during an action potential is carried predominantly by CA^{2+} ions, so that a change in spike duration is indicative of a change in CA^{2+} influx (15).

Our experimental protocol was similar to that described for the experiments demonstrating differential facilitation of EPSPs, except that we now (i) measured the durations of the action potentials in the sensory neurons instead of the amplitudes of the EPSPs in the motor neuron, (ii) carried out both training and testing with the abdominal ganglion (which contains the siphon sensory neurons) bathed in seawater containing 50mM TEA, and (iii) increased the number of training trials from 5 to 15. We found that additional training trials were necessary to maximize the differential effect under these conditions, perhaps because the presence of TEA in the abdominal ganglion altered the efficacy of the CS or the US, or both, during training. As in the postsynaptic potential experiments, two arbitrarily selected siphon sensory neurons were stimulated intracellularly, causing them to fire action potentials once every 5 minutes. Stimulation of one sensory neuron immediately preceded tail shock, whereas stimulation of the other neuron was specifically unpaired with tail shock (24). Five to 15 minutes after a series of 15 training trials, the action potential in the paired neuron was significantly broadened compared to its pretraining duration, while the action potential in the unpaired neuron was not. In 21 experiments, the mean ± S.E.M. was 123 ± 9 percent of pretraining control for the paired neurons ($t_{20} = 2.45$, $P < .05$) and 98 ± 5 percent for the unpaired neurons. Moreover, the percent change in the duration of the action potential in the paired neuron was significantly greater than that for the unpaired neuron ($t_{20} = 3.15$, $P < .01$). This differential broadening of action potentials was maintained for at least 3 hours after training in the 12 experiments in which both the paired and unpaired neurons were held that long ($t_{11} = 2.31$, $P < .05$) (Fig. 2, A_1 and B). The action potentials in both neurons continued to broaden during the 3 hours after training: this parallel results from behavior experiments on conditioning of the withdrawal reflex (5, 6, 25). When we blocked Ca^{2+} current by bathing the ganglion in 15 mM $CoCl_2$ after training, the durations of the spikes in both neurons were greatly reduced, confirming that the inward current during the late phase of the action potential is carried by Ca^{2+} ions (Fig. $2A_2$). These results are consistent with the hypothesis that activity-dependent amplification of facilitation is presynaptic in origin and involves a differential increase in spike duration and Ca^{2+} influx in paired versus unpaired sensory neurons.

An increase in spike duration (and hence in Ca^{2+} influx) may have as its primary cause

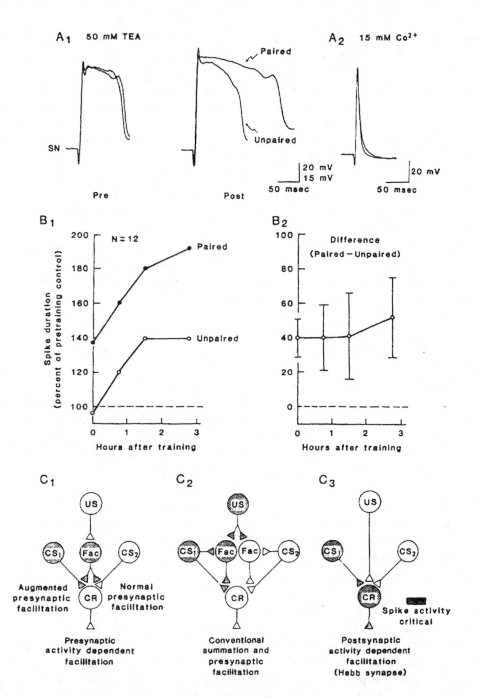

FIGURE 2 Differential broadening of the action potentials in two sensory neurons in the presence of 50 m*M* (tetraethylammonium (TEA). (A_1) Examples of the action potentials in a paired and unpaired sensory neuron before (*Pre*) and 3 hours after training (*Post*). The action potentials in the two neurons have been superimposed. Broadening of the action potential in the paired neuron is greater than that of the action potential in the unpaired neuron in the same experiment. (A_2) The action potentials in paired and unpaired neurons with 15 m*M* $CoCl_2$ added to the bath after the 3-hour posttest, from another experiment with action potentials similar to those shown in (A_1). (B_1 and B_2) Average differential spike broadening and time course of retention in 12 experiments in which both neurons were held for at least 3 hours after training. (B_1) Average spike broadening in the paired and unpaired neurons. (B_2) Average difference between the spike broadening in the paired neuron and that in the unpaired neuron in the same experiment (from the experiments shown in B_2). Bars indicate S.E.M. (C_1, C_2, and C_3) Diagram of activity-dependent presynaptic facilitation and two other possible cellular mechanisms of classical conditioning. These mechanisms require the occurrence of temporally paired spike activity in the shaded neurons. In (C_2), paired activity in neurons CS_1 and US causes firing of the left (but note the right) facilitator neuron. See text for discussion.

either an increase in Ca^{2+} conductance or a decrease in K^+ conductance. Klein and Kandel (16) found that presynaptic facilitation underlying sensitization of the withdrawal reflex is due to a decrease in K^+ conductance, which is reflected in a decrease in outward current elicited by depolarizing pulses in voltage-clamp experiments (with five training trials in normal seawater), we found a significantly greater decrease in the outward current in paired than in unpaired sensory neurons under voltage clamp (26). This result supports the conclusion from the spike broadening experiments that activity-dependent amplification of facilitation has a presynaptic mechanism. Since the pulse parameters used in this experiment were chosen to maximize the contribution of the K^+ conductance that is modulated during normal presynaptic facilitation, this finding also suggests that the mechanism of differential spike broadening is a differential decrease in K^+ conductance in paired versus unpaired sensory neurons, although it does not rule out the possibility of a differential increase in Ca^{2+} conductance.

The results of these experiments suggest that activity-dependent amplification of presynaptic facilitation (Fig. $2C_1$) is a mechanism of classical conditioning of the withdrawal reflex. However, at least two other types of cellular mechanisms could also explain conditioning of this reflex. First, the CS and US pathways might converge on facilitator neurons in such a way that paired presentations of the CS and US produces substantially greater firing of the facilitators and therefore greater presynaptic facilitation than unpaired presentation of the two stimuli (Fig. $2C_2$). That it is possible to produce differential facilitation of two arbitrarily chosen siphon sensory neurons makes this mechanism unlikely, since it would require a separate facilitator neuron for each sensory neuron. Furthermore, in experiments in which recorded from identified facilitator neurons in a semi-intact preparation, we found that paired presentation of the CS and US produced no more total firing of the facilitators than did unpaired presentation of the two stimuli (27). Thus our evidence does not support a summation mechanism, although we cannot rule out the possibility that summation in interneurons might contribute to the behavioral conditioning. A second mechanism that might explain the temporal specificity of conditioning was first proposed by Hebb (28). In the Hebb model (Fig. $2C_3$), the strength of a particular synaptic connection is increased if use of that synapse contributes to the occurrence of an action potential in the post synaptic (CR) neuron. Thus, if stimulation of a CS neuron is immediately followed by a US that causes neuron CR to fire, the CS-CR synapse will be strengthened. This mechanism is not necessary for conditioning to occur in our system, since in some of our experiments the postsynaptic neuron was held at a hyperpolarized level and did not fire any action potentials in response to the US. Furthermore, this mechanism is not sufficient, since intracellular stimulation of the postsynaptic neuron does not serve as an effective US (29).

Our experiments indicate that the mechanism of classical conditioning of the withdrawal reflex may simply be an elaboration of the mechanism of sensitization of the reflex, namely, presynaptic facilitation caused by an increase in action potential duration and Ca^{2+} influx in the sensory neurons. These experiments also suggest that the pairing specificity characteristic of classical conditioning results from amplification of the facilitation by temporally paired spike activity in the sensory neurons. We do not know which aspect of the action potential in a sensory neuron interacts with the process of presynaptic facilitation to amplify it. Four possibilities are depolarization, Na^+ influx, Ca^{2+} influx, and K^+ efflux. We also do not know which step in biochemical cascade leading to presynaptic facilitation is sensitive to one or more of these aspects of the action potential. As a working hypothesis we propose that the influx of Ca^{2+} with each action potential may provide the signal for activity and that it may interact with the serotonin-sensitive adenylate cyclase in the terminals of the sensory neuron so that the cyclase subsequently produces more cyclic AMP in response to serotonin (30). Alternatively, the catalytic unit of the cyclase, the regulatory unit (which couples the catalytic unit to the serotonin receptor) and the receptor itself, all of which are membrane voltage changes that occur during an action potential.

An attractive feature of the hypothesis that activity-dependent presynaptic facilitation is a mechanism of conditioning is that it is a type of mechanism which could be very general, for three reasons. First, it requires little special circuitry since the mechanism of pairing specificity is intrinsic to neurons in the CS pathway. The minimum requirements of this model are (i) facilitatory neurons, such as the L29 cells, which are excited by motivationally significant stimuli and which may project very diffusely (in principle, a single L29 neuron that produced facilitation in all of the sensory neurons would be sufficient to explain our results) and (ii) differential activity in the neurons that receive facilitatory input. We do not feel that there is anything unique about the siphon sensory neurons and believe that this mechanism is likely to operate throughout the nervous system wherever these two requirements are satisfied. Indeed, Walters and Byrne (31) report independent and similar results in another group of neurons in *Aplysia*. This mechanism may also operate in the vertebrate nervous system, with the diffusely projecting aminergic or cholinergic systems playing the rule that the L29 neurons play in the abdominal ganglion of *Aplysia*.

Second, the mechanism that we propose underlies activity dependence of presynaptic facilitation is amplification of a cyclic AMP-dependent decrease in K^+ conductance by voltage or ion fluxes that occur during an action potential. If the same mechanism occurred in locations other than the terminals of the sensory neurons, it could produce other aspects of learned behavior—for instance, if it occurred in the integrative region of interneurons or motor neurons it could produce features of operant conditioning (32). This speculation is rendered more plausible by the fact that cyclic nucleotides and decreases in K^+ conductance have been implicated in both classical and operant conditioning in other preparations (4,33). Of particular relevance are experiments on *Drosophila* which show that both sensitization and avoidance conditioning are affected by mutations that alter cyclic AMP metabolism (34).

Finally, the aspects of a mechanism of associative learning that are most likely to be general phylogenetically are those at the funda-mental molecular and biophysical level. Activity-dependent amplification of presynaptic facilitation probably involves the same cascade of biochemical and biophysical processes that mediate conventional presynaptic facilitation at the sensory neuron synapses: cyclic AMP-dependent protein phosphorylation and decreased ionic conductance. These processes are widespread phylogenetically and seem to be highly conserved (35). It thus sees possible that activity-dependent amplification of these processes may have similar generality. If so, it could provide a mechanism of conditioning in a wide range of species, including vertebrates.

∾

REFERENCES AND NOTES

1. J. Olds. J. F. Disterhoft, M. Segal, C. L. Kornblith, R. Hirsh, *J. Neurophysiol.* 35, 202 (1972); C. D. Woody and P. Black-Cleworth, *ibid*, 36, 1104 (1973); T. W. Berger, B. Alger, R. F. Thompson, *Science* 192, 483 (1976); C. M. Gibbs and D. H. Cohen, *Soc. Neurosci. Abstr.* 6, 424 (1980); D. A. McCormick, G. A. Clark, D. G. Lavond, R. F. Thompson, *Proc. Natl. Acad. Sci. U.S.A.* 79, 2731 (1982).
2. J. H. O'Brien, M. B. Wilder, C. D. Stevens, *J. Comp. Physiol. Psychol.* 91, 918 (1977); W. B. Levy and O. Steward, *Brain Res.* 175, 233 (1979) A. Baranyi and O. Feher, *Nature (London)* 290, 413 (1981).
3. W. J. Davis and R. Gillette, *Science* 199, 801 (1978); T. J. Chang and A. Gelperin, *Proc. Natl. Acad. Sci. U.S.A.* 77, 6204 (1980); T. J. Carew, E. T. Walters, E. R. Kandel, *Science* 211, 501 (1981).
4. G. Hoyle, *Neursci. Res. Prog. Bull.* 17, 577 (1979); T. J. Crow and D. L. Alkon, *Science* 209, 412 (1980); D. L. Alkon, I. Lederhendler, J. J. Schoukimas, *ibid.* 215, 693 (1982).
5. T. J. Carew, E. T. Walters, E. R. Kandel, *J. Neurosci.* 1, 1426 (1981).
6. T. J. Carew, R. D. Hawkins, E. R. Kandel, *Science* 219, 397 (1983).
7. V. Castellucci, H. Pinsker, I. Kupfermann, E. R. Kandel, *ibid.* 167, 1745 (1970); J. Byrne, V. Castellucci, E. R. Kandel, *J. Neurophysiol.* 37, 1041 (1974).
8. I. Kupfermann, T. J. Carew, E. R. Kandel,

J. Neurophysiol. 37, 996 (1974); A. J. Perlman, *ibid.* 42, 510 (1979); C. H. Bailey, V. F. Castellucci, J. Koester, E. R. Kandel, *ibid.*, p. 530.

9. R. D. Hawkins, V. F. Castellucci, E. R. Kandel, *ibid.* 45, 304 (1981).

10. E. T. Walters, T. J. Carew, E. R. Kandel, *Soc. Neurosci. Abstr.* 7, 353 (1981); E. T. Walters, J. H. Byrne, T. J. Carew, E. R. Kandel, in preparation.

11. H. Pinsker, I. Kupfermann, V. Castellucci, E. Kandel, *Science* 167, 1740 (1970); H. M. Pinsker, W. A. Hening, T. J. Carew, E. R. Kandel, *ibid.* 182, 1039 (1973); R. D. Hawkins, V. F. Castellucci, E. R. Kandel, in preparation.

12. V. Castellucci and E. R. Kandel, *Science* 194, 1176 (1976).

13. R. D. Hawkins, V. F. Castellucci, E. R. Kandel, *J. Neurophysiol.* 45, 315 (1981); R. D. Hawkins, *Soc. Neurosci. Abstr.* 7, 354 (1981).

14. V. F. Castellucci, E. R. Kandel, J. H. Schwartz, F. D. Wilson, A. C. Nairn, P. Greengard, *Proc. Natl. Acad. Sci. U.S.A.* 77, 7492 (1980); V. F. Castellucci, J. H. Schwartz, E. R. Kandel, A. Nairn, P. Greengard, *Soc. Neurosci. Abstr.* 7, 836 (1981).

15. M. Klein and E. R. Kandel, *Proc. Natl. Acad. Sci. U.S.A.* 75, 3512 (1978); R. D. Hawkins, *J. Neurophysiol.* 45, 327 (1981).

16. M. Klein and E. R. Kandel, *Proc. Natl. Acad. Sci. U.S.A.* , 6912 (1980).

17. E. R. Kandel and L. Tauc, *J. Physiol. (London)* 181, 28 (1965).

18. *Aplysia californica*, weighing 100 to 300 g (supplied by Pacific Biomarine, Venice, Calif), were anesthetized with isotonic $MgCl_2$ (50 percent of body weight) before surgery. The central nervous system (the pedal, pleural, cerebral and abdominal ganglia and connectives) was dissected free from all of the body except the tail, to which it was left attached by the posterior pedal nerves. The tail was then separated from the rest of the body (which was discarded) by a transverse cut at the level of the posterior insertion of the parapodia. The abdominal ganglion, which contains the siphon sensory and motor neurons, was partially desheathed, and the preparation was thoroughly washed with normal artificial seawater (Instant Ocean) before the experiment was begun.

19. Standard electrophysiological techniques were used (7–9). Sensory neurons and motor neurons were impaled with single-barreled glass microelectrodes filled with 2.5*M* potassium chloride and beveled to a resistance of 10 to 20 megohms. A Wheatstone bridge circuit was used for recording while passing current either to depolarize neurons (the sensory cells) or to hyperpolarize them (the motor neuron). In experiments in which the motor neuron was hyperpolarized to prevent it from firing, it was held at the same level while testing the PSPs from the two sensory neurons before and after training.

20. W. N. Frost, V. F. Castellucci, E. R. Kandel, in preparation.

21. The siphon sensory neurons are a cluster of about 24 cells that have similar properties and synaptic connections (7). These cells do not receive conventional excitatory synaptic input from each other or from the US (tail shock). Two neurons were picked arbitrarily and assigned to be paired or unpaired in such a way as to balance the average amplitudes of the paired and unpaired EPSPs before training (4.2 ± 0.7 mV for the paired neurons and 4.9 ± 0.8 mV for the unpaired neurons). Typically each sensory neuron was made to fire a train of five action potentials by intracellular injection of 40- to 50-msec depolarizing current pulses at 10 Hz. Current intensity was adjusted so that each current pulse produced one action potential. Two types of US were used: either 1.5 seconds of 50 mA, 60-Hz, a-c shock delivered to the tail through bipolar capillary electrodes, or a 1.5 second, 10-Hz train of 3-msec pulses delivered to the posterior pedal nerves through bipolar Ag-AgCl electrodes. The intensity of the tail or posterior pedal nerve stimulation was sufficient to produce brisk firing in the postsynaptic neuron when it was not hyperpolarized.

Onset of the US coincided with offset of intracellular stimulation of the paired neuron and followed simulation of the unpaired neuron by 2.5 minutes.

22. The summary statistics given the means an standard errors of the means. In all cases statistical comparisons are t-tests for correlated means. Thus each experimental score was compared to a control value in the same experiment. For within-cell comparisons, the control value was the pretest score, while for between-cell comparisons, the control value was the score for th other cell in the experiment. The EPSPs from the paired and unpaired neurons were tested 2.5 minutes apart, either 5 or 15 minutes after the last US. The order in which the two PSPs were tested was counterbalanced. Only the monosynaptic component of the EPSP (as judged by short and constant latency and smooth rise) was measured, although additional changes were sometimes observed in the polysynaptic response.

23. The degree of correlation between the cellular data and the behavioral data is better than might be expected, since in one case we measured EPSP amplitude and in the other case we measured duration of siphon withdrawal. However, a good correlation between these two measures has also been observed in previous experiments (for example, T. J. Carew and E. R. Kandel, *Science* 182, 1158 (1973) and could be explained by several possible mechanisms: (i) Frost *et al.* (20) identified interneurons in the siphon withdrawal circuit that fire an extended train of spikes in response to brief excitatory synaptic input from the sensory neurons. An increase in the amplitude of synaptic potentials from the sensory neurons could produce an increase in the duration of the resulting train of spikes in some of these interneurons, thus producing an increase in the duration of siphon withdrawal. (ii) The same cellular change that underlies increased transmitter release form the sensory neurons (for example, a decrease in K^+ conductance) could also lead to repetitive firing of the sensory neurons in response to a brief tactile stimulus. (iii) The activity-dependent change that occurs in the sensory neurons could occur in some interneurons as well, and might prolong interneuronal firing in a similar fashion. These possibilities are neither mutually exclusive nor exhaustive.

24. The abdominal ganglion was placed in a small well and perfused with TEA solution while the rest of the preparation was perfused with normal seawater. The plural-abdominal connectives were led through a silicon grease seal under the walls of the well. Sensory neurons were assigned to be paired or unpaired in such a way as to balance the durations of their action potentials before training (71 ± 9 msec for the paired neurons and 77 ± 10 msec for the unpaired neurons). Intracellular stimulation consisted of a single 5-msec depolarizing pulse. This typically produced a burst of several spikes in the sensory neuron, of which only the first was measured. The value of the spike duration for the pretest and each of the posttests was the mean of three measurements taken at 5-minute intervals. The US was 1.5 seconds of 50 mA, 60-Hz a-c shock to the tail. Onset of the US followed intracellular stimulation of the paired neuron by 500 msec and followed stimulation of the unpaired neuron by 2.5 minutes.

25. Continued broadening of the action potentials may have a number of possible explanations including (i) the onset of a process of consolidation of the memory into a long-term form, (ii) recovery from spike narrowing caused by repeated stimulation of the sensory neurons during training, (iii) prolonged exposure of the neurons to TEA, or (iv) progressive deterioration of the preparation. Preliminary experiments indicate that US-alone training does not produce continued broadening, which suggests that it may be due to recovery from spike narrowing.

26. R. D. Hawkins, T. W. Abrams, T. J. Carew, E. R. Kandel, in preparation.

27. R. D. Hawkins, in preparation.

28. D. O Hebb, *Organization of Behavior* (Wiley, New York, 1949).

29. T. J. Carew, T. W. Abrams, R. D. Hawkins, E. R. Kandel, in preparation.

30. U. Schwabe and J. W. Daly, *J. Pharmacol. Exp. Ther.* 202, 134 (1977); M. A. Brostrom, B. McL. Breckenridge, D. J. Wolff, *Adv. Cyclic Nucleotide Res.* 9, 85 (1978); D. J. Wolff and C. O. Brostrom, *ibid*, 11, 27 (1979).

31. E. T. Walters and J. H. Byrne, *Science* 219, 405 (1983).

32. A synpatically induced long-lasting decrease in K⁺ conductance in an interneuron or motor neuron would lead to (i) a long-lasting increase in the ease with which the neuron could be excited by synaptic input (T. J. Carew and E. R. Kandel, *J. Neurophysiol.* 40, 72 (1977), and (ii) a long-lasting increase in the firing rate or bursting frequency of a spontaneously active neuron. A consequence of the mechanism we are proposing is that these increases would be amplified if the neuron happened to be firing action potentials at the time of the modulatory synaptic input. This result would correspond formally to (and could underlie) an increase in the probability, rate, or frequency of a behavior by contingent reinforcement of that behavior.

33. C. D. Woody, B. E. Swartz, E. Gruen, *Brain Res.* 158, 373 (1978); J. Acosta-Urquidi, D. L. Alkon, J. Olds, J. T. Neary, E. Zebley, G. Kuzma, *Soc. Neurosci. Abstr.* 7, 944 (1981).

34. Y. Dudai, Y.-N Jan, D. Byers, W. G. Quinn, S. Benzer, *Proc. Natl. Acad. Sci. U.S.A.* 73, 1684 (1976); D. Byers, R. L. Davis, J. A. Kiger, *Nature (London)* 289, 79 (1981); J. S. Duerr and W. G. Quinn, *Proc. Natl. Acad. Sci. U.S.A.* 79, 3646 (1982).

35. P. Greengard, *Cyclic Nucleotides, Phosphorylated Proteins, and Neuronal Function* (Raven, New York, 1978); H. C. Hartzell, *Nature (London)* 291, 539 (1981).

36. This work was supported by NIH fellowship 5T32NS07062-0-6 (to T.W.A.), by NIH career awards 5K02 MH0081 (to T.J.C.) and 5KO2 MH18558 (to E.R.K.), by NIH grants NS 12744 and 6M 23540, and by a grant from the McKnight Foundation. We thank J. H. Schwartz for helpful comments on an earlier draft of this manuscript, L. Katz and K. Hilten for illustrations, and H. Ayers for preparation of the manuscript.

❧ JOURNAL ARTICLE REVIEW FORM ❧

Name _____ Date _____

Article Name: _____

Article Authors: _____

1. Why did the authors perform this study? (What question(s) did the authors want to answer?)

2. Identify the IV(s) and the DV(s) used in this study (Note: there may be more than one of each).

3. How was the welfare of human subjects or animal subjects safeguarded?

4. What were the major findings of this study?

5. Why were these results significant?

6. What would be a good follow-up to this study? (What study should be done next?)

PRACTICE EXAM FOR PART FIVE

1. The long fiber that extends from cell body of the neuron allowing it to transmit messages to other neurons is the:
   a. axon
   b. dendrite
   c. nerve bundle
   d. cell membrane

2. The process of neurotransmission occurs when:
   a. an electrical impulse travels from the dendrite to the axon of a single neuron.
   b. an electrical impulse travels from the dendrite of one neuron to the axon of another neuron.
   c. a chemical message travels from the axon of one neuron to the dendrite of another neuron.
   d. a chemical message travels from the dendrite to the axon of a single neuron.

3. Neuroscientists refer to cells of the nervous system as
   a. nerves
   b. neurons
   c. soma
   d. neurotransmitters

4. The part of the brain that controls motivated behavior and probably governs the activity of the anterior pituitary is the:
   a. cerebral cortex
   b. medulla
   c. hypothalamus
   d. reticular formation

5. Which part of the autonomic nervous system allows you to calm down and resume normal functioning after an emergency is past?
   a. sympathetic
   b. parasympathetic
   c. interstitial
   d. endocrine

6. The first neurotransmitter discovered is used by the peripheral nervous system. It is known as:
   a. aceytlcholine
   b. dopamine
   c. serotonin
   d. noradrenaline

7. The best description of the electroencephalogram (EEG) is that it:
   a. is a measure of electrical activity of only the cerebral cortex.
   b. measures activation primarily of ancient hind brain regions.
   c. is a measure of electrical activity of the entire brain.
   d. changes with subtle emotional differences and allows for "lie-detection."
   e. all of the above.

8. A hugely obese "VMH rat":
   a. is a finicky eater
   b. will eat only soft, fatty food
   c. refuses to work hard for its food
   d. will lose weight if given only distasteful food
   e. all of the above

9. The average person will enter an REM stage of sleep once every:
   a. twenty minutes
   b. thirty minutes
   c. forty minutes
   d. ninety minutes

10. The "set point" hypothesis suggests that:
    a. our set point is likely inherited.
    b. our set point gradually changes as we get older.
    c. weight loss will be actively resisted by the body.
    d. our individual set point can be calculated as height (in centimeters) multiplied by two.

11. Laboratory rats lesioned in the LH will recover eating if given a special treatment regimen and will live a normal life span although as a "thin" body size. These findings suggest the following:
    a. LH is not part of the brain circuitry that establishes the set point.
    b. LH effects on body weight are via its control of body temperature.
    c. existence of other brain regions that can take over LH function.
    d. set point theory must be incorrect.
    e. None of the above.

12. Which of the following is NOT true of REM sleep?
    a. you dream during REM sleep
    b. your mind is very active but your body is so relaxed it is paralyzed
    c. REM is the deepest stage of sleep
    d. brain waves during REM most closely resemble those of a waking state

13. All drugs affect consciousness and behavior by:
    a. killing some of the brain's neurons
    b. causing overproduction of hormones
    c. affecting the neurotransmission process
    d. a process not yet discovered or understood

14. Match the scientific terminology to its more familiar meaning.

    _____ ontogeny   a. long-term
    _____ etiology   b. cause
    _____ quantify   c. development
    _____ chronic   d. count
                            e. consequence

15. Again, match the scientific terminology to its more familiar meaning.

    _____ pathology   a. personality
    _____ DSM   b. abnormal
    _____ kin selection   c. diagnose
    _____ retrieval   d. "altruism"
                            e. forgetting

EPILOGUE

It has been wryly noted that psychology has a long past but only a short history. The long past refers to speculations about human behavior dating to classical antiquity. The short history emphasizes that scientific psychology is little more than a century old.

Early in its development, at the close of the nineteenth century, modern psychology was most clearly associated with philosophy. Productive relations between the two disciplines were sought and praised. At the universities, both in Europe and America, psychologists held appointments as philosophers. Few people realized that psychology one day would emerge as a separate scientific enterprise.

By the turn of this century, the influence of philosophy had lessened in favor of a second element—experimentalism. The president of the American Psychological Association at that time observed: "Psychological theory is influenced to a large, and perhaps at times to an embarrassing, extent by points of view and forms of expression derived from the physical sciences" (Sanford, 1903). A growing number of psychologists were not embarrassed; they continued this trend, emulating the methods of the natural sciences. A few years later, a new president of the Association noted that psychologists were meeting that year in affiliation with naturalists, rather than philosophers. In the grand style of his era, he declared: "We are off with our old love, and on with a new" (Marshall, 1908).

A third clear trend in psychology's short history is its diversity, of which this book is a prime example. Beginning in midcentury, contemporary psychology has been marked by the steady development of specialized branches. Today the field is so diverse that it sometimes seems unlikely to continue as a whole. Psychological inquiry now takes place in all aspects of human endeavor, and as new needs arise, diversity and specialization will increase (Hilgard, Leary, & McGuire, 1991).

The most dominant figure in early American psychology represented all three of these trends. William James was a philosopher, at times an experimentalist, and certainly a man of diverse interests. A man for all seasons, James influenced enormously the psychologists under his tutelage and those who came after him.

One of them, Mary Calkins, cherished pleasant memories of studying with James, a relationship that was especially significant because she was the only woman in his course. In looking back on that first seminar, she wrote: "The other members of his seminary in psychology dropped away in the early weeks of the fall of 1890; and James and I were left not . . . at either end of a log but quite literally at either side of a library fire" (Calkins, 1930).

The log to which Mary Calkins refers is Mark Hopkins's metaphor for education. The teaching-learning process, he said, involves a log with a teacher on one end and a student on the other.

It is now my moment to step off that log. I have enjoyed this experience. Best wishes to you at both ends in the future.

LDF

lock-and-key hypothesis, 561

norepinephrine, 317,318,321,328,562

second messenger system, 317-318

neurosis, 394-395

norepinephrine (NE), 317,318,321,328,562

normal distribution, 80,342

norms, 39-40

object permanence, 268

observational learning, 152-153

obsessive-compulsive disorder, 398-399

occipital lobe, 573

Oedipus complex, 20

old age

Alzheimer's disease, 562

Parkinson's disease, 562

Olsen, Paul, 341

ontogeny

adolescence, 265

androgen, 265

attachment, 262

cephalocaudal development, 260

differentiation, 258

estrogen, 265

imprinting, 262

maturation, 264

proximodistal development, 260

puberty, 265

sensorimotor development, 259-260

teratogens, 258

oogonia, 298-299

operant behavior, 136-137

operant conditioning, 137-148

extinction, 141

generalization, 140

operant response, 139

principles, 140-146

suppression, 389

survey method, 44-48

sympathetic nervous system, 420,579

sympathetic & parasympathetic systems, 527

synapse, 559-560

tabula rasa, 5

tardive dyskinesia, 439-440

temporal lobe, 573

territoriality, 225-227

tests, psychological, 49-50

testosterone, 296,297,312,318,321,322,328

thalamus, 570

theories of intelligence, 347-352

theory of evolution, 7

thirst and the brain, 619

Thorazine® (chlorpromazine), 431,432,433,436,437

thymus gland, 322,329

thyroid gland, 321,324-326,581

thyroid-stimulating hormone (TSH), 321-326

thyroxin, 318,321,324-326,329

      evolution, 330

top-down processing, 597

Tourette's syndrome, 571

trace conditioning, 128

triangular theory of love, 509

unconditioned response, 127

unconditioned stimulus, 127

urethra, 295-297

vagina, 298,300,302

Valium® (diazepam), 422,426

variable-interval reinforcement, 144

variable-ratio reinforcement, 143

vas deferens, 295,296,297,307,308

vasectomy, 307,308